Clinical Methods in
OBSTETRICS AND GYNECOLOGY

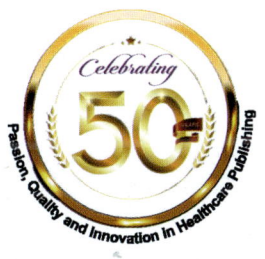

Clinical Methods in OBSTETRICS AND GYNECOLOGY

Second Edition

Manju Puri
MD (Obstetrics and Gynecology)
Director-Professor
Department of Obstetrics and Gynecology
Lady Hardinge Medical College
New Delhi, India

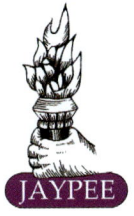

JAYPEE BROTHERS MEDICAL PUBLISHERS
The Health Sciences Publisher
New Delhi | London

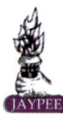 **Jaypee Brothers Medical Publishers (P) Ltd**

Headquarters

Jaypee Brothers Medical Publishers (P) Ltd
4838/24, Ansari Road, Daryaganj
New Delhi 110 002, India
Phone: +91-11-43574357
Fax: +91-11-43574314
E-mail: jaypee@jaypeebrothers.com

Overseas Office

JP Medical Ltd
83 Victoria Street, London
SW1H 0HW (UK)
Phone: +44 20 3170 8910
Fax: +44 (0)20 3008 6180
E-mail: info@jpmedpub.com

Website: www.jaypeebrothers.com
Website: www.jaypeedigital.com

© 2021, Jaypee Brothers Medical Publishers

The views and opinions expressed in this book are solely those of the original contributor(s)/author(s) and do not necessarily represent those of editor(s) of the book.

All rights reserved. No part of this publication may be reproduced, stored or transmitted in any form or by any means, electronic, mechanical, photocopying, recording or otherwise, without the prior permission in writing of the publishers.

All brand names and product names used in this book are trade names, service marks, trademarks or registered trademarks of their respective owners. The publisher is not associated with any product or vendor mentioned in this book.

Medical knowledge and practice change constantly. This book is designed to provide accurate, authoritative information about the subject matter in question. However, readers are advised to check the most current information available on procedures included and check information from the manufacturer of each product to be administered, to verify the recommended dose, formula, method and duration of administration, adverse effects and contraindications. It is the responsibility of the practitioner to take all appropriate safety precautions. Neither the publisher nor the author(s)/editor(s) assume any liability for any injury and/or damage to persons or property arising from or related to use of material in this book.

This book is sold on the understanding that the publisher is not engaged in providing professional medical services. If such advice or services are required, the services of a competent medical professional should be sought.

Every effort has been made where necessary to contact holders of copyright to obtain permission to reproduce copyright material. If any have been inadvertently overlooked, the publisher will be pleased to make the necessary arrangements at the first opportunity. The **CD/DVD-ROM** (if any) provided in the sealed envelope with this book is complimentary and free of cost. **Not meant for sale.**

Inquiries for bulk sales may be solicited at: jaypee@jaypeebrothers.com

Clinical Methods in Obstetrics and Gynecology

First Edition: 2015

Second Edition: **2021**

ISBN: 978-93-90020-67-6

Printed at: Samrat Offset Pvt. Ltd.

Dedicated to

*My parents
and
parents-in-law*

Contributors

Aimee Teong Chuin Ai MBBS
Medical Officer
Division of Obstetrics and Gynecology
KK Women's and Children's Hospital
Singapore

Anju Yadav MS
Fellowship in Reproductive
Medicine and Laparoscopy
Fertility Consultant
Cloudnine Hospital
Gurugram, Haryana, India

Anu Handa MS
Senior Resident
Department of Obstetrics and Gynecology
Lady Hardinge Medical College and
Smt Sucheta Kriplani Hospital
New Delhi, India

Anuja Rao MD DNB
Assistant Professor
Department of Dermatology
Santosh Medical College and Hospital
Ghaziabad, Uttar Pradesh, India

Anuradha Singh MD
Associate Professor
Department of Obstetrics and Gynecology
Lady Hardinge Medical College
New Delhi, India

Archana Kumari MS FICOG
Assistant Professor
Department of Obstetrics and Gynecology
All India Institute of Medical Sciences
New Delhi, India

Arpita De MS FMAS
Assistant Professor
Department of Obstetrics and Gynecology
Hamdard Institute of Medical Sciences and
Research
New Delhi, India

Aruna Nigam MS FICOG FMAS MNAMS
Unit Head (Endoscopy Unit)
Department of Obstetrics and Gynecology
Hamdard Institute of Medical Sciences and
Research
New Delhi, India

Asmita Kaundal MS DNB
Assistant Professor
Department of Obstetrics and Gynecology
Dr Baba Sahib Ambedkar Medical College
and Hospital
New Delhi, India

Deepika Meena MD
Associate Professor
Department of Obstetrics and Gynecology
Lady Hardinge Medical College and
Smt Sucheta Kriplani Hospital
New Delhi, India

GS Triveni MS DNB MNAMS
Assistant Professor
Department of Obstetrics and Gynecology
Lady Hardinge Medical College and
Smt Sucheta Kriplani Hospital
New Delhi, India

Harkiran Kaur Narang MS MRCOG
Specialty Trainee
Royal Alexandra Hospital
Castlehead, Paisley, Scotland

Harvinder Kaur MD DNB
Specialist Grade II
Department of Obstetrics and Gynecology
Deen Dayal Upadhyay Hospital
New Delhi, India

Indira Prasad MS DNB
Assistant Professor
Department of Obstetrics and Gynecology
All India Institute of Medical Sciences
New Delhi, India

Isha Khurana Vashisht MS DGO DNB PGDS
Fellowship in ART
Senior Consultant
Department of In Vitro Fertilization (IVF)
Apollo Fertility, New Delhi
Senior Consultant Obstetrician and Gynecologist
Kailash Nursing Home Pvt. Ltd.
New Delhi, India

Jasmeet K Monga
MD DNB FRCOG (UK) PGA (ART) (UK)
Consultant Obstetrician and Gynecologist
Clinic One
Gurugram, Haryana, India

K Aparna Sharma MD DNB
Additional Professor
Department of Obstetrics and Gynecology
All India Institute of Medical Sciences
New Delhi, India

Karishma Thariani MS DNB MNAMS
Fellowship Urogynecology and Pelvic
Reconstructive Surgery (AIIMS)
Consultant
Center for Urogynecology and Pelvic Health
New Delhi, India

Kazila Bhutia
MBBS MD MRCOG (London, UK) FAMS (S'Pore)
Consultant Obstetrician and Gynecologist
Department of Urogynecology
Division of Obstetrics and Gynecology
KK Women's and Children's Hospital
Singapore

Kirti Kishore Sharma DGO DNB MA
Fellowship in Fetal Medicine
Consultant Obstetrician and Gynecologist
Kalawati Hospital
Rewari, Haryana, India

Laxmi Goel MS (Obs & Gyne)
Consultant
Bloom Fertility Center
Fortis Escorts Hospital
Faridabad, Haryana, India

Manisha Bajaj MS FIAOG FMAS
Department of Obstetrics and Gynecology
ESI-PGIMER and ESIC Medical College and
Hospital
ODC EZ, Kolkata, West Bengal, India

Manisha Kumar MS FICOG
Professor
Department of Obstetrics and Gynecology
Lady Hardinge Medical College and
Smt Sucheta Kriplani Hospital
New Delhi, India

Meenakshi Singh MD DNB FICOG
Associate Professor
Department of Obstetrics and Gynecology
Lady Hardinge Medical College
New Delhi, India

Monika Bhatia MS DNB DCH MRCOG
Head and Senior Consultant
Department of Obstetrics and Gynecology
Venkateshwar Hospital
New Delhi, India

Monika Datta DGO MD (Ped)
Director
Directorate of Family Welfare
GNCTD
New Delhi, India

Monika Madaan MD DNB FICOG FMAS
Specialist Gr 1
Department of Obstetrics and Gynecology
ESIC Hospital
Manesar, Haryana, India

Namita Jain MS DNB MRCOG (UK)
IVF Fellowship (IFS)
Consultant
Department of Obstetrics and Gynecology
Paras Hospitals
Gurugram, Haryana, India

Neelam Jain MD (Radiodiagnosis)
Consultant Radiologist
Discovery Diagnosis and Jain Ultrasound Center
Jamshedpur, Jharkhand, India

Neha Gami MD DNB MRCOG FCLS
Diploma in Professional Ultrasound in
Obstetrics and Gynecology
Specialist, Obstetrics and Gynecology
Danat Al Emarat Hospital and Health Plus
Family Health Center
Abu Dhabi, UAE

Nidhi Malhotra MS
Consultant
Department of Obstetrics and Gynecology
Krishna Hospital
Ludhiana, Punjab, India

Nishtha Jaiswal MS DNB
Associate Professor
Department of Obstetrics and Gynecology
Lady Hardinge Medical College and
Smt Sucheta Kriplani Hospital
New Delhi, India

Pikee Saxena MD FICOG MNAMS PGCC
(Hospital Management) PGDCR (Clinical Research)
Professor
Department of Obstetrics and Gynecology
Lady Hardinge Medical College and
Smt Sucheta Kriplani Hospital
New Delhi, India

Pooja Dwivedi MS MRCOG FMAS
Consultant
Mother and Child Care Center
Guru Nanak Nagar, New Delhi, India

Prabha Lal MD FMAS FICOG
Professor
Department of Obstetrics and Gynecology
Lady Hardinge Medical College and
Smt Sucheta Kriplani Hospital
New Delhi, India

Prachi Dixit MS
Assistant Professor
Department of Obstetrics and Gynecology
NKP Salve Institute of Medical Sciences &
Research Center and Lata Mangeshkar Hospital
Nagpur, Maharashtra, India

Priyanka Arora MS DNB
Senior Resident
Department of Obstetrics and Gynecology
Lady Hardinge Medical College
New Delhi, India

Puneet K Kochhar MD DNB
MRCOG FICOG Diploma
Reproductive Medicine (Germany)
Diploma in Minimal Access Surgery
Consultant Gynecologist and IVF Specialist
Elixir Fertility Center
New Delhi, India

Raina Chawla MS
ESIC Medical College and Hospital
NIT, Faridabad, Haryana, India

*****Richa Aggarwal** DGO MS
Junior Consultant
Obstetrician and Gynecologist
Apollo Cradle Maternity and Children's Hospital
New Delhi, India

******Richa Aggarwal** MD DNB
Associate Professor
Department of Obstetrics and Gynecology
UCMS and GTB Hospital
New Delhi, India

Ritu Sharma MD
Associate Professor
Department of Obstetrics and Gynecology
Government Institute of Medical Sciences
Greater Noida, Uttar Pradesh, India

Sadia Mansoor MS DNB
Senior Resident
Department of Obstetrics and Gynecology
All India Institute of Medical Sciences
New Delhi, India

Sangeeta Gupta MD MRCOG
Director-Professor
Department of Obstetrics and Gynecology
Maulana Azad Medical College
New Delhi, India

Seema Singhal MS
Associate Professor
Department of Obstetrics and Gynecology
All India Institute of Medical Sciences
New Delhi, India

Shalini Malhotra MS DNB MNAMS MRCOG
Consultant Obstetrician and Gynecologist
Al Qassimi Women and Children Hospital
Ministry of Health
Sharjah, UAE

Shalini Singh MS
Associate Professor
Department of Obstetrics and Gynecology
MLN Medical College
Prayagrag, Uttar Pradesh, India

Shalini Warman MD
Specialist
Department of Obstetrics and Gynecology
Tata Main Hospital
Jamshedpur, Jharkhand, India

Sharda Patra MD DNB
Professor
Department of Obstetrics and Gynecology
Lady Hardinge Medical College and
Smt Sucheta Kriplani Hospital
New Delhi, India

Shilpa Dhingra MD FICOG
SMO, Civil Hospital Manimajra
Chandigarh, India

Shilpa Singla MD MICOG
Head
Department of Obstetrics and Gynecology
ESIC Model Hospital
Gurugram, Haryana, India

Shilpi Nain DGO DNB FICOG
Associate Professor
Department of Obstetrics and Gynecology
Lady Hardinge Medical College and
Smt Sucheta Kriplani Hospital
New Delhi, India

Sumi P Thampi DGO DNB
Consultant Gynecologist
Lisie Hospital Kaloor
Ernakulam, Kerala, India

Sumita Agarwal MD DNB
Goodwill Medical Centre
Tagore Garden, New Delhi, India

Swati Agrawal MBBS MD
Associate Professor
Department of Obstetrics and Gynecology
Lady Hardinge Medical College and
Smt Sucheta Kriplani Hospital
New Delhi, India

Tahmina S MS DNB
Professor
Department of Obstetrics and Gynecology
Melmaruvathur Adhiparasakthi Institute of
Medical Sciences and Research
Melmaruvathur, Tamil Nadu, India

Vibhu Mendiratta MD FIMSA
Director-Professor
Department of Dermatology
Lady Harding Medical College
New Delhi, India

Vidhi Chaudhary DGO DNB MRCOG
Associate Professor
Department of Obstetrics and Gynecology
Lady Hardinge Medical College
New Delhi, India

Vishrut Narang MS (Gen Surg) MCh (Ped Surg)
MRCS
Consultant Pediatric Surgeon
Child Care Centre
Sonipat, Haryana, India

Preface

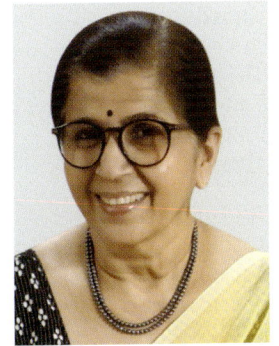

For a clinician to function effectively and appropriately, it is important to possess requisite knowledge, skills, attitude, values, and responsiveness. Clinical skills are a vital component of the competency set for budding clinicians. It includes eliciting a good history, conducting a thorough examination, effective interpretation, and integration of available data to generate differential diagnoses. It is important for the clinician to choose appropriate diagnostic tests and interpret these tests in the clinical context and plan the management of each patient.

The main objective of the second edition of *Clinical Methods in Obstetrics and Gynecology* is to facilitate honing of the clinical skills of students and clinicians in their day-to-day practice and stimulate their minds to think of differential diagnosis and systematically reach a final diagnosis.

The layout of the book is like the first edition. There are three sections: Obstetrics, Gynecology and General. The sections on Obstetrics and Gynecology have individual chapters dedicated to various complaints or conditions, the patients commonly present in the outpatient department. Each chapter begins with an introduction, a list of differential diagnoses followed by a discussion on history taking, examination of the patient and investigations as guided by the differential diagnoses. At the end of each chapter, there is additional information provided about the treatment and a list of latest guidelines from various societies to refer to. Some new chapters have been incorporated in the obstetric section. These include chapters on Pregnant women with multiple pregnancy, Rh-negative pregnancy, Decreased fetal movements, Positive aneuploidy test, and Suspected fetal growth restriction. In the General section, new topics include Cardiotocography, Endoscopic equipment and instruments, Minor procedures in the labor room and Government initiatives to improve maternal and neonatal health.

I hope this book will strengthen the foundation of students and clinicians by training them to make differential diagnoses, systematically evaluating each diagnosis based on history and examination, sharpening their analytical skills and planning appropriate management.

Manju Puri

Acknowledgments

I thank the almighty God for having bestowed upon me this opportunity to share my learnings and experiences with others through this book. This book is dedicated to all my teachers and mentors who moulded me to my present form. Prof Satish Sharma, my teacher from MLN College, Yamuna Nagar, Haryana, who taught me chemistry in pre-medical and gently nudged me to pursue the medical profession. A decision I have always cherished. Late Prof Sushila Rathee, former Head of the Department of Obstetrics and Gynecology at the Postgraduate Institute of Medical Sciences in Rohtak, Haryana played a pivotal role in my training as an Obstetrician and Gynecologist. The stimulating work environment and opportunities provided by Prof Shubha Sagar Trivedi, former Head of the Department of Obstetrics and Gynecology at Lady Hardinge Medical College, New Delhi, India, enabled me to thrive and grow to my fullest.

I am thankful for my students who clicked many of the photographs used in this book. I would also like to thank my colleagues from other specialties Dr Ashok Khurana, Dr Atul Kapila, Dr MK Narula, Dr Rama Anand, Dr Savita Nagpal and Dr Vibhu Mendiratta who generously provided photographs. My special thanks to Dr Roopali, Dr Indira and Ms Khusboo Saha for helping me with their photographic and sketching skills.

My students, colleagues and friends have contributed chapters and enriched this book with their ideas and suggestions. They have helped me make this book user friendly. I especially acknowledge Khushboo Kumari, Senior Resident in our department for her contribution for proofreading.

Blessings of parents and parents-in-law stay with you forever, I am fortunate to have these in abundance. I am very grateful for the support from my family—Dilip, Raghav and Madhavi. They have been patient, accommodative and caring. As a Psychiatrist, Dilip has helped me connect with my patients, allay their anxieties, and heal them instead of just treating them for which I shall always be indebted to him.

Finally, I am thankful to Shri Jitendar P Vij (Group Chairman), Mr Ankit Vij (Managing Director), Mr MS Mani (Group President), Ms Chetna Malhotra Vohra (Associate Director—Content Strategy), Ms Pooja Bhandari (Production Head), and Ms Nedup Denka Bhutia (Development Editor) of M/s Jaypee Brothers Medical Publishers (P) Ltd, New Delhi, India, for giving the go-ahead at the very beginning and helping me in every way possible to bring out this book.

Contents

Section 1: Obstetrics

1. **Approach to a Pregnant Woman Attending Antenatal Clinic** 3
   GS Triveni, Richa Aggarwal,* Pooja Dwivedi

2. **Approach to a Pregnant Woman Presenting with Bad Obstetric History** 25
   Monika Bhatia

3. **Approach to a Pregnant Woman Presenting with Bleeding in Early Pregnancy** 32
   Meenakshi Singh, Namita Jain

4. **Approach to a Pregnant Woman Presenting with Bleeding in Late Pregnancy** 40
   Namita Jain, Meenakshi Singh

5. **Approach to a Pregnant Woman Presenting with Abdominal Pain** 49
   Richa Aggarwal**

6. **Approach to a Pregnant Woman Presenting with Discharge Per Vaginum** 61
   Sharda Patra

7. **Approach to a Pregnant Woman Presenting with Vomiting** 72
   Puneet K Kochhar

8. **Approach to a Pregnant Woman Presenting with Diarrhea** 79
   Pikee Saxena, Priyanka Arora

9. **Approach to a Pregnant Woman Presenting with Fever** 85
   Shalini Malhotra

10. **Approach to a Pregnant or Puerperal Woman Presenting with Convulsions** 91
    Prachi Dixit

11. **Approach to a Pregnant Woman Presenting with Dyspnea** 100
    Richa Aggarwal**

12. **Approach to a Pregnant Woman Presenting with Pruritus** 111
    Ritu Sharma, Vibhu Mendiratta

13. **Approach to a Pregnant Woman with Decreased
    Fetal Movements** 122
    Deepika Meena

14. **Approach to a Pregnant Woman Presenting with a Positive
    Aneuploidy Screening Test** 127
    Manisha Kumar

15. **Approach to a Pregnant Woman with a Congenitally
    Malformed Fetus** 136
    Manisha Kumar

16. **Approach to a Pregnant Woman Presenting with Jaundice** 145
    Sharda Patra

17. **Approach to a Pregnant Woman Presenting with Pallor** 157
    Indira Prasad

18. **Approach to a Pregnant Woman Presenting with Hypertension** 169
    Shilpi Nain

19. **Approach to a Pregnant Woman Presenting with Heart Disease** 179
    Swati Agrawal

20. **Approach to a Pregnant Woman with Suspected Fetal
    Growth Restriction** 189
    Sangeeta Gupta

21. **Approach to a Pregnant Woman with Previous Cesarean Section** 201
    K Aparna Sharma

22. **Approach to a Pregnant Woman with Multiple Pregnancy** 209
    Shalini Warman, Neelam Jain

23. **Approach to a Pregnant Woman Presenting with Rh-negative
    Pregnancy** 219
    Sumita Agarwal

24. **Approach to a Pregnant Woman with Trauma** 226
    Prabha Lal

25. **Approach to a Pregnant Woman Brought in a Collapsed State** 234
    Aimee Teong Chuin Ai, Kazila Bhutia

26. Approach to a Postnatal Woman 240
    Sumi P Thampi, Anu Handa

27. Approach to a Woman with Specific Problems in Puerperium 250
    Priyanka Arora, Isha Khurana Vashisht

28. Approach to a Woman with Abnormal Behavior in Puerperium 269
    Jasmeet K Monga

Section 2: Gynecology

29. History Taking and Clinical Examination of a Woman Presenting with
    Gynecological Complaints 277
    Shalini Singh

30. Approach to a Woman Presenting with Vaginal Discharge 290
    Seema Singhal, Namita Jain

31. Approach to a Woman Presenting with Abnormal Uterine Bleeding 301
    Asmita Kaundal, Neha Gami

32. Approach to a Woman Presenting with Infertility 313
    Seema Singhal, Namita Jain

33. Approach to a Woman Presenting with Dysmenorrhea 328
    Manisha Bajaj

34. Approach to a Woman Presenting with Dyspareunia 334
    Manisha Bajaj

35. Approach to a Woman Presenting with Lower Abdominal Pain 342
    Manisha Bajaj

36. Approach to a Woman Presenting with Abdominal Lump 353
    Shilpa Dhingra

37. Approach to a Woman Presenting with Pelvic Organ Prolapse 360
    Nidhi Malhotra, Karishma Thariani

38. Approach to a Woman Presenting with Urinary Incontinence 374
    Nidhi Malhotra, Karishma Thariani

39. Approach to a Woman Presenting with Anal Incontinence 389
    Harvinder Kaur, Karishma Thariani

40. Approach to a Woman Presenting with Pruritus Vulvae 399
    Shalini Singh, Vibhu Mendiratta

41. Approach to a Woman Presenting with Vulvar Lesion 404
    Shilpa Singla, Anuja Rao

42. Approach to a Woman Presenting with Amenorrhea 414
    Ritu Sharma, Jasmeet K Monga

43. Approach to a Woman Presenting with Hirsutism 427
    Jasmeet K Monga

44. Approach to a Girl Presenting with Precocious Puberty 434
    K Aparna Sharma, Sadia Mansoor

45. Approach to a Girl Presenting with Delayed Puberty 442
    K Aparna Sharma, Sadia Mansoor

46. Approach to a Woman Presenting with Breast Lump 449
    Vishrut Narang

47. Approach to a Woman Presenting with Nipple Discharge 456
    Laxmi Goel

48. Approach to a Survivor of Sexual Assault 462
    Monika Madaan

Section 3: General

49. Minor Procedures in Gynecology 475
    Kirti Kishore Sharma, Richa Aggarwal*

50. Minor Procedures in Obstetrics 491
    Nishtha Jaiswal

51. Minor Procedures for Screening and Diagnosis of Cervical Cancer 501
    Tahmina S

52. Obstetrical and Gynecological Instruments 522
    Archana Kumari

53. Endoscopic Equipment and Instruments 548
    Aruna Nigam, Arpita De

54. **Cardiotocography** 564
    Vidhi Chaudhary, Shalini Malhotra

55. **Forceps and Ventouse** 575
    Anuradha Singh

56. **Contraception** 581
    Harkiran Kaur Narang, Anju Yadav

57. **Medical Termination of Pregnancy and Sterilization** 603
    Raina Chawla

58. **Government Initiatives to Improve Maternal and Neonatal Health** 626
    Monika Datta

Index *633*

Section 1

Obstetrics

- Approach to a Pregnant Woman Attending Antenatal Clinic
- Approach to a Pregnant Woman Presenting with Bad Obstetric History
- Approach to a Pregnant Woman Presenting with Bleeding in Early Pregnancy
- Approach to a Pregnant Woman Presenting with Bleeding in Late Pregnancy
- Approach to a Pregnant Woman Presenting with Abdominal Pain
- Approach to a Pregnant Woman Presenting with Discharge Per Vaginum
- Approach to a Pregnant Woman Presenting with Vomiting
- Approach to a Pregnant Woman Presenting with Diarrhea
- Approach to a Pregnant Woman Presenting with Fever
- Approach to a Pregnant or Puerperal Woman Presenting with Convulsions
- Approach to a Pregnant Woman Presenting with Dyspnea
- Approach to a Pregnant Woman Presenting with Pruritus
- Approach to a Pregnant Woman with Decreased Fetal Movements
- Approach to a Pregnant Woman Presenting with a Positive Aneuploidy Screening Test
- Approach to a Pregnant Woman with a Congenitally Malformed Fetus
- Approach to a Pregnant Woman Presenting with Jaundice
- Approach to a Pregnant Woman Presenting with Pallor
- Approach to a Pregnant Woman Presenting with Hypertension
- Approach to a Pregnant Woman Presenting with Heart Disease
- Approach to a Pregnant Woman with Suspected Fetal Growth Restriction
- Approach to a Pregnant Woman with Previous Cesarean Section
- Approach to a Pregnant Woman with Multiple Pregnancy
- Approach to a Pregnant Woman Presenting with Rh-negative Pregnancy
- Approach to a Pregnant Woman with Trauma
- Approach to a Pregnant Woman Brought in a Collapsed State
- Approach to a Postnatal Woman
- Approach to a Woman with Specific Problems in Puerperium
- Approach to a Woman with Abnormal Behavior in Puerperium

Approach to a Pregnant Woman Attending Antenatal Clinic

GS Triveni, Richa Aggarwal,* Pooja Dwivedi

INTRODUCTION

The aim of antenatal care (ANC) is to ensure that a normal pregnancy culminates in the delivery of a healthy baby from a healthy mother. The objectives of antenatal care are listed in Box 1. Early registration is required to help the woman recall the date of her last menstrual period (LMP), calculate expected date of delivery (EDOD), and offer medical termination of pregnancy if she does not wish to continue the pregnancy. It provides an opportunity to assess her health status, record baseline blood pressure (BP) and weight, screen for any preexisting diseases, and review any medications she is taking. It helps in building a rapport with the pregnant woman and start folic acid supplementation during the first trimester. However, a pregnant woman should be registered whenever she reports for her first time and is provided care.

HISTORY-TAKING

The aim of history-taking is to elicit an accurate account of the symptoms that represent the clinical problem and to set it against the background of the patient's life. The doctor must put the woman at ease and encourage her to talk freely.

During the first visit, a detailed history is taken to diagnose pregnancy, to identify any complications in previous pregnancies that may affect the outcome of present pregnancy, and to identify any medical or obstetric condition that may affect the present pregnancy.

For the purpose of record-keeping and reference for the subsequent visits, an antenatal card should be filled up for every registered pregnant woman and she should be asked to carry it with her for all successive visits as mentioned in Table 1.[1] The details to be asked and recorded in the antenatal card is as given below.

Name and Address

Name and address are asked to become familiar with the pregnant woman and establish a rapport with her. It helps to understand how far she stays from the medical facility and enables the healthcare provider to trace or contact her in the future, if required.

Box 1: Objectives of antenatal care.
- To screen and identify high-risk cases
- To prevent and detect complications at early stage for timely management
- To ensure continued medical surveillance and prophylaxis
- To educate the mother about the physiology of pregnancy, labor, and childbirth through demonstrations, charts, and diagrams
- To provide adequate psychological counseling to the mother and allay her fears
- To discuss the place, time, and mode of delivery with the couple
- To sensitize the couple about the need of family planning

Table 1: Schedule of antenatal visits.

Visit	Timing	Interval
First visit	First trimester	–
Second visit	18–20 weeks	6–8 weeks
Third visit	26 weeks	6 weeks
Fourth visit	30 weeks	4 weeks
Fifth visit	34 weeks	4 weeks
Sixth visit	36 weeks	2 weeks
Seventh visit	38 weeks	2 weeks
Eighth visit	40 weeks	2 weeks

Box 2: Dating of pregnancy.
- Relate her LMP to some major event or festival
- Date of quickening
- Date of any test done for confirmation of pregnancy: UPT, USG
- Any first-trimester USG
- Size of uterus on any prior pelvic or per abdomen examination

(LMP: last menstrual period; UPT: urine pregnancy test; USG: ultrasonography)

Age

Women <19 years of age or >35 years are at a higher risk of pregnancy-related complications.

Occupation

Knowing occupation helps in interpreting symptoms due to fatigue, understanding occupation hazards, and giving a reasonable and realistic antenatal advice to the woman.

Period of Gestation

The duration of pregnancy is to be expressed in terms of completed weeks. For calculating the weeks of gestation, counting is started from the first day of last menstrual period (LMP). The expected date of delivery (EDOD) is calculated using Naegele's formula in women with regular 28–30 days menstrual cycles before conception. The formula used is EDOD = LMP + 9 months + 7 days.

It is important to ensure that the last period was normal as some women may have implantation bleeding in first trimester, which is usually scanty, and the women may consider it as her LMP resulting in wrong dating and calculation of EDOD.

Dating of Pregnancy

Dating of pregnancy is important because many obstetrical interventions and decisions during pregnancy are based on the gestational age. In conditions such as fetal growth restriction, preeclampsia, premature rupture of membranes, and pregnancy with diabetes mellitus, termination of pregnancy is indicated before the EDOD.

First trimester is the best time to accurately date the pregnancy in women who are either not sure of dates or do not know or recall the date of their last menstrual period (DLMP). These are women who conceive in lactational amenorrhea, have delayed cycles, or conceive after stopping hormonal contraceptives such as depot medroxyprogesterone acetate (DMPA) or following abortion without resuming normal cycles. The various ways of dating of pregnancy are listed in Box 2.

Date of quickening, i.e., feeling the fetal movements for the first time, is helpful in dating pregnancy in women presenting for registration around 4–5 months of pregnancy. EDOD can be calculated by adding 22 weeks and 24 weeks to the date of quickening in primigravida and multigravida, respectively. Multigravida perceives quickening earlier than primigravida.

Ultrasonography is the most reliable investigation for dating of pregnancy. Its accuracy declines with successive trimesters. The accuracy of the assessment of period of gestation in first trimester is ± 1 week.[2] In second trimester, an average of two scans at

2–4 weeks' interval gives an accuracy of about ± 2 weeks.[3] Third-trimester scan is not a reliable method to date pregnancy. Its accuracy is ± 3 weeks.[4]

Complaints

The pregnant woman may present either for a routine antenatal checkup or may present with some specific complaint. The presenting complaint may be abdominal pain, bleeding or leaking per vaginam, loss of fetal movements, or swelling feet. While recording history of pregnant women admitted in the hospital, ask the woman about the reason for her admission and document.

In case there is a specific complaint, ask for the mode of onset, duration, progress, severity, any associations related to it, and any treatment received. If there is no specific complaint, start with the history of present pregnancy.

History of Present Pregnancy

The important symptoms that must be asked in each of the three trimesters are given in the following text:

First Trimester

It is important to find out whether pregnancy is planned or not? Whether it is spontaneous or assisted pregnancy, i.e., after treatment for infertility? Whether it was confirmed with urine pregnancy test or USG, if yes when? The reports should be reviewed to check for the accuracy of dating of pregnancy. Any exposure to irradiation should be noted. History of any bleeding per vaginam, excessive nausea or vomiting, or fever with or without rash is important. Any history of drug intake including folic acid intake should be elicited.

Second Trimester

History of quickening, tetanus toxoid (TT) immunization, intake of iron and calcium supplements, antenatal checkup, and USG should be elicited. The ultrasound report should be reviewed for number of fetuses, biometry, any gross congenital malformations, amount of liquor, and placental localization.

Third Trimester

Symptoms suggestive of preeclampsia such as headache, epigastric pain, blurring of vision, rapid gain of weight, swelling feet, and those suggestive of anemia—easy fatiguability, breathlessness, palpitations, generalized swelling, and passage of worms in stools—should be asked for. Any symptoms suggestive of urinary tract infection, i.e., burning micturition, lower abdominal or loin pain, increased frequency of micturition; and any history of watery or foul-smelling discharge per vaginam or any bleeding per vaginam is asked for. It is also important to find out if the woman is perceiving fetal movements.

Menstrual History

Age of menarche, duration and amount of blood flow, and length and cyclical pattern of the menstrual cycles should be recorded. The date of the LMP must be noted and EDOD calculated using the Naegele's formula. In case the menstrual cycles are irregular, EDOD must be corrected with the help of first-trimester USG.

Obstetric History

Gravidity and Parity

Gravidity is the number of times a woman has conceived including the present pregnancy, irrespective of the outcome of pregnancy. Parity refers to the number of times a woman has delivered a viable baby.

"Gravida" and "para" refer to pregnancies and not to babies. A woman who delivers twins in her first pregnancy is referred to as para one.

Primigravida, a woman with her first pregnancy, and grand multipara, a woman who has delivered more than four viable babies, are at a higher risk of pregnancy-related complications.

Obstetric history is relevant in multigravidae. Obstetric history is usually summarized as gravida, para, abortion, and live issues (GPAL).

It starts with inquiring how long the woman has been married and cohabiting followed by the details of her previous pregnancies including the antenatal, intranatal, and postnatal periods and the outcome of each pregnancy in chronological order.

The woman is asked in detail about each pregnancy as regards any antenatal complications such as abortion, ectopic pregnancy, molar pregnancy, preterm labor, hypertensive disorder of pregnancy (HDP), convulsions, gestational diabetes mellitus (GDM), malpresentation, and antepartum hemorrhage. Any intranatal or postnatal complications such as prolonged labor, obstructed labor, instrumental delivery, cesarean section, postpartum hemorrhage, stillbirth, neonatal death, and administration of Anti-D in case of Rh-negative woman are important as these may affect the outcome of the present pregnancy.

Details of the baby such as sex, birth weight, Apgar score, duration of breastfeeding, immunization status, milestones, and present condition must be recorded.

A detailed history of prior abortions, whether planned medical termination of pregnancy (MTP) or spontaneous abortion, is noted. In spontaneous abortions, it is important to know if the pregnancy was confirmed by urine pregnancy test or ultrasonography (USG), whether cardiac activity was documented or not, and whether it was followed by evacuation, dilatation and curettage, or medical abortion. Early pregnancy loss after the documentation of cardiac activity points toward a maternal cause of abortion whereas nonappearance of cardiac activity and/or fetal node implies a fetal cause of abortion. History of painless midtrimester expulsion of products of conception is suggestive of cervical incompetence.

The details of the postabortal period are important as regards any fever and persistent bleeding suggestive of complications such as postabortal sepsis and incomplete abortion. Any history of perforation or repeated dilatation and curettage can subsequently predispose a woman to morbidly adherent placenta.

Any old records, if available, should be reviewed.

The previous obstetric events are recorded chronologically as per the format given in Table 2.

Past Medical History

History of any systemic illness such as hypertension, diabetes mellitus, jaundice, tuberculosis, asthma, heart disease, renal disease, seizures, and blood transfusion is significant as preexisting medical disorders can worsen during pregnancy or influence the obstetric outcome necessitating management by a multidisciplinary team. One can ask the woman if she has had any prolonged illness, treatment, or hospitalization in past. History of any drug allergy or intake of any drug that may be potentially harmful for the fetus is important.

Table 2: Format for recording obstetric history, e.g., a multigravida with an obstetric formula $G_4 P_2 L_2 A_1$.

Date and year of obstetric event	Pregnancy events / Antenatal period	Labor events / Intranatal period/abortion events	Puerperium / Postnatal/post-abortal period	Family planning / Contraception	Outcome of the baby / Sex, birth weight, Apgar score, duration of breastfeeding, immunization status, and present condition
January 2013	Spontaneous abortion, 2-month gestation, confirmed by urine pregnancy test	Evacuation done at private nursing home	Uneventful	None	–
December 2014	Regular antenatal checkup; uneventful antenatal period	Uneventful Spontaneous term, normal vaginal delivery with episiotomy at private hospital	Uneventful	Barrier contraceptive condoms	2.6-kg girl cried at birth, breastfed till 1 year, immunized, attained normal milestones, alive and healthy
March 2017	Regular antenatal checkup; had preterm premature rupture of membranes (PPROM) at 32 weeks	Spontaneous preterm vaginal delivery at 33 weeks at private hospital	Uneventful	None	1.2-kg boy cried after resuscitation, kept in nursery for 5 days, breastfed for 15 months, immunized, attained normal milestones, alive and healthy

Past Surgical History

History of surgery on bowel or appendix may be associated with intra-abdominal adhesions. Previous surgeries such as classical cesarean, metroplasty, and myomectomy can cause adhesions. Women with classical cesarean section or myomectomy where the uterine cavity is opened during surgery are at an increased risk for uterine rupture in subsequent pregnancies or labor and are offered elective cesarean section. The surgical notes of the previous surgery should be reviewed.

Family History

Family history of hypertension or diabetes is important as it predisposes the woman to HDP and or GDM during pregnancy. Any history of repeated blood transfusions in the family is suggestive of thalassemia. Family history of multiple pregnancy, congenitally malformed children, or mentally retarded children is important as it increases the chances of same in the current pregnancy.

Personal History

Contraceptive practice prior to pregnancy must be inquired as use of oral pills or DMPA may delay ovulation and lead to wrong calculation of the EDOD. Ask for history of tobacco chewing, smoking, or alcohol consumption as these may harm the fetus and result in fetal growth restriction (FGR).

Socioeconomic History

Ask the woman about her education, occupation, husband's occupation, and per capita income and assess her socioeconomic status. Conditions such as prematurity, low birth weight, and anemia have been related to low socioeconomic status whereas GDM and obesity with high socioeconomic status.

Dietary History

A simple evaluation of diet is valuable in all pregnant women, especially those with anemia, diabetes mellitus, or FGR. Daily total caloric and protein intake can be estimated by 24-hour recall method. It is important to corroborate the dietary history with the nutritional status of the woman. In a well-nourished woman, if dietary history does not correlate with the nutritional status of women, it is likely to be inaccurate and needs to be elicited again.

CLINICAL EXAMINATION

A good physical examination requires a cooperative patient, a quiet, warm, and well-lit room. Daylight is better than artificial light, which may mask changes in skin color. The woman should be reassured and relaxed. The examination must be carried out as gently as possible. The woman is not exposed more than necessary.

General Physical Examination

The examination starts the moment a woman enters the room by observing her appearance, gait, demeanor, and responsiveness. The following parameters are considered for general physical examination:

Height

The woman is considered short statured in India if her height is <145 cm or 4'10" and is likely to be associated with a small pelvis.[5]

Weight

The weight must be measured at each visit on the same weighing machine. The baseline weight would be the weight during the first visit in first trimester. The body mass index (BMI) is calculated with prepregnant weight or first-trimester weight. BMI calculated later in pregnancy with the woman's weight at that time is not correct as the weight of the fetus and uterine contents add on to the maternal weight. Average weight gain during pregnancy is around 9–11 kg. After the first trimester, weight gain is around 2 kg every month or 0.5 kg per week. Rapid weight gain of >3 kg/month arouses suspicion of preeclampsia or multiple pregnancies. A low-weight gain is suggestive of FGR.

Pallor

Look at the lower palpebral conjunctiva (Figs. 1A and B), tongue (Figs. 2A and B), lips, oral mucosa, nails (Figs. 3A and B), and palmar creases (Figs. 4A and B) for its color and presence of pallor, which is indicative of anemia.

Jaundice

Look for any yellowness of the bulbar conjunctiva, undersurface of the tongue, hard palate, and skin.

Oral Cavity

Examine the tongue, teeth, gums, and tonsils. Presence of glossitis and stomatitis suggests malnutrition. Patients with poor oral hygiene,

Chapter 1: Approach to a Pregnant Woman Attending Antenatal Clinic 9

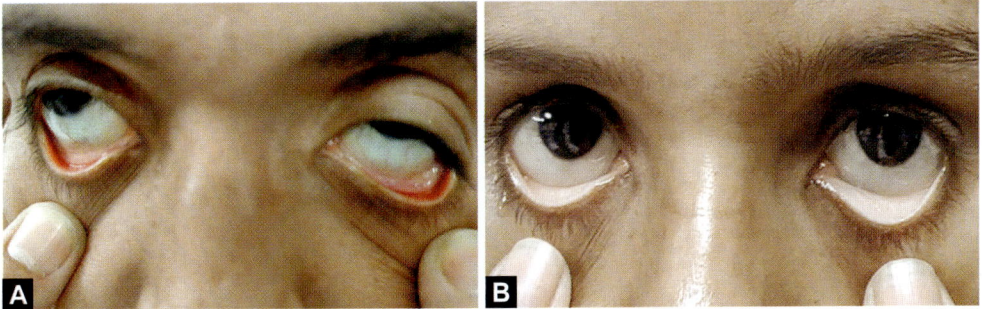

Figs. 1A and B: Inspection of conjunctiva for anemia. (A) Normal conjunctival color; (B) Women with conjunctival pallor.

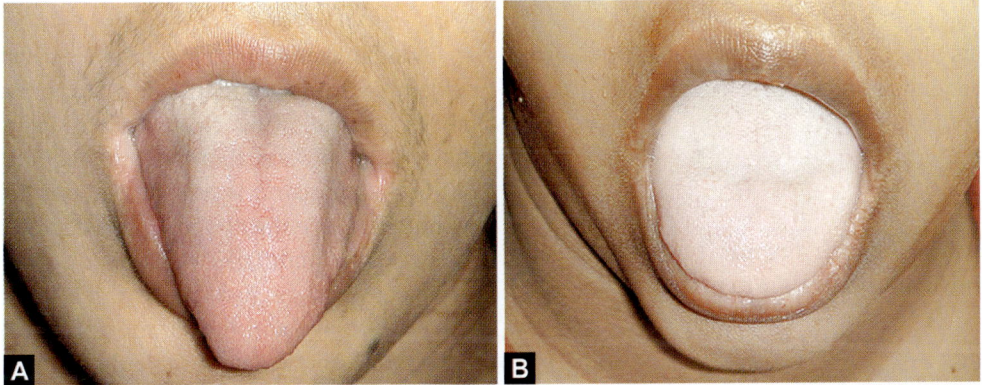

Figs. 2A and B: Inspection of tongue for anemia. (A) Tongue with normal color; (B) Pale tongue.

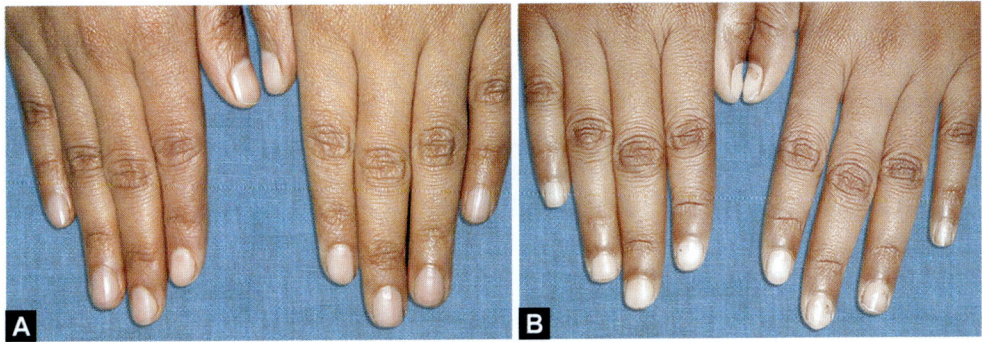

Figs. 3A and B: Examination of nails for anemia. (A) Normal nails; (B) Pale nails.

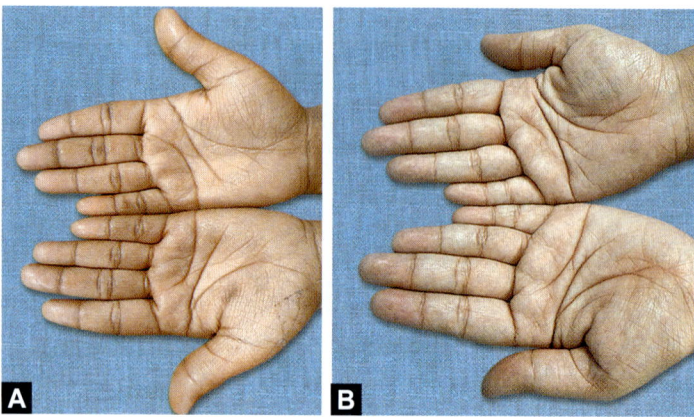

Figs. 4A and B: Examination of palm for anemia. (A) Normal palm; (B) Pale looking palm.

gingivitis, or dental caries should be referred to a dentist to minimize the risk of autoinfection.

Hair

Look at the hair texture; poor texture and brittle hair may be due to malnutrition.

Neck

Neck veins, thyroid gland, and lymph nodes are assessed for any abnormality. Examine the neck veins of the patient in good light. The woman is reclined at an angle of about 45° with neck supported to relax the neck muscles, especially the sternocleidomastoids. The vertical distance from the angle of Louis (sternal angle) to the imaginary line drawn from the upper end of jugular venous column gives jugular venous pressure (JVP), which is measured in centimeters. When JVP is raised 3 cm above the sternal angle or internal jugular vein is engorged above the level of clavicle, it is abnormal and suggestive of congestive heart failure (CHF), pericardial effusion, constrictive pericarditis, or any mediastinal mass.

Significant thyroid enlargement is usually evident on inspection. Thyroid gland always moves on swallowing. Normal thyroid gland may be palpable in thin patients. Palpation of the thyroid gland is best carried out from behind the patient with the fingers encircling the neck; the landmarks for palpation are the laryngeal cartilage, just below which are the cricoid cartilage and the isthmus of thyroid. If palpable, note whether the enlargement is diffuse and smooth or nodular.

Lymph Nodes

Examine for occipital, submandibular, cervical, supraclavicular, axillary, epitrochlear, inguinal, femoral, and popliteal groups of lymph nodes. If palpable, note the number, location, size, consistency, mobility, confluence, warmth, tenderness, and whether discrete or matted.

Pedal Edema

Patient is examined for pitting edema over the medial malleolus and anterior surface of lower one third of tibia that is shin. The area is pressed with thumb at least for 5 seconds

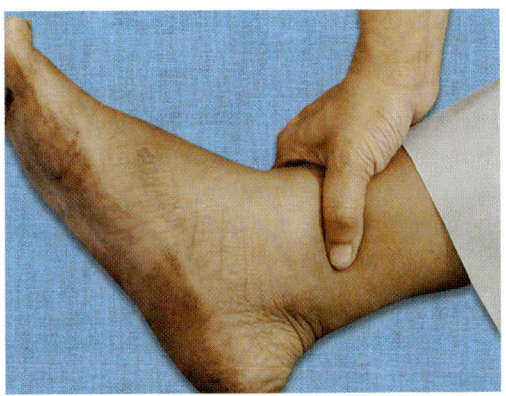

Fig. 5: Demonstration of pedal edema.

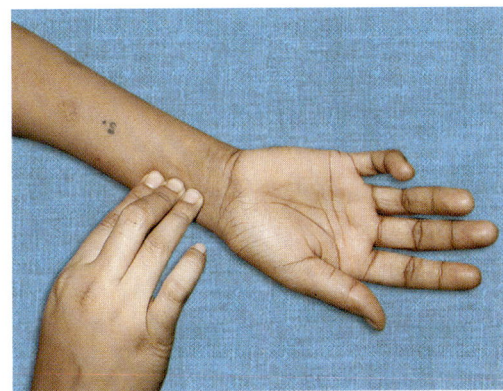

Fig. 6: Recording pulse rate.

to note whether the edema is pitting or not (Fig. 5).

Edema in pregnancy can be physiological or pathological. Physiological edema is due to the pressure of the gravid uterus on the common iliac vessels and pathological edema is a manifestation of disorders such as preeclampsia, anemia, hypoproteinemia, cardiac disease, or renal disease.

Varicosities

Note the presence of varicose veins and their distribution. Pregnancy tends to worsen them.

Temperature

The thermometer must be accurate and kept in position for a full minute. The temperature is usually taken in the mouth or in the axilla. The temperature of the mouth and rectum is generally at least half a degree higher than that of the axilla or groin.

Pulse

The presence or absence of the main peripheral arterial pulses should be noted. These include radial, brachial, carotid, femoral, popliteal, posterior tibial, and dorsalis pedis. The volume of each pulse is compared with that of the other side. The arterial pulses are detected by gently compressing the vessel against some firm underlying structure, usually bone. The radial pulse is felt with the tips of the fingers by compressing the radial artery against the head of the radius with patients' forearm slightly pronated and wrist slightly flexed (Fig. 6). Note the rate, rhythm, character and volume of the pulse, and presence or absence of any radiofemoral delay.

Blood Pressure

The blood pressure (BP) is measured at every visit. The BP should be measured with the patient sitting or lying laterally at ease with the manometer placed at the same level as the cuff on the patient's arm and the observer's eye (Fig. 7). All clothing should be removed from the arm. The cuff should be applied to the upper arm with the lower border of the cuff >2.5 cm from the cubital fossa. The cuff should be of appropriate size, i.e., 12.5–13 cm in width and 35 cm in length for an average adult. The first appearance of repetitive sounds or Korotkoff first sound is taken as the systolic pressure. Disappearance of sounds,

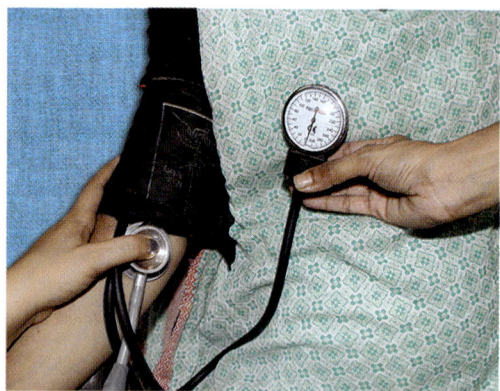

Fig. 7: Blood pressure measurement.

i.e., Korotkoff fifth rather than muffling of sounds or Korotkoff fourth sound are taken for measurement of diastolic pressure during pregnancy.

Breast Examination

Examination of the breasts is essential not only to note the changes of pregnancy but also to detect any abnormality, which can be timely corrected for successful breastfeeding. With the patient reclining, arms to the sides, inspect the shape and symmetry of breasts and nipples. Look for any reddening, ulceration or dimpling of the skin, retraction or cracking of the nipples, or any discharge. Palpate each breast with the flat of the fingers of both hands for any lump and if present, determine its situation, size, surface, edge, consistency, and mobility in relation to deep and superficial structures.

Respiratory System

Note the respiratory rate and inspect the exposed chest for its shape, symmetry, and movements. Palpate the chest for any swelling, tenderness, position of trachea and cardiac impulse. Percuss the chest and note its resonance to detect any area of dullness. Auscultate the chest for the intensity or loudness and quality of breath sounds, i.e., vesicular or bronchial, and presence of any adventitious sounds such as pleural rub, rhonchi, or crepitations. In a normal woman, bilateral vesicular breathing is heard all over the chest with no added sounds.

Cardiovascular System

Inspect the chest for any bulge, pulsations, dilated veins, and cardiac impulse. Locate the apex beat with the patient sitting or lying supine. Assess whether it is visible or not (look on both sides), its site whether shifted up, down, outward, inward or on right side, and character whether normal, feeble, tapping, heaving, and hyperkinetic. Apex beat is shifted to fourth intercostal space 2.5 cm outside the midclavicular line in pregnancy. Palpate for any thrill and note its site and timing. Thrill is associated with a murmur of grade IV or higher. Functional murmurs are never associated with a thrill. Auscultate the mitral, tricuspid, aortic and pulmonary areas, and look for intensity of heart sounds, splitting whether fixed or variable, third and fourth heart sounds, opening snap and additional sounds such as ejection systolic clicks, and murmurs. If murmur is present, evaluate its site of maximum intensity, grade, timing, character, quality, and radiation.

Abdominal Examination

Before inspecting the abdomen, make sure that the light is good, the room is comfortably warm, and there is adequate exposure. The patient should pass urine and lie comfortably in the supine position with the thighs slightly flexed and abducted to relax the abdominal muscles. The examiner stands on the right side of the patient. Ask about any tender areas on abdomen before starting the palpation and initiate palpation from the nontender areas. Comfort and gentleness can be enhanced by using the flat of the hand as well as the examining fingers.

Inspection

Note the uterine ovoid whether longitudinal, transverse, or oblique; contour of the uterus whether the fundus is convex or flattened or notched; shape of the uterus whether spherical or cylindrical; any undue enlargement of the uterus; any dilated veins, striae gravidarum, linea nigra, or scar marks of previous cesarean, or laparotomy; any evidence of ringworm or scabies infection and any visible fetal movements or peristalsis.

Palpation

Palpate for the presence of any uterine contractions, uterine tone, any tenderness, and fetal movements.

Fundal Height

Uterus remains a pelvic organ until 12th week of gestation and hence is usually not palpable in the first trimester. The ulnar border of the left hand is placed on the uppermost level of the fundus and an approximate duration of pregnancy is ascertained in terms of weeks of gestation (Fig. 8). In the later half of pregnancy, the uterus is centralized for assessing the fundal height in case it is deviated on one side usually on the right. The assessment of fundal height is as given in Table 3.

Alternatively, symphysis fundal height (SFH) can be measured more accurately with a tape. The upper border of the fundus is located by the ulnar border of the left hand and is marked after correcting the dextrorotation of the uterus. The distance from the upper border of the symphysis pubis up to the marked point is measured by a tape in centimeters (Figs. 9A and B). In a nonobese woman with singleton pregnancy in longitudinal lie, the SFH measured in centimeters corresponds to the number of weeks between 24 and 36 weeks. A variation of ±2 cm is accepted as normal. Variation, beyond the normal range, needs further evaluation.

The differential diagnosis of fundal height being more than or less than the period of gestation is listed in Table 4.

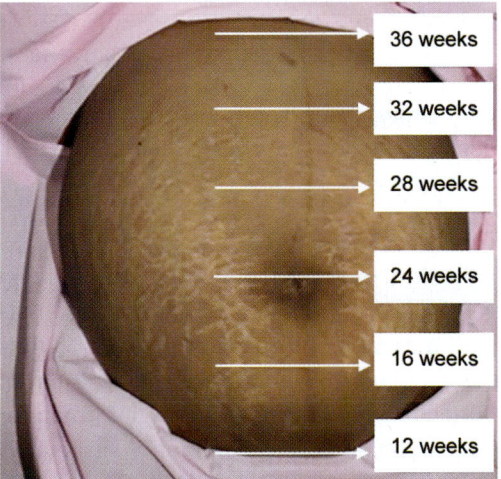

Fig. 8: Assessment of fundal height.

Table 3: Estimation of fundal height in weeks.

Weeks	Features
12	• Uterus is just palpable
16	• Fundus is equidistant from the symphysis pubis and the umbilicus
24	• Uterus reaches just above the level of umbilicus
30	• Uterus is equidistant from the xiphisternum and umbilicus
36	• Uterus reaches up to the level of xiphisternum
40	• Height is equivalent to 32–34 weeks, but flanks are full

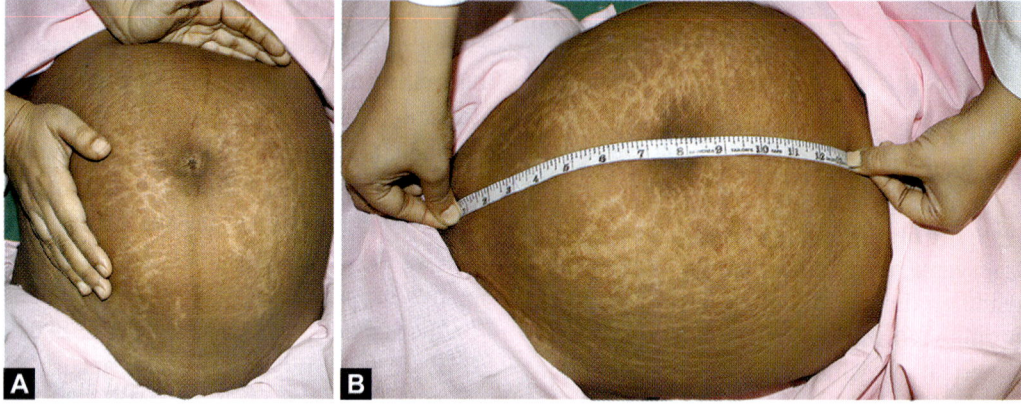

Figs. 9A and B: Measurement of symphysis-fundal height. (A) Marking the fundal height and correction of dextrorotation; (B) Measurement of distance between the fundus and the pubic symphysis.

Table 4: Causes of fundal height not corresponding to the period of gestation.

Fundal height more than the period of gestation	Fundal height less than the period of gestation
Wrong date of LMP	• Wrong date of LMP
Full bladder	• Missed abortion
Hydatidiform mole	• FGR
Multiple pregnancy	• Intrauterine death
Polyhydramnios	• Oligohydramnios
Pregnancy with pelvic mass (ovarian tumor or fibroids)	• Transverse lie
Concealed accidental hemorrhage	
Big baby	

(FGR: fetal growth restriction; LMP: last menstrual period)

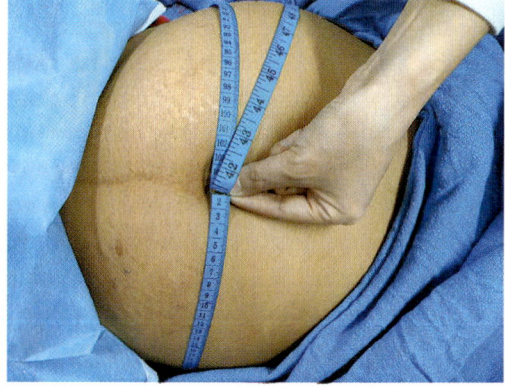

Fig. 10: Measuring abdominal girth.

Abdominal Girth

Abdominal girth is measured in inches by a tape at the level of the umbilicus (Fig. 10). Abdominal girth in inches corresponds to the period of gestation after 28 weeks and increases at the rate of 1 inch/week. At 40 weeks, the abdominal girth is 40" or 100 cm. It is better to record abdominal girth in inches and height in centimeters. Abdominal girth is more than the period of gestation in women with wrong dates, central obesity, transverse lie, multiple pregnancy, and hydramnios.

Obstetric Grips

Palpation must be conducted with utmost gentleness as clumsy and purposeless palpation is not only uninformative but may stimulate uterine contractions with resultant difficulty in getting satisfactory information. Palpation should be temporarily suspended in the presence of Braxton Hicks contraction or uterine contraction and resumed after the

Chapter 1: Approach to a Pregnant Woman Attending Antenatal Clinic   15

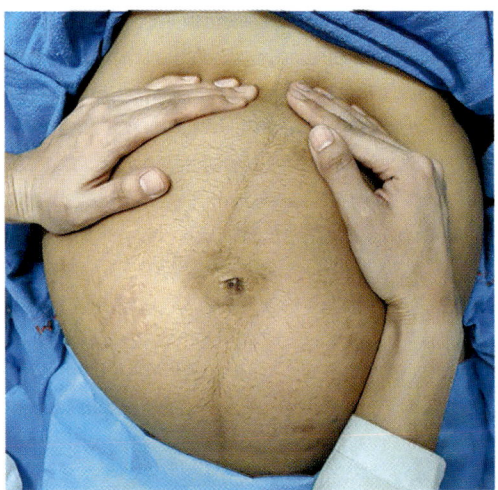

Fig. 11: Leopold's first maneuver.

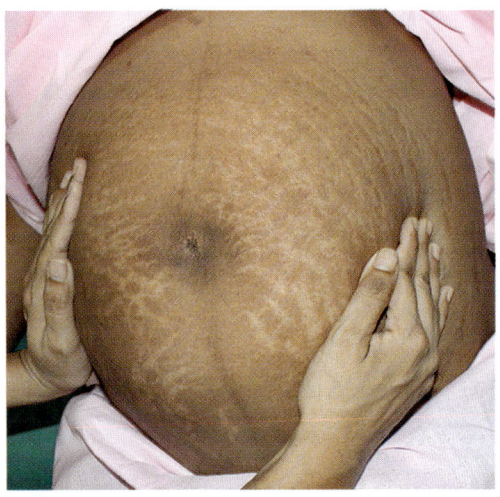

Fig. 12: Leopold's second maneuver.

contraction passes off. Abdominal examination is done using four maneuvers described by Leopold in 1894.[6] It may be difficult to perform and interpret the maneuvers in the presence of obesity, hydramnios, and anterior placenta. The first three maneuvers are done with the examiner facing the face of the pregnant woman whereas the fourth maneuver is performed with the examiner facing the woman's feet.

Leopold's Maneuvers

Leopold's first maneuver or fundal grip: The whole of the fundal area is palpated using both hands laid flat on it to identify the fetal pole occupying the uterine fundus—broad, soft, and irregular mass suggestive of breech or hard, globular, and ballotable mass suggestive of head (Fig. 11). In transverse lie, none of the fetal poles is palpable in fundal area.

Leopold's second maneuver or lateral grip: The hands are placed flat on either side of the umbilicus to palpate the sides and front of the uterus to locate the position of fetal back and limbs (Fig. 12). The back is suggested by smooth, curved, and resistant feel whereas the limbs feel small, knobby, and irregular. By noting whether the back is directed anteriorly, transversely, or posteriorly, the orientation and position of the fetus can be made out. To palpate one side, a hand on the other side stabilizes the uterus to facilitate palpation.

Leopold' third maneuver or superficial pelvic grip or Pawlik's grip: The overstretched thumb and four fingers of the right hand are placed over the lower pole of the uterus keeping the ulnar border of the palm on the upper border of the symphysis pubis (Fig. 13). When the fingers and the thumb are approximated, the presenting part is grasped distinctly, and side-to-side mobility of the presenting part can be assessed. If the presenting part is not engaged, a mobile mass head or buttocks will be felt. In transverse lie, this grip is empty. However, findings from this maneuver are simply indicative of the lower fetal pole presenting in the pelvis; the details are defined by the fourth maneuver.

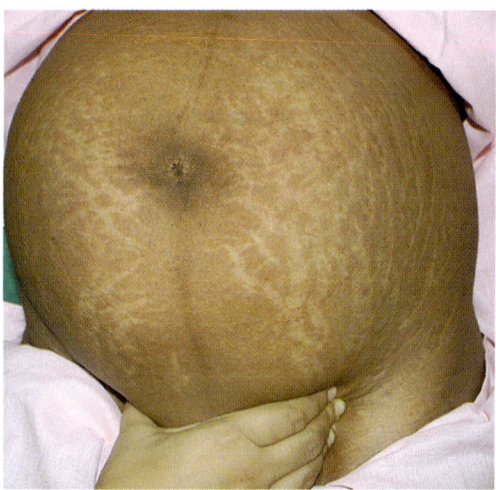

Fig. 13: Leopold's third maneuver.

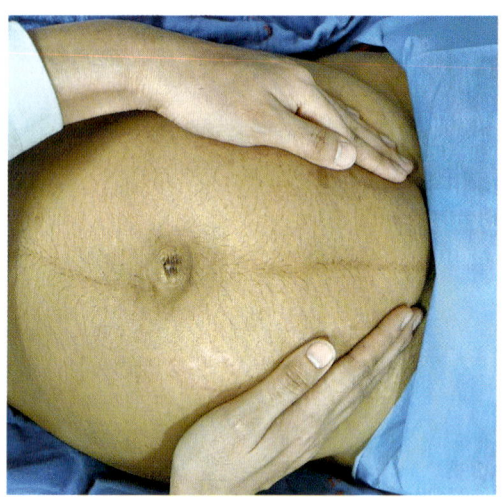

Fig. 14: Leopold's fourth maneuver.

Leopold's fourth maneuver or deep pelvic grip: With the examiner facing the feet of the patient, four fingers of both hands are placed on either side of the midline in the lower pole of the uterus and parallel to the inguinal ligament. The fingers are pressed downward and backward in a manner of approximation of fingertips to palpate the part occupying the lower pole of the uterus (Fig. 14).

The presenting part, attitude, and engagement in case of cephalic presentation can be commented on the fourth maneuver. This pelvic grip gives maximum information.

In vertex presentation, the cephalic prominence on the side of the back is the occiput and that on the side of limbs is the sinciput. The attitude of the head is inferred by noting the relative position of the sinciput and occiput. In well-flexed head, the sinciput is placed at a higher level, but in deflexed head, both the poles are at a same level. The engagement of the presenting part is ascertained by noting whether there is convergence or divergence of the fingertips during palpation. Divergence of the fingers indicates engaged head and convergence of the fingers indicates an unengaged head.

The amount of liquor is assessed by palpating in between the limbs. The fetal weight can be estimated either by clinical experience or by using Johnson's formula in cephalic presentation. Johnson's formula is estimated fetal weight in grams = symphysis fundal height in centimeters −12 (if head is not engaged) or 11 (if head is engaged) × 155.

Abdomen is then palpated gently to rule out any organomegaly. This is possible only in first half of pregnancy, when the uterus is small. Abdominal assessment of descent of the fetal head is done using "fifths" or Crichton's method. It is especially useful while monitoring progress of labor. Progress of labor is assessed per abdomen by descent of head, rotation of the anterior shoulder toward midline, and change in position of the fetal heart sound (FHS) downward and medially. Crichton used the "fifth" formula by estimating the number of "fifths" of the head palpable above the pelvic brim.[7] It is assessed in finger breadths that can be accommodated between the symphysis pubis and the groove

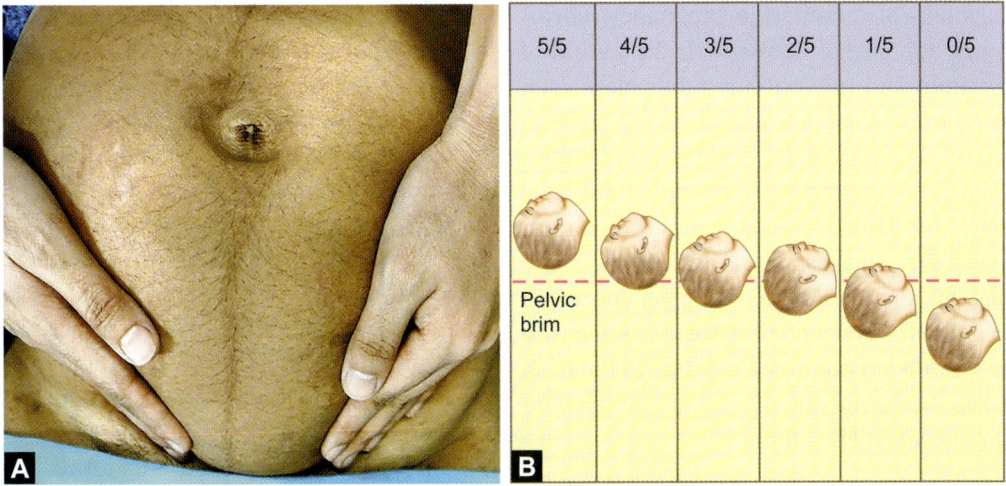

Figs. 15A and B: (A) Assessment of descent of fetal head; (B) Crichton's method.

of the neck of the fetus in suprapubic area. The head is engaged when either it is one fifth above the brim or is not palpable per abdomen (Figs. 15A and B).

Auscultation

Auscultation of distinct FHS helps in diagnosing a live fetus. The FHS can be heard after 24 weeks and are best audible through the back in vertex and breech presentation and through the fetal chest in face presentation. The site where it is best heard gives a clue to the likely presentation, position, and descent of head (Fig. 16). The maximum intensity of FHS is below the umbilicus in cephalic presentation and around the umbilicus in breech. In different positions of the vertex, the location of the FHS depends on the position of the back and the degree of the descent of the head. In the occipitoanterior position, the FHS is in the middle of the spinoumbilical line of the same side. In occipitolateral position, it is heard more laterally and in occipitoposterior position, it is heard toward the mother's flank on the same side. The rate

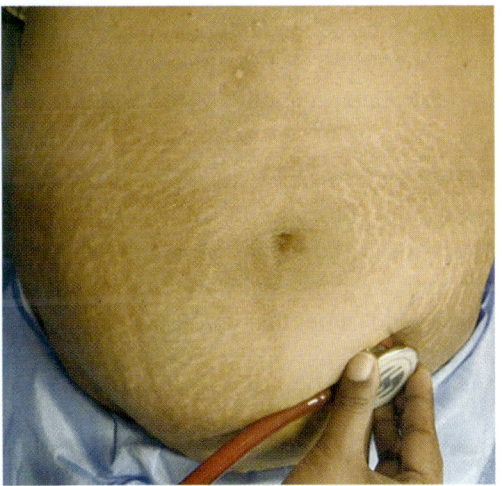

Fig. 16: Auscultation of fetal heart sounds.

and rhythm of the FHS is noted. The normal fetal heart rate ranges between 110 and 160 beats per minute.

Vaginal Examination

First Trimester

Vaginal examination is performed under all asepsis before 12 weeks to confirm the diagnosis of intrauterine pregnancy; corroborate the size of uterus with the period of gestation and rule out any other mass such as fibroid, ectopic pregnancy, or ovarian cysts. These days ultrasound examination has replaced routine internal examination as it is more informative in confirming pregnancy, its viability, and gestational age. However, one vaginal examination including per speculum examination is a good practice in women who have not been examined anytime in the past. A Pap smear may be offered in women who have never had it before.

Steps of vaginal examination: It is important to explain the procedure to the patient and a verbal consent is taken. The patient is asked to empty her bladder prior to examination and lie in dorsal position with legs flexed at hips and knees, and buttocks at the edge of the table. Before conducting the examination, the hands should be washed with soap and sterile gloves are worn.

Inspection: Look for any redness, swelling or ulceration of the vulva, perineum, or anus. Separate the labia using left thumb and index finger, and note the character of vaginal discharge, if any. Presence of cystocele, rectocele, or uterine prolapse is noted.

Speculum examination: The speculum should be warmed to body temperature and lubricated with a water-based jelly. Vulva is cleaned with antiseptic swabs, cleaning it from above downwards and discarding the swab. Cervix and vagina are examined with the help of good light source. Bluish discoloration of vagina and cervix is seen due to increased vascularity in pregnancy (Chadwick's sign). Cervical smear for exfoliative cytology is collected and a vaginal swab for culture sensitivity and a wet smear is prepared if there is abnormal discharge.

Bimanual examination: The examining fingers are lubricated with a water-based jelly and labia are gently parted with the index finger and thumb of the left hand, while index and middle fingers of right hand are introduced deep into the vagina. The left hand is now placed suprapubically; this provides gentle pressure to bring the pelvic viscera toward the vaginal fingers and serves to assess the size, mobility, and regularity of abdominopelvic masses in a bimanual manner. Gentle and systematic examination is done to feel the cervix for its direction, consistency, and any growth; uterus for its size, shape, position, consistency, and regularity; adnexa for any enlargement, mass, or tenderness. In pregnancy, the vaginal walls become soft and increased pulsations are felt through the lateral fornices (Osiander's sign). The pregnant cervix feels as soft as lips of the mouth compared to the feel of the tip of the nose in a nonpregnant uterus (Goodell's sign). The pregnant uterus also feels soft (Hegar's sign) and enlarged depending on the period of gestation. The size of a pregnant uterus corresponds to the size of a cricket ball at 8 weeks' gestation and fetal head size at 12 weeks' gestation.

Third Trimester

Per vaginal examination is indicated at term for assessment of the adequacy of pelvis. It is best done near the EDOD or at the onset of labor or before induction of labor. During labor, a digital vaginal examination is done to determine consistency and position of cervix, its effacement and dilation, the station and position of presenting part, presence or absence of amniotic membranes, degree of molding of the head, presence of caput succedaneum and shape, size, and adequacy of pelvis. Any history of vaginal bleeding

Table 5: Modified Bishop's score.

	0	1	2	3
Cervical position	Posterior	Central	Anterior	–
Cervical consistency	Firm	Medium	Soft	–
Cervical length (cm)	> 4	2–4	1–2	< 1
Cervical dilation (cm)	0	1–2	3–4	> 4
Station in relation to spine (cm)	–3	–2	–1 to 0	Below spines

Table 6: Features to be noted in pelvic assessment.

Inlet	Cavity	Outlet
Sacral promontory	Sacral curve	Subpubic angle
Diagonal conjugate	Side walls	Subpubic arch
Posterior surface of symphysis pubis	Ischial spines	Transverse diameter of outlet (TDO)
	Sacrosciatic notches	Sacrococcygeal joint

contraindicates vaginal examination. In a woman, who is planned for induction of labor, the cervix is assessed for its favorability for induction of labor. The various cervical and pelvic parameters are described collectively as Bishop's score (Table 5). The decision regarding method of induction is decided depending upon the Bishop's score.

The total score is 13, a score between 6 and 13 is favorable, and any score of <6 is unfavorable.

Assessment of pelvis: Clinical pelvimetry is usually performed at term in primigravida and in labor in multiparas. Delaying the assessment is useful due to progressive softening of the maternal tissues. The internal examination should be gentle, methodical, and purposeful.

The features to be noted during examination are as listed in Table 6.

Sacrum: Using two fingers of right hand, the length, breadth, and curvature of sacrum from below upward and side-to-side is noted. Normally, it is smooth, well curved, and usually inaccessible beyond lower three pieces. Any abnormal prominence of the sacrum is noted.

Sacrococcygeal joint: Its mobility and any forward projection of coccyx are noted.

Sacrosciatic notch: It is sufficiently wide to accommodate two fingers placed over the sacrospinous ligament covering the notch. Its configuration denotes the capacity of the posterior segment of the pelvis and the side walls of the lower pelvis.

Ischial spines: They are usually smooth, everted, and difficult to palpate simultaneously with maximally stretched index and middle fingers of pronated right hand. They may be prominent and encroach on to the cavity, thereby reducing the available space in the midpelvis (Fig. 17).

Iliopectineal lines: To note any beaking suggestive of narrow fore pelvis (android pelvis).

Side walls: They are usually divergent or parallel, convergent walls may suggest inadequate midpelvis or outlet.

Posterior surface of the symphysis pubis: It forms a smooth, rounded curve and any angulation or beaking suggests abnormality.

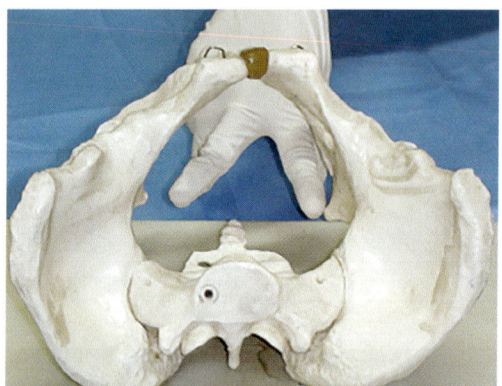

Fig. 17: Assessment of interischial diameter.

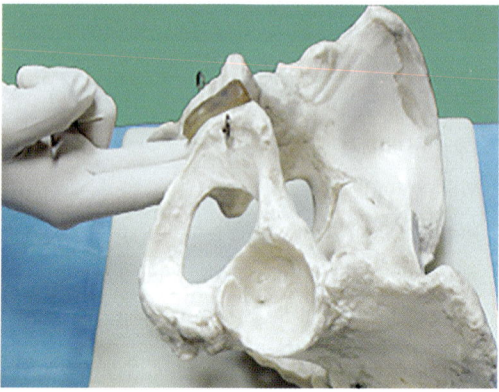

Fig. 18: Assessment of subpubic arch.

Subpubic arch: It is rounded and accommodates the palmar aspect of two fingers in a normal pelvis (Fig. 18).

Diagonal conjugate: The fingers are to follow the anterior sacral curvature. In normal pelvis, it is difficult to feel the sacral promontory or at best can be felt with difficulty. In order to reach the promontory, the elbow and the wrist are to be depressed sufficiently while the fingers are mobilized upward. The point at which the bone recedes from the fingers is the sacral promontory. The radial border of the fingers is then lifted to touch the lower border of symphysis pubis and a marking is placed over the gloved index finger. The distance between the marking and the tip of the middle finger gives the measurement of diagonal conjugate (Fig. 19). If the middle finger fails to reach the promontory or touches it with difficulty, it is likely that the conjugate is adequate for passage of an average size fetal head. Every obstetrician should know the distance between his/her tip of middle finger to the base of thumb and widely separated index and middle fingers of pronated dominant hand to measure the diagonal conjugate and interischial diameters.

Transverse diameter of the outlet: It is measured by placing the knuckles of first

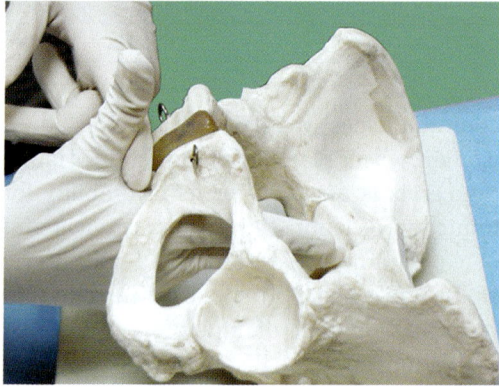

Fig. 19: Measuring diagonal conjugate.

interphalangeal joints or knuckles of the clinched fist between the ischial tuberosities. Normally, four knuckles can be easily placed in a normal pelvis (Fig. 20).

Pubic angle: The inferior pubic rami are defined on both sides and the angle roughly corresponds to the fully abducted thumb and index fingers. The angle is narrow in contracted pelvis.

INVESTIGATIONS

Most of the investigations are carried out in a pregnant woman during her first antenatal

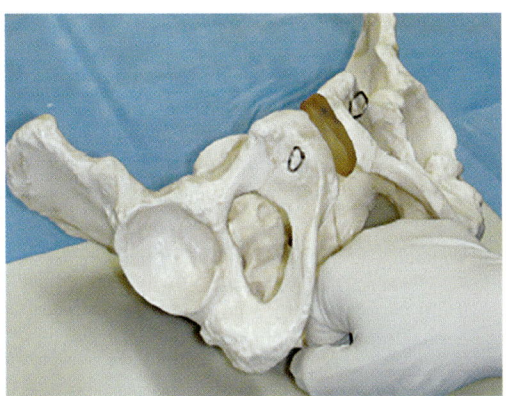

Fig. 20: Assessment of transverse diameter of outlet.

and sugar at each visit, screening for gestational diabetes by DIPSI at 24–28 weeks if it is normal at registration visit and an ultrasound examination to rule out congenital anomalies between 18 and 20 weeks is indicated.

Special Investigations

Special investigations are indicated in woman, who is at a high risk of certain disorders such as toxoplasmosis, rubella, cytomegalovirus, herpes simplex virus (TORCH) infections, thyroid disorders, thalassemia, and Down syndrome.

visit however there are others, which are gestation dependent.

At the first visit, investigations to be ordered are hemoglobin (Hb), ABO and Rh typing, venereal disease research laboratory (VDRL) test, human immunodeficiency virus (HIV) testing, hepatitis B surface antigen (HBsAg) and urine routine and microscopic examination. Hemoglobin level of >11 g/dL in first and third trimesters and >10.5 g/dL during the second trimester is considered normal in pregnancy.[8] Pregnant women with hemoglobin levels below this are diagnosed as anemia.

Given the increasing incidence of diabetes mellitus globally and pregnancy being a diabetogenic state, the International Association of Diabetes in Pregnancy Study Group has proposed first-trimester screening of pregnant women by offering glycated hemoglobin (HbA1c) levels or a fasting or random blood sugar levels. The Government of India recommends the DIPSI (Diabetes in Pregnancy Study Group India) test in all pregnant women on their registration visit. It is a 2-hour blood glucose testing after oral intake of 75 g glucose irrespective of their fasting status.

At subsequent visits, hemoglobin estimation at 28 and 36 weeks, urine for albumin

Screening for Thyroid Disorders

Considering the high incidence of maternal and perinatal morbidity, impaired neurological development of the offspring in pregnant woman with thyroid disorders, and selective screening by offering serum thyroid-stimulating hormone (TSH) is recommended in high-risk group (Box 3).

Screening for Thalassemia

The importance of recognizing thalassemia lies in the fact that the prenatal diagnosis and timely intervention can prevent birth of babies with thalassemia major and save the families of mental, emotional, and financial distress. Screening may be offered to those at higher risk due to their ethnic origin such as Sindhi and Punjabi populations or those with a family history of thalassemia or repeated blood transfusions. Red blood cell (RBC) indices mean corpuscular volume (MCV) <75 fL and mean corpuscular hemoglobin (MCH) < 27 pg and naked eye single tube red cell osmotic fragility test (NESTROFT) are simple screening tests. Further confirmation can be done by HbA2 estimation by high-performance liquid chromatography (HPLC)

Box 3: Women at high risk of thyroid disorder.	**Box 4:** Indications for offering TORCH serology.
• Women with history of thyroid disorder • Family history of thyroid disease • Presence of goiter • Presence of thyroid antibodies • Symptoms or clinical signs suggestive of thyroid dysfunction, i.e., excessive weight gain despite low appetite, anemia, elevated cholesterol, etc. • Women with type 1 diabetes or other auto-immune disorders • Women with previous therapeutic head or neck irradiation • History of recurrent miscarriages or preterm deliveries	• Women with fever, rash, lymphadenopathy • History of exposure or contact • *Women at high risk of infection*: Consumers of raw meat or unwashed fruits and vegetables, cat handlers, nonimmune to rubella, high-risk sexual behavior • *Evidence of ultrasound markers for congenital infections*: Unexplained fetal growth restriction (FGR), oligohydramnios, polyhydramnios, hydrocephalus or microcephaly

or Hb electrophoresis. If the mother is carrying thalassemia trait, husband should be screened and if the husband also tests positive for the thalassemia trait, prenatal diagnosis is offered to the couple.

Screening for TORCH Infections

Routine screening for TORCH infections is not recommended. The indications of maternal TORCH screen during pregnancy are as listed in Box 4.

Screening for Down Syndrome

Down syndrome is the most common chromosomal abnormality. Every woman is at risk for having an affected baby. In general population, the risk of giving birth to an affected baby is 1:800. The risk of having an affected baby increases with the maternal age from 1 in 1,500 at age of 25 years, 1 in 1,000 at 30 years, 1 in 417 at 33 years, 1 in 250 at 35 years, 1 in 69 at 40 years, and 1 in 19 at 45 years.[9] As majority of pregnancies occur in women <35 years of age, almost two thirds of Down syndrome babies are born to mothers <35 years of age. The background risk of a woman of carrying a fetus with Down syndrome depends upon her age and any past history of chromosomal defects. Although universal screening for Down syndrome is not a part of routine antenatal care, but it should be offered to all pregnant women after pretest counseling. Various methods of screening for Down syndrome are:

- Ultrasound for nuchal translucency (NT) at 10–14 weeks
- Fetal NT and first-trimester maternal serum screening [pregnancy-associated plasma protein-A (PAPP-A) and beta-human chorionic gonadotropin (β-hCG)] at 10–14 weeks
- Second-trimester maternal serum biochemical screening:
  – Triple test [β-hCG, maternal serum alpha-fetoprotein (MSAFP) and unconjugated estriol]
  – Quadruple test (triple test plus inhibin A).

Nuchal translucency is the measurement of the subcutaneous collection of fluid at the back of the fetal neck and is increased in Down syndrome. PAPP-A, MSAFP, and unconjugated estriol levels are reduced in Down syndrome, whereas β-hCG and inhibin A levels are raised in Down syndrome. Women are counseled regarding the interpretation of the test and need of further confirmation by diagnostic invasive tests.

ANTENATAL ADVICE

- Daily oral iron supplementation with 60 mg elemental iron and 0.4 mg folic acid is recommended from second-trimester to prevent anemia.
- Daily calcium supplementation of 1 g oral elemental calcium in two divided doses, preferably taken with meals, is recommended.
- Two doses of tetanus diphtheria Td toxoid 1 month apart during pregnancy with second dose given at least 2 weeks before delivery. In subsequent pregnancy of <3-year interpregnancy interval, women should receive single booster dose of tetanus toxoid.
- Counseling about optimal nutrition, healthy eating, avoiding alcohol, smoking, and health-affecting habits at every antenatal visit.
- She is advised to do moderate exercise throughout pregnancy and informed about the dangers of high impact sports involving the risk of trauma and scuba diving with resultant fetal birth defects and fetal decompression disease.
- Sexual intercourse in pregnancy is not known to be associated with any adverse outcomes except in conditions such as threatened abortion and placenta previa.
- *Each and every antenatal women should be made aware about the danger signs in pregnancy*: Severe abdominal pain, vaginal bleeding leaking per vagina, decreased, excessive or absent fetal movements, fever, foul smelling discharge, severe headache, blurring of vision, severe vomiting, difficulty in breathing, convulsions, loss of consciousness, and generalized swelling of body and facial puffiness.
- Pregnant women should be made aware of the importance of fetal movements in the third trimester and reporting the decreased fetal movements immediately to the healthcare provider. However, counting routine daily fetal movement is not recommended.
- Pregnant women should preferably be provided written information about the frequency, timing, and content of each antenatal appointment.

KEY POINTS

- Antenatal care is an opportunity for the healthcare providers to prioritize women's health by providing regular antenatal checkups, health promotion, nutritional intervention, prevention and early detection of pregnancy complications and concurrent diseases, family planning counseling, and information for positive perinatal and maternal outcome.
- The WHO recommends minimum of eight antenatal contacts with healthcare provider to improve women's experience of care and support, and an improved maternal and perinatal outcome.
- The first antenatal contact is recommended in the first trimester. Two antenatal contacts in second trimester at 20 and 26 weeks. Five antenatal contacts during third trimester at 30, 34, 36, 38, and 40 weeks of pregnancy.
- Accurate dating of pregnancy should be done preferably in first antenatal visit based on history, clinical examination, and sonological finding. It is crucial, especially in high-risk pregnancy for timing subsequent obstetrical interventions.
- At each subsequent visit, the weight, BP, urine albumin, and pedal edema is assessed and abdominal examination is conducted for assessing the fetal growth.

- Investigations such as Hb, ABO and Rh grouping, oral glucose tolerance test (DIPSI), VDRL, HIV, HBsAg testing, and routine urine analysis are advised on the first visit to all pregnant women.
- An ultrasound is advised at 18–20 weeks for ruling out congenital anomalies.
- Tests such as TSH and screening for Down's syndrome may be offered.
- Hb is repeated at 28 and 36 weeks of gestation.
- DIPSI is repeated at 24–28 weeks, if it is normal at the first antenatal visit.

REFERENCES

1. World Health Organization. (2016). New guidelines on antenatal care for a positive pregnancy experience. [online] Available from: http://www.who.int>news>antenatal-care. [Last accessed February, 2020].
2. Hadlock FP, Shah YP, Kanon DJ, Lindsey JV.. Fetal crown rump length: reevaluation of relation to menstrual age (5–18 weeks) with high resolution real time US. Radiology. 1992; 182(2):501-5.
3. American institute of Ultrasound in Medicine. AIUM practice guideline for the performance of obstetric ultrasound examinations. J Ultrasound Med. 2010;29(1):157-66.
4. Callen, Peter W. Ultrasonography in Obstetrics and Gynecology, 2nd edition. Philadelphia: WB Saunders;1988. pp. 47-64.
5. World Health Organization. (1978). Risk approach for maternal and child health care: a managerial strategy to improve the coverage and quality of maternal and child health/family planning services based on the measurement of individual and community risk. [online] Available from: https://apps.who.int/iris/handle/10665/37151. [Last accessed February, 2020].
6. Leopold J. Conduct of normal births through external examination alone. Arch Gynaecol. 1894;45:337.
7. Crichton D. A reliable method of establishing the level of fetal head in obstetrics. S Afr Med J. 1974;48:784-7.
8. Centers for Disease Control (CDC). CDC criteria for anaemia in children and childbearing-aged women. MMWR Morb Mortal Wkly Rep. 1989;38(22):400-4.
9. Corton MM, Leveno KJ, Bloom SL, Hauth J, Rouse D, Spong C. Prenatal diagnosis and fetal therapy. In: Cunningham GF, Lenevo, Gant FN (Eds). William Obstetrics, 25th edition. Mcgraw-Hill; 2018; pp. 277-9.

SUGGESTED READING

1. National Institute for Health and Care Excellence. (2008). Antenatal care for uncomplicated pregnancies. [online] Available from: https://www.nice.org.uk/guidance/cg62. [Last accessed February, 2020].

Approach to a Pregnant Woman Presenting with Bad Obstetric History

Monika Bhatia

INTRODUCTION

The term *"Bad Obstetric History* or BOH" is applied to mothers in whom a previous "poor" pregnancy outcome is likely to have a bearing on the prognosis of her present pregnancy. The previous pregnancy loss should be obstetrically related. Pregnancy loss is a devastating experience for the mother. Perinatal mortality remains a challenge in the care of pregnant women worldwide, particularly for those who had history of adverse outcomes in previous pregnancies. The obstetric disaster may be in the form of miscarriage, preterm birth, antepartum or intrapartum stillbirth, difficult delivery, birth asphyxia or early neonatal death consequent to intrapartum events. Depending on the nature of previous obstetric disasters, there can be various risk factors associated with it. A comprehensive work up of these women is indicated in the interval period to identify these risk factors and plan risk modification in the preconception period and during pregnancy. A detailed history and examination are followed by investigations in these women with the aim to identify the risk factors and initiate interventions to improve the outcome in index pregnancy.

DIFFERENTIAL DIAGNOSIS

Many obstetric disasters may have multiple causes. The differential diagnosis as regards the etiology of various obstetric disasters is as given in Box 1.

Box 1: Differential diagnosis of causes of bad obstetric history based on nature of previous obstetric disaster.

Recurrent abortions:
- *Anatomical*: Müllerian fusion abnormalities like septate uterus, cervical incompetence, intrauterine synechia, submucous fibroid
- *Immunological*: Antiphospholipid antibody syndrome, other immune disorders such as systemic lupus erythematosus (SLE)
- *Chromosomal*: Parental chromosomal abnormality like balanced translocations
- *Endocrinological*: Uncontrolled endocrine problems like diabetes and thyroid dysfunction
- *Others*: Thrombophilia

Previous intrauterine death:
- Chromosomal abnormalities
- Hypertensive disorders of pregnancy
- Uncontrolled endocrine problems such as diabetes mellitus, thyroid disorders
- Severe maternal systemic illness, renal disease, heart disease, SLE
- Maternal infections such as toxoplasmosis, *Cytomegalovirus* (CMV), syphilis, malaria
- Antiphospholipid antibody syndrome
- Thrombophilia
- Cholestasis of pregnancy
- Smoking
- Antepartum hemorrhage: Abruption

Previous hydrops:
- *Immune*: Rh incompatibility
- *Nonimmune infections*: Human parvovirus (HPV) B19, chromosomal abnormalities, cardiac causes, thoracic causes, hematologic causes—α-thalassemia, red cell enzyme defect, fetomaternal hemorrhage, metabolic disorders

HISTORY

To find the likely cause of mishap, it is important to take a detailed obstetric history of previous pregnancies. It includes the exact nature of disaster whether it was a miscarriage, intrauterine death, preterm delivery or difficult delivery.

In case of miscarriage, it is important to find out the gestation at which it happened, was the pregnancy confirmed by ultrasound or urine pregnancy test, was there any documentation of presence of fetal node and cardiac activity, was the pregnancy terminated by medical or surgical method, and whether the post abortion period was uneventful or did she have any problems such as fever, foul-smelling discharge per vaginam or bleeding per vaginam.

For late pregnancy mishaps, the duration of pregnancy and any significant antepartum or intrapartum events are recorded.

A descending pattern of adverse pregnancy outcomes such as a serial improvement with an increase in pregnancy order points toward syphilis which may be confirmed by Venereal Disease Research Laboratory (VDRL) and fluorescent treponemal antibody absorption (FTA-ABS). This is due to an increase in maternal antibodies. In women with uterine anomalies like unicornuate uterus the capacity of uterus increase with each pregnancy, hence a similar pattern.

An ascending pattern of adverse pregnancy outcome that is worsening of obstetric performance is suggestive of Rh isoimmunization, where the initial pregnancy outcome is good but it worsens with increase in pregnancy order due to Rh isoimmunization.

Antenatal Period

The details of antenatal period include whether previous pregnancy was booked or unbooked, whether there was any history of high blood pressure, swelling feet suggestive of pre-eclampsia, any bleeding per vaginam or abdominal pain suggestive of placental abruption, any itching especially on palms and soles suggestive of obstetric cholestasis. Any leaking per vaginam suggestive of some cord accident associated with ruptured membranes. Any fever with rash suggestive of infections like toxoplasmosis, varicella-zoster, parvovirus B19, rubella, Cytomegalovirus, or any lesions on the genitalia of parents suggestive of sexually transmitted infections (STIs). Any history suggestive of Rh isoimmunization such as receiving anti-D injection or repeated ultrasound examinations and intrauterine transfusions is asked. Any history suggestive of oligohydramnios or hydramnios is elicited.

Intrapartum Period

The details of the intrapartum period include the duration of labor whether spontaneous or induced, prolonged or precipitate, any rupture of membranes, cord prolapse, any bleeding per vaginam, presentation of the baby whether cephalic or breech; if breech, any difficulty or delay in delivery of the head of the baby, any instrumentation, any passage of meconium, any tight cord loops around the neck of the baby, weight of the baby whether it was very small suggestive of growth restriction or large as in diabetes mellitus. In case of a stillborn, it is important to know if it was a fresh stillborn as with abruptio placentae or macerated as with syphilis or swollen and hydropic as with Rh isoimmunization and parvovirus infection. It is important to find out if the baby had any gross congenital abnormality.

All these details are recorded systematically for each pregnancy.

The old records of the woman are reviewed to verify the facts furnished by the woman and review any investigations she has done for the fetal loss. Depending on the nature of the fetal loss according to obstetric history, certain points are elicited in the present and past medical and surgical history of the woman to identify the likely cause of the mishap (Table 1). Personal history is important in all women with bad obstetric outcome as smoking and drug abuse adversely affect the pregnancy outcome.

EXAMINATION

A detailed general and systemic examination may further help to shortlist the likely cause of BOH. These are then followed by a

Table 1: Detailed questions regarding specific etiologies to be elicited.

Relevant history	Disease
Previous history of genital ulceration, generalized rash or lymphadenopathy, gradually improving obstetric performance like late abortions, macerated stillbirth, fresh stillbirth, baby with congenital syphilis followed by birth of a healthy baby	Syphilis
Polyuria, polydipsia, polyphagia, polyhydramnios, large for date baby or fresh stillborn baby in previous pregnancy	Diabetes
Weight gain, lethargy, tiredness, dry skin, constipation, fluid retention, goiter, cold intolerance; untreated women may have increased risk of miscarriage, pre-eclampsia, abruption, low birth weight, stillbirth, impaired neurological development, and decreased intelligence quotient of offspring	Hypothyroidism
Weight loss, heat intolerance, palpitations, vomiting, emotional lability, recurrent fetal growth restriction with congenital goiter	Hyperthyroidism
Fever, fatigue, myalgia, lymphadenopathy, erythema over cheeks, photosensitivity, oral ulcers, small joint pain and swelling, seizures, headaches Increased risk of miscarriages, fetal growth restriction, fetal death and prematurity if active, disease is present at conception	Systemic lupus erythematosus
Venous or arterial thrombosis or pregnancy wastage in the form of three or more recurrent miscarriages before 10 weeks, one fetal death after 10 weeks, or one or more preterm births before 34 weeks due to placental insufficiency or pre-eclampsia	Antiphospholipid antibody syndrome
Breathlessness on exertion, chest pain, palpitations, syncope	Heart disease
Weakness, swelling over face or body, vomiting, decreased urine output	Renal disease
Painless cervical dilatation and rupture of membranes followed by expulsion of a live fetus in mid pregnancy Any history of trauma, cervical surgery like deep unrepaired cervical tear, conization, cervical amputation, etc.	Cervical incompetence
Recurrent preterm births and increasing mean gestational age at birth	Uterine anomalies
Worsening fetal outcome classically in the form of one or two uneventful births followed by neonatal death due to severe jaundice followed by stillborn hydropic baby	Rh-sensitized pregnancy
Recurrent abortions, early onset pre-eclampsia, fetal growth restriction and abruption	Thrombophilias: Inherited or acquired

Table 2: Physical examination and diagnosis.

General physical examination	Diagnosis
Generalized maculopapular rash involving palms and soles	Syphilis
Obesity, acanthosis nigricans	Diabetes
Bradycardia, delayed relaxation of deep tendon reflexes, goiter, carpal tunnel syndrome	Hypothyroidism
Tachycardia, goiter, palmar erythema, tremors, lid lag, lid retraction	Hyperthyroidism
Malar rash sparing nasolabial folds, discoid rash, arthritis	Systemic lupus erythematosus
Leg ulcers, hypertension, livedo reticularis	Antiphospholipid antibody syndrome
Cyanosis, clubbing	Heart disease
Pallor, facial puffiness, hypertension	Renal disease

per speculum and per vaginam examination if required.

The general physical examination is carried out as in any antenatal woman. The body mass index (BMI) of the woman is important as obesity is associated with poor obstetric outcome. Undernutrition and malnutrition also affect the pregnancy adversely. The findings on general physical examination suggestive of various diseases are as given in Table 2.

Systemic Examination

On respiratory system, look for any evidence of pleuritis or pericarditis, which are suggestive of systemic lupus erythematosus (SLE). In cardiovascular system, presence of any significant murmur that is any diastolic or loud systolic murmur grade 2 or more is suggestive of heart disease.

Pelvic Examination

Per speculum examination is important in pregnant women with history suggestive of incompetent os for any shortening of cervical length, any old healed cervical tears, ectropion, etc. In women with previous preterm birth, it is important to look for any vaginal discharge suggestive of bacterial vaginosis where the discharge is profuse homogenous and grayish white.

On per vaginum examination, any abnormality in the uterine contour, broad fundus or a marked deviation of uterus to one side may be suggestive of a uterine anomaly.

INVESTIGATIONS

Routine investigations are carried out for any antenatal woman as described in Chapter 1. Other investigations are based on the condition suspected on history and examination. But if no specific cause is suspected, then the woman has to be screened for all the likely causes. List of investigations depending upon the condition suspected to be the cause of loss is detailed in Table 3.

The clinical approach to a pregnant woman with a bad obstetric history is shown in Flowchart 1.

MANAGEMENT

Women with BOH are devastated and need reassurance and psychological support. Tender loving care should be given to all. The management is according to the cause identified. Table 4 lists the various treatment options according to the cause. However, the woman needs to be carefully monitored during her pregnancy.

Table 3: Investigations for a pregnant woman with bad obstetric history.

Investigations	Disease
Venereal Disease Research Laboratory, fluorescent treponemal antibody absorption test	Syphilis
Glucose tolerance test, glycated hemoglobin (HbA1c)	Diabetes mellitus
Free triiodothyronine (FT_3), free thyroxine (FT_4), thyroid-stimulating hormone	Thyroid disorders
Antinuclear antibody, anti-double-stranded DNA (anti-dsDNA) antibodies	Systemic lupus erythematosus
Lupus anticoagulant, Antiphospholipid antibody immunoglobulin G (IgG)/IgM, anti-β2 glycoprotein antibodies (documented twice 12 weeks apart)	Antiphospholipid antibody syndrome
Electrocardiogram, echocardiography, chest X-ray	Heart disease
Serum creatinine, blood urea, 24-hour urine protein estimation, urine microalbumin, GFR, USG for kidneys	Renal disease
Serial cervical length from 14 to 24 weeks for any shortening, or change in shape of cervical canal that is any funneling on transvaginal ultrasound	Cervical incompetence
High resolution ultrasound, three-dimensional (3D)-ultrasound, hysterosalpingography or hysteroscopy, or magnetic resonance imaging	Uterine anomalies
Blood group and Rh typing, titer of anti-D antibodies, Indirect Coombs' test	Rh-sensitized pregnancy
Thrombophilia screen (protein C, protein S, antithrombin 3)	Genetic thrombophilia

KEY POINTS

- A variety of causes are associated with recurrent poor pregnancy outcomes.
- Identification of various causes of adverse pregnancy outcomes can facilitate preconception and antenatal interventions to improve the perinatal morbidity and mortality in the index pregnancy.
- Some of the diseases may be identified with a specific pattern of presentation, others may present with overlapping pattern of abortions, preterm births, poor growth, fetal death, high blood pressure or abruption.
- In women with recurrent first trimester miscarriage, antiphospholipid antibody (APLA) syndrome and anatomical uterine anomaly may be specifically suspected.
- In women with recurrent second trimester miscarriage and preterm births, causes like cervical incompetence and uterine anomalies like Müllerian fusion defects are more likely.
- A descending pattern of adverse pregnancy outcomes such as a serial improvement with an increase in pregnancy order points toward syphilis or uterine anomalies like unicornuate uterus.
- An ascending pattern of adverse pregnancy outcomes that is worsening of obstetric performance is suggestive of Rh isoimmunization.
- Recurrent fetal growth restriction along with features of systemic disease may point toward heart or renal disease in the mother.
- Recurrent high blood pressure or placental abruption may be indicative of an underlying immune-mediated illness like SLE or APLA syndrome.

Section 1: Obstetrics

Flowchart 1: Algorithm for clinical approach to a pregnant woman with bad obstetric history.

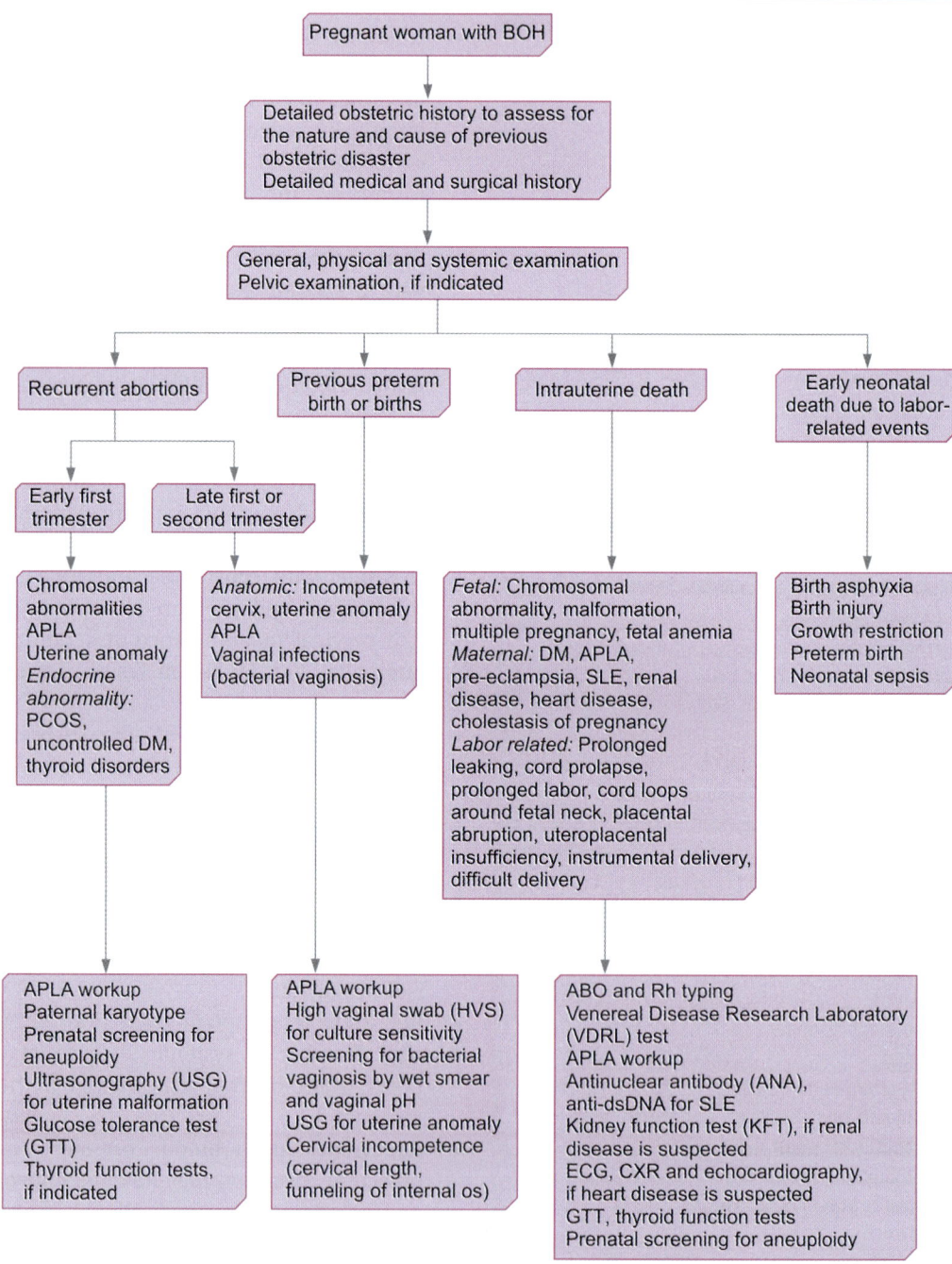

(APLA: antiphospholipid antibody; BOH: bad obstetric history; CXR: chest X-ray; DM: diabetes mellitus; dsDNA: double-stranded DNA; ECG: electrocardiography; PCOS: polycystic ovary syndrome; SLE: systemic lupus erythematosus)

Table 4: Interventions for women with bad obstetric history.

Condition	Interventions
Recurrent miscarriage: • Uterine septum • Cervical incompetence • Antiphospholipid syndrome • Parental karyotype abnormality • Uncontrolled DM/hypothyroidism	Tender loving care and lifestyle modification cessation of smoking, normalize BMI: • Hysteroscopic resection of uterine septum • Cervical cerclage • Aspirin + LMWH • Genetic counseling • Control with medications OHA/insulin, thyroxine
Preterm births	• Lifestyle modification cessation of smoking, normalize BMI • Treatment of asymptomatic bacteriuria • Avoid interpregnancy interval of <6 months preferably <12 months • Progesterone supplementation • Cervical cerclage in selected cases
Syphilis	• Benzathine penicillin 2.4 million units IM every week × 3 • Ceftriaxone 2 g IV every day × 10–14 days
Rh isoimmunization	• Assess fetal RhD genotype by fetal cf DNA after 10 weeks or from uncultured amniocytes by amniocentesis after 15 weeks • Follow maternal anti-D titers every month; if rising, then every 2 weeks till they reach critical value ≥10 IU/mL • Then follow with MCA-PSV • IUT if MCA-PSV ≥1.5 MOM Delivery 35–38 weeks
Recurrent anomalies	Genetic counseling

(LMWH: low-molecular-weight heparin; BMI: body mass index; DM: diabetes mellitus; OHA: hypoglycaemic agents; IUT: intrauterine transfusion; MOM: multiples of median; MCA-PSV: multiples of median middle cerebral artery peak)

SUGGESTED READING

1. American College of Obstetricians and Gynecologists (2018). Practice bulletin on early pregnancy loss. [online] Available from https://www.acog.org/Clinical-Guidance-and-Publications/Practice-Bulletins/Committee-on-Practice-Bulletins-Gynecology/Early-Pregnancy-Loss?IsMobileSet=false [Last accessed March, 2020].
2. European Society of Human Reproduction and Embryology (ESHRE). (2017). Clinical practice guideline on recurrent pregnancy loss, version 2.
3. National Institute for Health and Clinical Excellence (2015). Interventional procedures guidance. Hysteroscopic metroplasty of a uterine septum for recurrent miscarriage. [online] Available from https://www.nice.org.uk/guidance/ipg510 [Last accessed March, 2020].
4. National Institute for Health and Clinical Excellence (2019). Interventional procedures guidance. Laparoscopic cerclage for cervical incompetence to prevent late miscarriage or preterm birth. [online] Available from https://www.nice.org.uk/guidance/ipg639/resources/laparoscopic-cerclage-for-cervical-incompetence-to-prevent-late-miscarriage-or-preterm-birth-pdf-18998740516507141 [Last accessed March, 2020].
5. Royal College of Obstetricians and Gynaecologists (RCOG) (2010). Late intrauterine fetal death and stillbirth (Green-top Guideline No. 55). [online] Available from https://www.rcog.org.uk/en/guidelines-research-services/guidelines/gtg55/ [Last accessed March, 2020].
6. Royal College of Obstetricians and Gynaecologists (RCOG) (2011). Green-top Guideline No. 17. The investigation and treatment of couples with recurrent first trimester and second trimester miscarriage. [online] Available from https://www.rcog.org.uk/globalassets/documents/guidelines/gtg_17.pdf [Last accessed March, 2020].

3
Approach to a Pregnant Woman Presenting with Bleeding in Early Pregnancy

Meenakshi Singh, Namita Jain

INTRODUCTION

Pregnancy is characterized by amenorrhea. Any vaginal bleeding during pregnancy provokes anxiety and must be addressed at the earliest. The cutoff for pregnancy to be qualified as early or late pregnancy ranges from 20 to 28 weeks. In first few weeks of pregnancy, about 25% of all pregnant women experience spotting or bleeding and half of those who bleed miscarry. Other causes for bleeding in early pregnancy are ectopic pregnancy, hydatidiform mole, and benign or malignant lesions of cervix and vagina. According to the National Center for Health Statistics and Center for Disease Control and Prevention, abortion is defined as loss or termination of pregnancy before 20 weeks of gestation or fetus weighing <500 grams. However, it is important to note that fetal weight at 20 weeks is 320 grams and it is 500 grams at 22–23 weeks. Hence, recently the World Health Organization (WHO) defined abortion as loss or termination of pregnancy before 22 weeks of gestation.[1] Abortions included in early pregnancy loss are first trimester losses up to 12 + 6 weeks gestation and early second trimester pregnancy loss from 13 weeks onward.[2,3]

DIFFERENTIAL DIAGNOSIS

The differential diagnosis of a pregnant woman presenting with bleeding per vaginum is different in early and late pregnancy. The various causes of bleeding per vaginum in early pregnancy are listed in Box 1.

Box 1: Causes of bleeding in early pregnancy.
- *Abortion*:
  - Threatened
  - Inevitable
  - Incomplete
  - Complete
  - Missed
- Ectopic pregnancy
- Implantation bleeding
- Gestational trophoblastic disease
- Cervical/vaginal infections
- Cervical erosion/ectropion
- Cervical/vaginal tumors

HISTORY

History of Presenting Complaint

A detailed history of the presenting symptom, i.e., bleeding per vaginum, is important.

It includes details such as onset, duration, and amount of bleeding, whether mild, moderate, or severe. It is also important to know if this is the first episode or there have been previous episodes of bleeding per vaginum in the current pregnancy. Any factor which might have provoked bleeding, such as trauma or sexual intercourse, should be enquired. The amount of bleeding can be assessed by enquiring about the number of pads used and extent of soakage of pads, whether partially soaked or fully soaked.

The history of passage of clots or flooding implies heavy bleeding. The color of blood lost is important; bright red-colored bleeding indicates fresh blood as is seen in woman with threatened, inevitable, or incomplete abortion, whereas dark altered blood indicates old blood as is seen in woman with missed abortion.

Presence of any associated pain, its onset, duration, location, and severity are also important in early pregnancy. In ectopic pregnancy, the pain usually precedes bleeding per vaginum, whereas in abortions, bleeding is followed by intermittent pain due to uterine contractions.

Any history of passage of products of conception should be elicited, which is suggestive of incomplete or complete abortion. The patient usually describes the products of conception as fleshy white mass. It should be differentiated from passage of clots, which are dark or bright red in color and friable. History of passage of grape-like vesicles, severe nausea, and vomiting are suggestive of molar pregnancy.

Any history of fever, chills, abdominal or pelvic pain, and mucopurulent discharge is suggestive of septic abortion. History of use of any abortifacient, trauma, or surgical intervention suggests septic-induced abortion.

Symptoms such as dizziness, light headedness, or syncope may be present in ectopic pregnancy consequent to hypovolemia, or in septic abortion due to septic shock.

Menstrual History

The length of menstrual cycle, duration of bleeding, and date of last normal menstrual period (DLMP) are important. The importance of knowing whether the last menstrual period was normal or not lies in the fact that sometimes the woman may have cyclic spotting or scanty periods for the first 2-3 months of pregnancy and reports the date of spotting or scanty periods as her LMP with resultant miscalculation of period of gestation (POG).

Obstetric History

Obstetric history includes gravidity, parity, and a detailed outcome of previous pregnancies. (Refer to Chapter 1 section on obstetric history page no. 5)

Past Medical/Surgical History

In woman with bleeding per vaginum in early pregnancy, history of infertility, ovulation induction, pelvic inflammatory disease (PID) or sexually transmitted disease (STD) is important as it is associated with an increased risk of ectopic pregnancy. History of tubal sterilization or tubal reconstructive surgery such as recanalization, fimbrioplasty, or salpingoneostomy also increase the risk of ectopic pregnancy. History of autoimmune disorders such as systemic lupus erythematosus and antiphospholipid syndrome can cause recurrent abortions.

Personal History

Cigarette smoking doubles the risk of abortion compared to nonsmokers.[4] Alcohol abuse increases the risk of abortion. The risk seems to be related to the frequency and the amount of alcohol ingested.[5] Radiation exposure and chemotherapy particularly, methotrexate, may increase the risk of abortion. Any history of surgery in the present pregnancy should be elicited as early removal of corpus luteum, while removing an ovarian cyst, may result in abortion.

EXAMINATION

The examination of a pregnant woman presenting with bleeding per vaginum includes an assessment of general condition of the patient followed by a systemic examination with special emphasis to abdominal and pelvic examination. In woman with bleeding in first half of pregnancy, a pelvic examination including a per speculum and a bimanual vaginal examination are indicated to make a provisional diagnosis, decide a plan of action, and to identify women requiring prompt surgical intervention.

General Physical Examination

The physical examination includes assessment of the general condition of the woman—orientation, vitals, pulse, temperature, blood pressure, respiratory rate, and hydration status. An assessment of the amount of blood lost is important and is reflected by the pulse rate, blood pressure, and degree of pallor. Hypotension with tachycardia suggests hypovolemic shock, which can be due to ectopic pregnancy-related hemoperitoneum or excessive blood loss per vaginum as in incomplete or inevitable abortion or molar pregnancy which is in the process of expulsion. Restlessness, cold clammy extremities, poor skin perfusion, and piloerection response indicate hypovolemic shock due to excessive bleeding. Shock may be neurogenic due to dilation of cervix by products of conception or septic as in septic-induced abortion. The patient looks toxic in septic shock.

Systemic Examination

Thorough evaluation of cardiovascular, respiratory, and neurological systems should be done. Breast examination should be routinely carried out to palpate for any lump in the breast or discharge from the nipples.

Per Abdomen Examination

In woman with bleeding per vaginum in early pregnancy, the abdomen is essentially normal on inspection, but occasionally it may be distended because of intraperitoneal bleeding or distended bowel. Rarely, Cullen's sign—bluish discoloration of the periumbilical skin or Grey Turner's sign—bluish discoloration in iliac fossa may be seen in a woman with ruptured ectopic pregnancy. If anemia is out of proportion to obvious vaginal blood loss, ruptured ectopic pregnancy should be suspected as abdominal distension may not be clinically evident till significant hemoperitoneum is there.

On palpation, presence of generalized or localized tenderness, muscle guarding, rigidity or rebound tenderness suggest intra-abdominal bleeding as with ectopic pregnancy or peritonitis as with septic abortion. The uterus is palpable per abdomen if uterine size is more than 12 weeks. There may be a discrepancy in the calculated period of gestation and the estimated period of gestation. The size may be large for dates as in molar pregnancy or small for dates as in intrauterine demise, incomplete or complete abortion, and sometimes even with molar pregnancy. Uterus should be assessed for any uterine contractions in case it is palpable per abdomen. Abdomen should be percussed for any fluid thrill or shifting dullness suggestive of intra-abdominal hemorrhage seen with ruptured ectopic pregnancy. The bowel sounds may be absent in the presence of peritonitis or bowel injury in septic abortion.

Local Examination

Local vulvar inspection should be done to assess the amount of blood loss, whether bleeding is continuing or has stopped.

Per Speculum Examination

In bleeding per vaginum in early pregnancy, note if any clots are present and if there is any bleeding through cervical os, whether the os is closed (as in threatened abortion) or open (as in inevitable or incomplete abortion) or if any products of conception (incomplete abortion) or grape-like vesicles (molar pregnancy) are seen coming out through os or lying in vagina. Look for any local lesions such as vaginitis, cervical polyp, cervical erosion, cervical or vaginal growth, vulvovaginal varicosity, and any vaginal tears. The color of the vaginal mucosa is reflective of the hemoglobin status of the patient in the absence of vaginitis. In women with septic abortion, blood mixed foul-smelling purulent discharge could be seen.

Per Vaginal Examination

In woman with bleeding per vaginum in early pregnancy, a bimanual per vaginum examination is done to assess the uterine size, its position, consistency, any tenderness, status of internal os whether open or closed, if open whether any products are felt through it or does the uterine cavity appear empty, any palpable adnexa or mass in any of the fornices and cervical motion tenderness. The uterine size as determined by bimanual examination is compared with the period of gestation. It is smaller than the period of gestation in missed abortion, incomplete abortion, and ectopic pregnancy and more than the period of gestation in case of molar pregnancy and multiple pregnancy. In molar pregnancy, it may correspond to or sometimes be smaller than the period of gestation. In complete mole, 50% of the patients have uterine size large for gestational age, 25% correspond to gestational age, and rest 25% are small for gestational age.[6] The status of internal os helps to differentiate between different types of abortions. It is open in inevitable, incomplete, and sometimes in a recent complete abortion, whereas it is closed in threatened, missed, and complete abortion. The consistency of uterus is soft or firm in ectopic pregnancy and abortions, soft in intrauterine pregnancy, and doughy in molar pregnancy. The presence of cervical motion tenderness is suggestive of ectopic pregnancy or septic abortion. Unilateral tender adnexal mass or mass in pouch of Douglas (POD) is suggestive of ectopic pregnancy and pelvic hematocele. Restricted mobility and tenderness of uterus, thickening, induration and tenderness in fornices, bilateral masses in the fornices, and/or mass in POD are suggestive of septic abortion.

INVESTIGATIONS

Investigations should be done along with resuscitation and stabilization of the patient. These are guided by the clinical history and examination findings. In hemodynamically unstable patients two large-bore intravenous cannulae should be inserted and blood sample drawn for blood grouping and crossmatching, complete hemogram, coagulation profile, liver function test (LFT), and kidney function test (KFT). Thyroid function tests are ordered in case molar pregnancy is suspected as clinically evident hyperthyroidism is noted in 7% of the women with complete molar gestation.

Ultrasonography (USG) of abdomen and pelvis is done in all hemodynamically

Condition	Findings
Intrauterine pregnancy	• Confirmed by presence of yolk sac within the gestational sac (by 5.5 weeks) measuring around 2–5 mm in diameter; • Rate of growth of a normal gestational sac is 1 mm/day • Presence of cardiac activity at a crown-rump length (CRL) of 5 mm or more (Fig. 1)
Abortion	• Yolk sac > 5.6 mm in diameter is suggestive of impending miscarriage • Gestational sac > 20 mm without a visible yolk sac • Gestational sac > 25 mm without a visible fetus • An embryo > 5 mm without cardiac activity suggestive of abortion (Figs. 2 and 3)
Ectopic pregnancy	• An extrauterine tubal ring, either empty or containing a yolk sac and/or a fetal node with or without cardiac activity • A ruptured ectopic showing unilateral adnexal mass and free fluid or hematocele in pouch of Douglas (Figs. 4A and B)
Molar pregnancy	• Characteristic snow-storm pattern, fine vesicular, or honeycomb appearance • Large theca lutein cysts as a result of excessive beta-human chorionic gonadotropin (β-hCG) (Fig. 5)

Table 1: Characteristic ultrasonological findings of various conditions causing bleeding per vaginum in the first trimester.

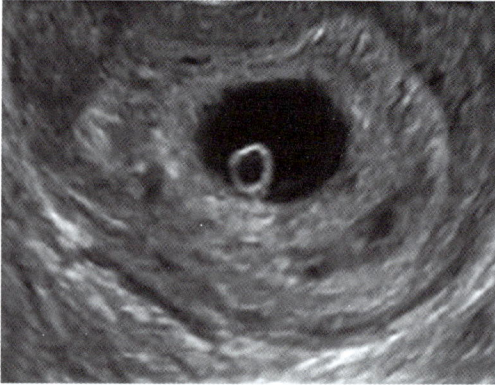

Fig. 1: Ultrasound image showing early intrauterine pregnancy with yolk sac.

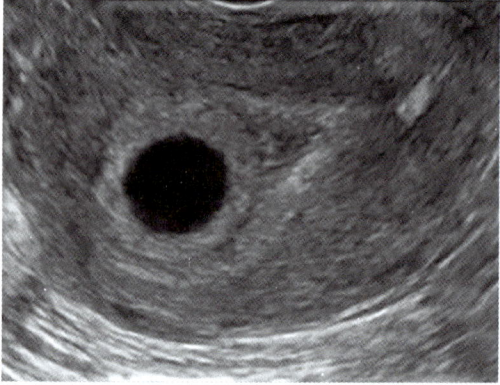

Fig. 2: Ultrasound image of blighted ovum.

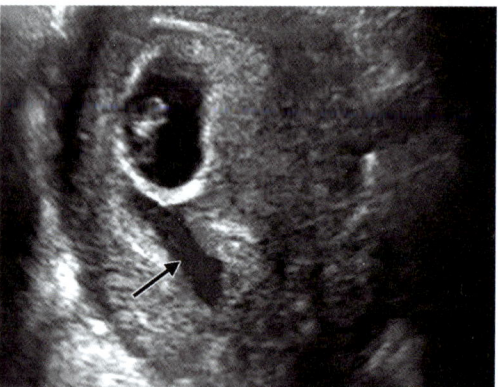

Fig. 3: Ultrasound image of early pregnancy with intrauterine gestational sac and fetal node with subchorionic bleed.

stable patients at the earliest to confirm the diagnosis and plan the management, whereas in hemodynamically unstable patients, it is done once the patient is stabilized. USG shows specific characteristics for different causes of bleeding as depicted in Table 1. Women with a nondiagnostic USG examination result, i.e., inability to localize the pregnancy either inside or outside, requires further evaluation including serial measurements of serum beta-human chorionic gonadotropin (β-hCG) levels.

The "discriminatory zone" of serum β-hCG is that level of β-hCG, at which an intrauterine

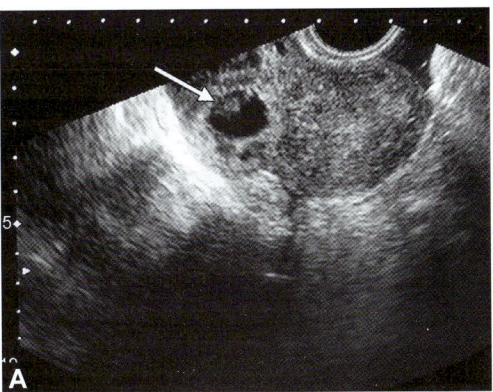
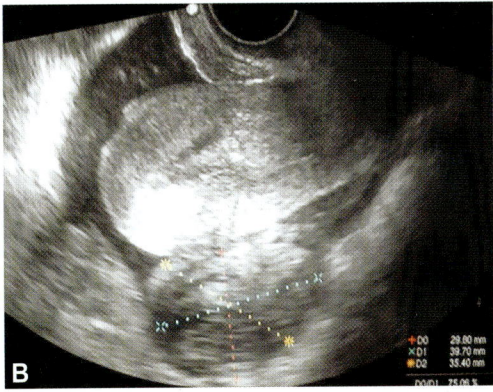

Figs. 4A and B: (A) 4A : Ultrasound image of adnexal mass of unruptured tubal ectopic pregnancy of 7 weeks gestation; (B) Heteroechoic adnexal mass with free fluid around uterus (a case of ruptured ectopic).

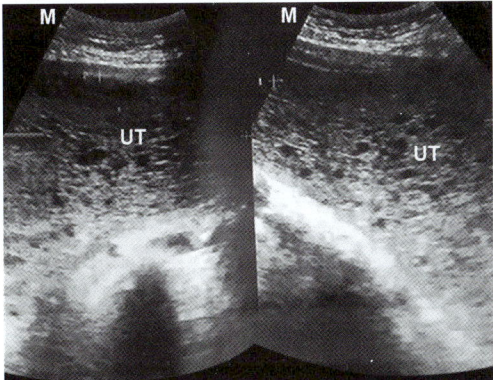

Fig. 5: Molar pregnancy on ultrasonography.

gestational sac can be seen on ultrasound. It is 1,500 mIU/ mL with transvaginal USG and 6,500 mIU/mL with transabdominal USG.[7] In early pregnancy, an increase in serum β-hCG of <53% in 48 hours confirms an abnormal pregnancy with a sensitivity of 99%. Determination of serum progesterone levels may help in confirming the abnormal pregnancy. Serum progesterone and serum β-hCG levels are independent of each other. An abnormal serum progesterone level is consistent with an abnormal or failing pregnancy but does not identify the site of the pregnancy whether it is failed intrauterine or ectopic pregnancy. Serum progesterone level of <5 ng/mL confirms an abnormal pregnancy with 100% specificity.[8] Serum progesterone level with most ectopic pregnancies is associated with a level between 10 and 20 ng/mL, hence not very useful clinically Serial serum β-hCG is indicated in woman with suspected ectopic pregnancy. In women with a normally growing intrauterine pregnancy, serum β-hCG levels double every 48 hours.

A systematic approach to the workup of a pregnant woman presenting with bleeding per vaginum in early pregnancy is summarized in Flowchart 1.

MANAGEMENT

The treatment of a woman with bleeding in early pregnancy is based on the clinical condition, diagnosis, and availability of facilities and expertise. In a clinically unstable patient, it is important to stabilize the patient and institute definitive treatment or refer to a suitable facility. Use of oxytocic agents in actively bleeding patient as in incomplete abortion and molar pregnancy can be lifesaving. Refer to Flowchart 2 that summarizes the management principles based on the differential diagnosis.

Flowchart 1: Algorithm for clinical approach to a woman with bleeding per vaginum in early pregnancy.

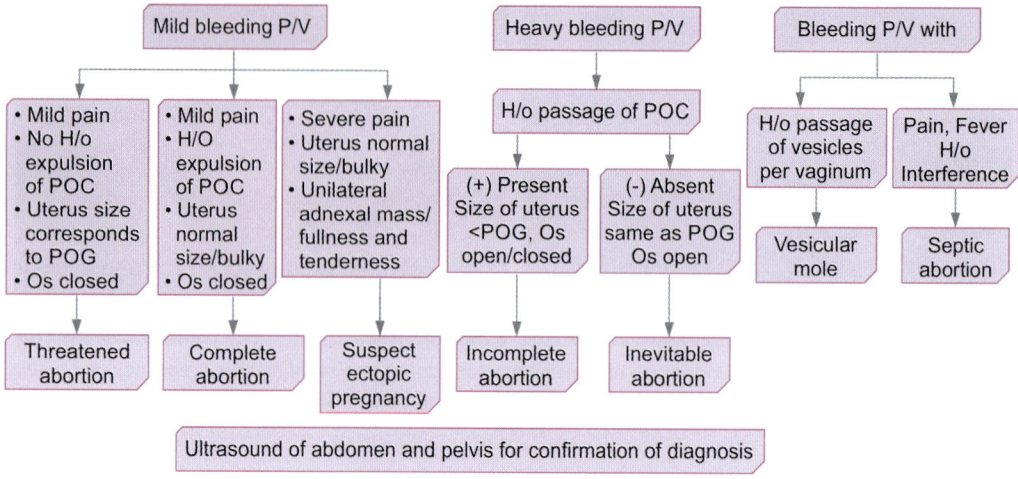

(H/o: history of; POC: products of conception; POG: period of gestation; P/V: per vaginum)

Flowchart 2: Algorithm for management of woman with bleeding per vaginum in early pregnancy.

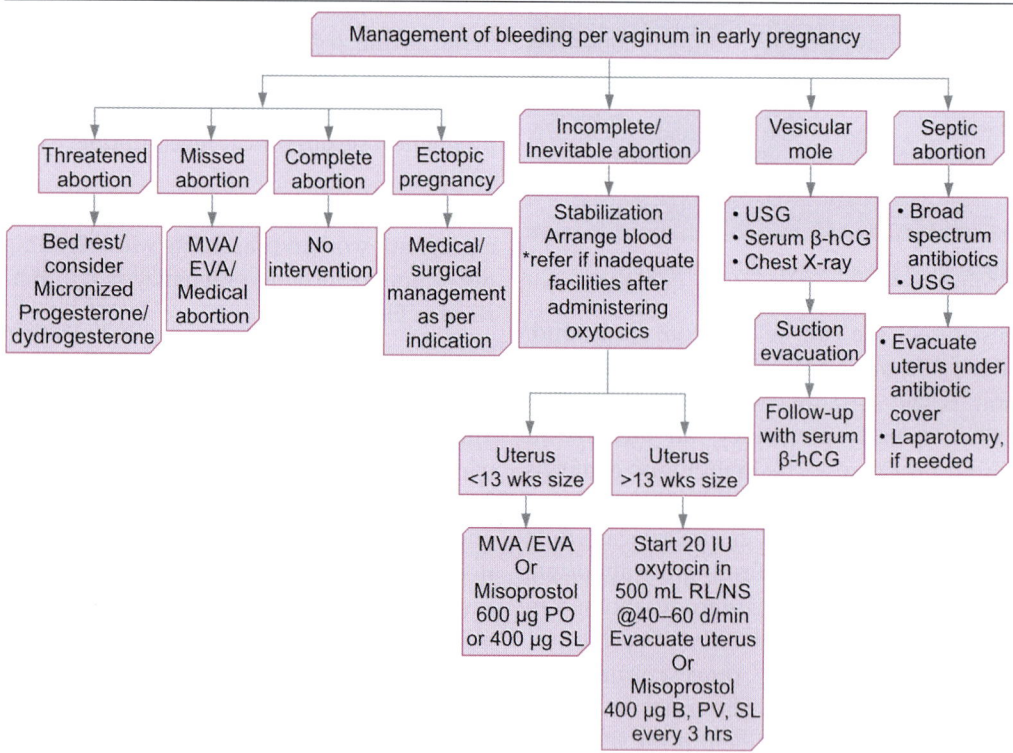

(β-hCG: beta-human chorionic gonadotropin; EVA: electric vacuum aspiration; MVA: manual vacuum aspiration; NS: normal saline; RL: Ringer's lactate; USG: ultrasonography)

KEY POINTS

- Any amount of vaginal bleeding during early pregnancy calls for assessment by a detailed history and examination.
- Most women with bleeding in early pregnancy will reach to term but some will miscarry.
- Pelvic ultrasound plays an important role in confirmation of diagnosis in bleeding in early pregnancy.
- A systematic workup and diagnosis is required for optimal management of these women.

REFERENCES

1. World Health Organization. (2019). Adaptation of WHO safe abortion guidelines in India. [online] Available from https://www.who.int/reproductivehealth/guideline-medical-abortion-care/en/. [Last accessed January, 2020].
2. ACOG Practice Bulletin No. 135: Second-trimester abortion. Obstet Gynecol. 2013; 121(6):1394-406.
3. ACOG Practice Bulletin No. 200 Summary: Early Pregnancy Loss. Obstet Gynecol. 2018; 132(5):1311-13.
4. Pineles BL, Park E, Samet JM. Systematic review and meta-analysis of miscarriage and maternal exposure to tobacco smoke during pregnancy. Am J Epidemiol. 2014;179 (7):807-23.
5. Maconochie N, Doyle P, Prior S, Simmons R. Risk factors for first trimester miscarriage—results from a UK-population-based case-control study. BJOG. 2007;114(2): 170-86.
6. Berkowitz RS, Goldstein DP. Current advances in the management of gestational trophoblastic disease. Gynecol Oncol. 2013; 128(1):3-5.
7. Connolly A, Ryan DH, Stuebe AM, Wolfe HM. Reevaluation of discriminatory and threshold levels for serum beta-hCG in early pregnancy. Obstet Gynecol. 2013;121(1): 65-70.
8. Mesen TB, Young SL. Progesterone and the luteal phase: A requisite to reproduction. Obstet Gynecol Clin North Am. 2015;42(1): 135-51.

SUGGESTED READING

1. ACOG Practice Bulletin No. 193. Tubal ectopic pregnancy. Obstet Gynecol. 2018;131(3): e91-103.
2. National Institute for Health and Care Excellence (NICE) (2019). NICE Guideline: Ectopic pregnancy and miscarriage: Diagnosis and initial management. [online] Available from https://www.nice.org.uk/guidance/ng126/resources/ectopic-pregnancy-and-miscarriage-diagnosis-and-initial-management-pdf-66141662244037. [Last accessed January, 2020].
3. Royal College of Obstetricians and Gynaecologists. (2010) Gestational Trophoblastic Disease (Green-top guideline no. 38). [online] Available from https://www.rcog.org.uk/en/guidelines-research-services/guidelines/gtg38/. [Last accessed January, 2020].
4. World Health Organization. (2018). Medical management of abortion. [online] Available from https://apps.who.int/iris/bitstream/handle/10665/278968/9789241550406-eng.pdf?ua=1. [Last accessed January, 2020].

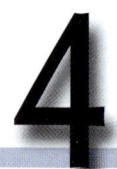

Approach to a Pregnant Woman Presenting with Bleeding in Late Pregnancy

Namita Jain, Meenakshi Singh

INTRODUCTION

Antepartum hemorrhage (APH) is defined as bleeding from or into the genital tract, occurring anytime from 24 + 0 weeks of pregnancy that is the period of viability till the birth of the baby.[1] Excessive bleeding occurring after the birth of the baby but before the delivery of placenta is known as third-stage postpartum hemorrhage. APH complicates 3–5% of pregnancies and is the major cause of perinatal and maternal mortality worldwide.[1] The cutoff for defining abortion is 20 weeks and the period of gestation between 20 and 24 weeks is a gray zone for fetal viability. The American Academy of Pediatrics and the American College of Obstetricians and Gynecologists consider the period between 20 and 23 weeks as previable and do not recommend neonatal resuscitation but recommend that resuscitation may be considered between 23 + 1 and 24 weeks.[2] As far as management is considered, the period between 20 and 24 weeks is managed as antepartum hemorrhage. A systematic assessment and triage in patients with antepartum hemorrhage is important for optimizing the outcomes. The most common causes for bleeding in late pregnancy are mostly placental—placenta previa and placental abruption. Both may be associated with significant hemorrhage and increased risk to the lives of both the mother and the baby, hence warranting immediate clinical attention, assessment, and timely management. Major degree of abruption is life threatening and is the most common obstetrical cause for consumptive coagulopathy.

DIFFERENTIAL DIAGNOSIS

The various causes of bleeding per vaginum in late pregnancy are listed in Box 1.

Box 1: Causes of bleeding after 28 weeks' of gestation.

Antepartum hemorrhage:
- Placental causes:
  - Placenta previa
  - Placental abruption
- Nonplacental causes:
  - Tumors of cervix and vagina
  - Cervical erosion/ectropion
  - Varicosities
  - Excessive show during labor
  - Ruptured vasa previa
  - Rupture uterus
- Nonvaginal source:
  - Anal canal/rectum like hemorrhoids
  - Urinary tract (e.g. vesical calculi)

HISTORY

History of Presenting Complaint

A detailed history of the presenting symptom, i.e. bleeding per vaginum, is important. It includes onset, duration, and amount of bleeding. There is no consistent definition of severity of APH; however, the Royal College of Obstetricians and Gynaecologists (RCOG) defines the severity of hemorrhage as spotting, minor (<50 mL), major (50—1,000 mL without signs of shock), and massive hemorrhage (>1,000 mL and/or signs of shock) depending upon the blood loss.[1] The amount of bleeding can be assessed by enquiring about the number of pads used and extent of soakage of pads—whether partially soaked or fully soaked. History of passage of clots or flooding implies heavy bleeding. The color of blood lost is important; bright red-colored bleeding indicates fresh blood as is seen in women with placenta previa and revealed abruption, whereas dark altered blood indicates old blood as is seen in women with concealed placental abruption. It is important to know if the bleeding is continuous or in bouts. Bleeding in placenta previa occurs in bouts whereas it is continuous in placental abruption.

It is also important to know if this is the first episode or there have been previous episodes of bleeding per vaginum in current pregnancy. Any factor which might have provoked bleeding, such as trauma or sexual intercourse, should be enquired.

Any associated feature such as abdominal pain, whether intermittent or continuous, is important. Intermittent pain associated with hardening of the uterus is suggestive of uterine contractions and continuous pain is suggestive of placental abruption. Pain also helps in differentiating placenta previa from placental abruption. Bleeding in placenta previa is mostly painless but may be sometimes followed by intermittent abdominal pain due to uterine contractions initiated as a result of release of prostaglandins consequent to some placental separation occurring due to the process of formation of lower uterine segment or cervical effacement and or dilatation. Blood mixed mucoid discharge associated with uterine contractions is suggestive of excessive bloody show.

It is important to ask whether the woman is perceiving normal fetal movements or not; perception of normal fetal movements suggests fetal well-being. Any symptoms suggestive of preeclampsia such as swelling of feet, tightening of rings due to fluid retention, epigastric pain, visual disturbances, or high blood pressure records may point toward preeclampsia, which is often associated with placental abruption.

Any history of leaking per vaginum followed by bleeding is suggestive of placental abruption. This association is common in women with hydramnios due to sudden decompression of the uterine cavity and in women with preterm premature rupture of membranes on conservative management.

Any history of trauma or procedures such as external cephalic version is important as these can result in placental abruption. There is a risk of fetomaternal hemorrhage if abruption is consequent to external abdominal trauma.

Any history of low-lying placenta on previous ultrasound scans or recurrent episodes of painless, causeless bleeding suggests placenta previa. History of in vitro fertilization is associated with an increased incidence of vasa previa (1/300).[3] If the bleeding episode is associated with spontaneous or artificial rupture of the fetal membranes and acute fetal distress ruptured vasa previa should be suspected.

History of any previous cervical smear is important to assess the possibility of any neoplastic lesion of the cervix as the cause of bleeding per vaginum. These women usually present with postcoital bleeding.

Menstrual History

Accurate dating is required to tailor the management of women with APH. Refer to Chapter 1 section on dating of pregnancy for further details.

Obstetric History

Obstetric history includes the number of years the woman had been married and number of years she has been cohabiting. Any history of treatment taken for infertility, the gravidity, parity, and outcome of previous pregnancies should be enquired. Refer to Chapter 1 section on obstetric history for further details.

The risk of placenta previa increases with increasing age and parity. Previous cesarean sections predispose to low-lying placenta, morbid adherence of placenta, and scar rupture; both these conditions may be associated with APH in subsequent pregnancies. Previous cesarean delivery increases the risk of occurrence of placenta previa from 0.65% after one cesarean to 10% after four or more caesarean sections.[4] Any history of perforation or repeated dilatation and curettage is important as it can subsequently predispose a woman to morbidly adherent placenta.

The risk of placental abruption is more in women belonging to black race. The risk increases with rise in age and parity. Multiple pregnancy and uterine fibroids may be associated risk factors for abruption.

History of APH in previous pregnancies increases its risk in future pregnancies. The recurrence risk of abruption is 6–17% after previous one abruption and 25% after previous two abruptions.[5]

Past Medical/Surgical History

In woman with bleeding in late pregnancy, any history of previous surgery such as myomectomy, metroplasty, or cesarean section increases the chances of morbidly adherent placenta.

Personal History

Cigarette smoking and cocaine abuse increase the risk of placental abruption.[6]

EXAMINATION

The examination of a pregnant woman presenting with bleeding per vaginum includes assessment of general condition of the patient followed by a systematic examination with special emphasis to abdominal examination. A per vaginum examination should not to be done without ruling out placenta previa on ultrasound to avoid the risk of provoking a life-threatening hemorrhage in cases of placenta previa. A careful gentle per speculum examination may be done to rule out any local lesion.

General Physical Examination

Physical examination includes assessment of the general condition and vitals of the woman. An assessment of the amount of blood loss is important and is reflected by the pulse rate, blood pressure, and degree of pallor. Hypotension with tachycardia suggests hypovolemic shock consequent to excessive blood loss which may be revealed or concealed. Restlessness, cold clammy extremities, poor skin perfusion, and piloerection response also suggest hypovolemic shock. If the shock is out of proportion to the visible blood loss, it is suggestive of concealed hemorrhage as in placental abruption or hemoperitoneum due to scar rupture or ruptured uterus.

Per Abdomen Examination

In woman with bleeding per vaginum in late pregnancy, a careful per abdomen examination includes inspection for any abdominal scars and a detailed obstetric examination. This includes assessment of fundal height, contour of the uterus, its tone, any area of tenderness, presentation of the fetus, whether the presenting part is free floating or deviated to one side or engaged, and presence or absence of uterine contractions.

The uterine contour is lost and fetal parts are felt superficially in uterine rupture. In women with a previous uterine scar, it is important to elicit any scar tenderness. The flanks are percussed for any shifting dullness suggestive of intraperitoneal collection. Flanks are usually resonant due to displacement of bowel loops laterally but may be dull in case of intraperitoneal hemorrhage consequent to rupture of uterus.

The fetal heart sound (FHS) is heard. It is absent in woman with severe abruption, uterine rupture, and placenta previa in shock.

The clinical signs that help in differentiating two common clinical conditions resulting in APH—placenta previa and placental abruption are listed in Table 1.

It is important to note that if the placental abruption is mild or predominantly revealed or if the placenta is located posteriorly then the abdominal signs such as tenderness and rigidity may not be very well appreciated.

Local Examination

Local vulval inspection should be done to assess the amount of blood loss, any clots in vagina, whether bleeding is continuing or has stopped.

Per Speculum Examination

A gentle speculum examination can be done in case of mild bleeding to rule out any

Clinical features	Placenta previa	Placental abruption
History	Painless, causeless, bright red bleeding in bouts	• Usually painful dark-colored continuous bleeding • History suggestive of preeclampsia
General physical examination	• Pallor proportionate to blood loss	• Pallor usually out of proportion to blood loss, especially with concealed abruption, but proportionate to blood loss with revealed abruption
	• Blood pressure (BP) normal or low if in shock	• BP may be high, normal, or low depending upon the presence of preeclampsia or hypovolemic shock
	• Features of fluid retention absent	• Features of fluid retention may be present such as facial puffiness, swelling feet, hands, etc., due to coexistent preeclampsia
Per abdominal examination	• Height of the uterus corresponds to the period of gestation	• The findings depend upon the degree of separation and whether abruption is revealed, or concealed • Height of the uterus may either correspond to the period of gestation (POG) as with revealed abruption or is more than POG as in concealed abruption
	• Uterus is soft, nontender	• The tone of the uterus is increased, and it may be hard and tender in concealed abruption
	• The fetus presents as either breech or transverse lie or oblique. In case it is cephalic, it is free floating usually deviated to one side	• Fetal parts are felt with difficulty
	• Fetal heart sound (FHS) is present and regular	• FHS is usually absent

Table 1: Clinical features differentiating placenta previa from placental abruption.

local cause of bleeding per vaginum, while it should not be done in woman presenting with severe bleeding.

Per Vaginal Examination

Per vaginum examination is contraindicated in woman presenting with bleeding per vaginum in late pregnancy as it can provoke severe hemorrhage in woman with placenta previa. It is postponed till the placenta is localized on ultrasonography (USG), and decision regarding termination of pregnancy is taken. Digital cervical examination, if necessary, should be performed only in an operating room with full preparation of cesarean delivery (double setup examination).

INVESTIGATIONS

Investigations should be done along with resuscitation and stabilization of the patient. These are guided by the clinical history and examination findings. In hemodynamically unstable patients, two large-bore intravenous cannulae should be inserted and blood sample should be drawn for blood grouping and crossmatching, complete hemogram, coagulation profile, liver function test (LFT), and kidney function test (KFT).

A transabdominal USG helps in localizing placenta, whether it is in lower uterine segment or upper uterine segment and detecting any retroplacental clot (Figs. 1 and 2). In addition, fetal presentation, fetal biometry, amount of liquor, estimated fetal weight, and any gross congenital fetal malformations should be commented upon on USG.

In case low-lying placenta is diagnosed, the findings should be confirmed by transvaginal USG which is more accurate (Fig. 3). Exact distance of the placental edge from the internal cervical os should be measured on transvaginal USG. Between 18 and 24 weeks' gestation in 2–4% women, the placental edge reaches or overlaps the internal cervical os on transvaginal scan (TVS) examination. A follow-up examination for placental location in the third trimester is recommended in these women. Overlap of >20 mm at 26 weeks is associated with an increased likelihood of persistence of placenta previa at term.[7] The sensitivity and specificity of TVS in

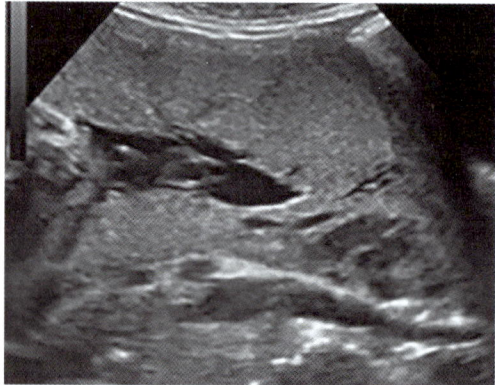

Fig.1: Placenta previa on transabdominal ultrasonography.

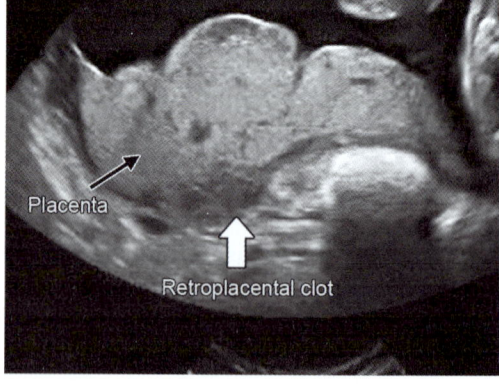

Fig. 2: Late pregnancy placental abruption on transabdominal ultrasonography.

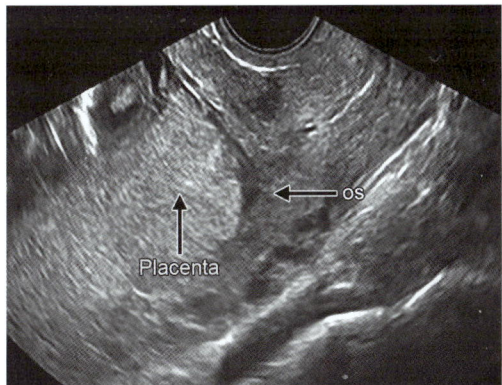

Fig. 3: Placenta previa on transvaginal scan (TVS).

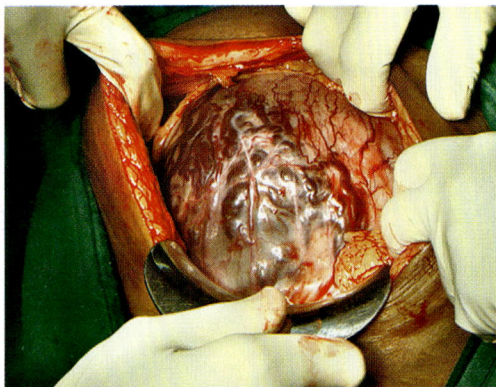

Fig. 4: Morbidly adherent placenta (perioperative).

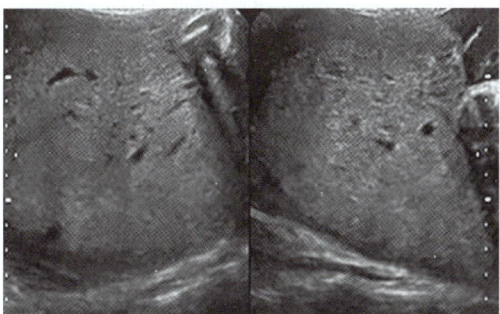

Fig. 5: Morbidly adherent placenta with lacunae on ultrasonography grayscale.

Table 2: Ultrasonographic features of morbidly adherent placenta previa.	
Gray scale ultrasound	• Loss of retroplacental sonolucent zone • Presence of an irregular retroplacental sonolucent zone • Disruption or thinning of the hyperechoic serosa-bladder interface • Invasion of the urinary bladder by focal exophytic masses • Presence of abnormal placental lacunae (Fig. 5)
Color Doppler	• Markedly dilated vessels over subplacental zone • Vascular lakes with turbulent flow • Hypervascularity of serosa–bladder interface (Fig. 6)

localization of placenta are 87.5% and 98.8%, respectively. The positive predictive value is 93.3% and negative predictive value is 97.6% with a false negative rate of 2.33%. In women with placenta previa, placental cord insertion should be evaluated. In case it is velamentous or marginal, possibility of vasa previa should be kept. The risk of velamentous insertion is also increased with a bilobate or succenturiate placenta. Woman with previous history of lower segment cesarean section and anterior low-lying placenta should be carefully examined for any evidence of morbid adherence of placenta to the scar (Figs. 4 and 5). USG criteria for diagnosis of adherent placenta are as given in Table 2. In doubtful cases, especially with posteriorly located placenta, magnetic resonance imaging (MRI) is useful to rule out morbidly adherent placenta.

Flowchart 1 depicts an algorithm showing a systematic workup of a pregnant woman presenting with bleeding per vaginum in late pregnancy and Flowchart 2 outlines the management.

Cardiotocograph (CTG) or handheld Doppler is useful for assessment of fetal well-being.

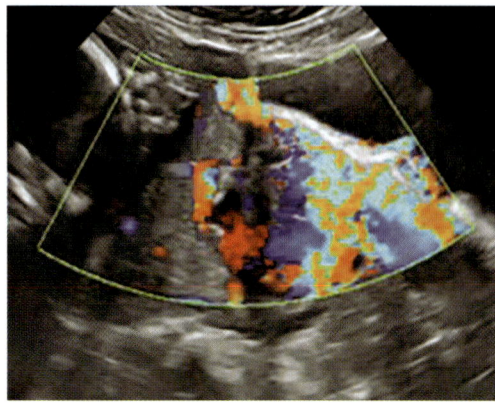

Fig. 6: Morbidly adherent placenta on color Doppler.

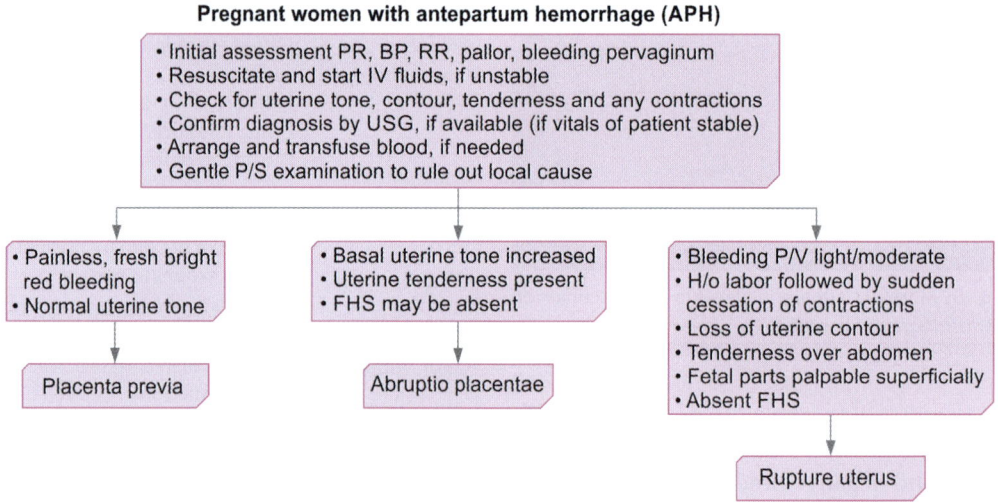

Flowchart 1: Algorithm for clinical approach to a woman with bleeding per vaginum in later half of pregnancy.

(BP: blood pressure; FHS: fetal heart sound; H/o: history of; IV: intravenous; PR: pulse rate; P/S: per speculum; P/V: per vaginum; RR: respiratory; USG: ultrasonography)

KEY POINTS

- Any amount of vaginal bleeding during pregnancy calls for rapid evaluation of the woman for amount of blood loss and workup for cause of bleeding.
- Bleeding in later half of pregnancy is mostly due to placental causes; placenta previa and placental abruption.
- USG for placental localization plays a significant role in diagnosing placenta previa and TVS is more sensitive and specific compared to transabdominal scan (TAS).
- USG is not a reliable method to diagnose placental abruption.
- A systematic workup and diagnosis is required to manage these women optimally.

Chapter 4: Approach to a Pregnant Woman Presenting with Bleeding in Late Pregnancy

Flowchart 2: Algorithm for management of woman with bleeding per vaginum in later half of pregnancy.

Pregnant women with antepartum hemorrhage (APH)

- **Placenta previa**
  - Heavy bleeding irrespective of gestational age
  - Term pregnancy ≥37 weeks
  - Patient in labor
  - Fetal distress
  - Malformed baby
  - Dead baby

  ↓

  Active management: Termination of pregnancy
  LSCS
  - If placenta is type II post III, IV
  - Patient in shock
  - Malpresentation
  - Fetal distress
  - Any other obstetric indication
  Double set-up examination in OT ARM and induction of labor

  - Light bleeding
  - POG <37 weeks
  - Live baby, no gross fetal anomaly
  - Patient not in labor

  ↓

  Expectant management:
  - Hospitalize
  - Build-up patient
  - Arrange blood
  - Fetomaternal surveillance
  - Steroids (if POG <34 weeks)

  ↓

  Active management:
  - If ≥37 weeks
  - Repeated bouts or heavy bleeding

- **Placental abruption**
  - Unstable patient
  - Heavy bleeding P/V and vaginal delivery not imminent
  - Fetal distress with a viable fetus

  ↓

  LSCS

  - Patients vitals stable
  - Bleeding P/V light/Moderate
  - FHS normal
  - Dead fetus

  ↓

  - Induction of labor
  - ARM + OXYTOCIN deliver in 6–8 hrs
  - Careful monitoring of abdominal girth, urine output and coagulation profile

- **Rupture uterus**

  Laparotomy followed by repair of uterus or hysterectomy

(ARM: artificial rupture of the membranes; FHS: fetal heart sound; LSCS: lower segment cesarean section; POG: period of gestation; P/V: per vaginum; POG: period of gestation)

REFERENCES

1. Royal College of Obstetricians and Gynaecologists. (2011). Antepartum haemorrhage (Green-top Guideline no. 63). [online] Available from https://www.rcog.org.uk/en/guidelines-research-services/guidelines/gtg63/. [Last accessed January, 2020]
2. Raju TN, Mercer BM, Burchfield DJ, Joseph GF. Periviable birth: executive summary of a joint workshop by the Eunice Kennedy Shriver National Institute of Child Health and Human Development, Society for Maternal-Fetal Medicine, American Academy of Pediatrics, and American College of Obstetricians and Gynecologists. J Perinatol. 2014; 34(5):333-42.
3. Swank ML, Garite TJ, Maurel K, Das A, Perlow JH, Combs CA, et al. Vasa previa: Diagnosis and management. Am J Obstet Gynecol. 2016; 215(2): 223.e1-6.
4. Klar M, Michels KB. Cesarean section and placental disorders in subsequent pregnancies–a meta-analysis. J Perinat Med. 2014; 42(5):571-83.
5. Tikkanen M. Etiology, clinical manifestations, and prediction of placental abruption. Acta Obstet Gynecol Scand. 2010;89(6):732-40.
6. Arnold DL, Williams MA, Miller RS, Qiu C, Sorensen TK. Iron deficiency anemia, cigarette smoking and risk of abruptio placentae. J Obstet Gynaecol Res. 2009;35(3): 446-52.
7. Creasy RK, Resnik R, Iams J, Lockwood C, Moore T, Greene M. Placenta previa, placenta accreta, abruptio placentae, and vasa

previa. Creasy and Resnik's Maternal-Fetal Medicine: Principles and Practice, 7th edition. Philadelphia, PA: Saunders; 2014. pp. 732-42.

SUGGESTED READING

1. American College of Obstetricians and Gynecologists (ACOG) and Society for Maternal-fetal Medicine (SMFM) Obstetric Care Consensus on Placenta Accreta Spectrum (2018).
2. International Federation of Gynecology and Obstetrics (FIGO): Consensus guidelines on placenta accreta spectrum disorders (2018).
3. Royal College of Obstetricians and Gynaecologists (2018). Placenta Praevia and Placenta Accreta: Diagnosis and Management (Green-top Guideline No. 27a). [online] Available from: https://www.rcog.org.uk/en/guidelines-research-services/guidelines/gtg27a/. [Last accessed January, 2020].
4. Royal College of Obstetricians and Gynaecologists (2018). Vasa Praevia: Diagnosis and Management (RCOG Green-top Guidelines No. 27b). [online] Available from: https://www.rcog.org.uk/en/guidelines-research-services/guidelines/gtg27b/. [Last accessed January, 2020].

5 Approach to a Pregnant Woman Presenting with Abdominal Pain

*Richa Aggarwal**

INTRODUCTION

Abdominal pain in pregnancy is a common complaint, which presents a unique clinical challenge due to altered natural history and clinical presentation of abdominal disorders in pregnancy. This is consequent to the anatomical, physiological, and biochemical changes in pregnancy. Moreover, the interests of both the mother and fetus need to be considered during management.

Though the management is essentially similar to that of a nonpregnant woman, certain aspects need to be kept in mind while evaluating a pregnant woman presenting with abdominal pain. Pregnancy is associated with a number of physiological and anatomical changes that can cause abdominal pain. The enlarging uterus can displace intra-abdominal organs, masking the symptoms, and altering the localizing signs of various diseases. Progesterone decreases lower esophageal sphincter pressure leading to heartburn, gastroesophageal reflux, and even stricture formation. Delayed gastric emptying leads to nausea and vomiting and slow colonic transit time may lead to constipation and abdominal pain. Pain from stretching of uterine ligaments and subluxation of pubic symphysis can be severe and often confused with nonobstetric causes.[1]

Physiological changes in laboratory values during pregnancy such as mild leukocytosis, dilutional anemia, increased alkaline phosphatase, hyponatremia, hypercoagulability, fasting hypoglycemia, and postprandial hyperglycemia can make the diagnosis difficult.[2,3]

Most radiographic or invasive diagnostic procedures carry little risk to the mother or fetus and should be performed, if considered necessary. Radiation damage is the most important risk factor and is worse in first trimester. Exposure of >15 rads (150 mGy) during second and third trimesters or >5 rads (50 mGy) in the first trimester should be of concern because of an association of increased risk of chromosomal and fetal abnormalities and childhood malignancies. Diagnostic studies such as intravenous pyelogram (IVP) and barium enema typically expose the fetus to ≥1 rad and 2–4 rads, respectively. Computed tomography (CT) abdomen exposes the fetus to 3.5 rads of ionizing radiations.[4]

DIFFERENTIAL DIAGNOSIS

The causes of abdominal pain in a pregnant woman can be broadly divided into three categories: Physiological causes, pathological conditions related to pregnancy, and pathological conditions incidental to pregnancy. The differential diagnosis is listed in Table 1.

Although diagnosing the cause of abdominal pain during pregnancy can be perplexing, a careful history and physical

Section 1: Obstetrics

Table 1: Differential diagnosis of abdominal pain in a pregnant woman.

Physiological	Pathological conditions related to pregnancy	Pathological conditions incidental to pregnancy

• Round ligament stretch
• Braxton Hicks contractions
• Gastritis due to vomiting
• Heartburn due to relaxed sphincter
• *Constipation*: Progesterone induced
	• *First trimester*:
	  - *Miscarriage*: Threatened, inevitable, and incomplete septic abortion
	  - *Vesicular mole*: In the process of expulsion
	  - Ectopic pregnancy
	  - Ruptured corpus luteum hematoma/cyst
	  - Acute urinary retention due to retroverted gravid uterus or impacted ovarian cyst
	• *Second trimester*:
	  - Mid-trimester abortion
	  - Angular pregnancy or rupture of a rudimentary horn pregnancy
	  - Red degeneration of fibroid
	  - Torsion of pedunculated myoma
	  - Torsion of ovarian or paraovarian cyst
	• *Third trimester*:
	  - Placental abruption
	  - Rupture uterus
	  - Scar dehiscence
	  - *Severe preeclampsia*: Subcapsular hepatic hematoma
	  - Spontaneous rupture of liver
	  - Acute fatty liver of pregnancy
	  - Acute hydramnios
	  - Chorioamnionitis
	  - Preterm labor pains
	  - Labor pains
	• *Miscellaneous*:
	  - Acute cystitis
	  - Acute pyelonephritis
	  - Acute cholecystitis or gallstones
	  - Rectus muscle hematoma
		• *Gastrointestinal causes*:
		  - Peptic ulcer
		  - Pancreatitis
		  - Acute appendicitis
		  - Acute gastroenteritis
		  - Acute diverticulitis
		  - Acute intestinal obstruction
		  - Intestinal volvulus
		  - Inflammatory bowel disease
		  - Strangulated hernia
		  - Hepatitis
		  - Hepatic rupture
		  - Splenic rupture
		• *Genitourinary causes*:
		  - Adnexal torsion
		  - Ureteric/renal calculi
		• *Respiratory causes*:
		  - Basal pneumonia
		  - Pleuritis
		• *Miscellaneous*:
		  - Vascular accidents, e.g. superior mesenteric artery syndrome, thrombosis/infarction
		  - Diabetic ketoacidosis
		  - Sickle cell crisis
		  - Ruptured spleen or splenic aneurysm
		  - Abdominal trauma
		  - Porphyria
		  - Acute myocardial infarction
		  - Any related causes

examination can enable the physician to formulate a working differential diagnosis (Flowchart 1). Prompt and appropriate management can then follow. A rapid initial assessment of the overall condition is the first step to determine the pace of further diagnostic and ultimately therapeutic interventions.

If the patient is in shock, she must be first stabilized. Shock in pregnancy is usually caused by hemorrhage and/or sepsis. Causes of hemorrhagic shock include acute ruptured ectopic pregnancy, ruptured corpus luteum, traumatic rupture of spleen, and gastrointestinal hemorrhage due to ulcer disease. Causes of sepsis during pregnancy include untreated pyelonephritis or chorioamnionitis.

Establishing the gestational age early in the evaluation is essential because the likelihood of different etiologies at different gestational ages, and to make an appropriate

Flowchart 1: Algorithm for clinical approach to a pregnant woman with abdominal pain.

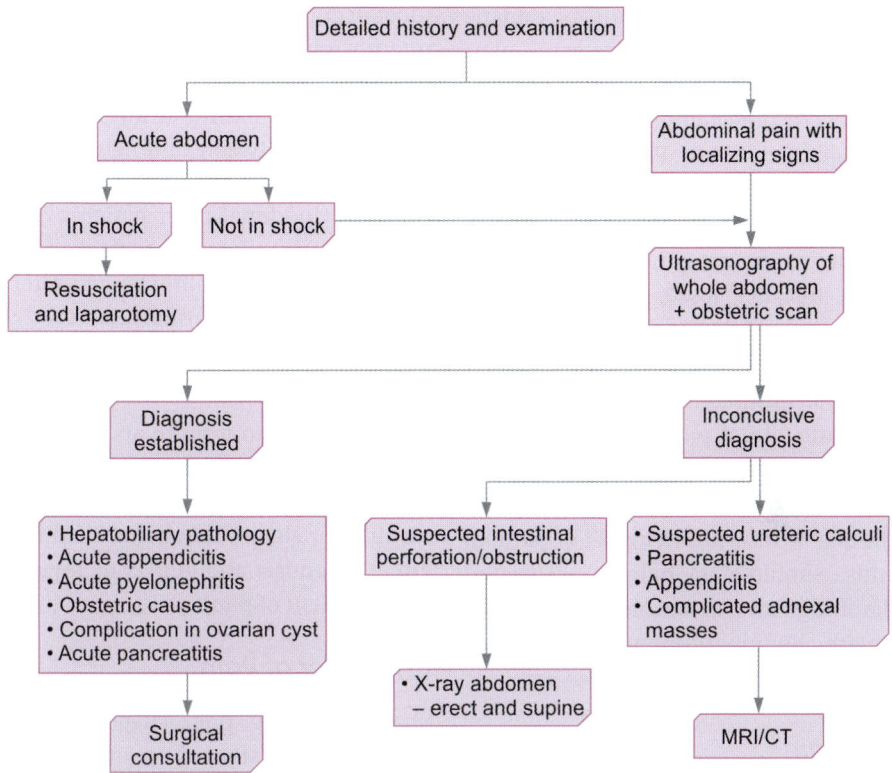

(CT: computed tomography; MRI: magnetic resonance imaging)

decision regarding fetal viability and the need for fetal evaluation.

HISTORY

History of Present Illness

A careful detailed history with respect to the presenting symptom is essential to establish the cause of pain and includes site, onset, duration, intensity, character, radiation, any associated symptoms, and aggravating or relieving factors.

Site of Pain

The patient is asked to indicate the site of pain with the fingertip (pointing test). If the pain is diffuse, the patient will use her whole hand instead of one finger. It is evaluated in relation to the period of gestation. The pain from appendicitis will localize to right lower quadrant in early pregnancy, but in the last trimester, due to the growing uterus and displacement of appendix, it is localized to the upper quadrant.

Pain related to foregut visceral structures (mouth to proximal duodenum including gall bladder) is generally felt in the upper abdomen, while that associated with midgut structures (distal duodenum to mid-transverse colon) is felt around the umbilicus. Hindgut structure (remaining colon and rectum) pain is generally felt in the lower abdomen.

Pain in right upper quadrant may be caused by cholecystitis, hepatitis, or hepatic rupture. Epigastric pain suggests acute pancreatitis, peptic ulcer, and hepatic involvement in severe preeclampsia or acute fatty liver of pregnancy (AFLP). Periumbilical pain is usually due to intestinal pathology. Pain arising from diseases of lower urinary tract or reproductive organs generally localize to suprapubic area, iliac fossa, or flanks.

Generalized abdominal pain suggests diffuse peritonitis as in cases of appendiceal perforation or intra-abdominal hemorrhage.[5] Shifting of the site of pain should be asked for as in appendicitis, the pain first appears around the umbilicus, but later on, it shifts to the right iliac fossa with the onset of parietal peritonitis. Shoulder-tip pain is associated with diaphragmatic irritation and is associated with hemoperitoneum or visceral perforation.

Onset of Pain

It is important to find out if the onset was sudden or insidious. Pain of sudden onset suggests rupture of abdominal organs such as perforation of duodenal ulcer or rupture of ectopic pregnancy, ovarian cyst, or uterus. Pain due to torsion of ovarian cyst or adnexa or due to intestinal or ureteric colic is also sudden in onset. Pain building slowly over a period of time indicates inflammatory or obstructive process.

Duration of Pain

Whether the pain was present before pregnancy or not helps in finding out whether the pain is pregnancy related or not. Duration can also help to differentiate an acute from a chronic process. Similar type of pain with varying intensities appearing off and on in the right lower abdomen is suggestive of appendicitis. The typical pain in duodenal ulcer occurs 2–3 hours after a meal and is frequently relieved by antacids or food, whereas in gastric ulcer, discomfort may be precipitated by food. Pain that awakes the patient from sleep (between midnight and 3 AM) is the most discriminating symptom, with two thirds of duodenal ulcer patients describing this complaint. Recurrent attacks of pain are usually caused by urolithiasis or ureteric colic or sometimes torsion of ovarian cyst.

Intensity of Pain

It is important to inquire about the intensity of pain. Is it dull aching, mild, moderate, or severe in intensity? Is it intense enough to disturb her sleep? This helps us in the differential diagnosis and guides us regarding the management of pain.

Character of Pain

Sharp, stabbing pain suggests perforation of a viscus, torsion of an ovarian cyst or a localized inflammatory process, while dull periodic pain usually suggests obstructive process.[2] Colicky pain is a sharp intermittent pain occurring in obstructive pathology. Constant burning pain is a feature of peritonitis as in cases of ruptured ectopic. Throbbing pain is suggestive of inflammation, e.g., hepatic or appendicular abscess. Diffuse third trimester discomfort is caused by abdominal wall distension, vigorous fetal activity, engagement of fetal head, and pressure effect of fetal head in breech presentation.

Radiation of Pain

This denotes extension of pain to another site, while the pain persists at the original site also. Pain radiating to flanks suggest a renal pathology as in case of urolithiasis, while pain of pancreatitis radiates to back.

Referred Pain

When the pain is felt at a distance from its site of origin with no pain at its original site, it is called referred pain. This occurs when the central nervous system (CNS) fails to differentiate between somatic and visceral impulses from the same segment. In renal colic, pain is referred from loin to groin and inner aspect of thigh along the distribution of genitofemoral nerve.

Precipitating or Relieving Factors

Knowledge about whether the pain gets worse or better by any factor such as food, posture, or movement is useful in differential diagnosis. Pain of acute pancreatitis is relieved by leaning forward. Round ligament pain is often felt in lower quadrants and is worsened by movement and turning sideways in bed in lying down position. In peritonitis, pain is slightly relieved if the patient lies still. Gastritis-induced pain is relieved by vomiting. Relation of pain with meals, whether it occurs before or after meals or is it relieved by meals is also important. Pain of gastritis usually increases after meals and is relieved by taking antacids.

Associated Symptoms

Pain associated with nausea, vomiting or diarrhea generally suggests gastrointestinal pathology. Absolute constipation is the usual accompaniment of intestinal obstruction. Presence of jaundice with pain suggests cholecystitis or hepatitis. Nausea and vomiting with severe right upper quadrant or epigastric pain may be the presenting complaints in AFLP. Painful, intermittent jaundice is very characteristic of common bile duct stone.[5] Flank pain associated with dysuria, urgency, or hematuria indicates urolithiasis.

History of trauma followed by acute pain suggests rupture of ovarian cyst, liver, spleen, or aneurysm or formation of rectus muscle hematoma. Early pregnancy with urinary retention is most commonly caused by retroverted gravid uterus. Pain with vaginal bleeding in early pregnancy is caused by abortion or ectopic pregnancy, while in late pregnancy, it suggests abruption, preterm labor, or uterine rupture. History of leaking per vaginum should be elicited as fever with leaking and pain suggests chorioamnionitis.

History of any surgical intervention such as dilatation and curettage in early pregnancy should be sought as it can lead to septic abortion.

Menstrual History

It is important to ask the date of last menstrual period (LMP) to ascertain the period of gestation. History of amenorrhea if present suggests pregnancy-related problem. Prior history of menorrhagia may suggest presence of uterine fibroids, which can cause pain by torsion, red degeneration, or causing abruption.

Obstetric History

In women who have conceived after treatment of infertility or have undergone tubal surgery for blocked tubes, presenting with pain in early pregnancy, ectopic pregnancy should always be ruled out. History of previous lower segment cesarean (LSCS), dilatation and curettage, or grand multiparity predisposes a woman to uterine rupture or scar rupture. Women conceived with ART may have pain due to ovarian hyperstimulation syndrome.

History of Past Illness

History of previous pelvic or abdominal surgery raises the possibility of intestinal obstruction or ectopic pregnancy due to adhesions. History of appendicitis, renal or biliary colic and peptic ulcer is important as these conditions may recur. History of any chronic illness such as tuberculosis, diabetes, and sickle cell disease should be inquired to rule out intestinal obstruction, diabetic ketoacidosis, and sickling crisis, respectively as a cause of pain. Any history of irritable bowel syndrome should be elicited. Rarely, if a patient is a known case of porphyria, acute exacerbation should be suspected. However, it may present for the first time in pregnancy.[6]

Personal History

History of domestic violence or marital disharmony should be elicited to rule out psychological or traumatic cause of abdominal pain. Any woman reporting a high number of ailments during antenatal care may be in the need of psychological support.

Dietary History

Acute gastroenteritis and hepatitis have a fecal–oral route of transmission and hence, it is important to elicit dietary history as well as similar history in other family members. Peptic ulcer also has diet-related precipitating factors, which should be enquired into. Spicy foods, alcohol, coffee, tobacco smoking, and non-steroidal anti-inflammatory drugs (NSAIDS) often precipitate pain of peptic ulcer, while high-fiber diet and probiotics have a protective effect.

EXAMINATION

General Physical Examination

A complete general physical examination is performed systematically and includes the following parameters.

Attitude

In colic, the patient is usually tossing in bed or doubled up, or rolls in agony seeking a position of comfort. Patients with peritonitis usually lie very still and do not move, because movement aggravates pain.

Vitals

In internal hemorrhage, pulse rate is fast, thin, and thready. In early stage of certain abdominal conditions such as peptic perforation and acute intestinal obstruction, the pulse remains normal, but with the spread of peritonitis, it becomes rapid and low volume.

Pain with high blood pressure (BP) records may be caused by placental abruption, AFLP, or hepatic rupture, though later, the BP may fall following excessive internal or external hemorrhage. Increased respiratory rate with movements of alae nasi points toward lungs as the seat of disease or peritonitis. In infective conditions, the patient may be febrile. Presence of high-grade fever indicates chorioamnionitis, pyelonephritis, or appendicitis, while low-grade fever may be associated with pancreatitis, degenerating myoma, or abdominal or genital tuberculosis.

Tongue

It is an index of state of hydration, vitamin deficiencies, and anemia. A dry tongue signifies dehydration. It is dry and brown in cases of septicemia.

Anemia, Cyanosis, and Jaundice

Obvious pallor is seen in hemorrhagic conditions such as ruptured ectopic gestation. Presence of icterus should be looked for as it points toward hepatitis, cholecystitis, and rarely pancreatitis. Cyanosis is noted in acute hemorrhagic pancreatitis.

Per Abdomen Examination

Inspection

A careful abdominal examination should begin with an overall inspection. The presence of abdominal scars indicate previous surgery, which raises the possibility of intestinal obstruction secondary to surgical adhesions or uterine rupture consequent to previous surgery on uterus such as cesarean section or myomectomy. In early pregnancy, the abdomen can be evaluated for distension, but in advanced pregnancy, the enlarged uterus may obscure this sign. Localized limitation of respiratory excursion is indicative of subjacent inflammation.

Palpation

It should be performed carefully and methodically, as it usually yields maximum diagnostic information. Diffuse peritonitis is manifested by pain with movement of the patient or movement of any intra-abdominal organ, particularly the uterus. A rigid abdomen usually accompanies peritonitis and indicates a true surgical emergency.

The location of tenderness helps in determining the etiology of the pain. It is usually best to begin palpation at the least tender area and move to the area of greatest tenderness. When performing a physical examination of the gravid abdomen, it is essential to remember the change in position of intra-abdominal organs at different gestational ages. Upper abdominal pain can be due to gallbladder disease, peptic ulcer disease, pancreatitis, or high-level intestinal obstruction. Upper abdominal pain may also be present in pulmonary disease such as pneumonia or pleural irritation. Disease of the appendix, colon, urinary tract, or reproductive organs may all produce lower abdominal pain. Tenderness over the area of round ligaments suggests round ligament pain. Tenderness over pubic symphysis indicates separation of pubic symphysis in pregnancy.

Rebound tenderness, a sign of peritonitis, occurs due to inflammation of parietal peritoneum secondary to underlying inflamed organ. Muscle guarding is another excellent indicator of irritation of parietal peritoneum either due to inflammation or presence of blood within parietal peritoneum. Both these peritoneal signs may be masked or delayed in pregnancy due to enlarged uterus and lax abdominal wall.

Palpation also allows the physician to estimate uterine size and gestational age. In early pregnancy, abdominal masses can be palpated easily, but as the pregnancy advances, masses other than the uterus are difficult to assess. Uterine tenderness may be present with abortion, red degeneration of fibroid, abruption, uterine rupture, chorioamnionitis, or uterine torsion, while uterine contractions indicate labor. To help distinguish extrauterine tenderness from uterine tenderness, performing the examination with the patient in right or left decubitus position, thus displacing the gravid uterus to one side, may be helpful.

When the fetus is considered viable, a thorough fetal evaluation is a must. Note the fetal heart rate and uterine tone. Fetal tachycardia is present in chorioamnionitis, while fetal heart sound is absent in uterine rupture or severe placental abruption. A nonreassuring fetal heart trace or evidence of fetal distress may suggest an obstetric etiology, e.g., placental abruption or uterine rupture.[2]

Auscultation

Hypoactive bowel sounds are indicative of ileus, which can be caused by a diffuse inflammatory process or advanced obstruction. Absent bowel sounds suggest paralytic ileus due to generalized peritonitis. Hyperactive bowel sounds can be heard in early intestinal obstruction.

Pelvic and Rectovaginal Examination

Pelvic and rectovaginal examination must be performed in all pregnant patients with abdominal pain, except those with third-trimester bleeding. However, it is very useful in early pregnancy to differentiate a pregnancy-related etiology from an incidental cause of abdominal pain. Bimanual examination will help to determine the presence of an adnexal mass. A unilateral mass with tenderness is suggestive of ectopic pregnancy, torsion, or ovarian abscess. Cervical motion tenderness is another sign suggestive of a pelvic inflammatory disease or an ectopic pregnancy. Rectovaginal examination allows the physician to evaluate the pouch of Douglas or cul-de-sac better.

INVESTIGATIONS

Hematological

Baseline laboratory data useful in evaluating a pregnant woman with abdominal pain include a complete blood count, blood glucose, serum electrolytes, serum amylase, liver function tests (LFT), blood urea nitrogen, serum creatinine, and urinalysis.

Complete blood count with peripheral smear is a very important investigation and provides information on degree and type of anemia, which may be either pre-existing or sudden in onset due to hemorrhage. Sickle cell anemia can be diagnosed on peripheral smear and can manifest as abdominal pain in sickle cell crisis. Leukocytosis is seen in the presence of an inflammatory pathology such as septic abortion, chorioamnionitis, appendicitis, cholecystitis, etc. Physiological leukocytosis of pregnancy (normal: 5.9–15.6 × 10^9/L) can mimic an acute intra-abdominal inflammatory process.[7] The white blood cell counts usually revert to the nonpregnant levels by the sixth postpartum day. C-reactive protein (CRP) is a useful marker of underlying infection and inflammation and its upper limit in pregnancy is suggested as 20 mg/L;[6] a serial rise in CRP levels is considered more reliable as a marker of infection than a one-off raised value. Lactate is also used in the recognition of sepsis and response to treatment: a level > 4 mmol/L is a marker of severe sepsis and indicates the need for goal-directed sepsis therapy.

Thrombocytopenia with deranged coagulation profile may be seen in AFLP and hemolysis, elevated liver enzymes and low platelets in HELLP syndrome.

Blood group is important during pregnancy, especially in situations with acute hemorrhage where urgent transfusion is required. The LFT and serum amylase are useful in patients with upper abdominal pain, where a hepatobiliary or pancreatic etiology is suspected. LFT is deranged in acute viral hepatitis, AFLP, or sometimes in cholecystitis. In AFLP, serum bilirubin is generally in the range of 2–10 mg/dL and liver enzymes are <1,000 IU/mL, while in viral hepatitis, bilirubin levels are higher (10–30 mg/dL) and enzymes are markedly raised to more than 1,000 IU/mL. Kidney function tests (KFTs) are important in woman with pyelonephritis or sepsis and also as a baseline if the patient is to be started on aminoglycosides.

Random blood sugar should be ordered to rule out diabetes mellitus. It is low in woman with acute fatty liver of pregnancy (AFLP).

Urine Examination

Urinalysis is required to rule out urinary tract infection (UTI) and severe renal disease. Other laboratory tests should be individualized according to the specific clinical situation.

Radiological

Conventional radiography, USG, and CT scan, all can be used for evaluating pregnant women.

X-rays

Plain flat and upright abdominal films can detect free air under the diaphragm, denoting a ruptured viscus.[8] The intestinal gas pattern can show the presence or absence of obstruction. When pulmonary or thoracic disease is suspected, chest films can be obtained with abdominal shielding.

Ultrasonography and Color Doppler

Perhaps the most useful and safest imaging technique that can be used during pregnancy is USG. This is very useful in the diagnosis of gallstones or subcapsular hemorrhage (Figs. 1A and B). This technique allows the kidneys and ureters to be imaged quite clearly. Fluid collection in the abdominal wall or abdominal cavity such as abscess, hematoma, and hemoperitoneum can be readily identified (Figs. 2A and B). In patients with antepartum hemorrhage, USG can detect any retroplacental collection and localize the placenta (Figs. 3A and B). Presence of any fibroid or adnexal mass can also be diagnosed on ultrasound (Fig. 4). The use of USG is also essential for fetal evaluation. USG helps to establish gestational age and fetal viability, excludes congenital anomalies, and assesses amniotic fluid volume and fetal well-being. This information may become critical later in the management of a gravid patient with an acute abdomen, when decisions regarding timing and mode of delivery and the use of tocolytics and steroids are to be made. The character of adnexal masses (cystic or solid) can be determined. Color Doppler may help to diagnose adnexal torsion by demonstrating absent ovarian flow in the central ovarian parenchyma.[2]

Computed Tomography

Computed tomography is the most sensitive and specific modality for the investigation

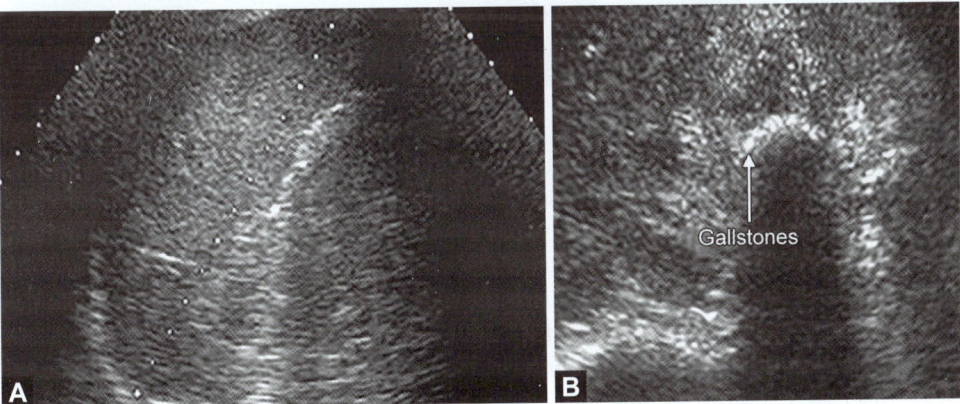

Figs. 1A and B: Ultrasonography. (A) Subscapular hematoma of liver; (B) cholelithiasis or gallstones.

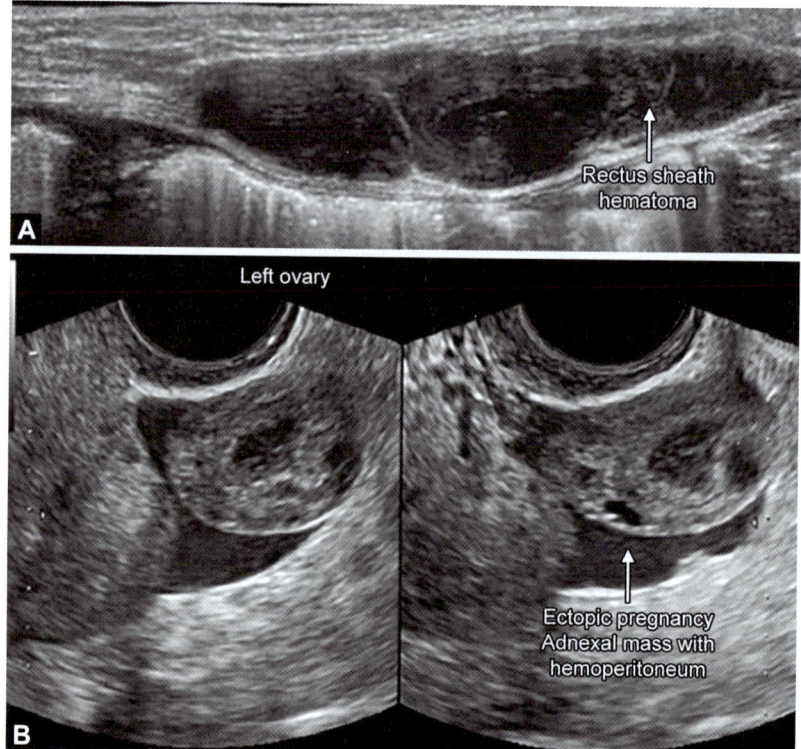

Figs. 2A and B: Ultrasonography. (A) Rectus sheath hematoma; (B) Hemoperitoneum.

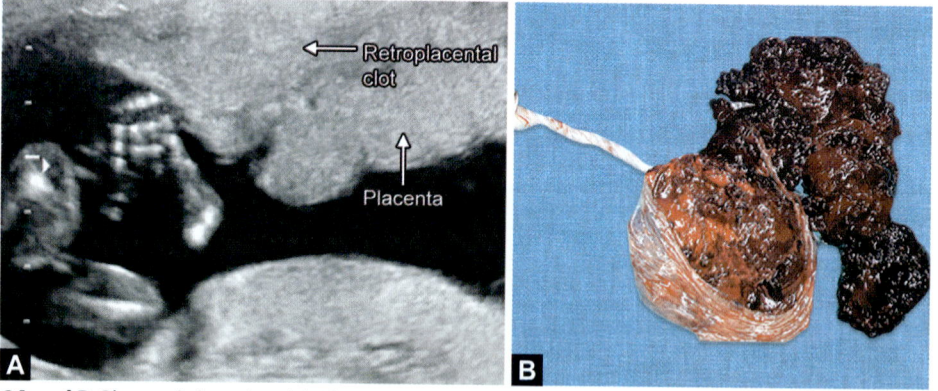

Figs. 3A and B: Placental abruption. (A) Ultrasonography placental abruption; (B) Placental specimen with retroplacental clots.

of abdominal pain but exposes the fetus and mother to ionizing radiations, which must be discussed. The usual fetal radiation dose for a routine CT of the abdomen and pelvis is around 25 mGy, which can be reduced to about 13 mGy with the use of automated exposure control facility in modern CT scanners.

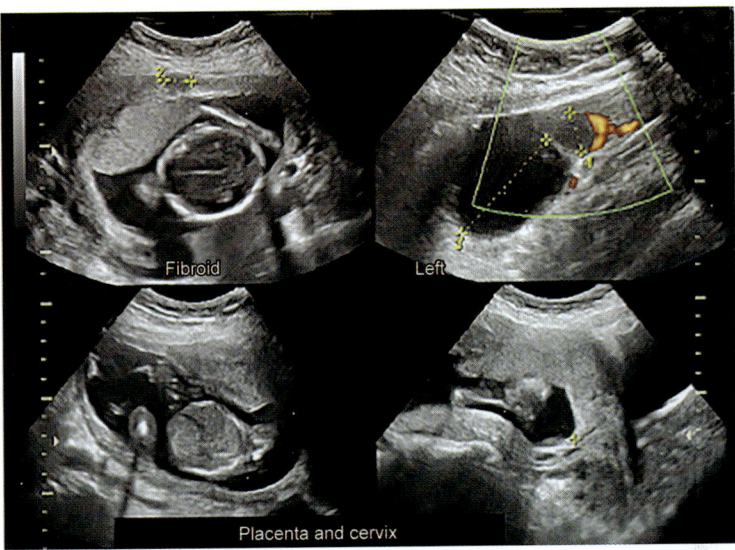

Fig. 4: Ultrasonography—pregnancy with fibroids.

Magnetic Resonance Imaging

Magnetic resonance imaging (MRI) is preferable to CT during pregnancy as it provides excellent soft-tissue imaging without the risk of ionizing radiation. MRI at 1.5 T or less has been shown to be safe in all trimesters of pregnancy. Pregnant women should, therefore, be imaged at 1.5 T or less. The safety of MRI at 3 T for pregnant women has not yet been proven.[9] Rapid-sequence MRI is preferable to conventional MRI. The possibility of adverse effects to the fetus due to the acoustic noise has not been established.

Endoscopy

Endoscopy can be done safely in pregnancy for diagnosing inflammatory bowel disease or peptic ulcer.

Others

If sickling crisis is suspected, hemoglobin (Hb) electrophoresis should be done to detect HbS to confirm the diagnosis of sickle cell anemia. Increased urinary levels of porphobilinogen and δ-aminolevulinic acid are diagnostic for acute intermittent porphyria.[4]

MANAGEMENT

The initial goal of management is to identify patients having a life-threatening or serious condition requiring urgent intervention. These include women presenting with moderate-to-severe pain with vomiting, fever, history of trauma, bleeding per vaginum, new-onset hypertension, or in shock.

The definitive management is directed according to the final diagnosis.

There are some red flag clinical indicators which prompt evaluation by an experienced clinician (Box 1). These need to be identified and appropriately addressed.

Box 1: Clinical red flags.
• Readmission or multiple admissions for abdominal pain • Repeated doses of analgesics without a cause for pain being established • New-onset anxiety and confusion being attributed to a psychiatric cause rather than underlying (undiagnosed) organic disease

KEY POINTS

- Abdominal pain in pregnancy is a common complaint with diverse obstetric, gynecologic, surgical, medical, and psychiatric causes.
- A clear understanding of the anatomical and physiological changes in pregnancy along with a careful history and methodical examination aided by selective investigations will usually reveal the cause of pain in most cases.
- Numerous physiological changes that occur in pregnancy may affect the presentation of abdominal pain in pregnancy.
- Nonionizing investigations are preferred as the first line of radiological investigation. However, investigations using ionizing radiations, such as X-ray and CT scan, are generally safe and should not be withheld if there is a definite clinical indication and there is no other alternative, especially in life-threatening conditions.
- Diagnosis of some conditions such as appendicitis can be delayed or missed during pregnancy; a high index of suspicion with knowledge of the ways in which different pathologic conditions present in pregnancy is needed.
- Because of the complexities involved in evaluating both mother and fetus, and the potential for severe complications associated with delay in diagnosis and treatment, a multidisciplinary approach is indispensable for timely diagnosis and treatment of these patients.

REFERENCES

1. Kilpatrick CC, Monga M. Approach to acute abdomen in pregnancy. Obstet Gynecol Clin North Am. 2007;34(3):389-402.
2. Boothby R. Acute abdominal pain in pregnancy. In: Benrubi GI (Ed). Obstetric and Gynecologic Emergencies. Philadelphia: Lippincott company; 1994.
3. Rubin S. Acute abdominal pain in pregnancy. In: Benrubi GI (Ed). Obstetric Emergencies. New York: Churchill Livingstone; 1990.
4. Ratnapalan S, Bona N, Chandra K, Koren G. Physicians' perceptions of teratogenic risk associated with radiography and CT during early pregnancy. AJR Am J Roentgenol. 2004;182(5):1107-9.
5. Mahomed K. Abdominal Pain. In: James D, Steer PJ, Weiner CP (Eds). High Risk Pregnancy: Management Options, 4th edition. St Louis, Missouri: Reed Elsevier India; 2011. pp. 13-26.
6. Woodhead N, Nkwam O, Caddick V, Morad S, Mylvaganam S. Surgical causes of acute abdominal pain in pregnancy. The Obstetrician & Gynaecologist. 2019;21:27-35.
7. Woodfield CA, Lazarus E, Chen KC, Mayo-Smith WW. Abdominal pain in pregnancy: diagnoses and imaging unique to pregnancy—review. AJR Am J Roentgenol. 2010; 194(6 Suppl): S42-5.
8. Devarajan S, Chandraharan E. Abdominal pain in pregnancy: a rational approach to management. Obstetrics, Gynaecology & Reproductive Medicine. 2011;21(7):198-206.
9. Zachariah SK, Fenn M, Jacob K, Arthungal SA, Zachariah SA. Management of acute abdomen in pregnancy: current perspectives. International Journal of Women's Health 2019;11:119-134.

SUGGESTED READING

1. Committee on Obstetric Practice. Committee Opinion No. 723: Guidelines for diagnostic imaging during pregnancy. Obstet Gynecol. 2017;130(4):e210-6.

Approach to a Pregnant Woman Presenting with Discharge Per Vaginum

Sharda Patra

INTRODUCTION

Vaginal discharge is a common problem for which a pregnant woman often seeks medical advice. Vaginal discharge can be physiological or pathological. It is usually physiological, when it occurs during pregnancy (Fig. 1) due to increased vascularity and hormonal influence which increases the vaginal transudate resulting in excessive discharge. Vagina harbors both aerobic and anaerobic organisms in close symbiosis in women who are in the reproductive age group. The acidic environment in the vagina due to presence of lactobacilli suppresses the growth of pathogenic organisms. However, when this acidic environment is disturbed, there is overgrowth of local flora resulting in infection and discharge per vaginum. However, any discharge that is watery, wets the underclothes of the pregnant women, or is associated with symptoms such as itching or foul smell is pathological and should be evaluated. Most often, watery discharge is due to preterm or term premature rupture of membranes (PPROM or PROM) before the onset of labor. However, the vaginal discharge could also be a manifestation of conditions such as vaginitis due to infective causes or sometimes stress urinary incontinence. The most common cause of abnormal vaginal discharge in pregnancy is candidiasis. However, trichomoniasis and bacterial vaginosis are other common causes.[1,2]

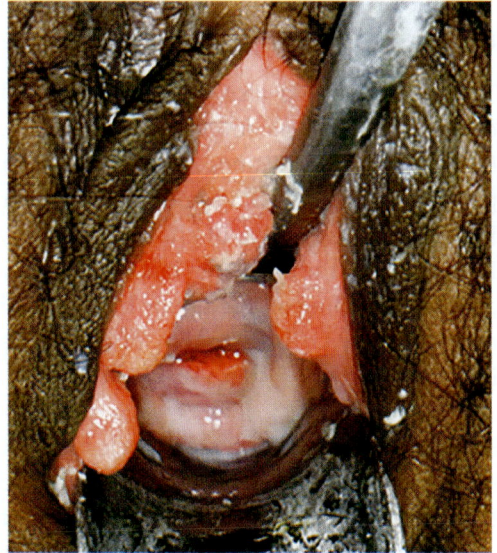

Fig. 1: Normal vaginal discharge of pregnancy.

DIFFERENTIAL DIAGNOSIS

The differential diagnosis of vaginal discharge in pregnancy is listed in Table 1.

Nonpregnant women with vaginal discharge are often treated empirically with a syndromic approach without being fully investigated. However, in pregnancy, it is important to make a definite diagnosis and institute appropriate management. A careful history and detailed examination backed up with relevant laboratory tests help to reach a definitive diagnosis.

Table 1: Causes of vaginal discharge in pregnancy.[1,2]

Infective (nonsexually transmitted)	Infective (sexually transmitted)	Noninfective
• Bacterial vaginosis • Candidiasis	*Infection with*: • *Trichomonas vaginalis* • *Chlamydia trachomatis* • *Neisseria gonorrhoeae*	• Preterm or term premature rupture of membranes (PROM) • Urinary incontinence, stress urinary incontinence (SUI), fistula • Cervical polyps and erosion • Genital tract malignancy • Foreign bodies (e.g. tampons and condoms)

HISTORY

Onset and Duration of Complaint

One must enquire about the onset of discharge, whether it was sudden or insidious. Woman with PPROM and PROM present with sudden gush of fluid wetting her undergarments and thighs. In such cases the discharge is thin, watery, copious in amount, and odorless.

If the vaginal discharge is thin, watery, odorless, starting insidiously and is intermittent, the possibility of high rupture of membranes with slow leak should be kept in mind.

Whenever the duration of the symptom is long with gradual onset, one must ask the woman if the discharge is related to an increase in intra-abdominal pressure such as coughing or sneezing, stress urinary incontinence is suspected.

Character of Discharge

The character of the discharge should also be asked. Is the discharge mucoid in nature and nonirritating, colorless or white? Whether it is odorless or has mild odor or is foul smelling? Mucoid, odorless discharge is usually physiological. In case the discharge is associated with pruritus and irritation, possibility of an infectious cause like candidiasis and/or trichomoniasis should be suspected. In trichomoniasis, the discharge is characteristically profuse, thin, greenish in color, and is associated with itching. If the discharge is thick, curdy white, appears like cottage cheese, and associated with itching, *Candida* infection is suspected. Excessive, watery thin, gray or white discharge with a fishy or foul odor is characteristic of bacterial vaginosis.[3] This fishy odor increases after sexual intercourse. Uriniferous odor is present in women with urinary incontinence.

Associated Complaints

The history should also include associated complaints such as fever and/or malaise. Fever indicates infection, if associated with prolonged leaking per vaginum (PPROM or PROM) it is suggestive of chorioamnionitis. In such cases, the discharge is usually scanty and foul smelling as the liquor has drained and is infected. The duration of leaking is important.

Presence of risk factors such as polyhydramnios or multiple pregnancies should be asked for in women with discharge due to rupture of membranes. Any history of cervical cerclage in the current pregnancy is also a risk factor for PPROM.[4]

Obstetrical History

Obstetrical history includes previous history of giving birth to big babies, hydramnios, or deranged sugars suggestive of diabetes mellitus which is associated with *Candida* infection.

Past History

Past history including any history of diabetes mellitus or any other chronic illness and intake of broad-spectrum antibiotics or steroids, which predispose to vaginal candidiasis, is elicited. Any past history of PPROM or preterm birth is important as both can give rise to PPROM in subsequent pregnancies. A history of pelvic infection or urinary tract infection (UTI) in the past points toward the likelihood of vaginitis, cervicitis, or UTI as a cause of discharge or leaking per vaginum due to PROM or PPROM.

EXAMINATION

While examining the patient, her general condition should be assessed. Woman might appear uncomfortable due to prolonged discharge, wetting of underclothes and due to itching in the vulvovaginal area. She may appear toxic, if chorioamnionitis has set in. In such cases, woman may have high-grade fever and tachycardia.

Obstetrical examination should be done to assess the fundal height. In PROM, the fundal height is less than the period of gestation, consequent to drainage of liquor. However, this finding may not be appreciable in multiple pregnancies and polyhydramnios. However, if the discharge is due to vaginitis or cervicitis, the height of uterus corresponds to the period of gestation.

On palpation, the uterus may feel tense or tender in case of chorioamnionitis. The lie, presentation, and fetal heart should be examined. The fetal heart rate (FHR) may be increased in women with chorioamnionitis. In case of PROM, the liquor appears reduced on palpation.

Genital Examination

Local examination of external genitalia is done to see the vulva for any moistness, fluid discharge, redness, and excoriation marks.

Per Speculum Examination

The vagina and cervix are inspected with a speculum. Look for the presence of any discharge, foreign body (tampons and condoms), cervical polyp, cervical erosion, or any other lesions in the vagina or on the cervix. In case of PROM, clear fluid can be observed escaping through the external os of cervix (Fig. 2). In case there is no fluid seen escaping, the woman can be asked to either cough or do Valsalva maneuver and observed for escape of fluid through cervical os. Woman

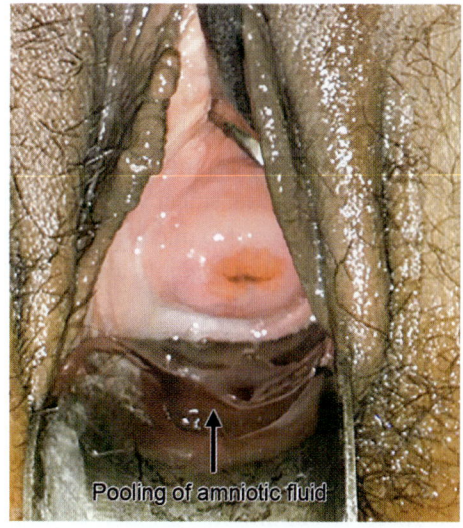

Fig. 2: Demonstration of leaking on speculum examination.

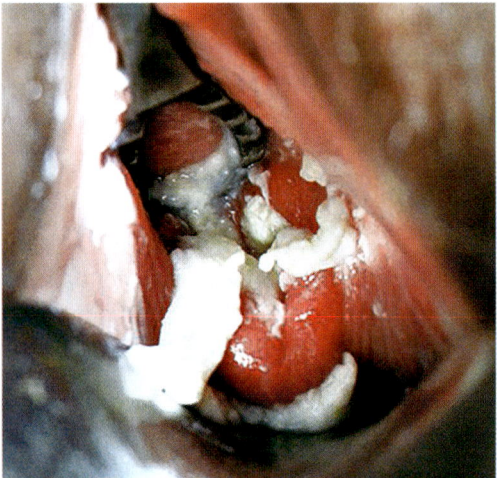

Fig. 3: Thick curdy white clumpy discharge in candidiasis.

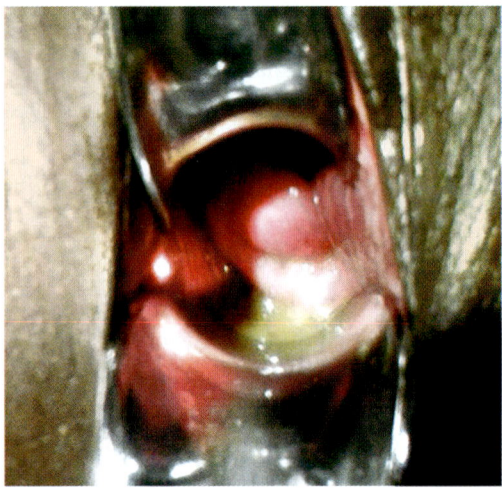

Fig. 4: White, yellow, or green frothy discharge with erythema of cervix and vagina in trichomoniasis.

can be observed for any escape of urine from urethral opening at the same time.

The discharge is observed for its color, consistency, amount, and odor. Thick, clumpy, curdy white discharge adherent to the vaginal walls with erythema and edema of vagina and vulva indicates candidiasis (Fig. 3), whereas an off white or yellow, frothy discharge with erythema of vagina and cervix (strawberry cervix) is characteristic of trichomoniasis (Fig. 4). Creamy white or gray, thin, copious discharge with a fishy odor is likely to be bacterial vaginosis (Fig. 5). It is important to collect the discharge, prepare a wet smear with saline and 10% KOH, and subject it to microscopic examination for *Trichomonas vaginalis* and *Candida albicans*.

A mucopurulent discharge from the cervix points toward chlamydial/gonococcal infection. Ammonia-like odor may be observed if the discharge is urine as in women with urinary incontinence or urinary fistula. In case there is continuous urinary dribbling in the absence of straining, then one should look for any fistulous opening.

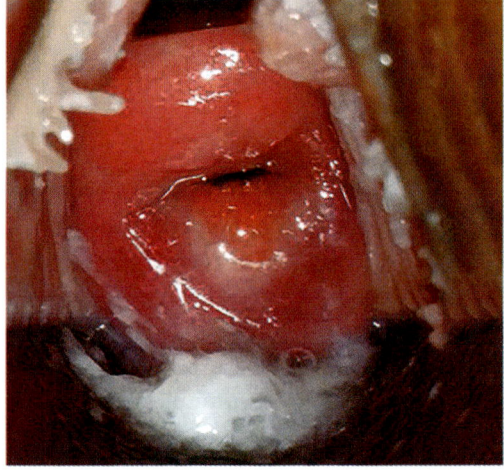

Fig. 5: Copious grayish white discharge in bacterial vaginosis.

INVESTIGATIONS

The various investigations, which are useful for confirmation of the cause of vaginal discharge are:[3-5]

- pH of discharge
- Wet mount
- Whiff test
- Gram stain

Table 2: Differential diagnosis of vaginal discharge in pregnancy based on clinical characteristics.

Clinical characteristic	Premature rupture of membranes (PROM)	Candidiasis	Bacterial vaginosis	Trichomoniasis
Signs and symptoms	Sudden escape of watery fluid from vagina	Scanty, thick, white, odorless (cottage cheese) discharge with severe itching	Excessive, thin, gray/white discharge with a fishy/foul odor	Copious, malodorous, thin, frothy greenish discharge associated with itching and vaginal irritation
Physical examination	Direct visualization of escape of watery fluid from the cervix	Inflammation of the vulva and vagina, thick, white curdy discharge that adheres to vaginal walls	Creamy white or gray, thin, copious discharge with a fishy odor	Off white or yellow, frothy discharge with erythema of vagina and cervix (strawberry cervix)

- High vaginal swab for presence of any pathogenic organism and culture sensitivity

For suspected cases of PROM, although per speculum examination clinches the diagnosis, sometimes in doubtful cases, especially some bedside tests can be done to confirm the diagnosis, namely pH of discharge, nitrazine test, and fern test (Table 2).

An algorithmic workup of a pregnant woman with discharge per vaginum is given in Flowchart 1.

pH of Discharge

The vaginal pH in pregnancy is acidic and ranges from 3.8 to 4.2. However, the pH of amniotic fluid is alkaline ranging from 7.0 to 7.7. A pH > 6.5 is diagnostic of leaking of amniotic fluid due to ruptured membranes.

Determination of pH of the Discharge

In bacterial vaginosis and trichomoniasis, the pH of the discharge is >4.5 whereas in candidiasis, it remains unchanged.

Wet Smear Preparation

For this, a drop of vaginal discharge is placed on a glass slide along with a drop of normal saline and covered with a cover slip. The slide is seen under microscope first under low power and then high power. Look for leukocytes, clue cells, motile flagellated trichomonads, lactobacilli, and yeast cells. In normal wet mount, one sees epithelial cells and lactobacilli (Fig. 6).

Whiff Test/KOH Slide

One drop of vaginal discharge is placed on a glass slide along with a drop of 10% KOH solution and it is covered with a cover slip. A fishy amine odor is characteristic of bacterial vaginosis and referred as a positive Whiff test. When the KOH preparation is seen under the microscope, presence of pseudohyphae, budding yeast indicates candidiasis (Table 3).

Gram Stain of Vaginal Discharge

Normally, it shows gram-positive lactobacilli in the vaginal discharge (*see* Fig. 6). Based on the Gram's stain various criteria such as Nugent's, Hay and Ison's, Spiegel's, Amsel's, are there to diagnose bacterial vaginosis (Box 1 and Table 4).[6-9]

Other Tests

Nitrazine Test

In nitrazine test, paper impregnated with nitrazine is soaked with vaginal fluid and

Section 1: Obstetrics

Flowchart 1: Algorithm for workup of a pregnant woman with discharge per vaginum.

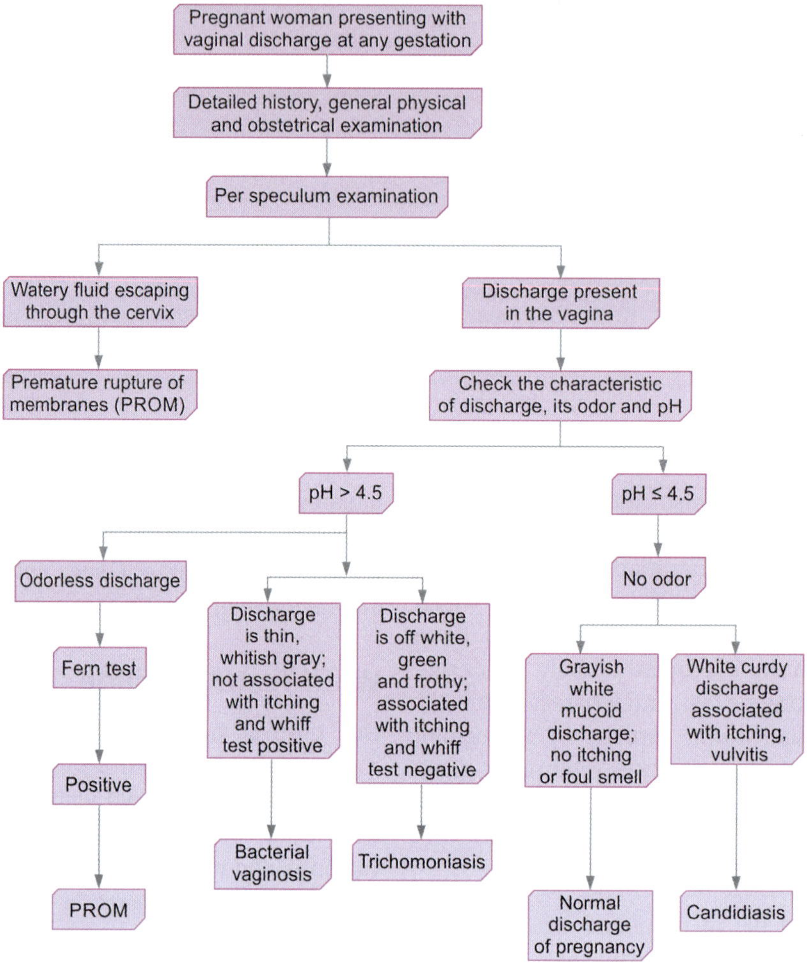

```
Pregnant woman presenting with
vaginal discharge at any gestation
             │
             ▼
Detailed history, general physical
and obstetrical examination
             │
             ▼
   Per speculum examination
         ┌───┴───┐
         ▼       ▼
Watery fluid     Discharge present
escaping through in the vagina
the cervix            │
    │                 ▼
    ▼         Check the characteristic
Premature     of discharge, its odor and pH
rupture of         ┌──────┴──────┐
membranes          ▼             ▼
(PROM)          pH > 4.5      pH ≤ 4.5
```

- **pH > 4.5** branch:
  - Odorless discharge → Fern test → Positive → PROM
  - Discharge is thin, whitish gray; not associated with itching and whiff test positive → Bacterial vaginosis
  - Discharge is off white, green and frothy; associated with itching and whiff test negative → Trichomoniasis

- **pH ≤ 4.5** branch (No odor):
  - Grayish white mucoid discharge; no itching or foul smell → Normal discharge of pregnancy
  - White curdy discharge associated with itching, vulvitis → Candidiasis

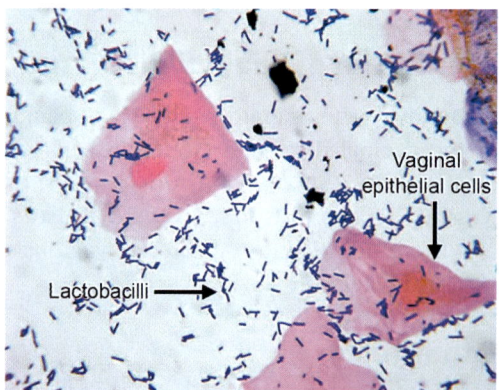

Fig. 6: Gram-stained normal smear showing lactobacilli.

compared with standard color chart. Nitrazine test is positive when a yellow nitrazine paper turns blue on contact with amniotic fluid. The test can be false positive when there is coexistent blood, semen, or bacterial vaginosis and false-negative, if discharge is scanty.

Fern Test

The fern test is based on the principle of crystallization of amniotic fluid to form a fern-like pattern due to relatively high concentration of sodium chloride in it. Few drops of fluid are collected from the posterior

Chapter 6: Approach to a Pregnant Woman Presenting with Discharge Per Vaginum

Table 3: Differential diagnosis of vaginal discharge in pregnancy based on laboratory tests.				
Investigation	PROM	Candidiasis	Trichomoniasis	Bacterial vaginosis
Vaginal pH	Elevated (7–7.3)	Normal (≤ 4.5) 4.0–4.5	Elevated (> 4.5) 5.0–6.0	Elevated (> 4.5)
Nitrazine test	Positive	Negative	Negative	Positive
Wet smear	Ferning	• Budding yeast cells • Pseudohyphae (Fig. 7)	• Motile flagellated protozoa • Many WBCs	• Clue cells (vaginal epithelial cells with obscured margins due to adherent bacteria) • Few lactobacilli • Occasional motile, curved rods
Whiff test/KOH	Negative	Negative	Positive	Positive
Gram stain		• Budding yeast cells • Pseudohyphae Many WBCs (Fig. 8)	• Flagellated protozoa • Many WBCs (Fig. 9)	• Clue cells • Decreased lactobacilli • Predominant gram-negative curved bacilli and coccobacilli (Fig. 10)

(PROM: premature rupture of membrane; WBCs: white blood cells)

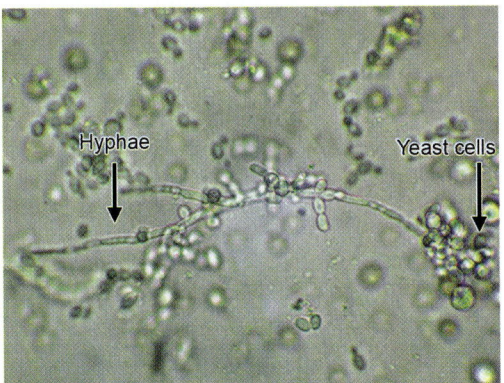

Fig. 7: Wet smear *Candida*.

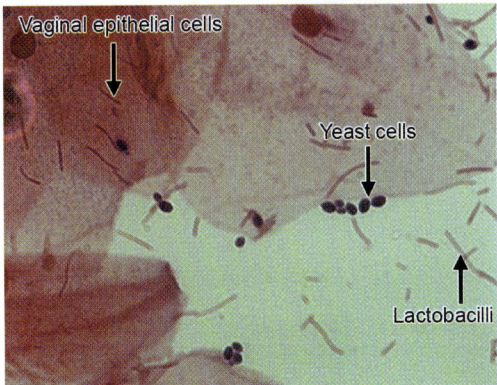

Fig. 8: Gram stain candidiasis.

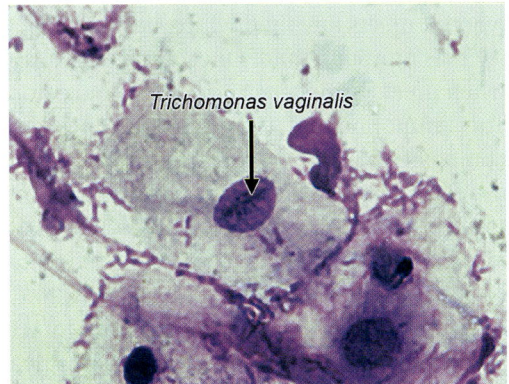

Fig. 9: Gram stain trichomoniasis.

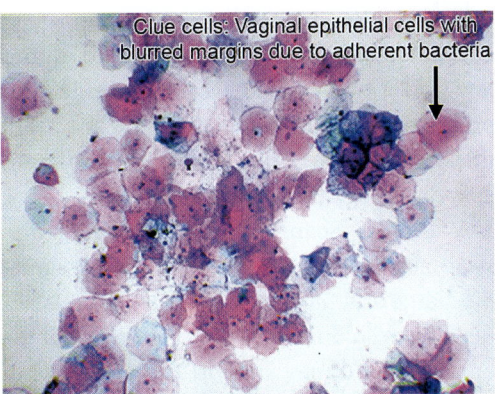

Fig. 10: Gram stain bacterial vaginosis; absence of lactobacilli.

> **Box 1:** Diagnosis of bacterial vaginosis (Amsel's criteria).[9]
> - White discharge
> - pH >4.5
> - *Positive whiff test*: Fishy odor with addition of 10% KOH to discharge
> - Presence of clue cells

Note: Three out of the four features are conclusive of bacterial vaginosis.

Table 4: Diagnosis of bacterial vaginosis (Nugent's criteria).[6]

Types of bacterial morphotypes scored	Average number of each morphotype per oil immersion field under microscope	Interpretation: Total score—sum of A, B, and C
A. *Lactobacillus acidophilus* (0–4) B. *Gardnerella vaginalis* and *Bacteroides* species (0–4) C. *Mobiluncus* species (0–2)	Scoring for each of the bacterial morphotypes except lactobacilli is: 0 = No morphotypes 1 = 0–1 morphotypes 2 = 1–4 morphotypes 3 = 5–30 morphotypes 4 = > 30 morphotypes Lactobacillus 0 = 4+ 1 = 3+ 2 = 2+ 3 = 1+ 0 = 0	• 0–3: Normal flora • 4–6: Indeterminate flora • 7 or higher is diagnostic of bacterial vaginosis

vaginal fornix and spread on a clean glass slide. It is air dried and examined under low-power microscope. Dried amniotic fluid produces a delicate fern pattern in contrast to thick and wide arborization fern pattern from a well-estrogenized cervical mucus (Figs. 11A and B). Scanty amniotic fluid on the swab and heavy contamination with vaginal discharge and blood, all can result in a false-negative result. Presence of oligohydramnios on ultrasound may support the diagnosis of PROM in woman with prolonged leaking per vaginum.

Indigo Carmine Test

In this diluted indigo carmine (1 mL in 9 mL of sterile saline) is instilled into the amniotic cavity under ultrasound guidance. A tampon is placed in the vagina. Blue staining of tampon after 1½ hours of instillation of dye indicates rupture of membranes.

Newer Tests

Tests based on detection of amniotic fluid proteomic markers such as placental α1-microglobulin,[5] insulin-like growth factor binding protein, placental protein 12 (PP12), and alpha-fetoprotein (AFP) are commercially available. These are highly sensitive and indicated as supplementary to the standard methods of diagnosis namely sterile speculum examination, pH test, and Fern test.

Noninvasive Absorbent Pad[10]

It is a new evidence-based test which is as accurate as standard methods of diagnosis. It is indicated in pregnant women with unexplained vaginal wetness and those with small leaks at frequent intervals difficult to be detected clinically. It uses a pH-dependent color changing strip on an absorbent pad that changes color from yellow to blue or green when it meets any fluid which has a pH >6.5 such as amniotic fluid. Once dried, this strip when meets urine reverts to its original color. The ammonium in the urine detaches the conjugate-based nitrazine molecules, hence the color reverts. Each pad can be worn for up to 12 hours and can detect as little as 2 drops of amniotic fluid. The sensitivity and specificity of pad test is 100% and between 65–90%, respectively. A negative result indicates intact membranes in 99% of cases and a positive result suggests a 70% chance of ruptured membranes hence requires confirmation.

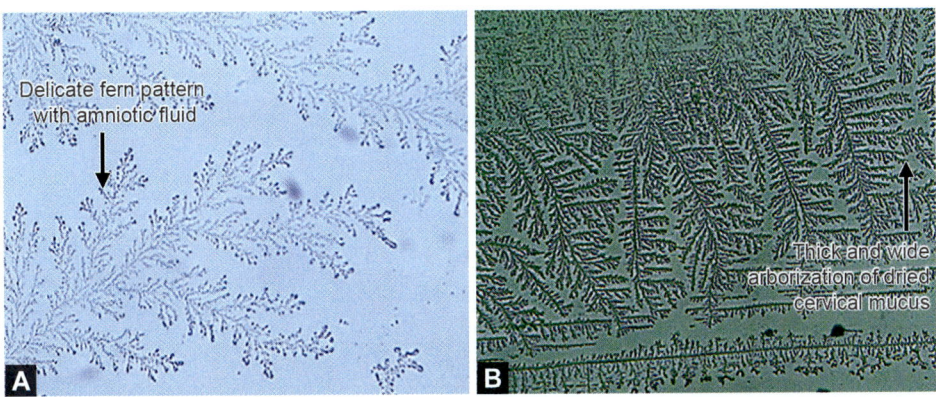

Figs. 11A and B: Fern test. (A) Fern pattern with amniotic fluid; (B) Fern pattern with cervical mucus.

All these tests are approved by the Food and Drug Administration (FDA); however, the management of women with rupture membranes should be solely based on clinical and other findings such as concomitant documentation of decreased liquor amnii on USG as the false-positive rates of these tests are high.

MANAGEMENT OF VAGINAL DISCHARGE IN PREGNANCY

Management depends on the cause of vaginal discharge.

The drug treatment of vaginal candidiasis, BV, and TV during pregnancy is described in Table 5.

The management of pregnant women with leaking per vaginum depends upon the gestational age and fetomaternal condition. Flowchart 2 outlines the management.

KEY POINTS

- The diagnostic approach to a pregnant woman with vaginal discharge should include a careful history, examination and laboratory tests.
- Most common cause of vaginal discharge in pregnancy is premature rupture of membrane (PROM), which is characterized by a sudden gush of watery fluid from vagina.
- Among the infective causes, candidiasis is the most common cause of abnormal discharge in pregnancy.
- Drugs prescribed for vaginal infections should be safe in pregnancy.
- The initial management of a woman presenting with suspected PROM should focus on confirming the diagnosis,

Table 5: Drug treatment of vaginal candidiasis, bacterial vaginosis (BV), and trichomonal vaginosis (TV) during pregnancy.[11]

Infection	First trimester
Candidiasis	• Topical clotrimazole vaginal pessary (100 mg) × 6 days or (200 mg) × 3 days or 500 mg stat • Oral fluconazole is avoided in pregnancy
Trichomoniasis	• Both oral and topical therapies can be used but oral more effective • Metronidazole 500 mg twice a day for 7 days or 2 g stat dose • Both partners to be treated
Bacterial vaginosis	• Oral or topical therapy • Metronidazole 500 mg twice a day for 7 days • Clindamycin 300 mg twice a day for 7 days

Section 1: Obstetrics

Flowchart 2: Management of PROM in pregnancy.

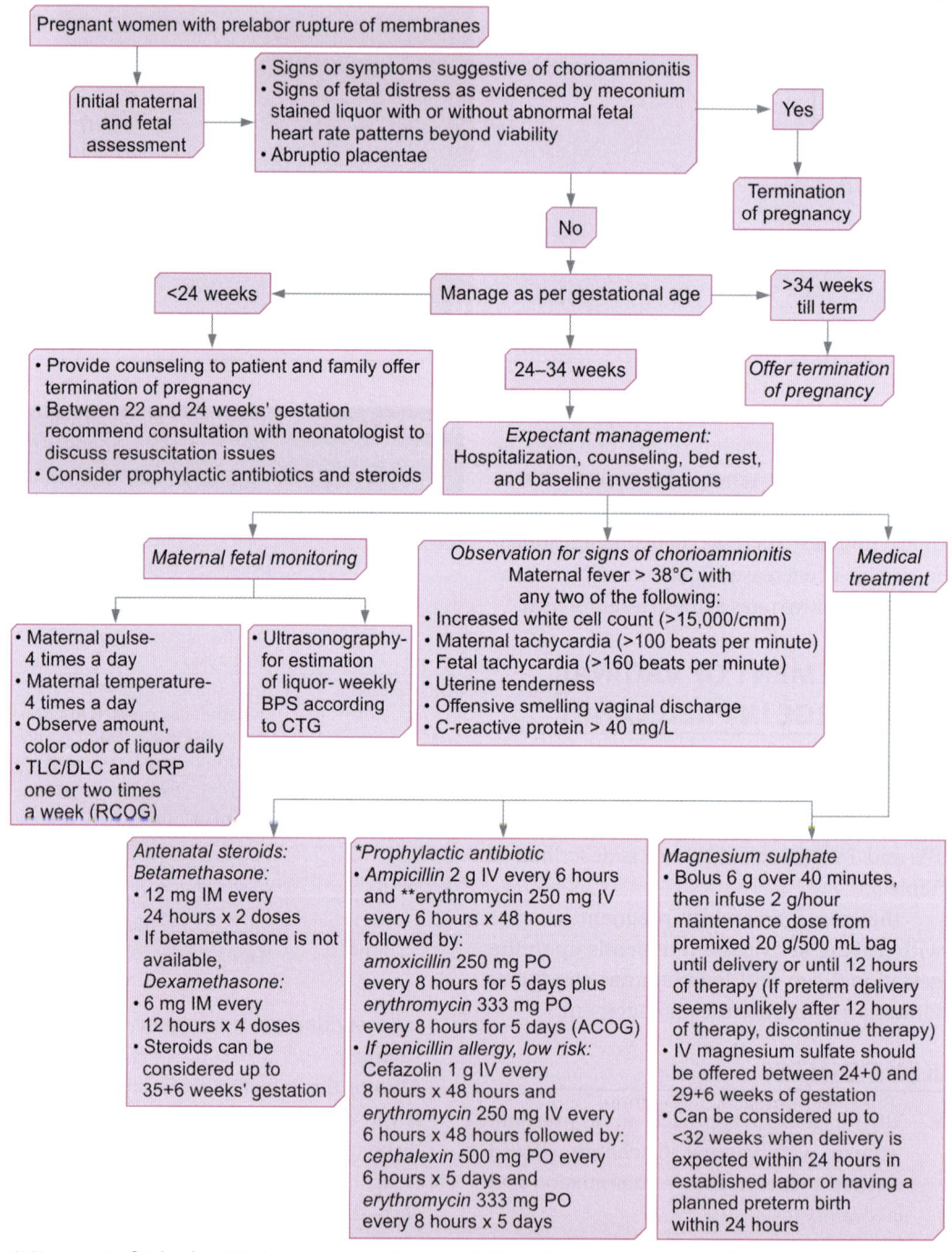

(AFI: amniotic fluid index; BPS: biophysical profile score; CTG: cardiotocography; DLC: differential leukocyte count; IM: intramuscular; IV: intravenous; PO: per oral; TLC: total leukocyte count)
*Alternate regime: Erythromycin 250 mg 4 times a day orally for 10 days or till woman goes in labor.
**IV and oral Erythromycin may be replaced by tab Azithromycin 1 gm orally at admission.

documenting correct gestational age, assessing fetal well-being, and deciding on the plan of management.
- Management options in preterm PROM between 24–37 weeks include admission to hospital, fetomaternal monitoring, administration of antenatal corticosteroids, and broad-spectrum antibiotics, if indicated.
- Traditionally, in the absence of fetal or maternal compromise, delivery should be accomplished after completing 34 weeks.
- Women with preterm PROM before 32 weeks of gestation who are thought to be at risk of imminent delivery should be considered for intravenous magnesium sulfate for fetal neuroprotection.
- Digital vaginal examinations should be avoided with PROM, unless the patient in labor or induction of labor is planned.

REFERENCES

1. Puri KJ, Madan A, Bajal K. Evaluation of causes of vaginal discharge in relation to pregnancy status. Indian J Dermatol Venereol Leprol. 2003;69(3):129-30.
2. Levett PN. Etiology of vaginal infections in pregnant and non-pregnant women in Barbados. West Indian Med J. 1995;44(3):96-8.
3. Anderson B, Gaitanis M. Non-viral infectious disease in pregnancy. In: de Swiet M, Powrie R, Greene M, Camann W (Eds). Medical Disorders in Obstetric Practice, 5th edition. Oxford: Blackwell Science; 2010. pp. 405-29.
4. Patra S. Premature rupture of membranes. In: Trivedi SS, Puri M, Aggarwal S (Eds). Management of High Risk Pregnancy: A Practical Approach, 2nd edition. New Delhi: Jaypee Brothers Medical Publishers (P) Ltd.; 2016. pp. 63-74.
5. Caughey AB, Robinson JN, Norwitz ER. Contemporary diagnosis and management of preterm premature rupture of membranes. Rev Obstet Gynecol. 2008;1(1):11-22.
6. Nugent RP, Krohn MA, Hillier SL. Reliability of diagnosing bacterial vaginosis is improved by a standardized method of Gram stain interpretation. J Clin Microbiol. 1991;29:297-301.
7. Spiegel CA, Amsel R, Holmes KK. Diagnosis of bacterial vaginosis by direct Gram stain of vaginal fluid. J Clin Microbiol. 1983;18:170-7.
8. Ison CA, Hay PE. Validation of a simplified grading of Gram stained vaginal smears for use in genitourinary medicine clinics. Sex Transm Infect. 2002;78:413-5.
9. Amsel R, Totten PA, Spiegel CA, Chen KC, Eschenbach D, Holmes KK. Nonspecific vaginitis diagnostic criteria and microbial and epidemiologic associations. Am J Med. 1983;74:14-22.
10. Mulhair L, Carter J, Poston L, Seed P, Briley A. Prospective cohort study investigating the reliability of the AmnioSens method for detection of spontaneous rupture of membranes. BJOG. 2009;116:313-8.
11. Workowski KA, Bolan GA. Centers for Disease Control and Prevention sexually transmitted diseases treatment guidelines, 2015. MMWR Recomm Rep. 2015;64(RR-03):1.

SUGGESTED READING

1. American Congress of Obstetricians and Gynecologists (ACOG) Committee on Practice Bulletins-Obstetrics. ACOG Practice Bulletin No. 188: Prelabor Rupture of Membranes. Clinical Management Guidelines for Obstetrician-Gynecologists. Updated 2018. Obstet Gynecol. 2018;131(1): e1-14.
2. Department of AIDS Control, Ministry of Health and Family Welfare, Government of India. (2014) National guidelines on prevention, management and control of reproductive tract infections and sexually transmitted infections. [online] Available from http://naco.gov.in/sites/default/files/National%20RTI%20STI%20technical%20guidelines%20Sep2014_0.pdf. [Last accessed January, 2020].
3. Paladine HL, Desai UA. Vaginitis: Diagnosis and treatment. Am Fam Physician. 2018;97(5): 321-9.
4. Royal College of Obstetricians and Gynaecologists. Care of women presenting with suspected preterm prelabour rupture of membranes from 24 + 0 weeks of gestation. BJOG. 2019;126:e152-66.

7

Approach to a Pregnant Woman Presenting with Vomiting

Puneet K Kochhar

INTRODUCTION

Nausea and vomiting accompany about 50–90% of all pregnancies.[1] The symptoms usually start at 5 weeks of gestation, peak at 9 weeks, and subside by 16–18 weeks of gestation. However, symptoms may continue till the third trimester in 15–20% and till delivery in 5%.[2] Majority 60% are asymptomatic within 6 weeks from onset of nausea.[2] If nausea and vomiting of pregnancy (NVP) or emesis gravidarum does not affect the routine day-to-day activity of the pregnant woman, it is of no pathological significance and is commonly known as morning sickness. The symptoms may occur at any time of day and often persist throughout the day. In 0.3–2%, it is severe and is known as hyperemesis gravidarum (HG).[3]

Although there is no clear demarcation between nausea and vomiting during pregnancy and HG, the latter is typically characterized by protracted vomiting leading to dehydration, dyselectrolytemia, nutritional deficiency, weight loss of >5% of the prepregnancy body weight and ketonuria unrelated to other causes and often leading to hospitalization.[4] Vomiting persisting even after delivery should be investigated for other causes (Flowchart 1).

DIFFERENTIAL DIAGNOSIS

Nausea and vomiting of pregnancy is diagnosed based on the history of onset in

Flowchart 1: Algorithm for clinical approach to a pregnant woman presenting with vomiting.

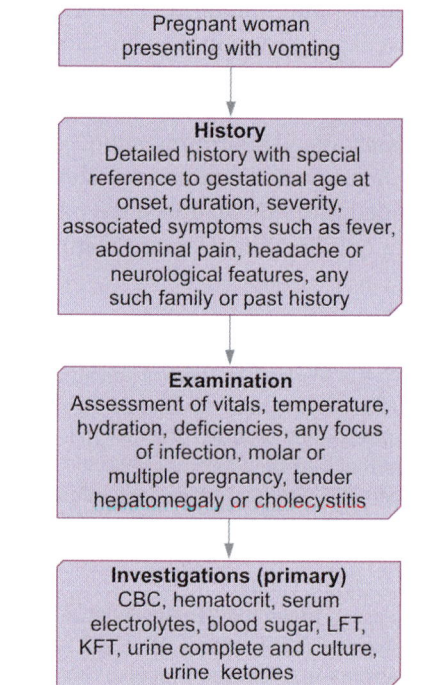

(CBC: complete blood count; KFT: kidney function test; LFT: liver function test).

early pregnancy mostly before 9 weeks of gestation. It is a diagnosis of exclusion. Other causes of persistent nausea and vomiting should be excluded. Some of these are listed in Box 1.

The presence of associated symptoms, such as fever, abdominal pain, and diarrhea, and neurological symptoms suggests other

Box 1: Differential diagnosis of nausea and vomiting during pregnancy.[5,6]

- *Gastrointestinal causes*:
  - Gastroenteritis
  - Reflux esophagitis
  - Gastroparesis
  - Achalasia
  - Diaphragmatic hernia
  - Biliary tract disease
  - Cholecystitis
  - Hepatitis
  - Pancreatitis
  - Appendicitis
  - Intestinal obstruction
  - Ileus
  - Peptic ulcer disease
  - Crohn's disease
  - Gastric malignancy
- *Metabolic causes*:
  - Addison's disease
  - Diabetic ketoacidosis
  - Porphyria
  - Hyperthyroidism/hypothyroidism
  - Hypercalcemia
- *Neurological causes*:
  - Psychiatric problems
  - Korsakoff psychosis
  - Migraine
  - Vestibular disorders
  - Wernicke encephalopathy
  - Pseudotumor cerebri
  - Tumors of the central nervous system (CNS)
  - Meningitis
- *Pregnancy associated*:
  - Acute fatty liver of pregnancy
  - Emesis gravidarum (<5 vomiting/day)
  - Hyperemesis gravidarum (>5 vomiting/day)
  - Multiple pregnancy
  - Preeclampsia
  - HELLP (hemolysis, elevated liver enzyme, and low platelet level) syndrome
  - Premature contractions
- *Urogenital causes*:
  - Pyelonephritis
  - Uremia
  - Ovarian torsion
  - Renal stones
  - Degenerating uterine leiomyoma
- *Other causes*:
  - Drug toxicity or intolerance
  - Food poisoning
  - Medications, e.g., iron, steroids, digoxin, theophylline and nonsteroidal anti-inflammatory drugs
  - Inferior myocardial infarction or ischemia
  - Peritonitis
  - Acute hemolysis

causes related to gastrointestinal, genitourinary, or central nervous system.

HISTORY

History of Present Illness

Clinical symptoms of NVP are usually nonspecific. Commonly reported symptoms are fatigue, exhaustion, and indisposition. Aversion or craving to certain foods is common. Woman may complain of excessive salivation. There may be increased fatigue and irritability.

Women with HG may report a variety of symptoms such as hematemesis, muscle pains, and decreased urine output, and neurological symptoms such as ataxia, confusion, weakness of limbs, and squint, indicating increased severity of illness and related complications such as Wernicke encephalopathy and pontine myelinolysis.

Obstetrical History

Any history of NVP in a previous pregnancy predisposes a woman to develop it again in subsequent pregnancies.

Socioeconomic History

A detailed socioeconomic history is important as an unfavorable or adverse socioeconomic situation may subject the woman to psychological stress and manifest as emesis gravidarum.

Personal History

Women with history of nausea and vomiting with combined oral contraceptive pills, motion sickness, migraine, etc., are at increased risk of development of emesis gravidarum.

Dietary History

Absence of multivitamin supplementation makes women prone to NVP.

Family History

There is a significantly higher risk of NVP in women whose sister or mother experienced the disorder.

Based on the history, severity of the condition can be assessed by various scoring systems such as Pregnancy-Unique Quantification of Emesis and Nausea (PUQE) scoring index and the Rhodes Index.[7] These indices use a point system to assign points for the number of hours each day the woman feels nauseated (1 = not at all to 5 = >6 hours), the number of times she vomits (1 = none to 5 = 7 or more times), and the number of times she has retching or dry heaves (1 = none to 5 = 7 or more times). A total score of <6 is considered mild nausea and vomiting, 7–12 moderate, and >13 severe. A high score indicates the patient should be evaluated for dehydration and her serum electrolyte levels should be checked.

Recently another scoring system, Hyperemesis Impact of Symptoms (HIS) Questionnaire, has been developed that takes into account psychosocial factors in addition to physical symptoms.[8]

EXAMINATION

Examination is guided by the history but essential aspects are as described below.

General

- *Vitals*: Check for temperature, pulse, blood pressure, and respiratory rate.
- *Assess for level of consciousness*: Extreme dehydration may lead to drowsiness, confusion, and delirium.
- Presence of acetone-like breath is suggestive of metabolic ketoacidosis.
- Assess for hydration status and presence of jaundice and pallor.
- *Systemic examination*: Look for any signs of systemic infection such as chest infection.
- *Assessment of weight*: Continuous loss of weight may be associated with hyperemesis gravidarum.

Per Abdomen

A detailed abdominal examination should be done including inspection, palpation, and auscultation to determine whether the uterine size is corresponding to the weeks of gestation to ensure fetal viability and to rule out other causes of vomiting. This will include palpation for any areas of tenderness, rebound tenderness, guarding, hepatomegaly.

Bimanual Pelvic Examination

Bimanual pelvic examination should be routinely done in cases with NVP in first trimester to determine the uterine size and look for any adnexal mass or tenderness, especially where molar pregnancy, multiple pregnancy, or ectopic pregnancy is suspected. Vaginal examination is also indicated in a laboring patient or when induction of labor is required.

INVESTIGATIONS

Most cases of nausea and vomiting do not require laboratory testing. In cases of severe NVP or if the diagnosis is not clear after history and physical examination, laboratory investigations are indicated. These can be classified into:

- *Primary tests*: Done to diagnose NVP, its severity, and associated conditions (Box 2)

Box 2: Primary tests for a pregnant woman presenting with vomiting.

- *Complete blood count (CBC)* including hematocrit and white blood cell count: An increase in hematocrit indicates hemoconcentration due to plasma volume depletion.
- *Serum electrolytes* to diagnose electrolyte derangements such as hypokalemia and metabolic alkalosis.
- *Blood glucose*: Hyperglycemia may indicate overt diabetes; hypoglycemia may occur secondary to nausea and vomiting of pregnancy (NVP).
- *Renal function tests (RFTs)*: Elevated blood urea nitrogen (BUN) indicates dehydration.
- *Liver function tests (LFTs)*: Liver enzymes are mildly elevated in 50% of patients with hyperemesis; higher values may suggest primary hepatic pathology. Alanine aminotransferase (ALT) is typically elevated to a greater degree than aspartate aminotransferase (AST). Values for both are usually mildly elevated, i.e. in the low hundreds, and rarely as high as 1,000 U/L. Hyperbilirubinemia can also occur, but rarely exceeds 4 mg/dL. The degree of abnormality in liver tests correlates with the vomiting; the highest elevations are seen in patients with the most severe NVP. Abnormal LFT resolves promptly upon resolution of vomiting.
- *Urinalysis*: For any pus cells, pH, presence of ketone bodies, increased specific gravity indicate dehydration and ketoacidosis.
- *Ultrasound* to exclude multiple pregnancy and trophoblastic disorders.

Box 3: Secondary tests for a pregnant woman presenting with vomiting.

- *Thyroid function tests*: Thyroid-stimulating hormone (TSH) suppression or even elevated serum free T_4 concentrations may be present suggesting mild hyperthyroidism, possibly due to high serum concentrations of human chorionic gonadotropin (hCG), which has thyroid-stimulating activity
- *Serum amylase* may increase as much as five fold as opposed to a 5–10 fold increase in acute pancreatitis
- *Serum calcium*: Hypercalcemia due to hyperparathyroidism may contribute to the vomiting
- Stool for occult blood, white blood cells, stool culture to rule out gastroenteritis
- Upper gastrointestinal (GI) series or upper endoscopy
- Abdominal ultrasound to rule out gallbladder/renal calculi, neoplasia, and other intra-abdominal pathology
- Electrocardiogram

Box 4: Tertiary tests for a pregnant woman presenting with vomiting.

- Lower gastrointestinal (GI) endoscopy
- Computed tomography or magnetic resonance imaging studies
- Urine toxicology
- Urine porphyrins

- *Secondary tests*: Done to rule out other common causes of vomiting in pregnancy (Box 3)
- *Tertiary tests*: To diagnose rarer causes of vomiting in pregnancy (Box 4)

Transient hyperthyroidism of HG can be differentiated from hyperthyroidism of other causes by absence of symptoms such as heat intolerance, muscle weakness, tremors, goiter, and ophthalmopathy. In addition, both serum free T_3 and T_4 concentrations are raised in true hyperthyroidism compared to minimally elevated serum T_4 and normal serum T_3 concentrations in women with HG.

Treatment of hyperthyroidism should not be initiated without clear evidence of a primary thyroid disorder such as goiter, elevated free serum free T_3 and T_4 concentration, or elevated levels of thyroid antibodies.

MANAGEMENT

Treatment of NVP is guided by severity of symptoms, impact on the woman's life and safety profile. Flowchart 2 depicts an algorithm for step-wise management of patients presenting with NVP. Dietary advice, lifestyle modifications, and nonpharmacological

Section 1: Obstetrics

Flowchart 2: Algorithm for step-wise management of NVP.

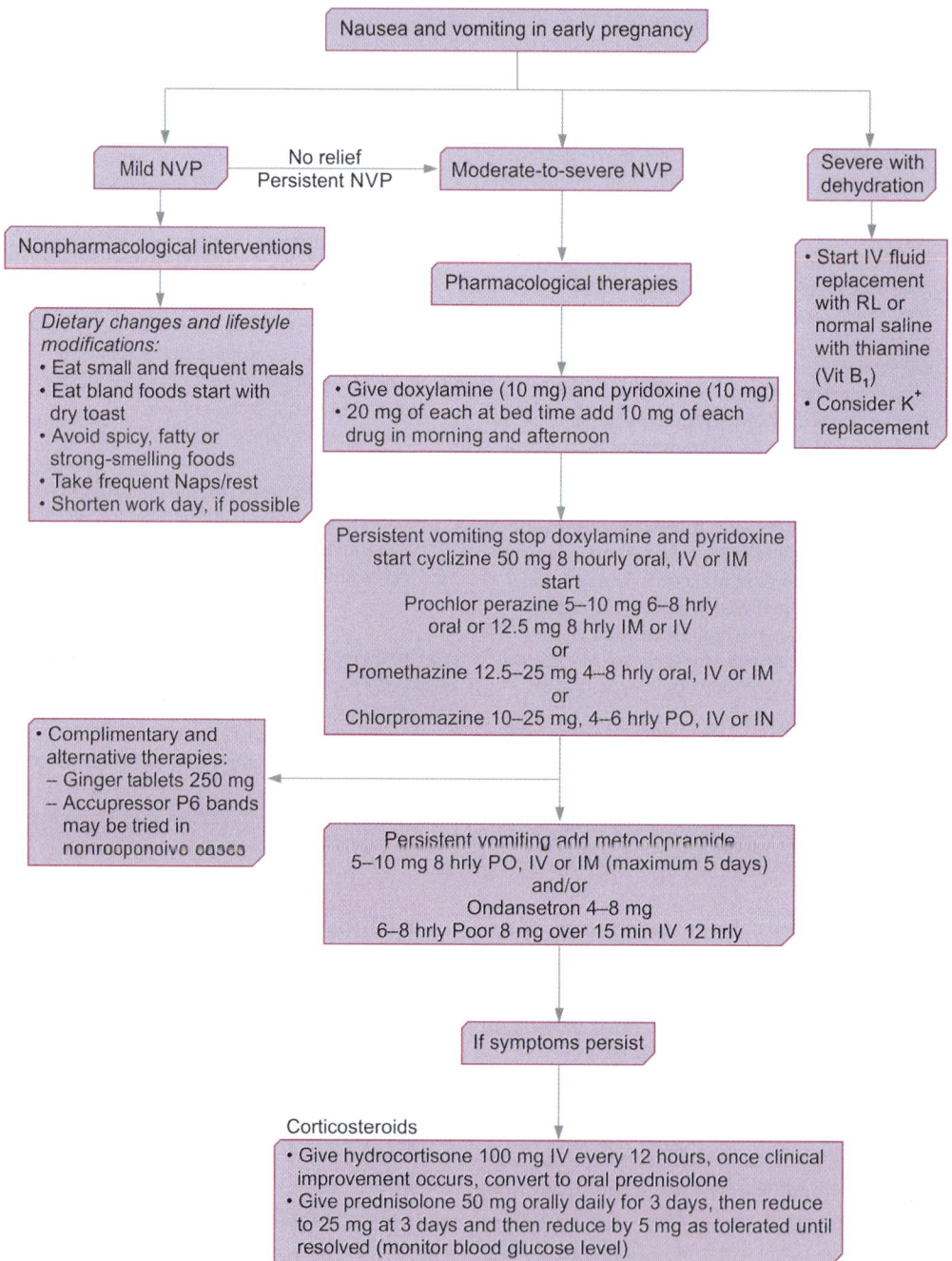

(IM: intramuscular; IV: intravenous; NVP: nausea and vomiting of pregnancy)

> **Box 5:** Complications of hyperemesis gravidarum.
>
> - *Maternal complications*:
>   - Dehydration
>   - Starvation ketosis
>   - Increased risk of thromboembolism
>   - Electrolyte imbalance—hypokalemia, hyponatremia, and hypochloremic alkalosis
>   - Wernicke's encephalopathy—due to thiamine deficiency
>   - Protein–energy malnutrition
>   - Folate deficiency leading to anemia
>   - Thyroid dysfunction
>   - Renal dysfunction
>   - Hepatic dysfunction
>   - Ulcerative esophagitis and Mallory–Weiss tears
>   - Psychological effects
> - *Fetal complications*:
>   - Fetal growth restriction
>   - Fetal loss
>   - Chronic illness in adult life of offspring (due to intrauterine undernutrition)

interventions (such as ginger) are the first line for management. Since iron tablets may exacerbate symptoms of NVP, withholding iron tablets is advisable. These interventions may relieve milder cases of NVP, but pharmacological agents are usually needed for more severe cases.

A pregnant woman with HG should be carefully observed for fetal and maternal complications listed in Box 5.

KEY POINTS

- Nausea and vomiting of pregnancy or morning sickness is a common problem related to pregnancy with the onset in the first trimester.
- HG is diagnosed when persistent vomiting unrelated to any other cause is associated with a weight loss of >5% of prepregnancy body weight, dehydration, electrolyte imbalance, and ketonuria in the first trimester.
- The initial evaluation includes measurement of weight, pulse and blood pressure, hydration status, serum electrolytes, and urine ketone.
- An ultrasound examination is indicated to exclude gestational trophoblastic disease and multiple gestations.
- Fever, abdominal pain, headache, or neurological symptoms and signs may indicate vomiting due to other causes.
- Women with mild NVP should be managed on outpatient basis with antiemetics.
- Inpatient management is recommended for:
  - Continued nausea and vomiting and inability to keep down oral antiemetics
  - Continued nausea and vomiting associated with ketonuria and/or weight loss (>5% of body weight), despite oral antiemetics
  - Suspected comorbidity (such as urinary tract infection and inability to tolerate oral antibiotics).

REFERENCES

1. Gadsby R, Barnie-Adshead AM, Jagger C. A prospective study of nausea and vomiting during pregnancy. Br J Gen Pract. 1993; 43(371):245-8.
2. Goodwin TM. Hyperemesis gravidarum. Obstet Gynecol Clin North Am. 2008;35(3): 401-17.
3. Bailit JL. Hyperemesis gravidarium: Epidemiologic findings from a large cohort. Am J Obstet Gynecol. 2005;193(3 Pt 1):811-4.
4. Davis M. Nausea and vomiting of pregnancy: an evidence-based review. J Perinat J Neonatal Nurs. 2004;18(4):312-28.
5. Jueckstock JK, Kaestner R, Mylonas I. Managing hyperemesis gravidarum: a multimodal challenge. BMC Med. 2010;8:46.
6. Ebrahimi N, Maltepe C, Einarson A. Optimal management of nausea and vomiting of pregnancy. Int J Womens Health. 2010;2: 241-8.

7. Lacasse A, Rey E, Ferreira E, Morin C, Bérard A. Validity of a modified Pregnancy-Unique Quantification of Emesis and Nausea (PUQE) scoring index to assess severity of nausea and vomiting of pregnancy. Am J Obstet Gynecol. 2008; 198(1):71.e1-7.
8. Power Z, Campbell M, Kilcoyne P, Kitchener H, Waterman H. The Hyperemesis Impact of Symptoms Questionnaire: development and validation of a clinical tool. Int J Nurs Stud. 2010;47(1):67-77.

SUGGESTED READING

1. ACOG Practice Bulletin No. 189: Nausea and vomiting of pregnancy. Obstet Gynecol. 2018;131(1):e15-30.
2. Institute of Obstetricians and Gynaecologists, Royal College of Physicians of Ireland and the Clinical Strategy and Programmes Division, Health Service Executive. (2018). Clinical Practice Guideline – Hyperemesis and Nausea/ Vomiting in Pregnancy. [online] Available from https://www.hyperemesis.ie/documents/Guidelines-Ireland-HyperemesisNauseaVomitinginPregnancy.pdf.
3. Royal College of Obstetricians and Gynaecologists (2016). The management of nausea and vomiting of pregnancy and hyperemesis gravidarum (Green-top Guideline no. 69). [online] Available from https://www.rcog.org.uk/en/guidelines-research-services/guidelines/gtg69/. [Last accessed January, 2020].

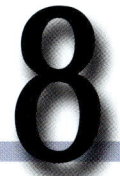

Approach to a Pregnant Woman Presenting with Diarrhea

Pikee Saxena, Priyanka Arora

INTRODUCTION

The World Health Organization (WHO) defines diarrhea as passage of three or more loose or watery stools per day.[1] It is consequent to either decreased absorption or increased secretion of water by intestinal mucosa with resultant increase in water content of stools. Diarrhea is usually a symptom which may be associated with fever, abdominal pain, loss of appetite, nausea, vomiting, and weakness. Invasive diarrhea or dysentery is loose stools with mucus and or blood and is usually associated with fever and or abdominal pain.

It may cause dehydration, electrolyte imbalance (sodium, chloride, potassium, and bicarbonate), hypovolemic shock, metabolic acidosis, low blood glucose levels, and uremia. Electrolyte imbalance can manifest as cramps, irritability, confusion, or even convulsions. It can precipitate preterm labor and premature rupture of membranes. Severe diarrhea may be life threatening, particularly in pregnant women who are malnourished or have impaired immunity.

CAUSES OF DIARRHEA

Diarrhea may be caused by damage to the lining of the gastrointestinal tract by viral, bacterial, protozoal, or fungal pathogens, so that the intestines are unable to absorb fluid with resultant secretory diarrhea. If excessive fluid is secreted into the bowel it is often a sign of bacterial infection. In diarrhea induced by anxiety or drugs, bowel contents move through the digestive system too quickly, so that the intestines do not have enough time to absorb fluid from the bowel contents. Food, such as lactose, if not absorbed properly, cause water to move out of the blood into the bowel, which dilutes the intestinal contents.[2] Presence of blood in the stools is an evidence of invasion of the bowel with pathogens and is known as dysentery.

Diarrhea may be classified depending on the duration of symptoms (Table 1).

The WHO classifies diarrhea as acute and persistent. However, the conventional classification has been acute and chronic diarrhea, where chronic diarrhea is defined as diarrhea persisting for >30 days.

DIFFERENTIAL DIAGNOSIS

The causes of diarrhea are as listed in Table 2. These are categorized according to the type

Table 1: Classification of diarrhea.

Types of diarrhea	Characteristics
Acute diarrhea	Starts suddenly and may continue for several days (usually ≤14 days)
Persistent diarrhea	Starts like acute diarrhea, but lasts for >14 days but ≤30 days
Dysentery	Blood and mucus mixed with stools
Chronic diarrhea	Diarrhea persisting for >30 days

Table 2: Causes of diarrhea.

Acute diarrhea	Persistent diarrhea	Dysentery
• *Infectious diarrhea*: Viral, bacterial, parasitic, and fungal • *Medications*: Antibiotics, nonsteroidal anti-inflammatory drugs (NSAIDs), laxatives, iron preparations, and antacids with magnesium • Emotional or anxiety induced • Pelvic abscess or collection in the pouch of Douglas	• *Inflammatory*: Ulcerative colitis, Crohn's disease, radiation colitis • *Osmotic*: Celiac sprue • *Secretory*: Carcinoid syndrome • *Altered motility*: Irritable bowel syndrome (IBS) • *Factitious*: Laxative abuse	*Infections*: • Shigella • *Entamoeba histolytica* • Campylobacter • Yersinia • Salmonella

of diarrhea, i.e., acute diarrhea, persistent diarrhea, and dysentery.

HISTORY

Detailed history may give insight into the cause and severity of illness. This includes history of presenting symptom, i.e., loose stools, its onset, frequency, duration, consistency, color, whether associated with blood, mucus, pain in abdomen, fever, nausea, and vomiting, and whether it is the first episode or there is a previous history of such episodes. Rice water stools are characteristic of cholera.

The history of intake of any drugs, such as iron preparations, broad-spectrum antibiotics such as ampicillin, and association of onset of the illness with the intake of drug, is important. The stools are usually passed frequently but are not too loose in drug-induced diarrhea. A detailed dietary history, travel history, and source of drinking water should be taken. Any history of similar illness in other members of the family or neighborhood points toward a possibility of consumption of contaminated food or water from a common source.

The history of any reduction in the volume of urine or passage of high-colored urine is suggestive of dehydration and poor renal perfusion consequent to it. History of irritability, confusion, lethargy, increased thirst, cramps, and convulsions suggest dehydration and electrolyte imbalance.

The history of perception of normal fetal movements implies fetal well-being. Any history of pain in abdomen with hardening of uterus should be elicited as other than intestinal cramps; intermittent colicky pain could be due to uterine contractions. Any history of watery discharge or leaking per vaginum should be enquired as it is suggestive of premature rupture of membranes.

Detailed menstrual, obstetrical, socioeconomic, and personal history should be taken as described in the Chapter 1 on the "Approach to a Pregnant Woman Attending Antenatal Clinic." The history of any prior treatment for the complaints should be elicited.

EXAMINATION

General Physical Examination

The vitals of the pregnant woman, pulse rate, pulse volume, blood pressure, and respiratory rate are recorded. The temperature is recorded for documentation of fever. Presence of pallor, icterus, or cyanosis is looked for.

It is important to assess the hydration status of the woman. For this, one looks at the tongue whether it is moist (Fig. 1), dry, or parched (Fig. 2). In mild dehydration, the tongue is dry, whereas in moderate and severe dehydration, the woman is restless, tongue is dry and parched, eyes are

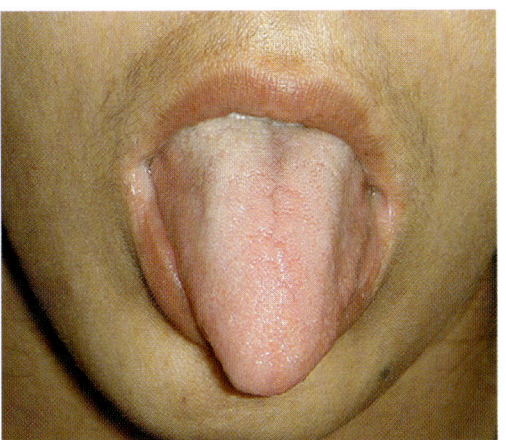

Fig. 1: Moist tongue.

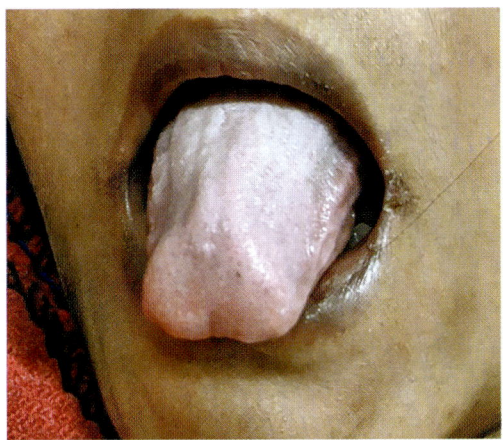

Fig. 2: Dehydrated dry tongue.

sunken, and the skin turgor is decreased. In severe dehydration, the woman may be in hypovolemic shock, with cold extremities, rapid and feeble pulse, low or unrecordable blood pressure, and peripheral cyanosis. The radial pulse may not be palpable sometimes. Rest of the general physical examination is conducted as described in the Chapter 1 on "Approach to a Pregnant Woman Attending Antenatal Clinic."

Systemic Examination

The breast examination, and cardiovascular, respiratory, and neurological examinations are carried out as described in Chapter 1.

Per Abdomen Examination

Per abdomen examination is important to assess for any abdominal signs such as distention, tenderness, rigidity, and rebound tenderness. Bowel sounds are heard; ileus is suspected if the bowel sounds are hypoactive.

A detailed obstetrical examination including assessment of fundal height, lie and presentation of the fetus, amount of liquor, any uterine contractions, and fetal heart rate is done in pregnant women in the last trimester. Fetal heart rate abnormalities and intrauterine death (IUD) are common in women with severe dehydration. Decreased liquor or oligohydramnios is often associated with dehydration.

Local Examination

Per speculum or per vaginal examination should be done as indicated in case the woman is having uterine contractions or complaining of leaking per vaginum. Per rectal examination or rectovaginal examination is useful to diagnose pelvic abscess in case it is suspected.

INVESTIGATIONS

In addition to the routine antenatal investigations such as hemoglobin, urine examination, and blood group and Rh typing, the patient is subjected to a complete blood count, serum electrolytes, renal and liver function tests. Enzyme-linked immuno-sorbent assay (ELISA) for human immunodeficiency virus (HIV) is done as a routine but is specifically indicated in pregnant women with persistent or chronic diarrhea.

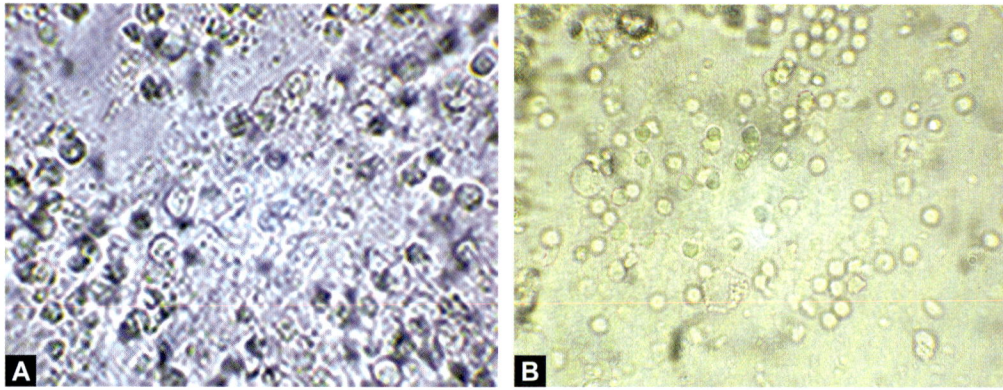

Figs. 3A and B: Stool microscopy. (A) Pus cells; (B) Blood cells.

Microscopic Examination of Stool

The microscopic examination of stool should be carried out for the presence of ova, cyst, pus cells, and blood (Figs. 3A and B). Stool may also be subjected to culture sensitivity. The stool is collected during acute stage before the initiation of the antibiotics. Contamination with urine or any other infective material should be avoided. Stool should be collected in a wide mouth, leakproof, screw capped, 25 mL container with a spoon taking care that the rim of the container is not soiled. Approximately 5 mL of liquid stool or pea size of formed stool should be collected to a maximum of three samples.

A wet mount can detect ova and trophozoites of parasites and white blood cells (WBCs) indicative of invasive pathogens. Phase-contrast microscopy helps in detection of *Campylobacter* and immune electron microscopy of viruses. Various stains can be used for enhancing the detection of ova and cyst of *Entamoeba histolytica*. *Vibrio cholerae* can be detected by an immobilization test and a hanging drop preparation, which shows active motility. A Gram stain test of *V. cholerae* will show curved gram-negative bacilli and catalase and oxidase test will show positive results.

Endoscopy

Endoscopy of lower gastrointestinal tract with or without biopsy may be required to confirm the diagnosis of inflammatory bowel disease.

Ultrasound Examination

Ultrasound examination of abdomen and pelvis may be required to diagnose any collection in the pelvis.

An obstetric ultrasound is indicated for confirming fetal maturity and assessing fetal well-being. The clinical approach to a pregnant woman presenting with diarrhea and persistent diarrhea is as given in Flowchart 1.

MANAGEMENT

The management of pregnant woman with acute diarrhea is predominantly symptomatic, major component being basic general measures such as fluid replacement and maintenance of nutrition with adjustments in diet if necessary.

Fluid replacement is the most critical step in managing diarrhea. The preferable mode of rehydration is the oral route, with solutions that contain water, salt, and sugar.

Flowchart 1: Algorithm for clinical approach to a pregnant woman presenting with diarrhea.

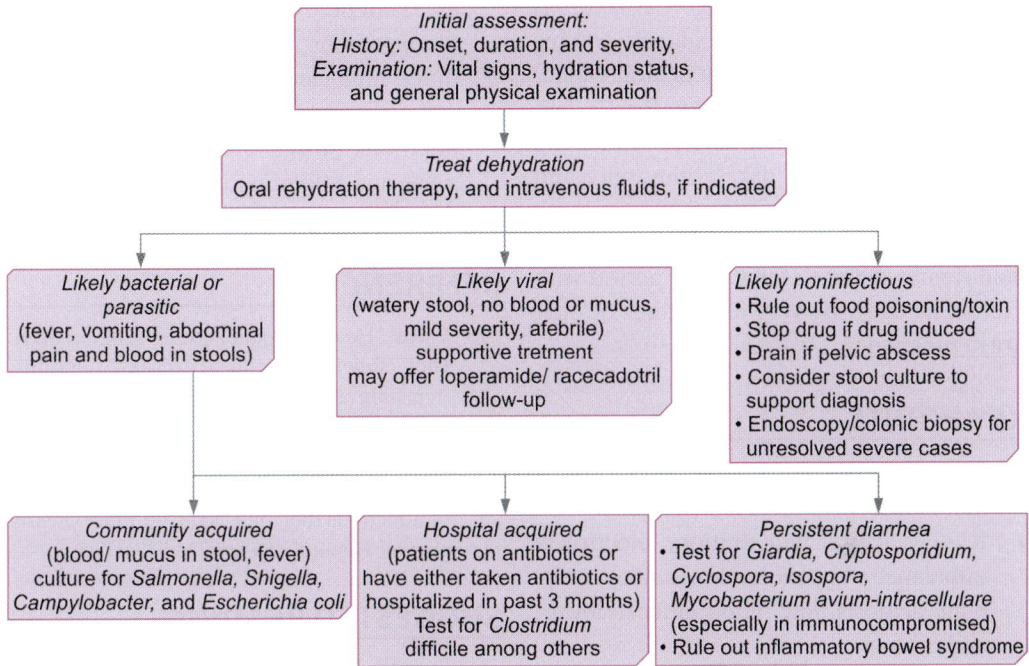

Oral rehydration solutions (ORS) by the WHO are appropriate. They should be used both to replete a depleted volume and to maintain adequate volume subsequently. Women with severe dehydration or severe hypovolemia should initially receive intravenous fluid repletion with normal saline or Ringer's lactate. In patients with hypovolemic shock as in cholera, initially rapid fluid replacement at the rate of 100 mL/kg should be given over 3 hours. Strict input output charting should be done to follow volume repletion.

Food advice includes bland diet containing boiled starches and cereals with salt such as potatoes, rice, and oats, soups, boiled vegetables, crackers, and bananas and avoidance of food with high-fat content.

Probiotics that assist in maintaining or recolonizing the intestine with nonpathogenic flora can be used as an alternative therapy.

Oral iron and calcium can cause gastric irritation and may worsen diarrhea, hence may be stopped temporarily till diarrhea resolves.

Antibiotic therapy is usually not indicated as mostly the diarrhea is caused by viruses and resolves spontaneously. It is recommended in severe symptomatic cases with symptoms and signs suggestive of invasive bacterial infection like dysentery or cholera. For cholera, oral azithromycin 1 g single dose or oral erythromycin 500 mg four times a day for 3 days is preferred and safer compared to oral doxycycline 300 mg single dose in pregnant women. The same regime can be used in women with dysentery. Quinolones, namely ciprofloxacin 500 mg twice daily for 3 days, should be avoided as most of the organisms are resistant to it and its safety in pregnancy is not proven although in therapeutic doses it does not seem to cause any harm to the fetus. For *Clostridioides* (formerly *Clostridium*) *difficile* infection, oral metronidazole 500 mg three times a day for 10 days or oral vancomycin 125 mg four times a day for 10 days is indicated. Drugs such as loperamide up to 4 mg four times a day (antimotility and antisecretory) and racecadotril 100 mg three times a day (antisecretory) may be used for noninvasive diarrhea for a short period with caution as there are very few studies of their use in pregnancy.

KEY POINTS

- Diarrhea is defined as passage of three or more loose or watery stools per day.
- It may cause dehydration, electrolyte imbalance, hypovolemic shock, metabolic acidosis, low blood glucose levels, and uremia.
- In pregnancy, it can precipitate preterm labor and premature rupture of membranes, oligohydramnios, and sudden IUD.
- It may be viral, bacterial, protozoal, non-infectious, iatrogenic, or due to irritable bowel syndrome.
- Initial assessment includes history of onset, duration, and severity of diarrhea, general physical examination including vital signs and hydration status, and fetal assessment.
- Management includes replacement of fluids and electrolytes orally and intravenously depending upon severity. Antimicrobial drugs are added rarely for suspected microbial infection. Supportive therapy remains the mainstay.

REFERENCES

1. World Health Organization. (2017). WHO Fact sheet: Diarrhoeal disease. [online] Available from https://www.who.int/news-room/fact-sheets/detail/diarrhoeal-disease. [Last accessed January, 2020].
2. Navaneethan U, Giannella RA. Mechanisms of infectious diarrhea. Nat Clin Pract Gastroenterol Hepatol. 2008;5(11):637-47.

SUGGESTED READING

1. Barr W, Smith A. Acute diarrhea. Am Fam Physician. 2014;89(3):180-9.
2. Kasper DL, Hauser SL, Loscalzo J, Longo DL, Jameson JL, Fauci AS. Chapter 55: Diarrhoea and Constipation. Harrison's Principles of Internal Medicine, 20th edition. United States: McGraw Hill Professional; 2018.
3. Operario DJ, Houpt E. Defining the etiology of diarrhoea: novel approaches. Current opinion in infectious diseases. 2011;24(5):464.

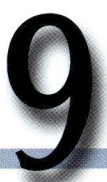

Approach to a Pregnant Woman Presenting with Fever

Shalini Malhotra

INTRODUCTION

Fever is a rise in core body temperature and is usually a sign of infection. The average body temperature is 98.6°F (37°C) and the range being 97°F (36.1°C) to 99°F (37.2°C). The rectal temperature is 0.2–0.3°C (0.5–0.7°F) more than oral temperature and axillary temperature is 0.55°C (1°F) less than oral. It tends to be lower in the morning and higher in the evening.

As per Mayo Clinic and John Hopkins, USA, the following thermometer readings generally indicate a fever:

- Rectal, ear, or temporal artery temperature of 100.4°F (38°C) or higher
- Oral temperature of 100°F (37.8°C) or higher
- Armpit temperature of 99°F (37.2°C) or higher

Fever is not uncommon in pregnancy. The consequences depend on the extent of temperature elevation, its duration, and the period of gestation at which it occurs. Mild exposures during the peri-implantation period and more severe episodes during the embryonic and fetal development often result in resorption of the embryo, fetal death, and structural and functional defects.[1] CNS is at maximum risk, as the surviving neuroblasts cannot replicate and make up for the lost neurons. Fever can lead to many potentially lethal defects related to CNS and other systems such as cleft lip and palate, micropthalmos, cataract, abdominal wall defects, and cardiovascular malformations such as atrial septal defect, hypoplastic left heart, and uterine contractility with resultant expulsion of the fetus at a nonviable gestation that is miscarriage or preterm birth.

Maternal fever in pregnancy also causes attention deficit hyperactivity disorder (ADHD), especially inattention problems, cerebral palsy, schizophrenia, and mental retardation.[2] The risk of ADHD is significantly increased with repeated episodes of fever, especially in the first trimester between 9 and 12 weeks of gestation.[3]

The MBRRACE-UK (Mothers and Babies: Reducing Risk through Audit and Confidential Enquiries) report, 2016 shows 14% mortality rate due to pneumonia or influenza in UK, a confirmation that fever in pregnancy can lead to serious outcomes, if not managed appropriately.[4]

DIFFERENTIAL DIAGNOSIS

The causes of fever in pregnancy are given in Table 1.

The clinical approach to a pregnant woman with fever is given in Flowchart 1.

HISTORY

It is important to elicit a detailed history to identify the cause of fever in a pregnant woman. The onset and duration of fever, its severity, whether continuous or intermittent,

Table 1: Causes of fever.

Pregnancy-related causes	Incidental causes
Septic abortion	*Respiratory tract infection*: COVID, swine flu, pneumonia, and tuberculosis
Sepsis after antenatal procedures such as chorionic villus sampling, cervical cerclage, and amniocentesis	*Urinary tract infections*: Cystitis and pyelonephritis
PROM with chorioamnionitis	*Gastroenteritis*
Group A streptococcal infections	*CNS infections*: Encephalitis, meningitis
	Viral illnesses: Rubella, CMV, varicella, herpes simplex, parvovirus, and HIV
	Parasitic infections: Malaria, dengue, chikungunya Q fever, and chlamydia trachomatis
	Rare causes: Appendicitis, tubo-ovarian abscess, pancreatitis and cholecystitis

(PROM: premature rupture of membranes; CNS: central nervous system; CMV: cytomegalovirus; HIV: human immunodeficiency virus)

Flowchart 1: Algorithm for clinical approach to a pregnant woman with fever.

History:
- Onset and duration of fever
- Severity of fever
- Pattern—continuous or intermittent
- Any diurnal variation
- Associated with chills and rigors
- Any localizing features such as cough or diarrhea
- History of systemic illness causing immunosuppression

General examination:
- *Vitals:* Pulse, blood pressure, respiratory rate, and temperature
- Level of consciousness
- Hydration
- Neck rigidity
- Any features of septic shock
- Look for any risk factors or localizing signs such as thrombophlebitis, subcutaneous/injection site induration/abscess

Systemic examination:
Any localizing signs and detailed systemic examination chest, CVS, abdomen, CNS
Obstetric examination:
Look for any signs of chorioamnionitis such as:
- Uterine tenderness
- Amount of liquor
- Fetal tachycardia
- Any vaginal loss of foul smelling liquor/abnormal discharge

any diurnal variation, and any association with rigors or chills are important as the pattern of fever varies with the condition the woman is suffering from.

Any localizing feature pointing to some infective focus is asked for such as cough, difficulty in breathing, urinary symptoms, vomiting, diarrhea, abdominal pain, any rash, vaginal discharge, or prolonged rupture of membranes. Any history of invasive procedure such as chorionic villus biopsy, amniocentesis, cervical cerclage, instrumentation, or intervention is asked for. If the woman has been in labor then detailed history of per vaginum examinations as regards to the number of examinations and whether done under aseptic precautions should be asked for.

Any history suggestive of diabetes mellitus, HIV infection or low immunity in the form of repeated infections is asked for.

It is imperative to take history of travel to any area with endemic diseases such as malaria and yellow fever.

Menstrual History

Date of onset of last normal menstrual period (LMP) and expected date of delivery are

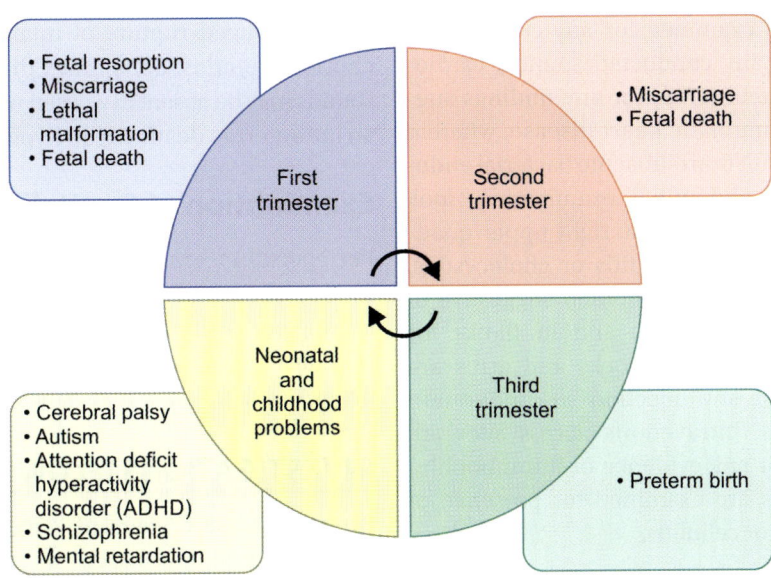

Fig. 1: Consequences of fever in pregnancy.

recorded and period of gestation is calculated. It is important to know the gestational age to predict complications and plan management.

Obstetric History

In addition to the detailed obstetric history, it is important to enquire about any intervention or instrumentation in the current pregnancy, any history of leaking per vaginum and any history of spontaneous or induced abortion.

Personal History

The socioeconomic status should be assessed as low socioeconomic status increases the likelihood of unhygienic living conditions, malnutrition, and predisposition to diseases such as malaria, tuberculosis, and dengue.

EXAMINATION

General Physical Examination

A physical examination includes the search for presence of risk factors for sepsis such as obesity, anemia, and malnutrition. The vitals such as pulse, blood pressure, respiratory rate, and temperature of the patient are recorded. The oxygen saturation is assessed with pulse oximeter. Her level of consciousness is noted as the woman may be disoriented in the presence of serious systemic infection, encephalitis, or cerebral malaria. Her state of hydration is assessed. Any neck rigidity is looked for as it is suggestive of meningitis. The woman may be in septic shock. Clinical features of septic shock are as shown in Box 1.

Systemic Examination

A detailed systemic examination is done for localizing signs of sepsis in all body systems.

Box 1: Clinical features of septic shock.

• Tachycardia
• Tachypnea
• Pyrexia
• Hypothermia
• Hypotension
• Poor peripheral perfusion:
  – Cold extremities
  – Oliguria

The chest is examined for any crepitations, rhonchi, or any conducted sounds, cardiovascular system (CVS) for any findings suggestive of rheumatic heart disease, wherein fever can result from subacute bacterial endocarditis. On abdominal examination, look for any tenderness in the right upper quadrant suggestive of hepatitis or cholecystitis, tenderness in lower abdomen suggestive of cystitis or appendicitis, and in flanks for pyelonephritis. The buttocks and arms are inspected for any injection site induration or abscesses. Intravenous access sites are inspected for any evidence of thrombophlebitis. Breasts are examined for presence of any mastitis or cellulitis.

Obstetric Examination

The uterus is examined for the presence of any tenderness, amount of liquor amnii, and fetal heart rate. Fetal tachycardia may be present in a febrile pregnant woman. The uterus is tender and liquor is reduced in women with prolonged rupture of membranes and chorioamnionitis. Sometimes the fetal heart sounds may be absent in women who have had an intrauterine death due to hyperthermia.

Examination of Genitalia

Per speculum examination is done to look for any abnormal or unhealthy discharge or leaking per vaginum. In many cases the fetus may have passed meconium due to maternal hyperthermia.

INVESTIGATIONS (FLOWCHART 2)

Pyrexia of >38°C warrants urgent investigations; these are based on history and examination findings and are as mentioned below (Flowchart 2):

- *Complete blood count*: White blood cells (WBCs) are usually increased, but may be normal or sometimes low in severe sepsis.
- *C-reactive protein (CRP)*: It is increased in sepsis.

Flowchart 2: Investigations in case of fever in pregnancy.

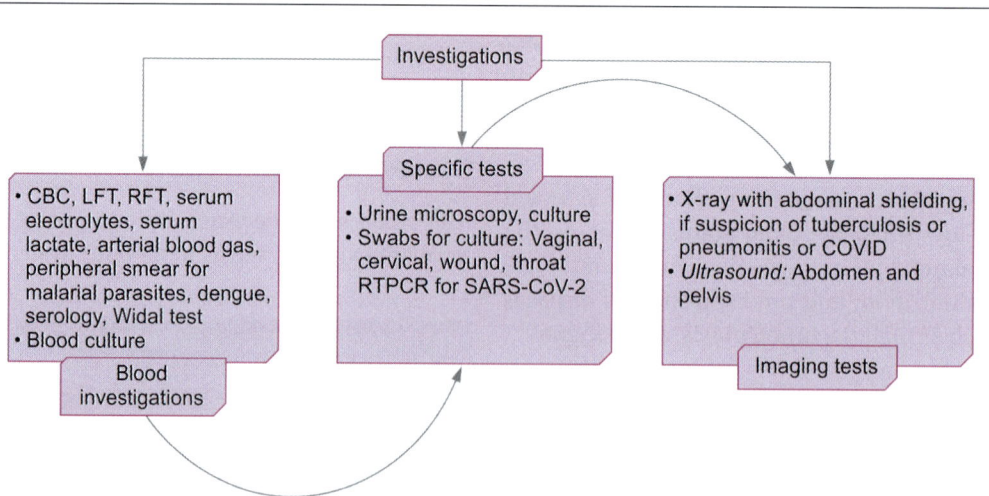

(CBC: complete blood count; LFT: liver function test; RFT: renal function test)

- *Liver function tests (LFTs) and renal function tests (RFTs)*: These are done to detect multiple organ involvement in women with severe sepsis.
- *Serum electrolytes*: These help to assess any associated dyselectrolytemia especially, if the woman is dehydrated due to vomiting or diarrhea. If present, it needs to be corrected urgently.
- *Serum lactate and arterial blood gas analysis*: It is done to detect any metabolic acidosis due to severe sepsis or septic shock and decide fluid replacement (Sepsis care bundle UK).[5]
- *Urine albumin, sugar, microscopy, and culture sensitivity*: It is done to rule out any urinary tract infection.
- *Vaginal, cervical, wound, throat swabs, and blood and urine cultures*: These are done to look for any focus of infection. It is best done before starting the antibiotics empirically.
- Throat swab for RTPCR SARS-CoV-2.
- *Microscopic examination of thick and thin films of blood*: This is carried out for detection of blood parasites such as Plasmodium, if suspected.
- *Widal test and blood culture*: These are ordered for the diagnosis of enteric fever.
- *Dengue serology*: It is done in woman where it is suspected.
- *Ultrasonography (USG) of abdomen and pelvis*: This is done for liver, gallbladder, kidneys, appendix, and pelvis.
- *X-ray chest*: It is done with abdominal shielding to look for any evidence of tuberculosis or pneumonitis or COVID.
- *Cardiotocography (CTG)*: It is done to assess the fetal condition, particularly at or near term as fever can result in fetal heart rate abnormalities.

MANAGEMENT

It is important to keep the temperature below 100°F with the help of antipyretics or hydrotherapy to reduce the fetal risks associated with hyperthermia.

The treatment is cause specific. If the fever is thought to be due to infection after sending the cultures, the woman is prescribed broad-spectrum antibiotics depending upon the likely site of infection and switched to specific antibiotic after culture sensitivity report is received.

Careful monitoring of fetal condition is indicated, particularly at or near term.

KEY POINTS

- In pregnant women presenting with fever, a detailed history followed by thorough examination should be done with the aim to find the cause of fever.
- The blood is sent for counts, smear, and culture.
- The woman is screened for COVID.
- Guided by the history and examination, appropriate investigations and cultures are sent for the presence of any pathogenic organisms and their sensitivity to specific antibiotics.
- Careful monitoring of maternal and fetal condition is indicated.

REFERENCES

1. Edwards MJ. Review: Hyperthermia and fever during pregnancy. Birth Defects Res A Clin Mol Teratol. 2006;76(7):507-16.
2. Gustavson K, Ask H, Ystrom E, Stoltenberg C, Lipkin WI, Surén P, et al. Maternal fever during pregnancy and offspring attentions deficit hyperactivity disorder. Sci Rep. 2019;9(1):9519.

3. Andrade C. Use of acetaminophen during pregnancy and the risk of attention-deficit/hyperactivity disorder in the offspring. J Clin Psychiatry. 2016;77(3):e312-4.
4. MBRRACE—UK. (2019). Saving Lives, Improving Mothers' Care. [online] Available from https://www.npeu.ox.ac.uk/downloads/files/mbrrace-uk/reports/MBRRACE-UK%20Maternal%20Report%202019%20-%20WEB%20VERSION.pdf. [Last accessed January, 2020].
5. Royal College of Obstetricians and Gynaecologists. (2012). Sepsis in Pregnancy, Bacterial (Green-top Guideline No. 64a). [online] Available from https://www.rcog.org.uk en/guidelines-research-services/guidelines/gtg64a/. [Last accessed January, 2020].

SUGGESTED READING

1. National Institute for Health and Care Excellence. (2016). Sepsis: recognition, diagnosis and early management. [online] Available from https://www.nice.org.uk/guidance/ng51. [Last accessed January, 2020].

10 Approach to a Pregnant or Puerperal Woman Presenting with Convulsions

Prachi Dixit

INTRODUCTION

A pregnant or puerperal woman presenting with convulsions in emergency is not uncommon. Convulsions are abnormal, involuntary, and unintended movements of body caused by excessive neuronal activation in cerebral cortex.

The most common cause of convulsions in pregnancy is eclampsia and all convulsions in pregnancy beyond 20 weeks of gestation should be treated as eclampsia until proved otherwise. Eclampsia is an important cause of maternal mortality in India and other parts of the developing world. Eclampsia may develop during pregnancy or postpartum period in patients with or without signs and symptoms of preeclampsia. However, in pregnant and postpartum women presenting without features of preeclampsia, other causes of convulsions should be ruled out.

According to a recent study, the incidence of eclampsia in India is constant since the last few decades at 1.5%[1] compared to a much lower incidence of 0.036 and 0.28%, respectively in UK and USA.[2,3] Epilepsy as a cause of convulsions in pregnancy has a prevalence of 0.5% of all pregnancies. Up to 10% of epileptic women may convulse during pregnancy due to causes such as noncompliance, decreased absorption due to vomiting, intake of antacids, increased requirement of antiepileptics due to weight gain, hemodilution, and pregnancy-related stress.[4] Subarachnoid hemorrhage is seen in 1 per 10,400 pregnancies, the most common cause of bleeding being ruptured berry aneurysm.[5] Pregnancy is a hypercoagulable state; cerebral vein thrombosis complicates 1 per 10,000 pregnancies more so in the postpartum period.[6] Amniotic fluid embolism is a rare life-threatening condition where patient has sudden onset of dyspnea, cyanosis, convulsions, and/or coma.

Convulsions can be partial (focal involvement of some part of body) or generalized. International League Against Epilepsy (ILAE) defines status epilepticus as a seizure lasting for 5 minutes or more or when 30 minutes or more of incomplete recovery of consciousness between ≥2 discrete seizures elapse.[7]

DIFFERENTIAL DIAGNOSIS

The initial management of any pregnant or puerperal woman presenting with convulsions is stabilization but for a definitive management, diagnosing the cause of convulsions is important. The differential diagnosis of a woman presenting with convulsions is as given in Box 1.

IMMEDIATE APPROACH TO A PREGNANT OR PUERPERAL WOMAN WITH CONVULSIONS

A quick history is taken, vitals are recorded, and measures to control convulsions are

> **Box 1:** Differential diagnosis of convulsions in pregnancy and puerperium.
>
> - Eclampsia
> - Epilepsy
> - *Cerebrovascular accident*:
>   - *Embolism*: Paradoxical embolism with rheumatic heart disease
>   - *Thrombosis*: Lateral or superior sagittal or cortical venous thrombosis in association with preeclampsia, sepsis or thrombophilia
>   - *Hemorrhage*: Ruptured berry aneurysm, arteriovenous (AV) malformation, and severe hypertension
> - *Metabolic disorder*: Consequent to renal or hepatic failure, hypocalcemia, hypokalemia, hypoglycemia, and hyponatremia
> - *Infections*: Meningitis, postinfectious encephalopathy, cerebral malaria, toxoplasmosis, pyogenic abscess, tuberculosis, HIV, and cysticercosis
> - Trauma
> - Tumor
> - *Inflammatory*: Systemic lupus erythematous (SLE) and multiple sclerosis
> - *Drugs*: Antibiotics such as penicillin and metronidazole, antimalarials, lignocaine, and oxytocin-induced water intoxication
> - *Drug abuse or poisoning*: Strychnine, organophosphorus, alcohol withdrawal
> - Amniotic fluid embolism
> - Psychogenic nonepileptic seizures

> **Box 2:** Immediate care of a woman presenting with convulsions.
>
> - Quick check on circulation, airway, breathing (CAB)
> - Keep the patient in dimly lit room to avoid stimulation
> - Give lateral decubitus position to prevent aspiration
> - Padded tongue blade/airway is inserted to prevent tongue bite or tongue rolling back
> - Oral suctioning
> - Railed cot is preferred to prevent accidental fall
> - Start oxygen at the rate of 6 L/min by mask
> - Establish intravenous access and collect blood for investigations
> - Magnesium sulfate or antiepileptic medication is administered as indicated
> - Fetal heart rate is recorded in antenatal women
> - After stabilization self-retaining urinary catheter is inserted and urine is checked for proteinuria and urinary output is monitored

undertaken after initial resuscitation (Box 2). In women presenting at a primary health facility, airway is cleared, precautions to prevent injury due to convulsions are taken, and patient is referred to a higher center with details of treatment given, if any. Magnesium sulfate (MgSO$_4$) is available in primary healthcare level and is administered for immediate control of eclamptic convulsions before referral to an appropriate facility.

HISTORY

Initially, a quick history is taken from the patient or from the attendants if the patient is in the postictal phase, disoriented, comatose, or sedated and the initial resuscitation in the form of establishing the CAB (circulation, airway, breathing) is started.[8] Patient is put in left lateral position, oxygen is started, and treatment for control of convulsions is instituted. Once patient has been stabilized, a detailed history is taken.

History of Present Illness

- This includes the duration of convulsions, frequency of convulsions, duration of each episode, and time since last convulsion. The attendant who had observed the convulsion is encouraged to narrate the sequence of events before, during, and after the convulsion.
- History of tongue bite, injury, and urinary or fecal incontinence is elicited as presence of these features rule out a functional cause of convulsions.
- History suggestive of preeclampsia in the form of high blood pressure records, swelling feet, headache, vomiting, pain in epigastric region, blurring of vision,

and decreased urine output is elicited. However, sometimes eclampsia may not be associated with any warning symptoms or signs.
- History of head injury or fall is important to rule out any trauma-related cause.
- History of fever is elicited. Fever may be high grade as in meningitis, encephalitis, malaria or abscess or low grade as in TB and HIV.
- History of jaundice or liver disorder is important as convulsions may be due to liver disease-related metabolic disorders or hepatic encephalopathy.
- History of renal disease is significant as convulsions may be due to uremia or hyponatremia consequent to renal disease.
- History of drug intake such as antimalarials and metronidazole should be elicited as they reduce seizure threshold. Although rare, history of prolonged use of oxytocin may suggest water intoxication as a cause for convulsions.
- History of perception of fetal movements should be asked for to ensure fetal well-being, if the patient is conscious as convulsions may be associated with placental abruption or intrauterine death.
- History of bleeding per vaginum may suggest complications such as abruptio placentae.
- This should be followed by a trimester-wise history and review of her antenatal records, if she is a booked patient. (Refer to chapter no 1 for trimester-wise history.)

Obstetric History

Gravidity is important as young primigravidae are at a higher risk of preeclampsia and eclampsia. In women presenting with convulsions in puerperium, it is important to look for presence of high risk factors which predispose a woman to thrombosis-like preeclampsia, prolonged rupture of membranes, prolonged labor, instrumental delivery, caesarean section, puerperal sepsis, and superficial thrombophlebitis.

Menstrual History

This is important to calculate the period of gestation. Eclamptic convulsions are typically seen after 20 weeks of pregnancy, if presenting earlier other causes of convulsions should be considered. Irregular ovulation and menstrual cycles are associated with an increased risk of hypertensive disorders of pregnancy.

Past History

History of epilepsy, details of intake of antiepileptic mediations, and compliance to treatment are taken. It is important to find out if the epileptic seizures were well controlled before pregnancy. History of diabetes mellitus, tuberculosis, hypertension, or heart disease is taken.

Family History

History of tuberculosis, diabetes mellitus, or hypertension in family is important. Presence of pets in home, especially cats, point toward toxoplasmosis as a possible cause for convulsions.

Personal History

Whether the woman is a vegetarian or nonvegetarian is asked for as nonvegetarians are more likely to be predisposed to neurocysticercosis as a cause of convulsions. History of alcohol or drug abuse is elicited as withdrawal of alcohol can result in convulsions.

EXAMINATION

Examination should be gentle but thorough which disturbs the patient no more than necessary.

General Physical Examination

Observe general appearance, and any injury marks on the face, head, or elsewhere on the body due to fall. Assess for the level of consciousness (Glasgow coma scale)[9] and the orientation of the patient.

Her pulse, blood pressure, and respiratory rate are assessed. The pulse may be irregular in atrial fibrillation which can result in paradoxical cerebrovascular embolism. High blood pressure may suggest eclampsia or essential hypertension as a cause for convulsions. However, normal blood pressure does not rule out eclampsia as the blood pressure may be normal or low due to hemorrhage associated with placental abruption in eclampsia. Hypotension and shock may be associated with amniotic fluid embolism and septic shock.

Temperature is recorded; high-grade fever is associated with an infectious pathology such as meningitis and malaria.

The oral cavity is inspected for tongue bite. The airway is then assessed for any obstruction and is cleared of the blood and secretions with the help of oral suction catheter and an oropharyngeal airway is inserted to prevent tongue bite and facilitate suction.

Both pupils are assessed for symmetry and pupillary reflex. Evidence of pallor, icterus, and cyanosis is looked for. Mild icterus is seen in women with HELLP (H = Hemolysis, EL = Elevated Liver enzymes, LP = Low Platelets) syndrome whereas deep jaundice may be seen in women with fulminant hepatic failure or hepatic encephalopathy. Cyanosis is seen in women with aspiration pneumonia, cyanotic heart disease, and pulmonary edema. The skin is looked for petechiae or ecchymosis as in HELLP, thrombotic thrombocytopenic purpura (TTP), disseminated intravascular coagulation (DIC), and sepsis.

Jugular venous pressure (JVP) may be raised in congestive cardiac failure associated with peripartum cardiomyopathy or rheumatic heart disease. Presence of pedal edema and/or vulvar edema is looked for. It may be associated with eclampsia and/or cardiac failure. Unilateral edema of the leg is often associated with deep vein thrombosis.

Neck rigidity is assessed with the patient lying supine. The neck is passively flexed to touch the chin to the chest. In meningitis, neck flexion causes pain and extensor muscles of neck resist the movement of the neck (Fig. 1).

Calf tenderness or Homan's sign is elicited in suspected deep vein thrombosis. In this, the patient perceives pain on dorsiflexion of foot with the patient lying supine. Kernig's sign is elicited with patient lying supine on bed with legs flexed. The patient's knee is passively extended with hips flexed at 90° angle (Fig. 2). This movement causes pain in hamstrings in women with meningitis affecting lower part of spinal subarachnoid space.

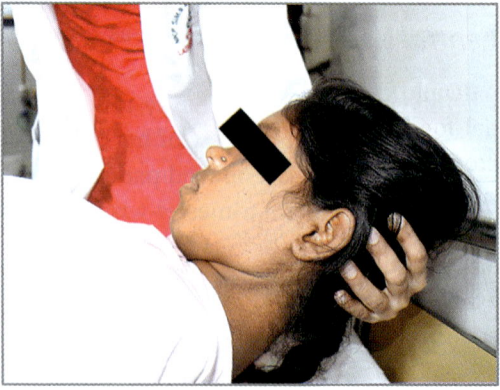

Fig. 1: Neck rigidity.

Chapter 10: Approach to a Pregnant or Puerperal Woman Presenting with Convulsions

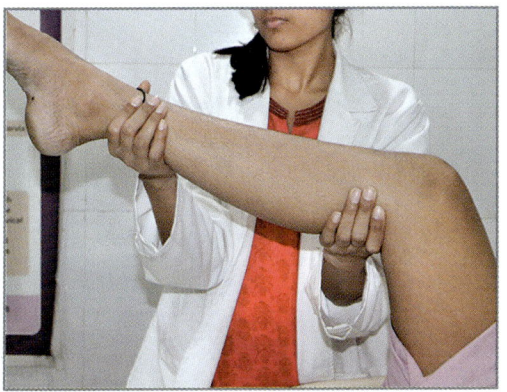

Fig. 2: Kernig's sign.

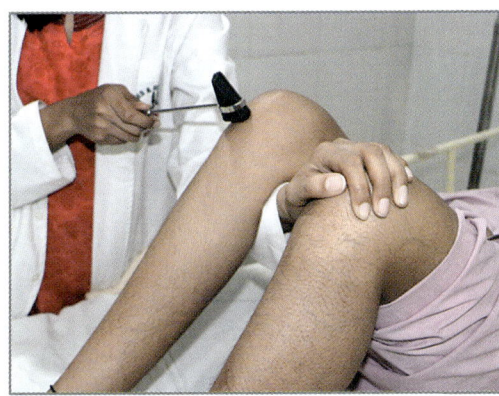

Fig. 3: Knee reflex.

Fundus examination is very useful in detecting the changes of hypertensive retinopathy, papilledema, or retinal detachment.

Systemic Examination

Respiratory System

Chest is auscultated for any crepitation or rhonchi suggestive of aspiration or pulmonary edema. Aspiration pneumonitis is common after convulsions.

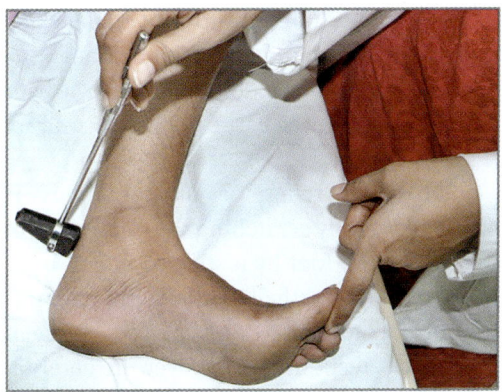

Fig. 4: Ankle reflex.

Cardiovascular System

Look for any evidence of valvular heart disease.

Central Nervous System

A detailed neurological examination is essential for making a diagnosis. This includes a gross motor examination for any weakness suggestive of some focal cerebral lesion.

Deep tendon reflexes including knee, ankle, and biceps jerks are tested. These are exaggerated in eclampsia because of cerebral edema effecting cortical neurons. Hyperreflexia is also seen in upper motor neuron corticospinal lesions.

Knee jerk: Contraction of quadriceps is seen when patellar tendon is tapped. Patient lies in supine position. Examiner's hand is passed under the knee to be tested and placed upon the opposite knee. Knee to be tested rests on the dorsum of observer's wrist. Patellar tendon is struck between its origin and insertion. In normal circumstances, a brief extension of the knee is seen (Fig. 3).

Ankle jerk: Place lower limb on the bed so that it lies everted and slightly flexed. Stretch the Achilles tendon by dorsiflexing the foot. Strike the tendon. Sharp contraction of calf muscles is seen (Fig. 4).

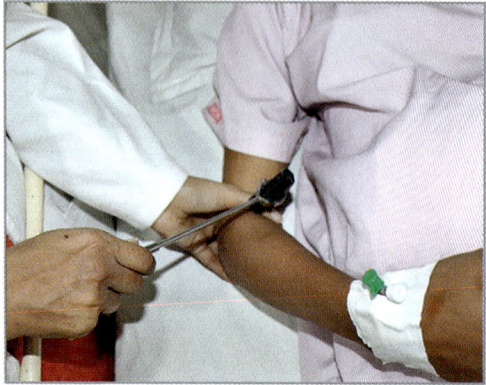

Fig. 5: Biceps reflex.

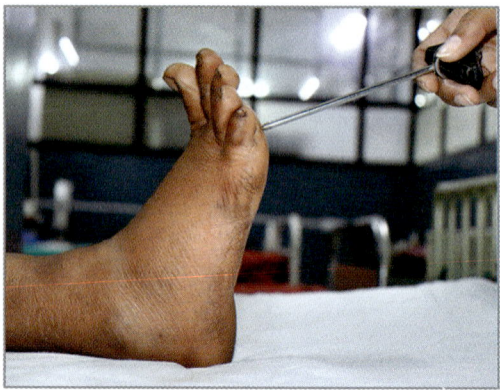

Fig. 6: Planter reflex.

Biceps jerk: Flex the elbow to right angle. Place forearm in semipronated position. Place your own thumb on biceps tendon. Strike it with hammer and biceps can be seen to contract (Fig. 5).

Superficial reflex or plantar reflex is elicited by gently scratching the outer edge of the sole of the foot by a stick or pencil from heel to toe medially along metatarsus. In normal adults, flexion of toes is seen (Babinski's response). However, in cerebral infarction or hemorrhage an extensor response may be seen (Fig. 6).

Abdominal Examination

This includes a complete obstetrical examination as described in the section on Approach to an Antenatal Woman in Chapter 1. The fundal height may be less than the period of gestation, suggestive of fetal growth restriction associated with severe preeclampsia or increased as in women with abruptio placentae. Evidence of tenderness or increase in tone of the uterus is suggestive of abruptio placentae. Fetal heart rate is auscultated as hypoxemia due to convulsions or abruption can cause fetal distress or intrauterine death. Persistence of fetal bradycardia, variable or late deceleration for 30 minutes after an episode of convulsion, may be observed due to seizure-related increased sympathetic tone.[10,11]

Pelvic Examination

Look for any bleeding per vaginum which is suggestive of placental abruption. Per vaginum examination is done only when the patient is stabilized and termination of pregnancy is contemplated.

INVESTIGATIONS

- *Complete blood count with peripheral smear*: Low hemoglobin diagnoses anemia and a raised total and differential leukocyte count points to presence of infection. Low platelet count is associated with DIC, HELLP syndrome, and TTP. However, thrombocytosis may be present in infections. A peripheral smear is helpful in identifying the type of anemia, any evidence of hemolysis, and presence of toxic granules in leukocytes.
- Coagulation profile includes prothrombin time (PT), international normalized ratio (INR), activated partial thromboplastin time (APTT), fibrinogen levels,

and fibrinogen degradation products (FDP) levels.
- Random blood sugar is indicated to rule out hypoglycemia as a cause of convulsions or support the diagnosis of acute fatty liver of pregnancy with encephalopathy.
- Serum electrolyte levels are estimated to rule out metabolic causes of convulsions, namely hyponatremia, hypokalemia, hypocalcemia, hypomagnesemia, and water intoxication.
- Liver and renal function tests are done to rule out any liver or renal dysfunction as a cause of convulsions. These are helpful in the diagnosis and management of conditions such as HELLP, hepatic encephalopathy, chronic hypertension, and preeclampsia.
- VDRL test, ELISA for HIV (enzyme-linked immunosorbent assay for human immunodeficiency viruses), and HBsAg (hepatitis B surface antigen) are offered for detecting neurosyphilis, HIV infection, and hepatitis B, respectively.
- Urine routine, microscopy, and culture sensitivity are done for the presence of albumin suggestive of preeclampsia, urinary tract infections, and/or renal disease.
- 24-hour urinary protein is done for the diagnosis of hypertension with significant proteinuria or preeclampsia.
- Pulse oximetry is important to assess oxygen saturation and if found deranged, arterial blood gas analysis is indicated.
- X-ray chest with abdominal shield is indicated, if pulmonary edema or aspiration is suspected.
- Electrocardiogram (ECG) and echocardiography are essential for suspected heart disease or long-standing hypertension to assess the cardiac size.
- USG is done for fetal biometry, placental localization, amniotic fluid index (AFI), placental grading, estimated fetal weight, and any congenital abnormalities. Known cases of epilepsy on antiepileptic drugs should be specifically screened for congenital anomalies in the fetus.
- Nonstress test is indicated for assessment of fetal well-being after 28 weeks of gestation.
- Electroencephalogram (EEG) may be suggested by a neurologist in women with intractable convulsions.
- Neuroimaging, including CT scan, MRI, and MR angiography, is indicated in suspected cases of trauma, hemorrhage, tumor, tuberculoma, and other space-occupying lesions. CT head shows abnormality in about 30% of women with eclampsia. CT shows hypodensities in cerebral cortex and subcortical white matter located in posterior parietal, occipital, and watershed regions between anterior, middle, and posterior cerebral artery.[12] MRI picks up changes in 46% of eclamptic women. MRI is useful in diagnosing conditions such as multiple sclerosis and cysticercosis whereas MR angiography is indicated in women with suspected cerebral vascular aneurysm or AV malformation.
- Lumbar puncture is indicated in suspected cases of infectious pathology of brain or subarachnoid hemorrhage which may be missed out on neuroimaging.

Neurology consultation should be taken whenever convulsions differ from typical eclamptic convulsion.

MANAGEMENT

The principles of management of eclampsia are given in Box 3.

> **Box 3:** Principles of management of eclampsia.
>
> - Resuscitation
> - General measures
> - *Control of convulsions*: Magnesium sulfate (MgSO$_4$), phenytoin
> - *Control of hypertension*: Labetolol, hydralazine, nifedipine
> - Strict input–output charting
> - Restrict fluid infusion rate to <80 mL/h to avoid pulmonary edema
> - Termination of pregnancy after stabilization

> **Box 4:** Principle of management of epilepsy.
>
> - Resuscitation
> - General measures
> - *Control of seizures*: Intravenous lorazepam 4 mg can be repeated after 15 minutes or phenytoin 20 mg/kg in normal saline over 30 minutes
> - *In pregnant women already on antiepileptics*:
>   - Check for compliance
>   - Readjust dose of antiepileptics
> - *In women with newly detected epilepsy*: Start antiepileptics in consultation with neurophysician. Lamotrigine or levetiracetam are preferred drugs and valproate should be avoided in all situations
> - Folic acid supplementation is continued throughout pregnancy
> - Pregnancy can be continued
> - Woman is warned against activities such as driving and swimming
> - Vitamin K should be given to mother before delivery to prevent hemorrhagic disease of newborn
> - Labor pain relief is important to prevent precipitation of seizures

Magnesium sulfate is drug of choice in the management of eclampsia. Phenytoin and benzodiazepines are considered only when MgSO$_4$ is unavailable or contraindicated as in myasthenia gravis, hypocalcemia, moderate-to-severe renal failure, cardiac ischemia, heart block, or myocarditis.

Magnesium sulfate is given either by Pritchard regime or Zuspan regime.

In Pritchard regime, a loading dose of 14 g is given, 4 g as 20% solution given slow intravenously at the rate of 1 g/min and 5 g as 50% solution deep intramuscular in each buttock followed by a maintenance dose of intermittent injections of 5 g as 50% solution every 4 hourly deep intramuscularly in alternate buttock.

In Zuspan regime, a loading dose of 4 g as 20% solution is given slow intravenously at the rate of 1 g/min followed by a maintenance dose of 1–2 g MgSO$_4$ as infusion.

MgSO$_4$ is continued till 24 hours after delivery or last convulsion, whichever is later.

Signs of MgSO$_4$ toxicity that is absence of deep tendon reflexes, depressed respiration RR < 16 and decreased urine output <25 mL/hr should be ruled out before giving maintenance intramuscular therapy.

The principles of management of epilepsy are given in Box 4.

KEY POINTS

- All women presenting with new onset convulsions in pregnancy after 20 weeks of gestation should be treated as eclampsia.
- Immediate stabilization and early initiation of treatment can prevent associated morbidity and mortality.
- Other causes of convulsions should be ruled out by proper history, clinical examination, and necessary investigations because many of the causes, if not diagnosed, can be life threatening.
- Magnesium sulfate remains the therapy of choice for eclampsia and termination of pregnancy is needed for definitive treatment.

REFERENCES

1. Nobis PN, Hajong A. Eclampsia in India through the decades. J Obstet Gynecol India. 2016;66(S1):S172-6

2. Mattar F, Sibai BM. Eclampsia VIII risk factors for maternal morbidity. Am J Obstet Gynecol. 2000;182(2):307-12.
3. Sibai BM. Prevention of preeclampsia: A major disappointment. Am J Obstet Gynecol. 1998;179:1275-8.
4. Brodie MJ. Management of epilepsy during pregnancy and lactation. Lancet. 1990; 336(8712):426-7.
5. Miller HJ, Hinkley CM. Berry aneurysm in pregnancy: a 10 year report. South Med J. 1970; 63(3):279.
6. Abraham J, Rios PS, Inbaraj SC, Shetty G, Jose CJ. An epidemiological study of hemiplegia due to stroke in south India. Stroke. 1970;1(6):477-81.
7. Trinka E, Cock H, Hesdorffer D, Rossetti AO, Scheffer IE, Shinnar S, et al. A definition and classification of status epilepticus—Report of the ILAE Task Force on Classification of Status Epilepticus. Epilepsia. 2015;56(10):1515-23.
8. ACLS algorithms. 2020, February 2011. ACLS Secondary Survey for a Patient in Respiratory Arrest. Available at: https://www.acls.net/acls-secondary-survey.htm
9. Teasdale G, Jennet B. Assessment of coma and impaired consciousness. A practical scale. Lancet. 1974;2(7872):81-4.
10. Paul RH, Kosh KS, Bernstein SG. Changes in fetal heart rate-uterine contraction patterns associated with eclampsia. Am J Obstet Gynecol. 1978;130(2):165-9.
11. Teramo K, Hiielesmaa V, Bardy A, Saarikoski S. Fetal heart rate during grand mal epileptic seizure, J Perinat Med. 1979;7(1):3-6.
12. Dahmus MA, Barton JR, Sibai BM. Cerebral imaging in eclampsia: magnetic resonance imaging versus computed tomography. Am J Obstet Gynecol. 1992;167(4 Pt 1):935-41.

SUGGESTED READING

1. AAN and AES: Practice parameter update—management issues for women with epilepsy: focus on pregnancy (an evidence based review) (2009, reaffirmed 2013).
2. ACOG practice bulletin number 202. Gestational hypertension and preeclampsia. Obstet Gynecol. 2019;133(1):e1-25.
3. Harden CL, Pennell PB, Koppel BS, Hovinga CA, Gidal B, Meador KJ, et al. Practice Parameter update: Management issues for women with epilepsy—focus on pregnancy (an evidence-based review): Vitamin K, folic acid, blood levels, and breastfeeding: report of the Quality Standards Subcommittee and Therapeutics and Technology Assessment Subcommittee of the American Academy of Neurology and American Epilepsy Society. Neurology. 2009;73(2):142-9.

11
Approach to a Pregnant Woman Presenting with Dyspnea

Richa Aggarwal**

INTRODUCTION

Dyspnea is common in pregnancy. It may be a normal physiological response to pregnancy or may result from an underlying or new, cardiac, or pulmonary disease. Physiological dyspnea of pregnancy occurs in 60–70% of healthy pregnant women presenting early in pregnancy and tends to improve toward term.[1] It is usually worse in the sitting position, not associated with or aggravated by exercise and does not interfere with routine activities of the pregnant woman. The exact cause of shortness of breath during normal pregnancy is not known; it may be due to increased progesterone levels stimulating the respiratory center leading to hyperventilation and an associated fall in arterial carbon dioxide tension (PCO_2). Studies have shown that dyspnea during pregnancy is common in women with a high baseline PCO_2 in nonpregnant state and a low PCO_2 during pregnancy.[2]

A comprehensive understanding of the pregnancy-induced physiological changes in cardiac and respiratory systems are important to differentiate between physiological or pathological causes in a woman presenting with breathlessness in pregnancy.

DIFFERENTIAL DIAGNOSIS

The causes of dyspnea in pregnancy can be broadly divided into three categories: Physiological dyspnea of pregnancy, pathological dyspnea due to conditions specific to pregnancy, and conditions incidental to pregnancy (Table 1).

HISTORY

A detailed history should be obtained from the pregnant woman complaining of breathlessness to establish whether the underlying cause is cardiac or pulmonary. This includes details regarding the onset, progression, timing, and any associated symptoms.

Onset of Breathlessness

If the onset of dyspnea is gradual and no other symptoms are present; it is probably physiological, while sudden-onset dyspnea accompanied with cough, chest pain, or wheezing is more likely to be pathological and requires a detailed evaluation. Conditions such as pulmonary embolism (PE), ischemic heart disease, aortic dissection or arrhythmias, anaphylaxis, pneumothorax, or amniotic fluid embolism present as sudden-onset breathlessness.

Progression of Symptoms

Breathlessness occurring at rest and not worsening with exertion is typical for dyspnea of pregnancy whereas symptoms that occur with exertion and progress on to symptoms at rest usually point toward some pathology.

Table 1: Differential diagnosis of breathlessness in pregnancy.

Physiological	Pregnancy-specific pathological conditions	Pathological conditions incidental to pregnancy

Physiological dyspnea of pregnancy	• Amniotic fluid embolism
	• Pulmonary edema
	• *Preeclampsia*: Uncontrolled hypertension or fluid overload
	• Tocolysis
	• Labor induction with oxytocin
	• Peripartum cardiomyopathy
	• Gestational trophoblastic disease
	• Hydramnios
		Respiratory causes:
		• *Acute pulmonary disease*:
		  – Pneumonia (COVID 19, bacterial)
		  – Pulmonary embolism (PE)
		  – Spontaneous pneumothorax
		  – Acute respiratory distress syndrome (ARDS) related to sepsis, aspiration pneumonitis, massive blood transfusion
		  – Upper airway obstruction as in anaphylaxis
		  – Pleuritis
		• *Chronic pulmonary disease*:
		  – Asthma
		  – Tuberculosis
		  – Cystic fibrosis
		  – Sarcoidosis
		Cardiac causes:
		• Ischemic heart disease
		• Valvular heart disease
		• Cardiomyopathy
		• Arrhythmias
		Hematological diseases:
		• Severe anemia
		Drug-related:
		• Nitrofurantoin
		• Aspirin
		• Cocaine
		Metabolic:
		• Diabetic ketoacidosis
		• Uremia
		• Thyrotoxicosis
		Psychological:
		• Anxiety
		Others:
		• Carbon monoxide poisoning
		• Chest trauma with rib fracture
		• Neuromuscular disease
		• Stroke
		• Ascitis

Timing of Breathlessness (in Relation to Gestation)

Breathlessness starting in early pregnancy and getting better towards term suggests dyspnea of pregnancy whereas that which starts in mid-trimester and progresses is likely to be due to cardiac disease or asthma. While breathlessness developing during labor or shortly after delivery suggests aspiration pneumonitis, PE, pulmonary edema, amniotic fluid embolism, or high-level epidural block.

Pneumothorax should be suspected if the pregnant woman develops severe chest pain and breathlessness in labor. If breathlessness first develops in last month of pregnancy or within 5 months postpartum, peripartum cardiomyopathy is a strong differential diagnosis.

Associated Symptoms

Cough

Acute cough usually indicates acute respiratory tract infection but may be an acute exacerbation of an underlying chronic obstructive pulmonary disease (COPD) or rarely PE. Chronic cough is often due to asthma or tuberculosis. It is important to know if the cough is productive or not. If productive, the nature of sputum needs to be asked. Copious frothy sputum is characteristic of pulmonary edema, while purulent sputum is present in infective etiologies such as bronchopneumonia, lung abscess, or bronchiectasis. Blood-stained sputum is suggestive of tuberculosis or pulmonary edema.

Wheezing

Cough and wheezing are common symptoms of asthma and cardiac disease with pulmonary venous hypertension.

Chest Pain

Presence of breathlessness and chest pain usually indicates cardiac disease including coronary artery disease, arrhythmias, or aortic dissection. Sudden-onset chest pain is also seen in spontaneous pneumothorax or PE.

Orthopnea

A certain degree of orthopnea is expected in late pregnancy due to diaphragmatic elevation. Progressive orthopnea associated with paroxysmal nocturnal dyspnea may be suggestive of left ventricular dysfunction or diaphragmatic dysfunction/paralysis.

Other History

History of palpitations and syncopal attacks, if present, indicates cardiac etiology of breathlessness. History of swelling over lower limbs or all over the body may be due to severe anemia with hypoproteinemia or congestive cardiac failure.

Past History

History of previous episodes of breathlessness and wheezing, especially with change in season, is typical of asthma. History of recurrent pulmonary infection and bronchiectasis is common in patients with cystic fibrosis. History of calf pain and swelling of lower limbs preceding breathlessness points toward deep vein thrombosis (DVT) as the possible etiology. History of massive blood transfusion raises the possibility of acute respiratory distress syndrome (ARDS). History suggestive of pyelonephritis should be sought, since as many as 10% of cases of pyelonephritis in pregnancy develop ARDS.[3,4]

Obstetric History

In a patient with history of high blood pressure (BP) records presenting with dyspnea, pulmonary edema should be strongly suspected as up to 3% of patients with preeclampsia develop pulmonary edema.[5]

Drug History

A careful drug history should be obtained because drug-induced pneumonitis is a rare but reversible cause of respiratory failure and has been reported to occur with nitrofurantoin.[6] Beta adrenergic agonists, ritodrine and terbutaline, used for tocolysis, especially in women with multiple pregnancy, might cause pulmonary edema in 0.3–9% of cases.[7] Administration of glucocorticoids in preterm labor can also result in fluid retention with resultant breathlessness.

Personal History

History of smoking and substance abuse, especially of cocaine and heroin, should be enquired. A vast majority of patients with cocaine-induced pulmonary edema develop severe pulmonary hypertension.

Family History

Family history of tuberculosis, asthma, and/or allergies should be elicited.

Occupational History

Occupational history should be asked in detail to find out the possible exposure to animal, mineral, or vegetable allergens.

EXAMINATION

A thorough physical examination can provide important clues to the etiology of breathlessness.

General Physical Examination

A complete general physical examination is performed, and it should include the following points:
- *Gait*: Patient's gait should be observed as kyphosis and/or scoliosis can cause respiratory failure due to decreased lung capacity, atelectasis, and fatigue of respiratory muscles due to overwork. Scoliotic pregnant woman with a primary curve of >25° may worsen in pregnancy, whereas those with lesser curves remain unaffected.[8]
- *Pulse*: Tachycardia is present in the setting of hypoxia associated with cardiac or pulmonary causes of dyspnea.
- *Respiration*: Presence of tachypnea, i.e. increased respiratory rate is suggestive of underlying cardiac, pulmonary, or neuromuscular disease. Presence of paradoxical breathing, i.e., breathing movements where all or part of the chest wall moves in during inspiration and out on expiration or the use of accessory muscles of respiration (sternomastoid, scalene, trapezius, and alae nasi) should be carefully looked for as it might suggest impending respiratory failure.
- *Temperature*: Fever, if present, suggests an infective etiology.
- *Blood pressure*: Dyspnea with high BP records suggests pulmonary edema secondary to preeclampsia.
- *Pallor*: Pallor should be looked for ascertaining anemia as the cause of breathlessness.
- *Cyanosis and clubbing*: These are seen in chronic cardiac or pulmonary diseases.
- *Jugular venous pressure (JVP)*: It is raised in normal pregnancy, fluid overload, or ventricular dysfunction.
- *Other general examination*: Neck should be observed for any thyroid swelling or any scars, or sinuses suggestive of tubercular lymphadenopathy. Presence of bilateral pedal edema is normal in the latter half of pregnancy, but it may be a sign of heart failure or hypoproteinemia.

Examination of the Respiratory System

Inspection

A careful examination of respiratory system should begin with an overall inspection. Shape of the chest should be observed, as kyphosis or scoliosis may decrease the size of the thoracic cavity and restrict lung movements. Normally, both sides of the chest wall move uniformly. Unilateral diminished movements are seen in obstruction to the main bronchus, consolidation, or fibrosis of the lung or massive lung collapse.

Percussion

Percussion should be performed carefully and methodically. Presence of impaired note on percussion suggests consolidation, infiltration, fibrosis, or collapse. The percussion note is hyperresonant in pneumothorax, emphysema, or a large cavity. Classically, the note is stony dull over pleural effusion.

Auscultation

Auscultation of the chest should be done to note the type of breathing and presence of any adventitious sounds. Normal breath sounds are vesicular in character. Bronchial breath sounds suggest underlying consolidation, cavity, or collapse. Rhonchi or wheezing may be present in cases of bronchial asthma, chronic bronchitis or cardiac failure. Crepts are heard in cases of pneumonia, pulmonary edema or pulmonary fibrosis. Fine basal crepts suggestive of pulmonary congestion are an early sign of pulmonary edema or left heart failure. Coarse crepts usually indicate presence of chest infection.

Examination of the Cardiovascular System

The diagnosis of heart disease in pregnancy is difficult as many physiological changes of normal pregnancy mimic heart disease. Signs such as systolic murmurs, accentuated respiratory effort, and pedal edema may occur in normal pregnancy. Clinical findings such as cyanosis, clubbing of nails, distended neck veins, presence of thrill, systolic murmur greater than grade 2/6, diastolic murmur, cardiomegaly, and persistent arrhythmia suggest heart disease.

INVESTIGATIONS

When clinical evaluation leads the clinician to suspect that a patient's breathlessness is due to more than just the pregnancy, the clinician should be confident that all the relevant diagnostic imaging procedures for investigating other causes of breathlessness can be safely performed during pregnancy. Flowchart 1 outlines the diagnostic approach to a pregnant woman presenting with breathlessness. Once the diagnosis is made proper management can be initiated at the earliest according to the etiology (Table 2).

To maintain a high standard of safety, particularly when imaging potentially pregnant patients, imaging radiation must be applied at levels as low as reasonably achievable (ALARA), while the degree of medical benefit must counterbalance the well-managed levels of risk. It is important to note that even a combination of chest radiography, lung scintigraphy (V/Q scan), computed tomographic (CT) pulmonary angiography, and traditional pulmonary angiography exposes the fetus to around 1.5 m Gy of radiation, which is well below the accepted limit of 50 mGy for the induction of detrimental effects in the fetus.

Complete Blood Count

Complete blood count is helpful in identifying cases of dyspnea attributable to severe anemia. Raised total leukocyte count and neutrophilia indicate an infective pathology such as pyelonephritis or pneumonia.

Kidney Function Tests

Kidney function tests are done to rule out renal failure or as baseline, if the woman must be prescribed aminoglycosides in the presence of infection.

Flowchart 1: Algorithm of clinical approach to a pregnant woman with dyspnea.

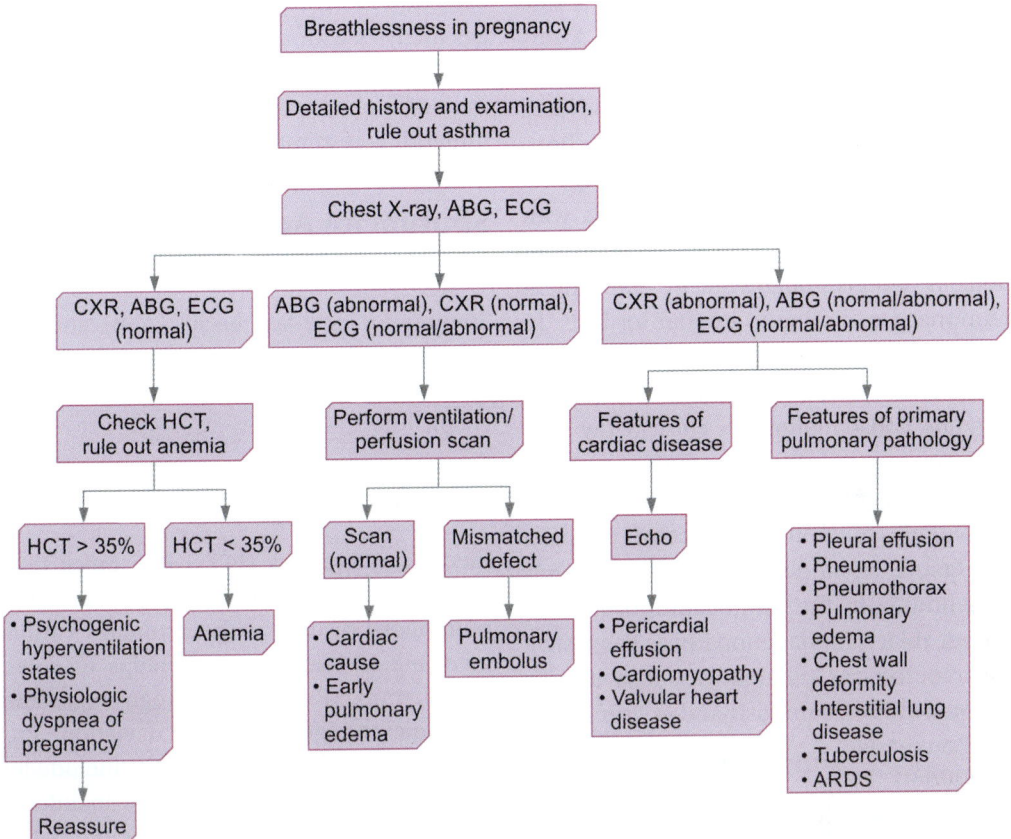

(ABG: arterial blood gas; ARDS: acute respiratory distress syndrome; CXR: chest X-ray; ECG: electrocardiography; Echo: echocardiogram; HCT: hematocrit)

Thyroid Function Tests

Thyroid function tests are carried out to rule out thyrotoxicosis, as breathlessness is a common symptom in patients of thyrotoxicosis.

Urine Examination

Urinalysis and urine culture are done, if breathlessness is associated with fever and urinary symptoms and pyelonephritis is suspected.

Oxygen Saturation Measurement

Oxygen saturation (SpO_2) measurement is the simplest and quickest test of oxygenation in the presence of breathlessness. Measurement of SpO_2 by pulse oximetry with moderate exertion can be used to rule out serious causes of dyspnea in pregnancy. If the SpO_2 remains normal (>95%) on exercise, it is unlikely that the patient has any major problem. Demonstration to the patient that her oxygenation is maintained, despite the feeling of dyspnea can also help alleviate patient's anxiety about her symptoms.

Chest X-ray

Chest X-ray should be done, if indicated with abdominal shield to protect the fetus from unnecessary exposure to irradiation. A radiation exposure of up to 5 rads is safe for the fetus and in a routine chest X-ray, it is 0.01 rads.[9] Radiographic changes in a normal pregnant woman include elevated diaphragmatic domes due to enlarged uterus, with upward and lateral displacement of the heart and short, wide lung fields with prominent vascular markings. The left upper cardiac border is straightened by a prominent pulmonary trunk due to lumbar lordosis. In the lateral view, there may be an increase in the anteroposterior diameter.[10]

Lung consolidation on chest X-ray suggests pneumonia. Pleural effusion may be present in conditions such as tuberculosis, pneumonia, pulmonary infarction, and cardiac failure. Small pleural effusion is a common finding in the immediate postpartum period. Hilar lymphadenopathy is suggestive of sarcoidosis or tuberculosis. It is usually symmetrical in sarcoidosis and asymmetrical in tuberculosis.

Spirometry

It is useful in the diagnosis of asthma and is safe in pregnancy. Improvement in airflow obstruction after administration of inhalational bronchodilators confirms the diagnosis of asthma.

Arterial Blood Gas Analysis

The arterial pH is slightly alkaline in pregnancy; it ranges between 7.40 and 7.47. This is consequent to progesterone-induced hyperventilation and respiratory alkalosis. The arterial pCO_2 falls and ranges between 27 and 32 mm Hg during pregnancy, whereas the arterial oxygen tension (pO_2) increases to 101–104 mm Hg in third trimester. Respiratory alkalosis is followed by compensatory renal excretion of bicarbonate. Therefore, a blood gas analysis with a PaO_2 of 80 mm Hg and a $PaCO_2$ of 40 mm Hg in a pregnant woman is markedly abnormal and can even represent impending respiratory failure.

Sputum for Acid-fast Bacilli and Culture

Sputum for acid-fast bacilli (AFB) and culture sensitivity is indicated in woman with breathlessness along with fever and productive cough.

Electrocardiography

Electrocardiography (ECG) is a quick noninvasive test performed to rule out cardiac or pulmonary disease with secondary cardiac involvement such as PE. It helps to detect rate, rhythm, ST or T wave changes suggesting ischemic changes, and axis deviation. Pregnancy-induced changes in ECG include left axis deviation, mild ST changes in inferior leads, and atrial and ventricular premature contractions.[11]

Two-dimensional Echocardiography

Two-dimensional echocardiography helps to diagnose cardiac disorders such as left or right ventricular dysfunction, cardiomyopathy, valvular or congenital heart disease, and pulmonary hypertension. Physiological echocardiographic findings in pregnancy include mild tricuspid regurgitation and significantly increased left atrial size and left ventricular outflow cross-sectional area, slight increase in systolic function, and small pericardial effusions.[12]

Plasma Brain Natriuretic Peptide or N-terminal pro-Brain Natriuretic Peptide

Brain natriuretic peptide (BNP) is useful in differentiating pregnant women with dyspnea due to cardiac cause from those with pulmonary cause. Its levels are not affected by pregnancy. The normal levels are <50 pg/mL. Its levels are raised in dyspnea due to heart failure usually to >400 pg/mL. Values of <100 pg/mL are associated with high negative predictive value.

D-dimer

D-dimer is used as a screening test for venous thromboembolism (VTE) in nonpregnant women and has a high negative predictive value. However, its levels are elevated in normal pregnancy and associated conditions such as preeclampsia; hence, it has limited utility in the diagnosis of PE in pregnancy.[13]

Proximal Vein Compression Ultrasonography (CUS)

This test is performed as the initial test if symptoms and signs such as pain, swelling, and redness in legs suggestive of deep vein thrombosis are present. A positive test is enough to stop any more evaluation and is an indication for initiating treatment for PE; however, a negative compression ultrasonography (CUS) indicates further imaging. This test has the advantage of avoiding exposure to radiation and administration of contrast in pregnant women.

Ventilation Perfusion Scan (Pulmonary Scintigraphy)

This is a reliable noninvasive test to diagnose PE if the chest X-ray is normal. V/Q scan result is stratified in to normal, low, moderate, or high probability of risk. Normal or high probability scans are considered reliable whereas low and moderate probability scans are indeterminate. Abnormal chest X-ray is an important cause for an indeterminate report of V/Q scan. The prevalence of PE in this group ranges from 21 to 40%.[14] Pulmonary angiography may be performed in these women to confirm the diagnosis. Perfusion scanning alone is recommended initially and the ventilation scan is added when perfusion defects are noted.

The major advantage of V/Q scan over CT pulmonary angiography is the lower radiation dose to the maternal breast; its major disadvantage is its inability to provide an alternative diagnosis in the absence of PE. Majority of V/Q scans in pregnant women (70–90%) are diagnostic.

Computed Tomography Pulmonary Angiography

Computed tomography pulmonary angiography (CTPA) is a sensitive and specific test for the diagnosis of PE. It is used to rule out PE and helps with the evaluation of pulmonary parenchyma. Additional advantage in cases of PE is that it provides clues of the clot burden and even some prognostic information about the right ventricle. CT chest helps in evaluating the mediastinum, the parenchyma and the airways. This is helpful in diagnosing lung and mediastinal masses as well as interstitial lung disease.

Pulmonary Angiogram

Pulmonary angiogram, although considered the gold standard for the diagnosis of PE but is rarely used now a days with the advent of CTPA.

Magnetic Resonance Imaging

Magnetic resonance (MR) imaging has potential advantages for imaging the pregnant population due to its lack of ionizing radiation and the absence of proven harmful effects to the mother or fetus. MR imaging may be valuable in pregnant women with known allergy to iodinated contrast material in whom a V/Q scan is interpreted as intermediate probability or when a low-probability study is coupled with a high clinical suspicion for PE. However, this investigation is not validated for pregnancy.

Pulmonary Function Testing

Pulmonary function testing (PFT) is a routine investigation in the management of chronic and acute asthma. Forced expiratory volume in 1 second (FEV1) and peak expiratory flow rate (PEFR) are two useful investigations to assess the severity of airway obstruction. FEV1 of < 1 L correlates with severe disease.[15] PEFR correlates very well with FEV1 and can be measured dependably with low-cost portable peak flow meters. FVC (forced vital capacity) increases significantly after 14–16 weeks of gestation and throughout pregnancy. PEF

Table 2: Management of common causes of acute dyspnea in pregnancy.

Disease	History	Laboratory	Interventions
Physiological dyspnea in normal pregnancy	• Needs to take a deep breath intermittently • Inability to get a deep enough breath • Not associated with wheeze or cough	Normal PO_2 and arterial pH value	Reassurance
Asthma/airway disease	• History of recurrent cough/dyspnea/ nocturnal dyspnea/ wheezing	• Spirometry, pre- and post- bronchodilator • Hypoxic or hypercapnic respiratory failure in severe cases	Inhalational beta 2 agonists ± inhalational steroids
Pulmonary edema	• Nocturnal dyspnea/ wheezing • Cardiomegaly/gallop rhythm/valvular disease • Tocolytic therapy	• *Chest X-ray*: Cardiomegaly, interstitial edema, perihilar consolidation • *Echocardiography*: Mitral or aortic valve disease, left ventricular dilation or hypertrophy, hypocontractile left ventricle (peripartum cardiomyopathy)	• Diuretics • Antihypertensives NTG infusion if high BP • Inotropes if cardiomyopathy
Pulmonary embolism	• Sudden onset of dyspnea/wheezing any trimester • May have associated features of DVT	• Arterial hypoxemia/ Abnormal perfusion on ventilation • Lower extremity Doppler • V/Q scan • Computed tomography pulmonary angiogram (CTPA)	Anticoagulation with injectable heparins in pregnancy, warfarin in the postpartum period
Amniotic fluid embolism	• Sudden onset dyspnea • History of delivery, CS, abortion in last 24–48 hrs • Bleeding from various sites	Disseminated intravascular coagulation/ demonstration of fetal elements in the maternal circulation	• Supportive
Cardiac disease Myocardial/Valvular dysfunction	• Sudden onset of dyspnea chest pain palpitations • Known case of valvular disease	ECG and echocardiogram	• Diuretics, beta-blockers as indicated • ACE inhibitors contraindicated in pregnancy

(PO_2: partial pressure of oxygen in arterial blood)

(peak expiratory flow) increases significantly during healthy pregnancies and should be interpreted cautiously in pregnant women with impaired lung function. Any change in FEV1 (forced expiratory volume in 1 second) during pregnancy however can be ascribed to the pulmonary disease, as FEV1 remains unchanged during a normal pregnancy.

MANAGEMENT

The management of common causes of acute onset breathlessness in pregnancy are described in Table 2.

KEY POINTS

- Breathlessness is a common symptom in pregnancy and is usually physiological.
- It may be insightful of some serious underlying cardiac or pulmonary pathology such as pulmonary edema, thromboembolism, pneumonia, and asthma associated with adverse fetomaternal outcomes.
- A thorough evaluation of a woman presenting with dyspnea is warranted to rule out all serious pathological conditions before attributing this symptom to normal physiological changes of pregnancy.
- Diagnostic imaging tests clearly play an important role in the evaluation of dyspnea in pregnant patients but should be performed with careful attention to minimize radiation risk. The treating physician should be familiar with the relative advantages and disadvantages of available imaging modalities, radiation risks, and risk management guidelines.
- Radiation doses resulting from most diagnostic procedures present no substantial risk of causing fetal death, malformation, or impairment of mental development.

REFERENCES

1. Gibson PS, Powrei RO. Respiratory disease. In: James D, Steer PJ, Weiner CP, Gonik B (Eds). High Risk Pregnancy: Management Options, 4th edition. St Louis: Elsevier; 2011. pp. 657-82.
2. Hytten FE, Leitch I. The Physiology of Human Pregnancy, 2nd edition. Oxford: Blackwell Scientific; 1971.
3. Goodrun LA. Pneumonia in pregnancy. Semin Perinatol. 1997;21(4):276-83.
4. de Veciana M, Towers CV, Major CA, Lien JM, Toohey JS. Pulmonary injury associated with appendicitis in pregnancy: Who is at risk? Am J Obstet Gynecol. 1994;171(4):1008-13.
5. Sibai BM, Mabie BC, Harvey CJ, Gonzalez AR.. Pulmonary edema in severe preeclampsia-eclampsia: analysis of thirty-seven consecutive cases. Am J Obstet Gynecol. 1987;156(5):1174-9.
6. Powrie RO. Acute lung injury. In: Lee RV, Rosene-Montella K, Barbour LA (Eds). Medical Care of the Pregnant Patient, 2nd edition. Philadelphia: American College of Physicians; 2000. pp. 397-411.
7. Bandi VD, Mannur U, Matthay MA. Acute lung injury and acute respiratory distress syndrome in pregnancy. Crit Care Clin. 2004;20:577-607.
8. de Swiet M. The respiratory system. In: Hytten FE, Chamberlain G (Eds). Clinical Physiology in Obstetrics, 2nd edition. Oxford: Blackwell; 1991. p.83.
9. ACOG Committee on Obstetric Practice. ACOG Committee Opinion. Number 299, September 2004 (replaces No. 158, September 1995). Guidelines for diagnostic imaging during pregnancy. 2004; 104(3):647-51.
10. Bourjeily G, Khalil H, Paglia MJ. Approach to shortness of breath in pregnancy. In: Powrie RO, Greene MF, Camann W (Eds). de Swiet's Medical Disorders in Obstetric practice, 5th edition. Oxford: Blackwell;2010. pp. 689-94.
11. Carruth JE, Mivis SB, Brogan DR. The electrocardiogram in normal pregnancy. Am Heart J. 1981;102:1075-8.

12. Yuan L, DuanY, Cao T. Echocardiographic study of cardiac morphological and functional changes before and after parturition in pregnancy-induced hypertension. Echocardiography. 2006;23(3):177-82.
13. Marik PE, Plante LA. Venous thromboembolic disease and pregnancy. N Engl J Med. 2008; 359(19):2025-33.
14. PIOPED investigators: Value of ventilation/perfusion scan in acute pulmonary embolism: Results of the Prospective Investigation of Pulmonary Embolism Diagnosis (PIOPED). JAMA. 1990;263(20):2753-9.
15. Noble PW, Lavee AE, Jacobs NM. Respiratory diseases in pregnancy. Obstet Gynecol Clin North Am. 1988;15(2):391-428.

SUGGESTED READING

1. Greer I, Thomson AJ. (2015). Thromboembolic disease in pregnancy and the puerperium: acute management (Green-top Guideline No. 37b). [online] Available from https://www.rcog.org.uk/globalassets/documents/guidelines/gtg-37b.pdf. [Last accessed January, 2020].
2. Grindheim G, Toska K, Estensin M, Rosseland I. Changes in pulmonary function during pregnancy: a longitudinal cohort study. BJOG. 2012;119:94-101.
3. Murphy VE. Managing asthma in pregnancy. Breathe (Sheff). 2015;11(4):258-67.
4. Regitz-Zagrosek V, Roos-Hesselink JW, Bauersachs J, et al. Guidelines for the management of cardiovascular diseases during pregnancy. Eur Heart J. 2018;39(34): 3165-241.
5. Wan T, Skeith L, Karovitch A, Rodger M, Gal GL. Guidance for the diagnosis of pulmonary embolism during pregnancy: Consensus and controversies. Thromb Res. 2017;157:23-8.

12. Approach to a Pregnant Woman Presenting with Pruritus

Ritu Sharma, Vibhu Mendiratta

INTRODUCTION

Pruritus or itching is the most common dermatological complaint in pregnancy with a reported prevalence of 14–20% in all pregnancies.[1] It may be physiological or pathological, signaling the onset of specific dermatoses of pregnancy or onset or exacerbation of coincidental or preexisting dermatoses which are not specific to pregnancy. Dermatosis specific to pregnancy are more common. The most common being atopic eruption of pregnancy (AEP) and most specific being pemphigoid gestationis (PG).[2,3] The preexisting skin diseases may either worsen (lupus erythematosus) or improve (psoriasis) due to pregnancy-related immunological and hormonal alterations. Some of the dermatoses are associated with fetal compromise. In case where all causes of pruritus have been ruled out, pruritus in pregnancy is labeled as physiological pruritus occurring as a result of abdominal stretching, edema of legs, and xerosis.

Table 1: Differential diagnosis of pruritus in pregnancy.[2-4]

Dermatosis specific to pregnancy	Dermatosis nonspecific to pregnancy
Physiological: • Xerosis • Stretching of skin • Edema *Pathological:* • Atopic eruption of pregnancy (AEP) • Polymorphic eruption of pregnancy (PEP) • Pemphigoid gestationis (PG) • Intrahepatic cholestasis of pregnancy (ICP)	*Preexisting dermatosis:* • Atopic dermatitis, lichen planus, lichen sclerosis, ichthyosis, urticaria, bullous pemphigoid, and psoriasis *Infections:* • Varicella, hepatitis A, B, C, vulvovaginal candidiasis, tinea, folliculitis *Infestations:* • Scabies, and pediculosis *Systemic diseases:* • Renal, diabetes, thyroid, anemia, malabsorption, malignancies, and liver diseases *Contact dermatitis:* • Allergic and irritant contact dermatitis • Drugs *Neurogenic:* • Peripheral neuritis, brain tumor • Psychogenic

DIFFERENTIAL DIAGNOSIS

Pruritus in pregnancy can be broadly divided into dermatoses specific to pregnancy or dermatoses nonspecific to pregnancy (Table 1). Pregnancy specific dermatosis includes four types: Pemphigoid gestationis (PG), polymorphic eruption of pregnancy (PEP), atopic eruption of pregnancy (AEP), and intrahepatic cholestasis of pregnancy (ICP).[2-4] PG is an autoimmune disorder caused by antibodies against bullous pemphigoid (BP) antigen or against collagen in the basement zone of skin and placental membranes. PEP is an inflammatory disorder caused by release of antigens due to the damage to the connective tissue in response to excessive stretching of abdominal wall. AEP is an immunological disorder flared up in pregnancy due to increase in T helper 2 to T helper 1 ratio. Etiology in ICP includes genetic, hormonal, and environmental factors. Raised estrogen levels lead to cholestasis. One must take proper history, do thorough examination, and order relevant investigations to reach the correct diagnosis (Flowchart 1).

HISTORY

Taking a detailed and focused history is very important as it can give important clues to clinch the diagnosis.

Flowchart 1: Algorithm for clinical approach to a pregnant woman with pruritus.

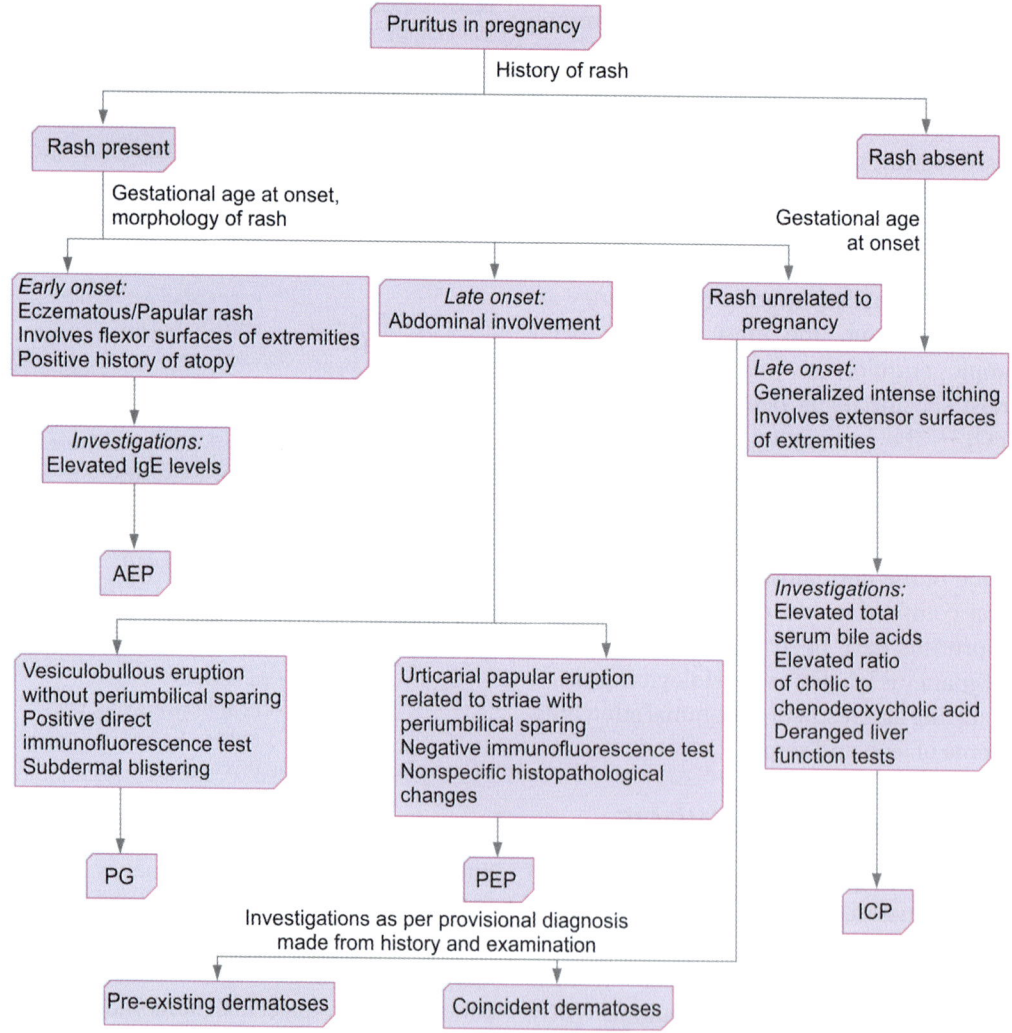

(AEP: atopic eruption of pregnancy; ICP: intrahepatic cholestasis of pregnancy; IgE: immunoglobulin E; PEP: polymorphic eruption of pregnancy; PG: pemphigoid gestationis)

Chapter 12: Approach to a Pregnant Woman Presenting with Pruritus

History of Present Illness

The following points need to be elaborated upon in the history of presenting complaint that is pruritus:

- *Time of onset*: Onset of symptoms in late pregnancy occurs in PG, PEP, and ICP, while AEP manifests in early pregnancy, i.e., before third trimester. In case of nonspecific dermatoses, lesions may be present before pregnancy or may appear at any time during pregnancy.
- *Presence of skin lesions*: Majority of dermatoses present with rash as a prominent feature, except ICP, where severe generalized itching without rash is characteristic. It is more at night involving extensor surfaces of extremities, especially palms and soles. Transient lesions without blistering are present in urticaria.
- *Site and spread of lesions*: Ask the pregnant woman regarding the initial site of onset and spread of rash, as different types of dermatoses are associated with definite patterns of rash (Table 2). Predominant abdominal involvement is there in case of PG and PEP, with periumbilical sparing in PEP. In AEP, trunk and flexor surfaces of limbs are involved including face and neck and in ICP, palms, soles, and extensor surfaces of the extremities are involved. Extremities are involved in insect bite, erythema nodosum, ICP, and AEP.
- *History of fever*: This gives a clue that the rash may be due to drug reaction or infection such as chickenpox.
- *Relation with weather*: Tiny vesicles on trunk and extremities appearing in hot weather are suggestive of miliaria.

Table 2: Characteristics of rash in various dermatoses.[4-8]

Pemphigoid gestationis (PG) (Figs. 1A and B)	Polymorphic eruption of pregnancy (PEP) (Figs. 2A and B)	Intrahepatic cholestasis of pregnancy (ICP) (Figs. 3A to D)	Atopic eruption of pregnancy (AEP) (Figs. 4A and B)	Others
Lesions: Prebullous stage: Urticarial, erythematous papules and plaques Bullous stage: Vesiculobullous eruption	Lesions: Initially urticarial papules appear followed by polymorphous features in >50% of patients (urticaria 49%, vesicles 17%, target lesions 6%, and eczema 22%)	Lesions: Initially generalized pruritus appears without primary lesions Secondary skin lesions due to scratching range from excavations to prurigo nodules	Lesions: About 20% present as exacerbated preexisting dermatitis and 80% present with onset for first time Two thirds have E-type or eczematous AEP; One third have P-type or papular AEP	Insect bite: Lesions are present on extremities Scabies: Linear papules appear in finger webs, elbows, areola, and genitals Pityriasis rosea: Herald patch (oval, slightly scaly plaque) on trunk
Site: Typical abdominal involvement including umbilical region, Face and mucus membranes spared	Site: Papules appear within striae gravidarum on the abdomen with periumbilical sparing, face, neck, palms, and soles are usually spared	Site: Typically involves palms, soles, and extensor surfaces of extremities; nocturnal pruritus is common	Site: Involve trunk, limbs (flexor surfaces), face, and neck	Chicken pox: Small red spots appear on face, scalp, chest, upper arm, and legs progressing to blisters and pustules followed by umbilication and scab formation

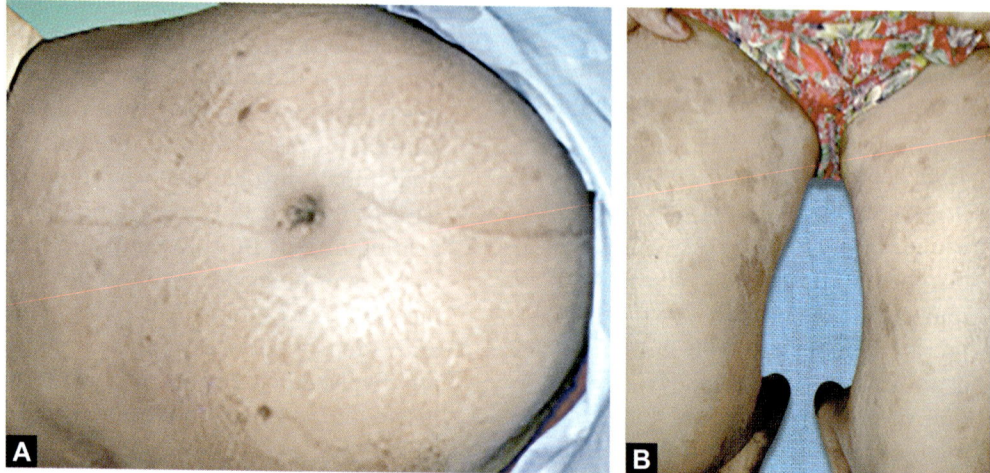

Figs. 1A and B: Pemphigoid gestationis. (A) Prebullous stage of pemphigoid gestationis involving umbilicus at 32 weeks' gestation; (B) Bullous stage of pemphigoid gestationis.

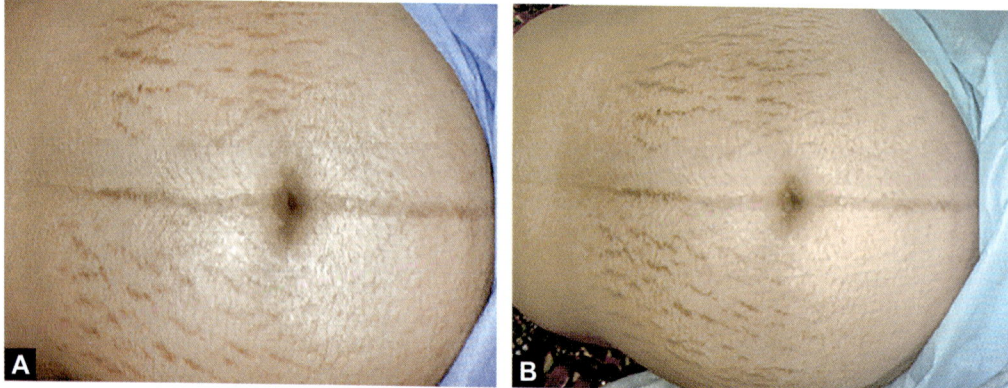

Figs. 2A and B: Polymorphic eruption of pregnancy at 37 weeks with dark red, urticated striae distensae with typical periumbilical sparing.

Psoriasis also shows seasonal variation becoming worse in winter. ICP in some studies has shown increased incidence in winter.
- *History of nausea and vomiting*: This may be associated with hyperemesis gravidarum, preeclampsia, ICP, and liver disorders.
- *History of hypertension*: This is associated with preeclampsia and deranged liver enzymes.
- *History of jaundice*: The patient should be asked about the color of urine and stool and yellowish discoloration of skin and mucous membranes. Positive history can be elicited in liver disorders coincidental with pregnancy and in 10–20% cases of ICP. Jaundice in ICP follows pruritus.
- *History of upper abdominal pain*: This may be present in women with preeclampsia, acute fatty liver of pregnancy, cholelithiasis, ICP, and bile duct obstruction.

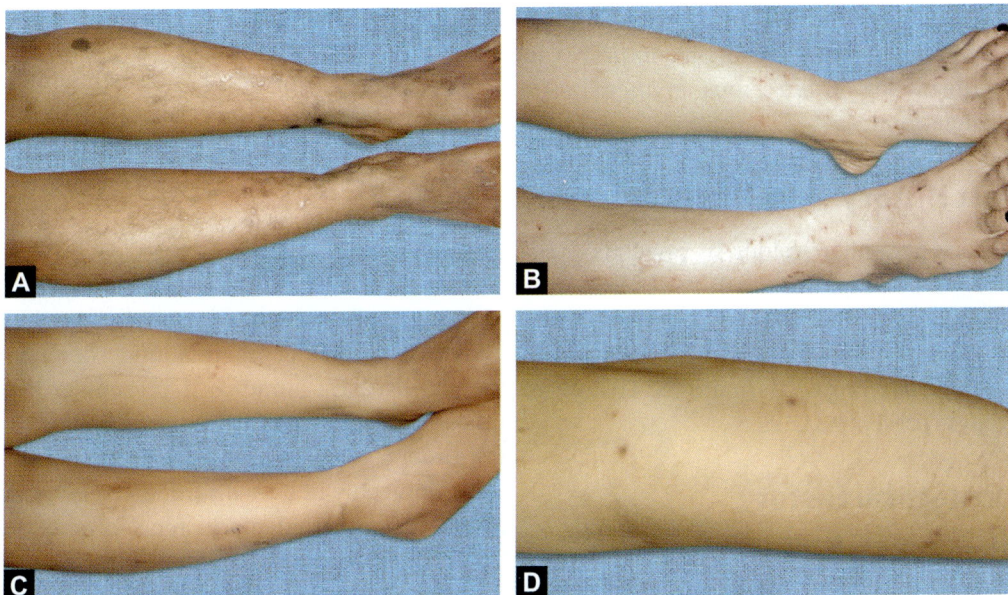

Figs. 3A to D: Intrahepatic cholestasis of pregnancy at 34 weeks' gestation with secondary skin lesions. (A and B) Secondary skin lesions ranging from excoriation to prurigo nodules on extensor surface of lower limbs; (C) Secondary lesions especially excoriation marks on extensor surface of lower limbs; (D) Secondary skin lesions (papules) on extensor surface of upper limbs.

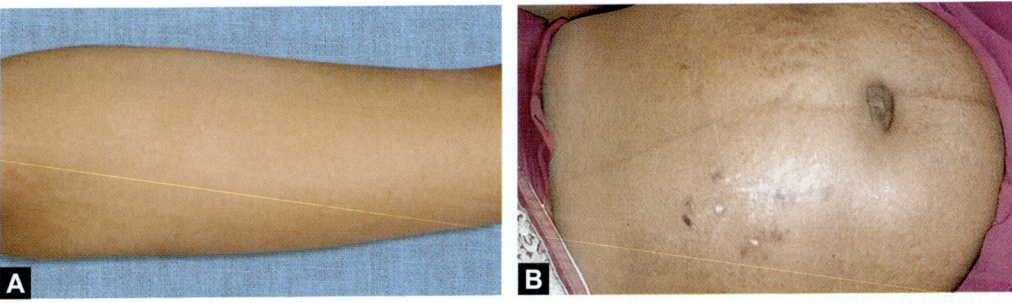

Figs. 4A and B: Atopic eruption of pregnancy (AEP). (A) With small papular eruptions and erythematous rash P-type AEP involving flexor aspect of upper limb; (B) With eczematous rash E-type AEP involving abdomen at 35 weeks' gestation.

- *History of insect bite*: This is suggestive of rash in response to the bite.
- *History of drug intake or contact to allergens*: This helps to diagnose drug-induced dermatitis and contact dermatitis, respectively.
- *History of passage of worms in stool*: Positive history may suggest pruritus in response to intestinal worm infestation.
- *Course of dermatoses*: It is important to note whether the pruritus and rash have improved or worsened with advancing gestation. The PG improves at term only to flare up at the time of delivery and resolves within weeks to months postpartum, whereas PEP resolves within 4–6 weeks after delivery. Pruritus in ICP resolves after delivery within few days

(usually within 1–2 days) and jaundice within 2–4 weeks. Psoriasis improves in pregnancy, while lupus erythematosus deteriorates.

Past History

History of similar lesions in previous pregnancy may be present in ICP, PG, and AEP. Positive history of similar lesions in past, irrespective of pregnancy, can be elicited in nonspecific chronic dermatoses. History of atopy is present in AEP.

Obstetrical History

Polymorphic eruption of pregnancy is common in primigravidae. PEP and ICP show an association with multiple pregnancy, whereas PG shows association with molar pregnancy.

Medical History

To rule out systemic diseases associated with pruritus, detailed history is required to find out the cause. Ask whether patient is a known case of diabetes mellitus, thyroid disorder, renal or liver disease, hypertension, or any malignancy. Otherwise, any history of bleeding disorders, weight loss or gain, palpitations, tremors, edema, and bowel and bladder symptoms should be elicited. Pruritus is a late manifestation of most chronic diseases. Pregnancy-specific dermatoses also show association with them, e.g., association of PG with Graves' disease has been observed.

Family History

A positive family history can be elicited in AEP and ICP. History of similar complaints in family can be present in scabies.

EXAMINATION

After a detailed history, a thorough general physical, local, and obstetrical examination is required. History and examination together can usually diagnose majority of the cases.

General Physical Examination

Look for pallor which is present in hemolytic anemia, pernicious anemia, and some systemic diseases; jaundice is present in liver disorders and ICP; thyromegaly in thyroid disorders; lymphadenopathy in lymphoma; hepatomegaly in liver disorders; facial puffiness and pedal edema in renal diseases or preeclampsia; and hypertension in preeclampsia. Look for personal hygiene and do psychological assessment.

Rash

Rash may or may not be present with pruritus. If present, the characteristics and distribution of rash can provide clues to the diagnosis (*see* Table 2).

Obstetrical Examination

Look for the fundal height, amount of liquor, and number of fetuses. Multiple pregnancy is associated with PEP and ICP. Association of fetal growth restriction and oligohydramnios has been observed with PG.

Per Speculum and Per Vaginal Examination

Per speculum and per vaginal examination are done if indicated as in preterm labor and vulval pruritus. Preterm labor is associated with PG and ICP. Vulval pruritus is a symptom of vaginal candidiasis.

INVESTIGATIONS

Based on the provisional diagnosis made on history and clinical examination, the relevant investigations required to confirm the diagnosis are advised.

Basic Investigations[1,5]

Basic investigations are done to rule out systemic causes of pruritus and have been tabulated in Table 3.

Specific Investigations[5-9]

Special investigations helpful in diagnosing specific dermatoses of pregnancy are as follows.

Immunofluorescence Tests

These are positive in PG and negative in rest all. Direct immunofluorescence test shows linear complement component 3 (C3) deposition along basement membrane zone of epidermis (Fig. 5), amnion, and chorion in

Table 3: Basic investigations to rule out systemic causes of pruritus.[1,5]

Investigations	Associated pathology
Complete hemogram: • Hemoglobin • Total leukocyte count • Eosinophilia • Erythrocyte sedimentation rate (ESR)	• Iron deficiency or megaloblastic anemia, chronic infections, malabsorption syndrome, and malignant and systemic diseases • Bacterial infections • Worm infestations • Raised in chronic infections, chronic skin and systemic diseases, and malignancies
Liver function tests (LFTs)	Liver disorders, intrahepatic cholestasis of pregnancy (ICP), preeclampsia and diabetes
Hepatitis serology	Viral hepatitis
Kidney function tests	Renal diseases, preeclampsia, and diabetes
Urine examination	Renal pathology, diabetes, preeclampsia, and urinary tract infection (ICP shows association with urinary tract infections)
Thyroid function tests	Thyrotoxicosis or myxedema (in thyrotoxicosis, pruritus is due to vasodilatation and activation of kinins secondary to increased tissue metabolism; whereas in myxedema, it is secondary to xerosis)
Parathyroid hormone levels	Chronic renal failure, hyperparathyroidism (chronic renal failure leads to hyperparathyroidism; hyperparathyroidism results in hyperphosphatemia which is pruritogenic)
Iron studies	Iron deficiency even in absence of anemia causes pruritus
Folic acid and vit B_{12} levels	Megaloblastic anemia
Blood sugar levels	Diabetes and liver disorders (diabetes cause pruritus secondary to infections, poor circulation, xerosis, and neuropathy)
Serum electrolytes	• Hyperphosphatemia, hypercalcemia, hypermagnesemia (increased divalent ions as in chronic renal failure, cause stimulation of free nerve endings resulting in pruritus) • Hypocalcemia (seen in impetigo herpetiformis) • Dyselectrolytemia (involving sodium, potassium, and chlorides and is associated with hyperemesis gravidarum)
Protein electrophoresis	• Hypoalbuminemia (seen in preeclampsia, ICP, and impetigo herpetiformis), • Elevation in alpha-2 and beta globulins (ICP)
Stool examination (ova, cyst, and occult blood)	Worm infestation

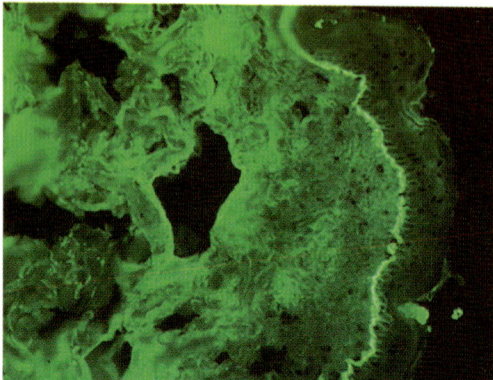

Fig. 5: Direct immunofluorescence test showing linear complement component (C3) deposition along basement membrane zone of epidermis in pemphigoid gestationis.

100% of cases. Indirect immunofluorescence detects immunoglobulin G (IgG) antibodies in patient's serum in 30–100% cases.

Histopathology of the Biopsy from the Skin Lesion

Histopathology of the biopsy from the skin lesion is specific in cases of chronic skin diseases. In pregnancy-specific dermatoses, characteristic changes are seen only in PG. Upper and mid-dermis edema is seen in prebullous stage followed by subdermal blistering in bullous stage of PG. In PEP, dermal edema with perivascular lymphocytic infiltrates superficial to mid-dermal level is present in early lesions, whereas nonspecific epidermal changes such as spongiosis, acanthosis, hyperkeratosis, and parakeratosis are present in late lesions.

Anti BP 180 NC16A

Pemphigoid gestationis is an autoimmune disorder caused by autoantibodies against bullous pemphigoid antigen 180, hence diagnosis of PG can be made by detecting anti BP180NC16A by ELISA.

Serum Bile Acid Levels

Total serum bile acid level of >11 µmol/L (normal range is 4.6–8.7 µmol/L) and cholic-to-chenodeoxycholic acid ratio of >1.5 (normal ratio 0.7–1.5) is diagnostic of ICP. The glycine-to-taurine ratio is decreased to <1 (normal is 0.9–2.0). As pruritus often precedes rise in bile acid levels by 3–4 weeks, the investigation is repeated weekly if initial levels are normal, despite clinical diagnosis.

Liver Function Tests

In ICP, elevated bilirubin level (predominantly direct bilirubin) ranging from 2 to 5 mg/dL is seen in 10–20% cases. Liver function tests (LFTs) are normal in 30% cases of ICP; raised aminotransferase levels [SGOT (serum glutamic oxaloacetic transaminase) and SGPT (serum glutamic pyruvic transaminase)] are seen in 20–60% of patients. Alpha-2 and beta globulin will be raised, and prothrombin time will be prolonged due to vitamin K deficiency.

Serum IgE Levels

Serum IgE levels are raised in 20–70% of women with AEP.

Ultrasonography

Obstetrical ultrasound is done to rule out molar pregnancy and fetal growth restriction, confirm number of fetuses and assess for fetal well-being. Abdominal ultrasonography is done to rule out any pathology in liver, gallbladder, kidneys, or any other abdominal organ.

Computed Tomography Scan/ Magnetic Resonance Imaging

Computed tomography (CT) scan or magnetic resonance imaging (MRI) may be required for diagnosis if any tumor is suspected (gastric tumor, pancreatic tumor, or brain tumor). In malignancy, release of toxins (e.g., serotonin in carcinoid syndrome and leukopeptidase and bradykinins in lymphomas) have been implicated for pruritus.

MANAGEMENT[10-14]

Early diagnosis and prompt management of the underlying etiology of pruritus in pregnancy are very important. ICP is associated with increased risk of preterm delivery, meconium stained liquor, still birth, and intrauterine death (IUD) due to arrhythmia and placental vasospasm secondary to accumulation of bile acids in amniotic fluid (especially if total serum bile acid levels are >100 μmol/L). PG is associated with FGR and oligohydramnios. Hence, management of pruritus in pregnancy requires a multidisciplinary approach involving obstetrician, neonatologist, and dermatologist (Flowchart 2).

Flowchart 2: Management of pruritus in pregnancy.

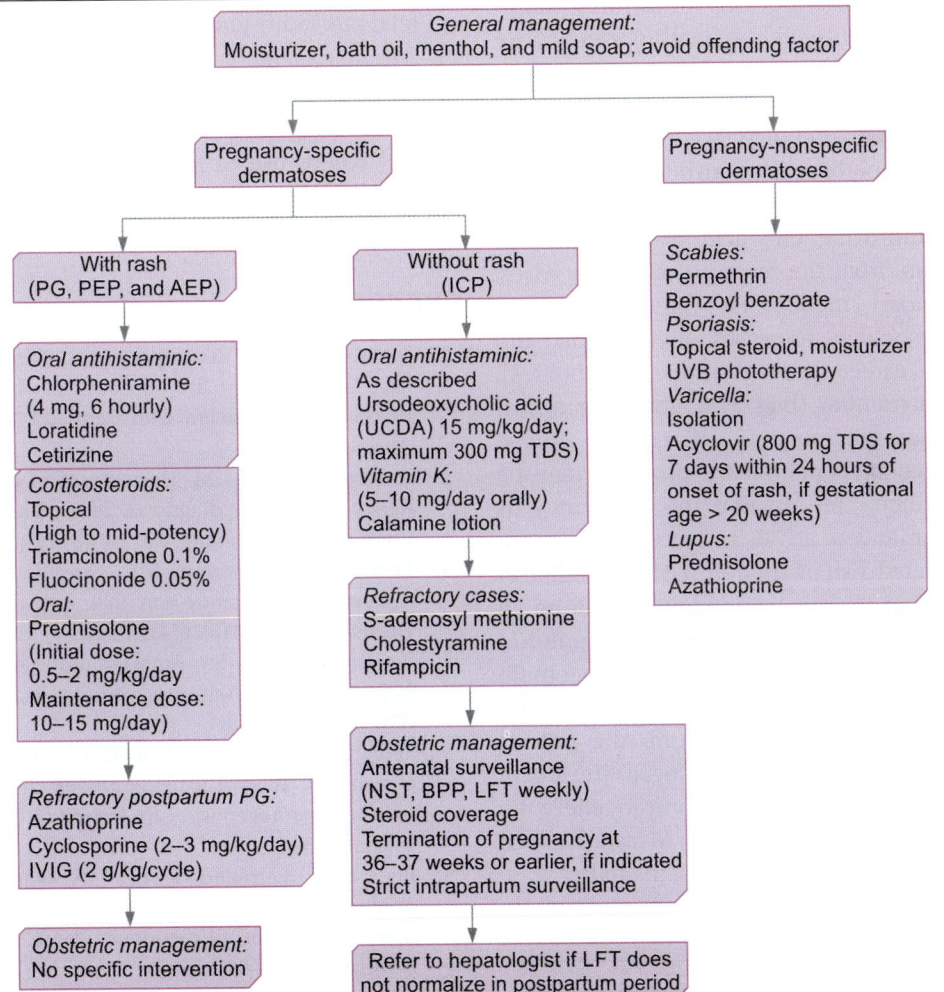

(AEP: atopic eruption of pregnancy; ICP: intrahepatic cholestasis of pregnancy; PEP: polymorphic eruption of pregnancy; PG: pemphigoid gestationis; NST: nonstress test; BPP: biophysical profile; LFT: liver function test)

In addition to the specific topical and systemic treatments for the underlying etiology, general pruritus-relieving measures and avoidance of precipitating factor, if any, are indicated. Management of most pregnancy-specific dermatoses, except ICP, include antihistaminic and corticosteroid usage. Recent studies have shown that oral corticosteroids are relatively safe in pregnancy without any increased risk of congenital malformations, though high dose is associated with slight increased risk of preterm delivery and fetal growth restriction. In refractory postpartum cases of PG, we can use immunosuppressants such as azathioprine, cyclosporine, and IV immunoglobulins.

In ICP, ursodeoxycholic acid (UDCA) is the treatment of choice. UDCA displaces more hydrophobic bile salts from bile acid pool, thus preventing hepatocyte membrane damage and improving bile acid clearance across placenta from the fetus. In refractory cases, s-adenosyl methionine (glutathione precursor which increases methylation and biliary excretion of hormone metabolites), cholestyramine (bile acid chelating agent) or rifampicin (pregnane X receptor agonist involved in hepatobiliary process) may be prescribed. Termination of pregnancy is recommended at 36–37 weeks because of associated risk of sudden IUD and stillbirth after that. Earlier termination is done in case of total bile acid levels > 100 μmol/L, jaundice, previous history of IUD before 36 weeks, or fetal compromise. If LFT does not return to normal postpartum, the patient should be referred to hepatologist. The aim of management should not be only to relieve the maternal discomfort but also to improve fetal outcome by timely delivery of the baby.

KEY POINTS

- Pregnancy-specific dermatoses remain the most prevalent cause of pruritus in pregnancy with AEP being the most common and PG being most specific.
- PG and ICP are associated with adverse fetal outcome.
- Diagnosis is usually made clinically though biochemical (e.g., total serum bile acids in ICP) and histopathological correlation (e.g., in PG) is required to confirm the diagnosis in some cases.
- Urgent evaluation of pruritus in pregnancy in consultation with other specialties is required not only to relieve maternal distress but also to decrease the fetal morbidity and mortality.
- The management in most of pregnancy-specific dermatoses includes use of antihistaminics and corticosteroids, except ICP where use of ursodeoxycholic acid and delivery at 36–37 weeks or earlier is recommended.

REFERENCES

1. Meta N, Chen K, Kroumpouzos G. Skin disease in pregnancy: the approach of obstetric medicine physician. Clin Dermatol. 2016; 34(3):320-6.
2. Ambros-Rudolph CM. Dermatoses of pregnancy - clues to diagnosis, fetal risk and therapy. Ann Dermatol. 2011;23(3):265-75.
3. Lehrhoff S, Pomeranz MK. Specific dermatoses of pregnancy and their treatment. Dermatol Ther. 2013;26(4):274-84.
4. Vaughan Jones S, Ambros-Rudolph C, Nelson-Piercy C. Skin disease in pregnancy. BMJ. 2014;348:g3489.
5. Sadik CD, Lima AL, Zillikens D. Pemphigoid gestationis: Toward a better understanding of the etiopathogenesis. Clin Dermatol. 2016; 34(3):378-82.
6. Regnier S, Fermand V, Levy P, Uzan S, Aractingi S. A case-control study of polymorphic eruption of pregnancy. J Am Acad Dermatol. 2008; 58(1):63-7.
7. Roth MM, Cristodor P, Kroumpouzos G. Prurigo, pruritic folliculitis, and atopic

eruption of pregnancy: Facts and controversies. Clin Dermatol. 2016;34(3):392-400.
8. Hillman SC, Stokes-Lampard H, Kilby MD. Intrahepatic cholestasis of pregnancy. BMJ. 2016; 353: i1236.
9. Manzotti C, Casazza G, Stimac T, Nikolova D, Gluud C. Total serum bile acids or serum bile acid profile, or both, for the diagnosis of intrahepatic cholestasis of pregnancy. Cochrane Database Syst Rev. 2019;7(7):CD012546.
10. Kirtschig G, Middleton P, Bennett C, Murrell DF, Wojnarowska F, Khumalo NP. Interventions for bullous pemphigoid. Cochrane Database Syst Rev. 2010;10: CD002292.
11. Chi CC, Wang SH, Wojnarowska F, Kirtschig G. Safety of topical corticosteroids in pregnancy. Cochrane Database Syst Rev. 2015;CD007346.
12. Bacq Y, le Besco M, Lecuyer AI, Gendrot C, Potin J, Andres CR, et al. Ursodeoxycholic acid therapy in intrahepatic cholestasis of pregnancy: Results in real-world conditions and factors predictive of response to treatment. Dig Liver Dis. 2017;49(1):63-9.
13. Chappell LC, Bell JL, Smith A, et al. Ursodeoxycholic acid versus placebo in women with intrahepatic cholestasis of pregnancy (PITCHES): A randomised controlled trial. Lancet. 2019;394 (10201):849-60.
14. Lambert J. Itch in Pregnancy Management. Curr Probl Dermatol. 2016;50:164-72.

SUGGESTED READING

1. ACOG Committee Opinion No 764: Medically indicated Late-Preterm and Early-term Deliveries. Obstet Gynecol. 2019;133(2):e151-5.
2. Royal College of Obstetricians and Gynaecologists (2011). Obstetric Cholestasis (Green-top Guideline No. 43). [online] Available from: https://www.rcog.org.uk/en/guidelines-research-services/guidelines/gtg43/.[Last accessed January, 2020].
3. Society for Maternal and Fetal Medicine. Understanding-intrahepatic-cholestasis-of-pregnancy. [online] Available from: https://www.smfm.org/publications/96-understanding-intrahepatic-cholestasis-of-pregnancy. [Last accessed January, 2020].
4. Weisshaar E, Szepietowski JC, Darsow U, Misery L, Wallengren J, Mettang T, et al. European Guideline on Chronic Pruritus. Acta Derm Venereol. 2012;92(5):563-81.

13. Approach to a Pregnant Woman with Decreased Fetal Movements

Deepika Meena

INTRODUCTION

Fetal movements have been defined as maternal sensation of any discrete kick, flutter, swish or roll.[1] Maternal perception of fetal movement is one of the first signs of fetal life and virtually provides reassurance of the integrity of the central nervous and musculoskeletal system of the fetus. Movements are first perceived by the mother between 18 and 20 weeks of gestation. Multiparous women may perceive fetal movements earlier than 18 weeks of gestation and primiparous women later than 20 weeks of gestation. The number of movements tends to increase till 32 weeks of gestation and then plateau. The usual alarm limit has been defined as 10 or more movements in 2 hours, felt by a woman when she is lying on her side and focusing on the movements[2] or 10 distinct movements felt within 12 hours of normal maternal activity (the Cardiff "count to ten" method).

The fetus adapts to chronic hypoxia by conserving energy and reducing oxygen consumption by moving less. Decreased fetal movements are regarded as a marker for suboptimal intrauterine conditions. Maternal perception of reduced fetal movements is associated with poor perinatal outcomes, including fetal death (Flowchart 1).

Daily fetal movement counting may be used routinely in all pregnant women or selectively in women who are at increased risk of adverse perinatal outcomes. It allows the clinician to make timely interventions to optimize outcomes. However, fetal movement counting may cause unnecessary anxiety to pregnant women, or trigger unnecessary interventions such as hospital admission, induction of labor, and cesarean sections.[3]

All clinicians involved in the care of pregnant women should understand the potential pregnancy factors and outcomes associated with decreased fetal movement (DFM).

The various factors contributing to DFM are listed in Box 1.

Box 1: Pregnancy factors associated with decreased fetal movements.

Fetal factors:
- Fetal sleep
- Fetal position (anterior spine)
- Congenital anomalies (neurological, musculoskeletal)
- Fetal growth restriction
- Intrauterine fetal death

Placental and amniotic fluid related factors:
- Anterior location of placenta
- Oligohydramnios
- Polyhydramnios
- Placental insufficiency

Maternal factors:
- Intake of sedative drugs alcohol, benzodiazepines, barbiturates
- Administration of antenatal steroids
- Cigarette smoking
- Preterm labor
- Intrauterine infections
- Maternal disease: anemia, diabetes mellitus, hypothyroidism

Chapter 13: Approach to a Pregnant Woman with Decreased Fetal Movements

Flowchart 1: Algorithm for approach to a pregnant woman presenting with decreased or absent fetal movements.

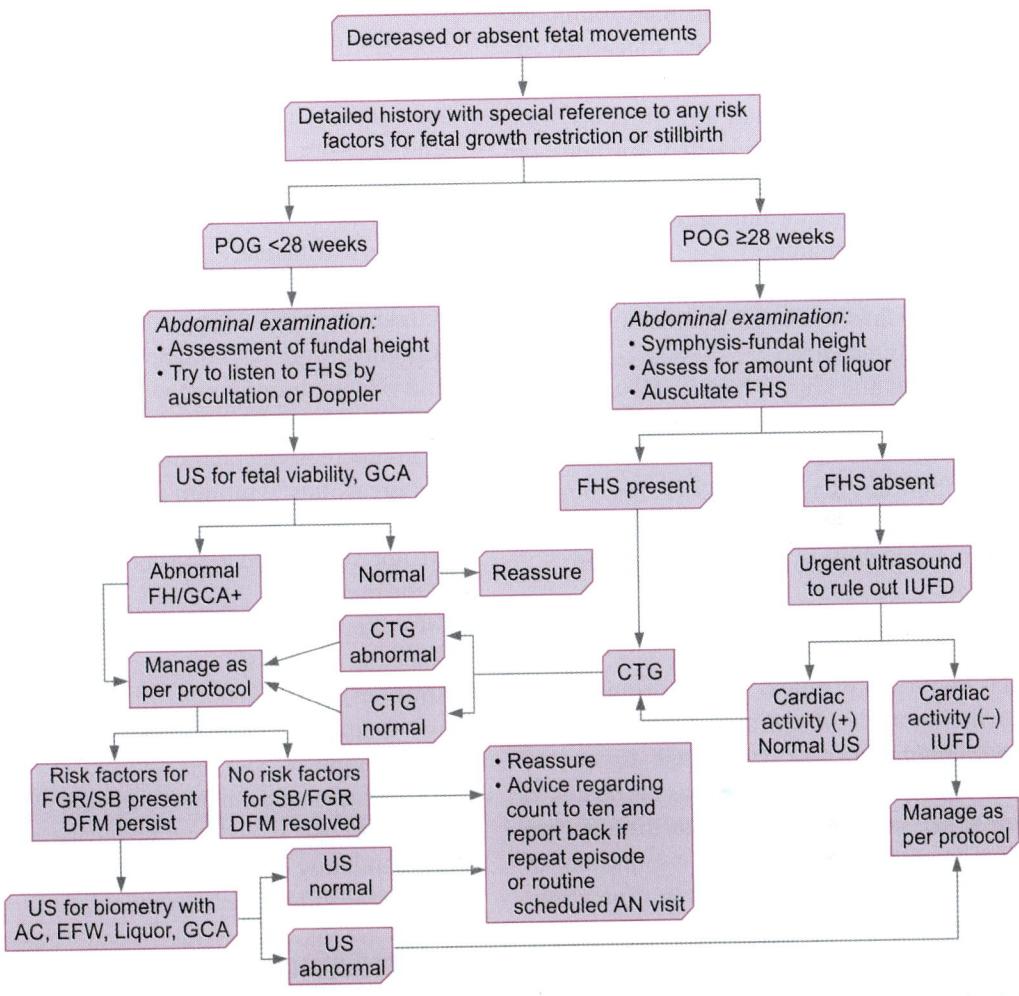

(POG: period of gestation; FHS: fetal heart sound; US: ultrasound; GCA: gross congenital anomaly; FH: fundal height; CTG: cardiotocography; IUFD: intrauterine fetal demise; FGR/SB: fetal growth restriction/still birth; DFM: decreased fetal movement; EFW: estimated fetal weight)

HISTORY

The initial aim of assessment of a woman presenting with decreased fetal movements is to rule out intrauterine fetal death and subsequently identify pregnancies at risk of fetal compromise and adverse outcomes.

History of Present Illness

This should include:
- The time since onset of DFM since fetus has sleep periods ranging between 20–90 min when there are no fetal movements.

- Whether the fetal movements are decreased or absent?
- Any history of trauma, fall, pain abdomen or bleeding per vaginum suggestive of placental abruption.
- Whether she has had any previous episodes of DFM as repeated episodes of DFM are more likely to be associated with adverse perinatal outcomes and need a detailed evaluation.
- Is there any history of intake of sedatives or administration of antenatal corticosteroids recently?
- Is there any known high-risk fetal factor present such as fetal anomaly, fetal growth restriction (FGR)?
- Is there any maternal high-risk factor present such as hypertension, diabetes, autoimmune disease, hypothyroidism, etc.

Obstetric History

It is important to note if she is a primigravida or multigravida. As primigravidae feel fetal movements late as compared to multigravidae. Any history of past adverse obstetric event like recurrent miscarriage, intrauterine fetal death, FGR, and stillbirth, is important as it increases the likelihood of adverse outcome in subsequent pregnancies.

Personal History

History of smoking and excess alcohol intake may be associated with decreased fetal movements.

EXAMINATION

General Physical Examination

A complete general physical examination is performed systematically with special reference to presence of obesity, anemia, hypertension and pedal edema.

Abdominal Examination

For detailed description of abdominal examination, refer to Chapter No. 1, page 12.

Special points to be focused on are:
- Assessment of fundal height on palpation and measurement of symphysis-fundal height to note any lag in fetal growth. It should be compared with any previous records if available.
- The fetal lie and presentation with special reference to the fetal spine, if it is anterior.
- Amount of liquor as both polyhydramnios and oligohydramnios may be associated with decreased fetal movements. Sometimes decreased fetal movements may be the presenting symptom in women with acute hydramnios as the fetal movements are not transmitted to the abdominal wall of the mother.
- Any uterine tenderness suggestive of placental abruption.
- Any uterine contractions.
- Any palpable fetal movements while examination.
- Auscultation of fetal heart sounds with a stethoscope or a Doppler device and differentiating it from maternal pulse by noting the difference between the two.

INVESTIGATIONS

Cardiotocography (CTG)

Cardiotocography should be performed for at least 20 minutes if the pregnancy is over 28 weeks of gestation. A reactive CTG is defined by two accelerations exceeding 15 beats per minute sustained for at least 15 seconds in a 20-minute period. However, between 28–32 weeks' gestation, accelerations of more than 10 beats per minute for 10 seconds may be considered normal.[4] A normal CTG represents a healthy fetus with a normal, functioning autonomic system.

Ultrasound

Ultrasonography is useful in confirming fetal viability and detection of conditions possibly contributing to DFM. Ultrasound assessment should include documentation of cardiac activity, fetal biometry including abdominal circumference and/or estimated fetal weight to detect FGR or macrosomia, assessment of amniotic fluid volume, placental grading and an anatomic survey for any gross congenital anomaly in the fetus. Doppler flow studies are indicated if FGR is suspected. Doppler of middle cerebral artery may be considered if an abnormal CTG is found but an ultrasound shows a normal fetus to rule out fetal anemia.[5]

Urgent ultrasound assessment should be considered in any woman presenting with DFM when FHR cannot be documented or CTG is abnormal. It is also indicated if the woman has persistent maternal perception of DFM despite a normal CTG or if there is suspected FGR. It should be done at the earliest and preferably not later than 24 hours.

Biophysical Profile

A modified biophysical profile (BPP) including nonstress test (NST) and amniotic fluid index (AFI) is usually adequate in assessing women reporting DFM. Biophysical profile may be used selectively in women with DFM especially in those with high-risk factors such as FGR. BPP in high-risk women has a good negative predictive value; as fetal death is rare in women in the presence of a normal BPP.

MANAGEMENT

Management strategies in response to perceived DFM include early delivery or expectant management with close fetal surveillance such as CTG, ultrasonography for fetal biometry, amniotic fluid volume, placental grading and Doppler flow studies. If investigations are abnormal then further management is decided accordingly. Decision whether or not to induce labor at term in a woman who present recurrently with DFM when the growth, liquor and CTG appear normal must be made after careful consultant led counseling of the couple including the pros and cons of induction of labor on individualized basis.

KEY POINTS

- Maternal perception of DFM is a common complaint and one of the most frequent cause of unplanned visit in pregnancy.
- Maternal concern and perceived reduction in fetal movements is more important than any definition of DFM based on movement counting.
- Women's perception of DFM is decreased with maternal obesity and if placenta is anterior in location.
- About 70% of pregnancies with a single episode of DFM have an uneventful outcome.
- All women with DFM should be assessed as soon as possible for risk factors of stillbirth.
- Evaluation for DFM should prompt review for predisposing factors, examination, CTG and an ultrasound.
- Early delivery is an option for DFM when the risks to the mother and baby have been weighed up appropriately.

REFERENCES

1. Royal College of Obstetricians and Gynecologists. (2011). Reduced fetal movements. [online]. Available from: https://www.rcog.org.uk/globalassets/documents/guidelines/gtg_57.pdf [Last Accessed January, 2020].
2. Hofmeyr GJ, Novikova N. Management of reported decreased fetal movements for improving pregnancy outcomes. Cochrane Database Syst Rev 2012;4:CD009148.

3. Flenady V, Macphail J, Gardener G, Chadha Y, Mahomed K, Heazell A, et al. Detection and management of decreased fetal movements in Australia and New Zealand: a survey of obstetric practice. Aust N Z J Obstet Gynaecol. 2009;49(4):358-63.
4. Antepartum fetal surveillance. Practice Bulletin No. 145. American College of Obstetricians and Gynecologists. Obstet Gynecol. 2014;124:182-92.
5. New South Wales Health Guideline (2011). Decreased Fetal Movements in Third Trimester (GL2011_012).

SUGGESTED READING

1. Fretts RC. Decreased fetal movements Diagnosis, evaluation and management. UpToDate. 2019.
2. Gardener G, Daly L, Bowring V, Burton G, Chadha Y, Ellwood D, et al. Clinical practice guideline for the management of women with decreased fetal movements. Australia and New Zealand Stillbirth Alliance (ANZSA). 2016.
3. Royal College of Obstetricians and Gynecologists. (2011). Reduced fetal movements. [online]. Available from: https://www.rcog.org.uk/globalassets/documents/guidelines/gtg_57.pdf [Last Accessed January, 2020].
4. World Health Organization. (2018). WHO recommendation on daily fetal movement counting. [online]. Available from: https://extranet.who.int/rhl/topics/preconception-pregnancy-childbirth-and-postpartum-care/antenatal-care/who-recommendation-daily-fetal-movement-counting [Last Accessed January, 2020].

14. Approach to a Pregnant Woman Presenting with a Positive Aneuploidy Screening Test

Manisha Kumar

INTRODUCTION

Chromosomal abnormalities affect approximately 0.4% of births (1/250) according to the population-based registries. These include live births, fetal deaths, and pregnancy terminations, of which Trisomy 21 accounts for >50%, Trisomy 18 for 15%, and Trisomy 13 for 5% (Fig. 1).[1] Due to the profound social and economic impact on the family, there is a great emphasis on early detection and counseling of the parents for the termination of pregnancy. The availability of high-definition ultrasound and serum markers for the screening of aneuploidies has revolutionized the concept of prenatal care with respect to aneuploidy screening but has also led to the availability of several options for the management of the screen-positive pregnant women. Therefore, there is a need to understand the algorithm to be followed when the screening test is positive.

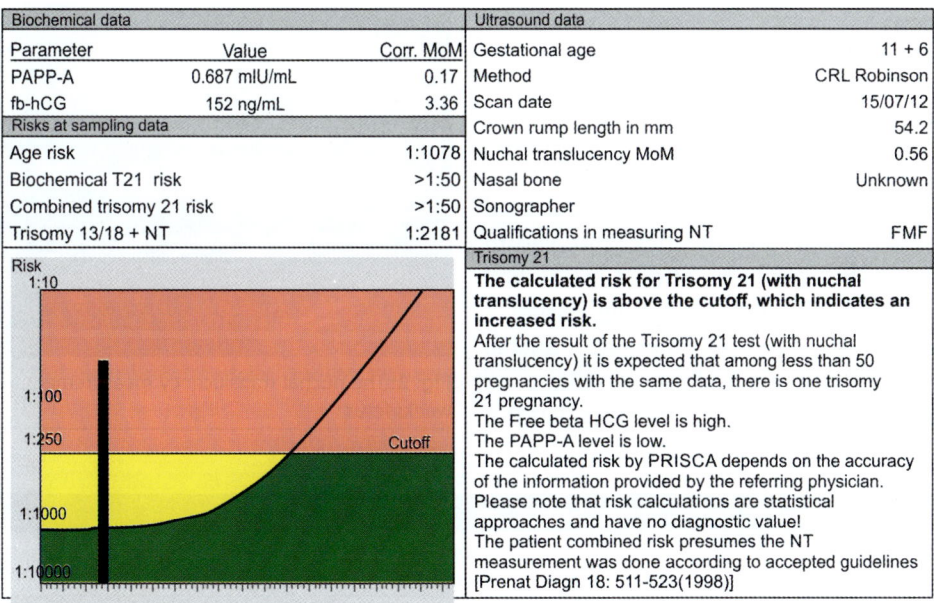

Fig. 1: Report of first trimester combined test showing risk of 1:50, therefore high risk of trisomy 21.
(fb-hCG: free beta-human chorionic gonadotropin; MoM: multiple of the median; NT: nuchal translucency; PAPP-A: pregnancy-associated plasma protein A)

PRENATAL SCREENING VERSUS PRENATAL DIAGNOSIS

The screening tests are done to assess whether a pregnant woman is at increased risk of having a fetus affected by aneuploidy. In contrast, the prenatal diagnosis is intended to determine, whether a specific condition is present in the fetus or not. Usually, a diagnostic test follows if the woman is at a high risk in a screening test. All pregnant women should be offered screening for aneuploidies after an informed counseling.[2] A discussion of the risks, benefits, and alternatives of the various prenatal diagnoses and screening options, including the option of no testing, should be undertaken with all pregnant women prior to any prenatal screening. Maternal age alone is a poor minimum standard for prenatal screening for aneuploidy, and it should not be used as a basis for recommending invasive fetal diagnostic testing when noninvasive prenatal screening for aneuploidy is available (Table 1).

First-trimester Screening

Screening test is done in the first-trimester between 11 and 13^{+6} weeks of gestation.

A combined screening by ultrasound markers nuchal translucency and serum biochemistry should be offered in the first trimester after pretest counseling. Figure 2 shows ideal view to measure nuchal translucency in fetus from 11-13w + 6 days. Serum biochemistry includes PAPP-A (pregnancy-associated plasma protein A) and free β-hCG (beta-human chorionic gonadotropin). This has a detection rate 80–85% with a false-positive rate of 5%.[3,4] The first trimester nuchal translucency should be interpreted for risk assessment only when measured by sonographers or sonologists trained and accredited for this fetal screening service and when there is ongoing quality assurance (Table 2).

Mandatory background information needed at the time of tests are ethnicity, maternal age (preferably date of birth), maternal weight, method of conception, diabetes, smoking, number of fetuses, and chorionicity.

The women are divided into groups depending upon their risk—if the risk is >1:250, it is considered high risk; if it is between 1:250 and 1:1500, it is considered intermediate risk; if it is <1:1500, it is considered low risk. Flowchart 1 summarizes the options according to the result of screening test.

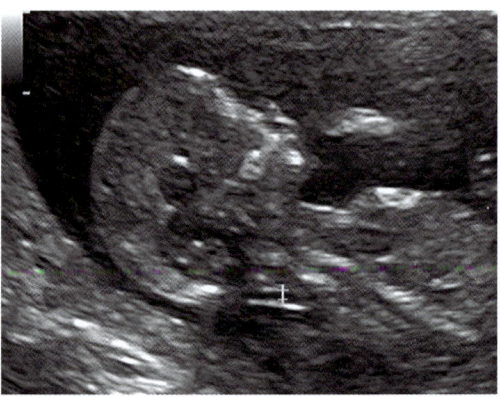

Fig. 2: The nuchal translucency measurement in a 12 weeks fetus.

Table 1: Bar showing degree of sensitivity of screening tests.[2]

Maternal age	Triple test	Quadruple test	Combined first trimester test	Integrated test including NT	NIPT
DR 44%	DR 71%	DR 77%	DR 83%	DR –87%	DR >99%
FPR 16%	FPR 7.2%	FPR 5.2%	FPR 5%	FPR 1.9%	FPR 0.1%

(DR: detection rate; FPR: false positive rate; NIPT: noninvasive prenatal testing; NT: nuchal translucency)

Table 2: The recommended options for aneuploidy screening with their detection rate (DR) and false-positive rate (FPR) and odds of fetus being affected given a positive result (OAPR).

Screening options	Markers	Trimester	Cutoff	DR%	FPR%	OAPR
First-trimester screening (FTS)	NT, PAPP-A, Free β hCG, Maternal (MA)	1st	1:325	83%	5%	1:27
Quadruple test	AFP, uE3, Free β hCG, inhibin MA	2nd	1:385	77%	5.2%	1:50
Integrated prenatal screening (IPS)	NT, AFP, PAPP-A, Free β hCG, total hCG, inhibin, MA	1st and 2nd	1:200	87%	1.9%	1:10
Serum integrated prenatal screening (IPS)	AFP, PAPP-A, Free β hCG, total hCG inhibin, MA	1st and 2nd	1:200	85%	4.4%	1:26

Flowchart 1: Management options according to first trimester screening results.

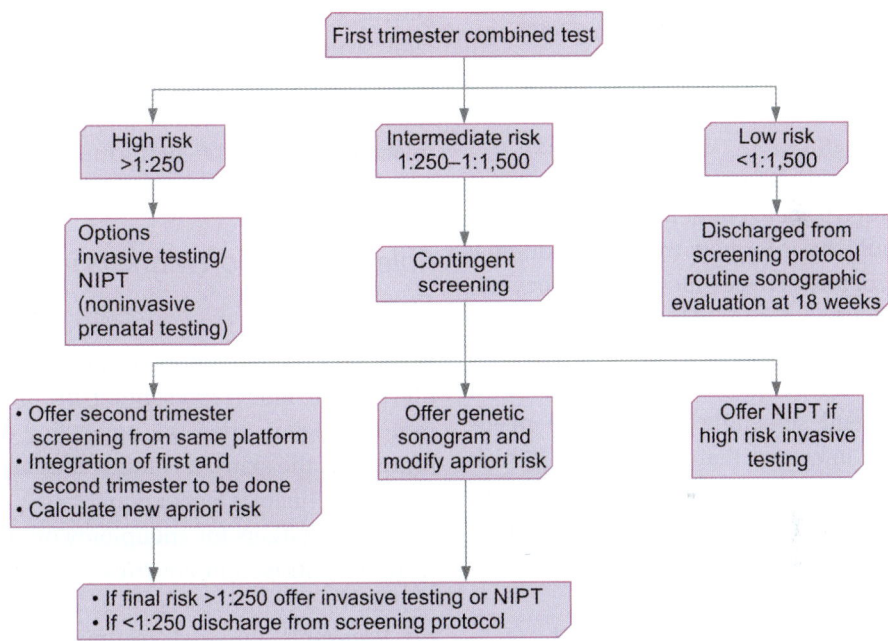

If the first trimester combined screening report is high risk or positive (risk >1:250), women should be referred for fetal medicine consultation (Table 3).[5]

If the First-trimester Combined Test Shows High-risk

A fetal medicine consultant can offer any of the following alternatives:

- *Invasive testing*: Chorionic villus sampling (CVS) or amniocentesis
  Both CVS and amniocentesis are diagnostic tests for aneuploidy in pregnancy. CVS, carried out to obtain placental villi for analysis, is usually performed between 11^{+0} and 13^{+6} weeks' gestation. Amniocentesis, performed to obtain amniotic fluid for analysis, is usually offered from

Table 3: Summary of options if the first-trimester screening is positive.

Test	Options if high risk/positive
FTS combined test/dual test positive	• Invasive test • NIPT • Contingent testing
NT >3.5 mm	• Invasive testing • TORCH serology • Parvovirus serology • Fetal echo at 18–20 weeks
Other soft markers present	• Risk can be adjusted taking apriori risk of combined test in consideration • Invasive test • NIPT • Contingent testing

[FTS: first trimester combined screening; NIPT: noninvasive prenatal testing; NT: nuchal translucency; TORCH: toxoplasma gondii, other viruses, rubella, cytomegalovirus and herpes simplex]

15^{+0} weeks. Informed written consent is advised prior to either procedure. Women should be informed that the additional risk of miscarriage following amniocentesis or CVS performed by a skilled operator is likely to be <0.5%.[6]

- *Noninvasive prenatal testing*: It is a high-end screening test. Couple needs to be informed that if the result is high risk or positive, then amniocentesis for diagnostic testing is further required for confirmation.

If First-trimester Combined Test Shows Intermediate Risk

The woman in this risk category can either be offered invasive testing or NIPT or offered contingent testing. The apriori risk is modified after a genetic sonogram is done. Further advice is based on the final risk.

The management is as per the Flowchart 1.

The combination of first and second trimester biochemical markers needs specialized accredited software and hence, integration is possible only if the biochemical markers are analyzed in both the first and the second trimesters on the same platform.[7]

If There is a Large Nuchal Translucency (>3.5 mm)

An increased nuchal translucency (>3.5 mm) is an indication for invasive testing to look for chromosomal abnormalities. Karyotype or preferably microarray testing should be advised, NIPT should not be offered. If karyotype is normal, further genetic counseling and ultrasonography for fetal structural abnormalities and detailed echocardiography for cardiac abnormalities is also required. Maternal screening for viral infections should be performed (including TORCH, Parvovirus, and Varicella).[8]

Role of Other Soft Markers in the First-trimester

Nasal bone is marked as present only when the bottom line (representing the bone) is more echogenic than the upper line (which represents the skin). It is marked as absent if the echogenicity is less or equal.[9]

Other markers for aneuploidy on the first trimester ultrasound are *tricuspid regurgitation* and *absent or reversed "a" wave in ductus venosus*.[10] Targeted scanning for these increases the detection rate of the first-trimester screening while decreasing the false positivity. Integration can be done using the specialized software to change the apriori risk.[1]

Second-trimester Aneuploidy Screening

The summary of second-trimester screening options, if the second-trimester screening test is positive, are given in Table 4.

Flowchart 2: Management options according to Quadruple test results.

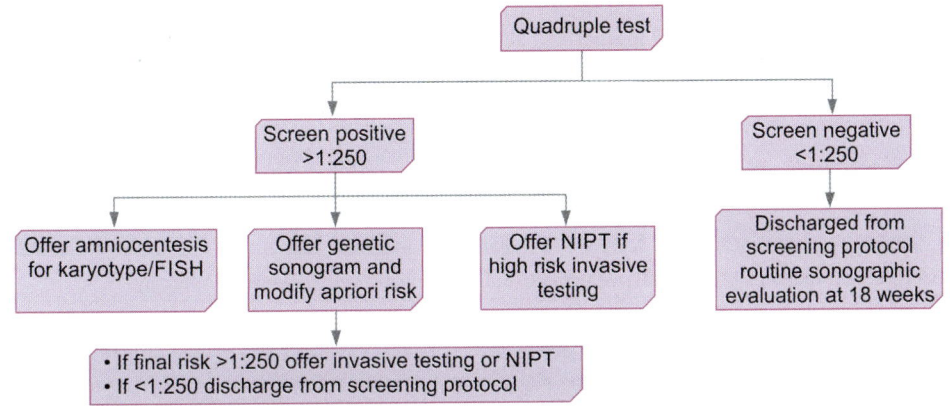

(FISH: fluorescence in situ hybridization; NIPT: noninvasive prenatal testing)

Table 4: Summary of options if the second-trimester screening test is positive.

Test	Options if high risk/positive
Quadruple test or Integrated test positive	• Invasive test • NIPT • Genetic sonogram: Risk can be adjusted taking apriori risk of Combined test in consideration
Soft markers present	
• Echogenic bowel • Increased nuchal fold thickness (NFT) • Ventriculomegaly • Absent/hypoplastic NB • Aberrant right subclavian artery (ARSA)	• Invasive testing • TORCH serology • Parvovirus serology • Fetal echo at 18–20 weeks • Follow-up ultrasound
• Short femur or humerus • Echogenic intracardiac focus (EIF) • Mild pyelectasis	• Risk can be adjusted taking apriori risk of combined test in consideration • *If risk is high*: NIPT/invasive testing • Follow-up ultrasound

(NIPT: noninvasive prenatal testing; NB: nasal bone; TORCH: toxoplasma gondii, other viruses rubella, cytomegalovirus, and herpes simplex)

If a pregnant woman presents for the first time in the second trimester, quadruple test should be offered between 15 and 20 weeks after counseling. The triple test should not be offered as it is suboptimal. The test needs correct dating and it also screens for open neural tube defects by measuring alpha fetoprotein level.[11]

If Quadruple Test is Positive

If the woman is found to be at high risk (>1:250) on quadruple test, she should be sent for the fetal medicine consultation, where NIPT or amniocentesis for karyotype/FISH may be offered. Screen negative or low risk woman (risk <1:250) can undergo detailed sonographic evaluation at 18–20 weeks (Flowchart 2).

If Soft Markers are Found in Anomaly Scan

All women should be offered a detailed ultrasound at 18–20 weeks to detect structural abnormalities. "Soft markers" can also be detected at the same time and they can be used to modify the apriori risk. The list of the relevant soft markers is given in Box 1. The soft markers are nonspecific, often transient, and can be readily detected during the second-trimester ultrasound. They may be seen in the normal fetus but have an increased incidence

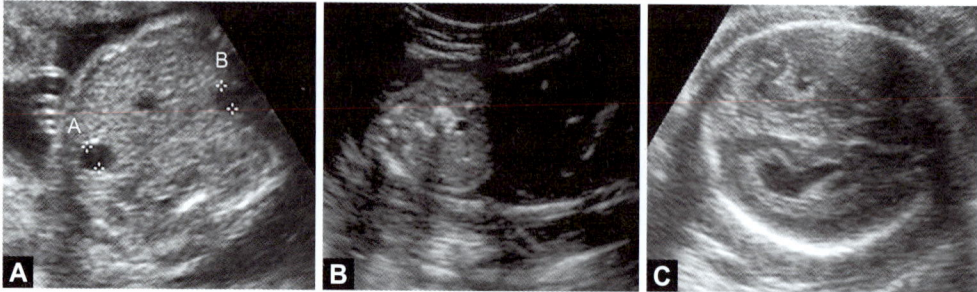

Figs. 3A to C: Soft markers. (A) Bilateral pyelectasis; (B) Echogenic bowel; (C) Ventriculomegaly.

Box 1: List of soft markers with their description.

- *Absent/hypoplastic nasal bone*: <5th centile for gestational age, or <3.8 mm at 18–20 weeks is considered short for Indian population[8]
- *Ventriculomegaly*: Lateral ventricle >10 mm at any gestational age
- *Increased nuchal fold*: >6 mm at 18–24 weeks
- *Mild hydronephrosis*: Unilateral or bilateral AP diameter of renal pelvis ≥4 mm
- *Echogenic intracardiac focus*: Equal to or brighter than bone in vicinity, may be single or multiple, in any ventricle
- *Echogenic bowel*: Brightness equal to or more than bone in vicinity
- *Short femur*: <5th centile for gestational age
- *Short humerus*: <5th centile for gestational age
- *Aberrant right subclavian artery*: Right subclavian artery originating from descending aorta and going behind the trachea
- There are other soft markers such as clinodactyly, sandal gap, short ear, wide iliac angle and so on which are poorly defined and are difficult to include in risk calculation.

---

in fetus with chromosomal abnormality (Figs. 3A to C).

Detection of a soft marker warrants looking for other soft markers and a detailed evaluation of the fetal anatomy and offering biochemical screen if not done already, in order to calculate a composite risk. Various soft markers have different associations with aneuploidy, hence the risk with each marker should be considered individually, as shown in the Box 1.

To make sure that the parents understand the results of the genetic sonogram, counseling is important after the ultrasound. The couple should preferably be referred to a Geneticist/ Fetal medicine specialist for risk calculation and counseling. Table 5 gives the likelihood ratios (LR) of the important soft markers and can be used to modify the apriori risk (Flowchart 3).

If a woman has undertaken either first trimester combined or quadruple test, the apriori risk will be the adjusted risk from previous screening. In case no previous screening has been done, the apriori risk will be age based. New risk will be calculated by multiplying the positive LR of the markers present and negative LR of markers absent. Short humerus and short femur have a high correlation so only one of the two is used for calculation of risk.

For example, a woman who had a risk of 1:2,500 from previous screening, and also has mild hydronephrosis and echogenic intracardiac focus, with all other markers absent, then her new risk will be

Chapter 14: Approach to a Pregnant Woman Presenting with a Positive Aneuploidy

Table 5: Likelihood ratios (LR) of soft markers for Trisomy 21.[12]

Marker	LR+	LR−	LR isolated*
Short femur	3.72	0.8	0.61
Short humerus	4.81	0.74	0.78
Echogenic intracardiac focus (EIF)	5.83	0.8	0.95
Mild pyelectasis	7.63	0.92	1.08
Echogenic bowel (EB)	11.44	0.9	1.65
Increased NFT	23.3	0.8	3.79
Ventriculomegaly (VM)	27.52	0.94	3.81
ARSA	21.48	0.71	3.94
Absent/hypoplastic NB	23.27	0.46	6.58

*Derived by multiplying the positive LR for the given marker by the negative LR of each of all other markers, except for short humerus.
(ARSA: aberrant right subclavian artery; EIF: echogenic intracardiac focus; NFT: nuchal fold thickness; NB: nasal bone)

Flowchart 3: Management in the presence of soft markers.

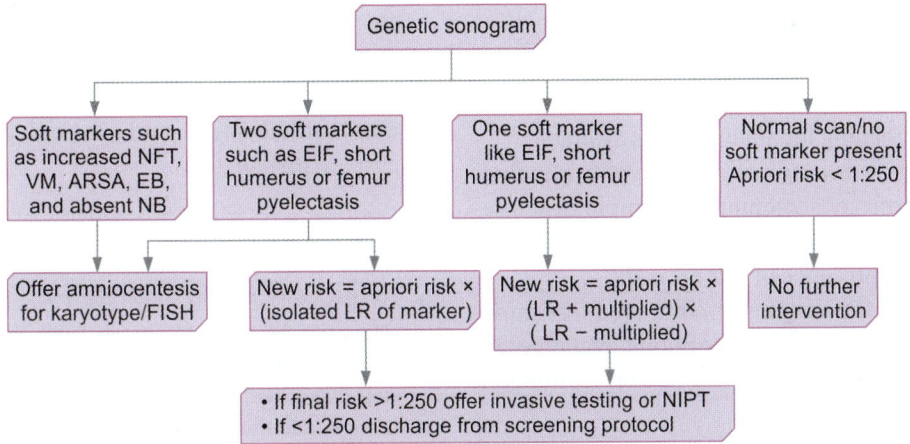

(ARSA: aberrant right subclavian artery; EB: echogenic bowel; EIF: echogenic intracardiac focus; LR: likelihood ratio; NB: nasal bone; NIPT: noninvasive prenatal testing; NFT: nuchal fold thickness)

(1/2,500)*7.63 (LR+ of mild hydronephrosis) *5.83 (LR+ of EIF)*0.94*0.8*0.9*0.74*0.71*0.46 (LR − of all other markers not found) = 1/343

If the estimated risk is >1:250 at term, invasive procedure should be offered.

If No Soft Markers are Present the Apriori Risk is reduced to Half (x 0.5)

See Box 2 on next page.

KEY POINTS

- All pregnant women, regardless of age, should be offered, through an informed counseling process, the option of a prenatal screening test for the most common fetal aneuploidies.
- Maternal age alone is a poor minimum standard for prenatal screening for aneuploidy, and it should not be used

> **Box 2:** Practice points in interpretation of soft markers.
> - Some soft markers such as increased nuchal fold thickness, ventriculomegaly, absent right subclavian artery, echogenic bowel, and absent nasal bone with high likelihood ratio may warrant an invasive test despite low risk on screening, hence should be referred for counseling to a Geneticist or a Fetal medicine specialist
> - If the above markers are absent but out of the rest two or more markers are present, invasive test should be offered
> - No additional evaluation is required if earlier screen is negative and single soft markers such as echogenic intracardiac cardiac focus, choroid plexus cyst are present
> - There is a role for modifying apriori risk after second trimester screen to reduce invasive procedures

as a basis for recommending invasive fetal diagnostic testing when prenatal screening for aneuploidy is available.

- *The screening options available are*: first-trimester screening, quadruple test, integrated screening, contingent screening, and presence of soft markers.
- If the first trimester combined test shows high risk (>1:250), options available are invasive testing, NIPT, or contingent screening.
- A large nuchal translucency (>3.5 mm) should be considered as a major marker for fetal chromosomal and structural anomalies and requires genetic counseling, an offer of invasive testing, and detailed second-trimester ultrasound follow-up.
- Women who are considering undergoing maternal plasma cell-free DNA (cfDNA) screening should be informed that all positive cfDNA screening results should be confirmed with invasive fetal diagnostic testing prior to any irrevocable decision.
- The screening test offered in the second trimester are quadruple test, integrated test, and identification of soft markers on genetic sonogram.
- If the quadruple test or integrated screening is positive, options available are invasive test, NIPT, or performing a genetic sonogram. After genetic sonogram risk can be adjusted, taking apriori risk of combined test in consideration depending upon the presence or absence of soft markers.
- Some soft markers such as increased nuchal fold thickness, ventriculomegaly, absent right subclavian artery, echogenic bowel, and absent nasal bone with high likelihood ratio may warrant an invasive test despite low risk on screening.
- No additional evaluation is required if earlier screening is negative and single soft markers such as echogenic intracardiac cardiac focus and choroid plexus cyst are present.

REFERENCES

1. Wellesley D, Dolk H, Boyd PA, Greenlees R, Haeusler M, Nelen V, et al. Rare chromosome abnormalities, prevalence and prenatal diagnosis rates from population-based congenital anomaly registers in Europe. Eur J Hum Genet. 2012;20(5):521-6.
2. Cartier L, Murphy-Kaulbeck L; Genetics Committee. Counselling Considerations for Prenatal Genetic Screening. J Obstet Gynaecol Can. 2012;34(5):489-93.
3. Malone FD, Canick JA, Ball RH, Nyberg DA, Comstock CH, Bukowski R, et al. First-trimester or second-trimester screening, or both, for Down's syndrome. N Engl J Med. 2005;353(19):2001-11.
4. Wald NJ, Rodeck C, Hackshaw AK, Walters J, Chitty L, Mackinson AM, et al. First and second trimester antenatal screening for Down's syndrome: the results of the Serum,

Urine and Ultrasound Screening Study (SURUSS). Health Technol Assess. 2003; 7(11):1-77.
5. Brigatti KW, Malone FD. First trimester screening for aneuploidy. Obstet Gynecol Clin N Am. 2004;31(1):1-20.
6. Royal College of Obstetricians and Gynaecologists. (2010). Amniocentesis and Chorionic Villus Sampling (Green-top Guideline No. 8). [online] Available from https://www.rcog.org.uk/globalassets/documents/guidelines/gtg_8.pdf. [Last accessed January, 2020].
7. Chitayat D, Langlois S, Wilson RD. No. 261-Prenatal screening for fetal aneuploidy in singleton pregnancies. Obstet Gynaecol Can. 2017;39(9):e380-94.
8. Committee on Practice Bulletins—Obstetrics, Committee on Genetics, and the Society for Maternal-Fetal Medicine. Practice Bulletin No. 163: Screening for Fetal Aneuploidy. 2016;127(5):e123-37.
9. Cicero S, Longo D, Rembouskos G, Sacchini C, Nicolaides KH. Absent nasal bone at 11–14 weeks of gestation and chromosomal defects. Ultrasound Obstet Gynecol. 2003;22(1):31-5.
10. Kagan KO, Valencia C, Livanos P, Nicolaides KH. Tricuspid regurgitation in screening for trisomies 21, 18 and 13 and Turner syndrome at 11+0-13+6 weeks of gestation. Ultrasound Obstet Gynecol. 2009;33(1):18-22.
11. Wald NJ, Kennard A, Hackshaw A, McGuire A. Antenatal screening for Down's syndrome. J Med Screen. 1997;4(4):18-246.
12. Agathokleous M, Chaveeva P, Poon LCY, Kosinski P, Nicolaides KH. (Meta-analysis of second-trimester markers for trisomy 21. Ultrasound Obstet Gynecol. 2013;41(3): 247-61.

SUGGESTED READING

1. Audibert F, De Bie I, Johnson J, Okun N, Wilson RD, Armour C, et al. No. 348- Joint SOGC-CCMG Guideline: Update on prenatal screening for fetal aneuploidy, fetal anomalies, and adverse pregnancy outcomes. J Obstet Gynaecol Can. 2017;39(9):805-17. 348, September 2017
2. Royal College of Obstetricians and Gynaecologists. (2019). Non-invasive Prenatal Testing (Green-Top Guideline No. 74). [online] Available from https://www.rcog.org.uk/en/guidelines-research-services/guidelines/gtg74/. Last accessed January, 2020].

15
Approach to a Pregnant Woman with a Congenitally Malformed Fetus

Manisha Kumar

Malformations are morphological defects that occur due to errors in the normal development and differentiation of embryo. The incidence of single minor malformation in newborns is approximately 14%, single major malformation is 3%, and multiple malformations is 0.7%.[1] In India, 8–15% of perinatal deaths and 13–16% neonatal deaths are due to congenital anomalies.[2]

Detection of congenital anomaly at any period of gestation is a matter of grief and concern to the family. After detection of malformation, there are two concerns that the couple has: (1) The prognosis of the defect and (2) the possibility of recurrence. Both prognosis and chances of recurrence can only be derived if the cause of malformation is known; therefore, all attempts must be made to find out the cause that has led to the malformation. For example, in case of duodenal atresia, which is surgically correctable after birth, the chances of chromosomal abnormality are 30%, so if the defect is associated with Down syndrome, the mental impairment will remain even after surgical correction.[3] The various causes of congenital anomalies, their incidence, and recurrence risk in next pregnancy are given in Table 1.

HISTORY

The detailed description of history taking in a pregnant woman is given in Chapter No. 1. In a pregnant woman presenting with the

Table 1: Causes and contribution of various causes to occurrence and recurrence of congenital anomaly.[4]

Cause	Incidence (%)	Risk of recurrence
Genetic:		
• Chromosomal	6	<1/100 in trisomy, varies in unbalanced translocation, 1–3% in males, 10–15% in female carriers
• Single gene	7.5	25% autosomal recessive, 50% autosomal dominant (if either parent not affected chances of recurrence is sporadic as it may be a new mutation)
Multifactorial	30–40	1–4%
Environmental	5–10	
Drugs and chemicals	2	Rare, if offending agent is not present
Infections	2	Rare
Maternal illness, diabetes, and pyrexia	2–5	Rare, if disease is controlled
Unknown	50	Unknown (very low)

diagnosis of a structurally malformed fetus on ultrasonography, certain specific points need to be elicited in the history:
- *Age of the parents*: Advanced age of the parents, especially of the mother, is associated with occurrence of congenital birth defects
- Exposure to irradiation, drugs, or fever with or without rashes in the first trimester
- History suggestive of diabetes mellitus
- *Exposure to infections*: As assessed by taking occupational history, travel history, and contact with children, pets
- *Obstetric history*: Any history of recurrent abortions or prior fetal losses
- *Family history*: Any history of consanguinity, mental retardation, or congenital anomalies should be elicited. Any family history of medical problems such as diabetes should be noted.[5]

EXAMINATION

Clinical features suggestive of an autosomal dominant trait in either parent must be looked for, e.g., microdeletion 22q11.2 may present as a heart defect in the fetus. Examination of parents may reveal the characteristic facial features such as periorbital fullness, narrow upslanted palpebral fissures, prominent nose with large tip and small nares, small mouth with everted upper lip, and small dysmorphic ears.

INVESTIGATIONS

Maternal investigations include:
- TORCH serology immunoglobulin G (IgG) and IgM (TORCH stands for toxoplasmosis, others like hepatitis, varicella zoster, human immunodeficiency virus, rubella, cytomegalovirus, herpes simplex)
- Venereal Disease Research Laboratory (VDRL) testing
- Glucose tolerance test (GTT) and glycosylated hemoglobin levels
- Ultrasound
- Parental genetic testing.

TORCH Serology

It is important to understand that the fetal infection and the subsequent damage can take place only when the mother has acute infection during pregnancy. Acute infection is diagnosed by seroconversion or a two- to four-fold rise in IgG titers over a period of 2–4 weeks and low IgG avidity testing.

Ultrasound Examination

Findings, which are known to be closely associated with intrauterine infections, are hydrocephalus, microcephaly, nonimmune hydrops, cardiac anomaly, intracranial or abdominal calcifications, and polyhydramnios.

A detailed scan needs to be done to look for other associated anomalies.[6] Fetal echocardiography is indicated as minor cardiac defects may be missed on routine scan and cardiac defects are the most common congenital defects. Finding other associated anomalies can help in reaching a diagnosis and may alter the fetal prognosis and the risk of recurrence.

For example, ventriculomegaly is generally multifactorial but may be associated with a genetic cause such as X-linked hydrocephalus. This X-linked recessive genetic disorder affects males and is associated with aqueductal stenosis and adducted thumb. The recurrence risk in next pregnancy would be 50% in male babies. Figures 1A to E show ultrasound and postdelivery picture of a stillborn baby boy with adducted thumb. As the risk of recurrence was up to 50% in males, the second baby also had the similar finding and the pregnancy was terminated at 17 weeks' gestation.

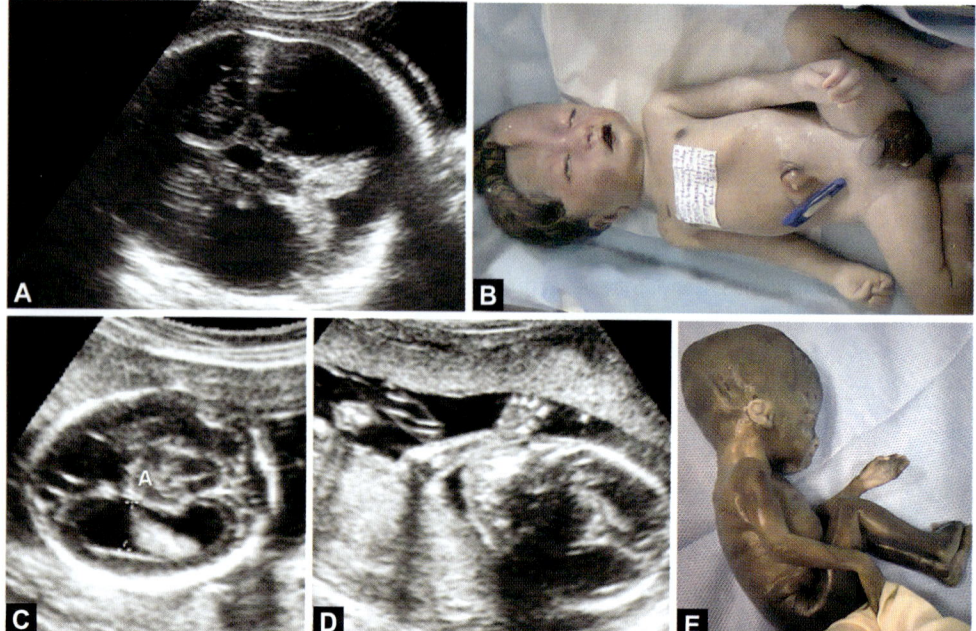

Figs. 1A to E: Ultrasound and postdelivery picture of stillborn baby boy with hydrocephalus and adducted thumb.

Minor defects such as cleft lip or polydactyly, if present in isolation, have good prognosis, but presence of other associated defects makes the prognosis grave.

Parental Testing

Parental genetic testing is valuable, if the fetal structural anomaly suggests genetic etiology. Parental genetic testing is helpful if a specific autosomal dominant or recessive disorder is suspected in the fetus. As shown in the ultrasonographic finding of meconium peritonitis on ultrasonography would prompt parental testing for *CFTR* mutation indicative of a likely diagnosis of fetal cystic fibrosis.[7]

Invasive Testing

Fetal Karyotyping

Karyotyping has been the gold standard for prenatal diagnosis of chromosomal abnormalities but has its limitations. It detects structural abnormality to the resolution of 5–10 Mb only; it is labor intensive, with a turnaround time of 14–21 days. The sample for karyotyping can be collected by invasive methods such as chorionic villus sampling (CVS), amniocentesis, or fetal blood sampling (cordocentesis) depending upon the gestational age at diagnosis. CVS is performed between 10 and 13 weeks and amniocentesis after 15 weeks. These are usually offered when the risk of aneuploidy is estimated to be >1 in 250 on prenatal screening, as the risk of complications associated with the invasive procedure is less than this.[7]

Fetal karyotyping can diagnose aneuploidy, polyploidy, deletions, duplications, and translocations. The risk of chromosomal anomaly varies with the type of malformation (Table 2). The risk is only 1% in gastroschisis, while it is up to 40% in omphalocele. Karyotype from amniotic fluid was done for a

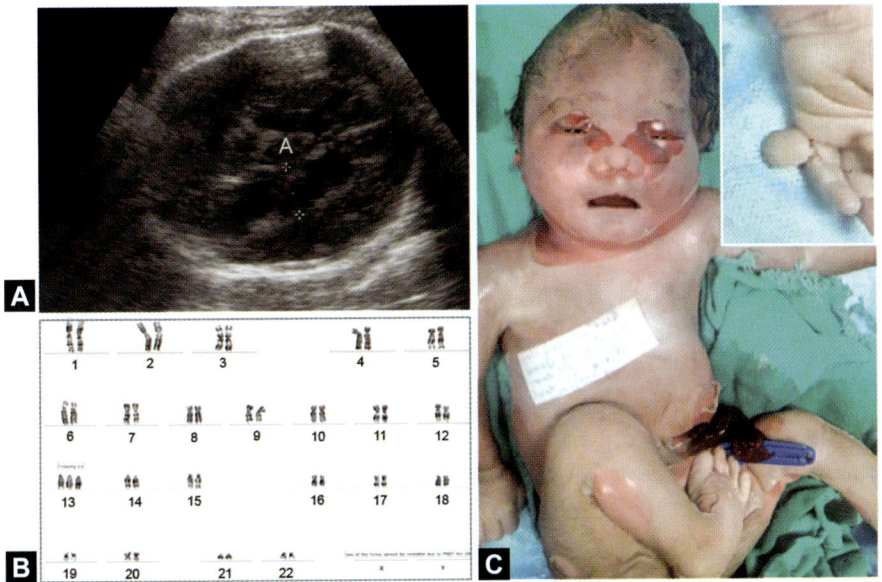

Figs. 2A to C: Case of mild ventriculomegaly on ultrasound, trisomy 13 on karyotype; after delivery polydactyly was additional finding.

Table 2: Risk of chromosomal anomaly with type of congenital malformation.[8]	
Anomaly	Chances of chromosomal anomaly
Cystic hygroma	70%
Holoprosencephaly	60%
Omphalocele	40%
Cardiac defect	30%
Duodenal atresia	30%
Dandy-Walker malformation	30%
Renal disease	30%
Spina bifida	10%
Hydrocephalus	10%
Diaphragmatic hernia	10%
Gastroschisis	<1%
Single umbilical artery	<1%

case of mild ventriculomegaly on ultrasound, which showed trisomy 13; after delivery additional finding of polydactyly was observed (Figs. 2A to C).

Fluorescence In Situ Hybridization

Fluorescence in situ hybridization (FISH) technique is a rapid and accurate test for detection of aneuploidies affecting chromosomes 13, 18, 21, X, and Y on uncultured cells within 24–48 hours. In FISH technique, a probe is used for a specific chromosomal region where the deletion or duplication is suspected. For example, in cases with cardiac defect, FISH test for 22q11.2 is indicated.

Chromosomal Microarray

Chromosomal microarray (CMA) is replacing fetal karyotype. It has the advantage of shorter turnaround time of 1 week as it does not require cell culture Moreover, it can detect smaller gain or loss of genetic material 10–100 kb as compared to 5–10 Mb by karyotyping.[8] However, it has the disadvantage of identifying background genetic variability not associated with anomalies. It is especially useful in intrauterine demise or stillbirth

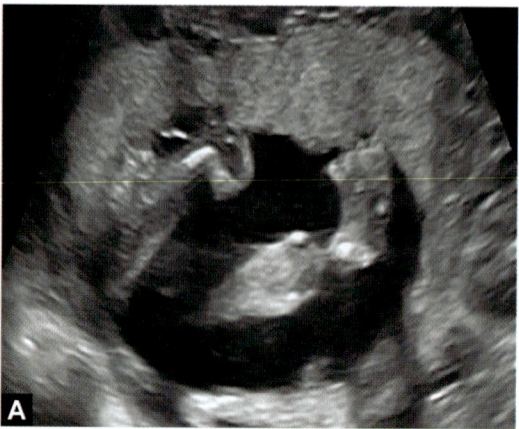
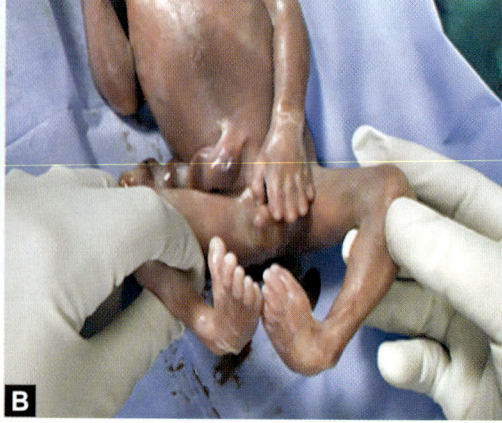

Test performed—Chromosomal microarray
Following clinically significant chromosomal abnormalities were found in the sample submitted for analysis.

CN State	Type	Chr. No	Cytoband start	Size (kbp)	Genes	Genomic coordinates	Interpretation
00	Loss	X	p22.31	1,620	7	arr[hg38] Xp22.31(6,568,448-8,188,133)x0	Pathogenic

Genes in the cytoband region Xp22.31: *PUDP, STS, MIR4767, VCX, PNPLA4, MIR651, VCX2*

Figs. 3A and B: Shows the antenatal ultrasound, post abortion photograph of the baby with bilateral talipes equinovarus the pathogenic microarray report at the bottom.

where there is an increased diagnostic yield of 12–15% with CMA compared to conventional karyotyping.[9] Prenatal CMA analysis is recommended for a patient with a fetus with one or more major structural abnormalities identified on ultrasonographic examination.

In the case shown in (Figs. 3A and B), the ultrasound at 19 weeks showed bilateral talipes. It can be an isolated defect or may be associated with a genetic defect or be a part of a syndrome. The parents were offered CMA test on amniotic fluid. The CMA showed pathogenic deletion in short arm of X chromosome. The report was available within a week, and the couple decided for a termination of pregnancy after counseling.

Gene Sequencing

This is indicated when the chromosomal analysis by karyotyping and CMA are normal or when certain specific genetic condition is suspected. This molecular genetic study can be performed on fetal DNA from cultured chorionic cells or amniocytes and sometimes can be collected directly from the chorionic sample or amniocytes without culture. This test may include targeted gene sequencing, i.e., of a single gene or gene panels or whole-exome sequencing. Single gene testing is offered based on family history or a previously identified mutation as in achondroplasia.

Whole-exome sequencing: Exome is the part of genome that encodes for proteins. It comprises only 1% of whole genome but contains 85% of all disease-producing mutations. The whole-exome sequencing is a broad molecular diagnostic approach to identify the etiology for fetal abnormalities. Whole-exome sequencing of fetal DNA obtained by amniocentesis, chorionic villi, or umbilical cord blood may be offered for specific clinical indications. There is no consistent data for prenatal whole-exome sequencing, although the potential for long turnaround time limits the use of whole-exome sequencing for prenatal diagnosis for reproductive decision-making. The second major limitation of this technology is the high number of variants of uncertain significance that are detected. Due to many complex issues that arise in use of whole-exome sequencing clinically, the College and the Society for Maternal–Fetal Medicine recommends that all patients considering whole-exome sequencing should receive counseling from a healthcare provider with expertise in genetics.

Figure 4A shows a case with massive abdominal distension due to polyhydramnios. The ultrasound showed consistent full bladder of baby in Figure 4B. The biochemical testing of amniotic fluid was suggestive of raised sodium and chloride in the amniotic fluid with the possibility of Bartter syndrome. The next-generation sequencing (NGS) was done from amniotic fluid which confirmed the deletion of *KCNJ1* gene, corresponding to Bartter's syndrome (Fig. 4C). The chance of recurrence in the next pregnancy would be up to 25% as it is autosomal recessive; it can be diagnosed early in the next pregnancy by CVS and molecular testing.

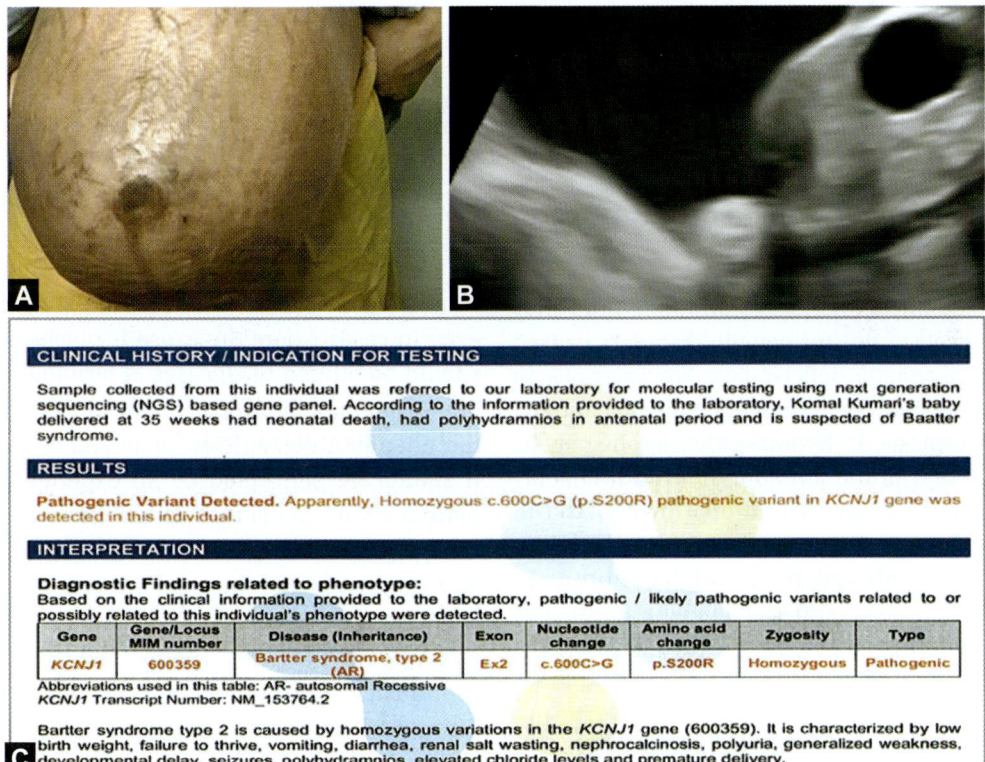

Figs. 4A to C: (A) shows a case with massive abdominal distension due to polyhydramnios; (B) The ultrasound showed consistent full bladder of baby. (C) The biochemical testing of amniotic fluid was suggestive of raised sodium and chloride in the amniotic fluid with the possibility of Bartter syndrome. The next-generation sequencing (NGS) was done from amniotic fluid which confirmed the deletion of *KCNJ1* gene, corresponding to Bartter's syndrome.

Flowchart 1: Algorithm for clinical approach to a pregnant woman presenting with a congenitally malformed fetus.

- Pregnant women presents with fetal anomaly on ultrasound in fetal medicine clinic
- *History:* Fever with rash, drug or X-ray exposure, and DM
- *Family history:* Consanguinity, developmental delay, congenital anomaly, and DM
- *Examination:* Clinical features of autosomal dominant trait in either parent
- *Investigations:* TORCH, VDRL, OGTT, targeted ultrasound, and fetal echo
- *Invasive tests:* Karyotype, FISH, CMA, NGS, enzyme studies, PCR for infection, and molecular tests for prenatal diagnosis
- Follow-up ultrasound at regular interval till delivery for evolution of other anomalies
- *Stillbirth:* Fetal autopsy
- Photograph, infantogram, external and internal examinations, karyotype, CMA HPE of relevant tissue
- Liveborn examined by pediatrician
- Referral to pediatric surgeon/specialist for expert follow-up care
- Couple called for counseling by geneticist/fetal medicine specialist after 4–6 weeks for counseling regarding future pregnancy and risk of recurrence

(DM: diabetes mellitus; CMA: chromosomal microarray; HPE: histopathological examination; NGS: next-generation sequencing; OGTT: oral glucose tolerance test; PCR: polymerase chain reaction; TORCH: for toxoplasmosis, others like hepatitis, varicella zoster, etc.; rubella, cytomegalovirus, and herpes simplex; VRDL; Venereal Disease Research Laboratory)

Biochemical Analysis of Amniotic Fluid

Biochemical analysis of amniotic fluid may be used to test for genetic disorders caused by enzymatic deficiencies. For example, in women with nonclassical congenital adrenal hyperplasia, 17-hydroxyprogesterone may be assessed in the amniotic fluid to prenatally diagnose congenital adrenal hyperplasia in the fetus. In fetuses with neural tube defect, components such as alpha-fetoprotein (α-fetoprotein) and acetylcholinesterase may be determined in amniotic fluid to assess if a neural tube defect is open or closed.

Polymerase Chain Reaction for Infectious Agents in Amniotic Fluid

Polymerase chain reaction (PCR) for DNA is done on amniotic fluid to diagnose congenital infections such as *Toxoplasma, rubella,* and cytomegalovirus.

Fetal Autopsy

Fetal autopsy is included in the basic protocol of investigation into a perinatal death even in cases where the cause is obvious. It should be offered to all cases of termination of pregnancy, stillbirth, or neonatal death by the attending obstetrician or neonatologist. It should be performed by an experienced perinatal or pediatric pathologist. Fetal autopsy is found to add to the diagnosis in 30–40% cases and thus aid in counseling regarding risk of recurrence in future pregnancy.[9] In investigating a perinatal death, the coordinated effort of obstetrician, neonatologist, and pathologist is required. The basic elements of autopsy are photograph, infantogram, external and internal examinations of the baby, and the karyotype.

The detailed workup of a pregnant woman with fetal anomaly is described in Flowchart 1.

Chapter 15: Approach to a Pregnant Woman with a Congenitally Malformed Fetus

Flowchart 2: Management of fetal anomaly and their counseling regarding risk of recurrence.

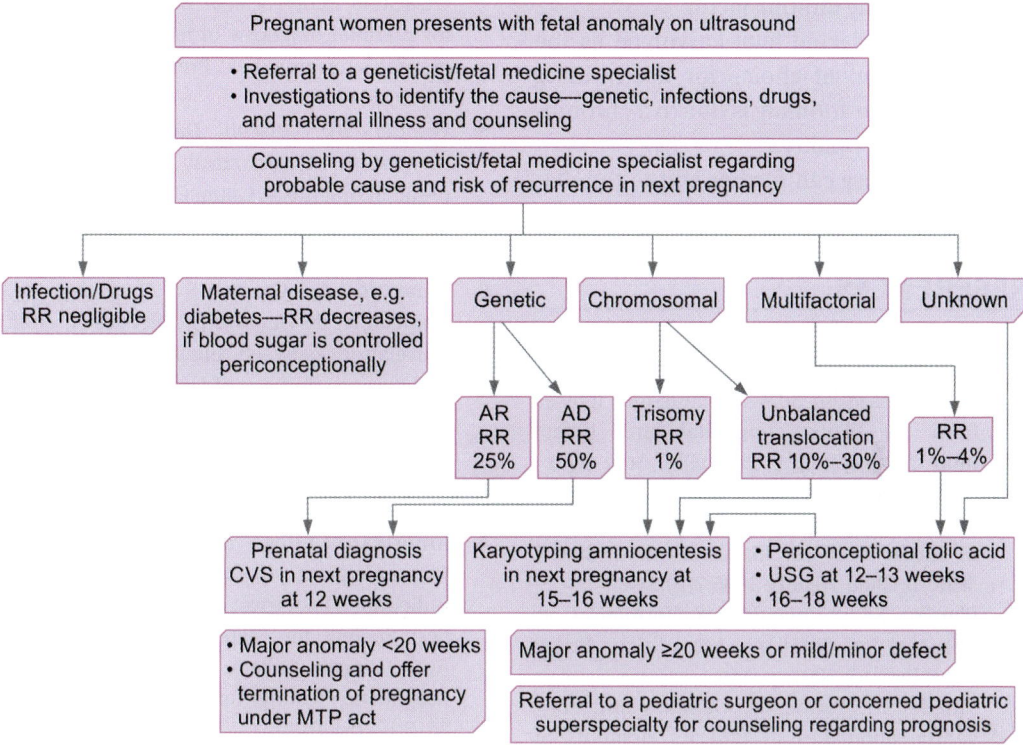

(AR: autosomal recessive; AD: autosomal dominant; CVS: chorionic villus sampling; MTP: medical termination of pregnancy; RR: recurrence risk)

MANAGEMENT

The management of a pregnant woman presenting with a malformed fetus depends upon the gestational age, type of anomaly—minor or major, any associated chromosomal anomaly, and the wish of the parents.

Flowchart 2 describes the management in detail.

KEY POINTS

- If a pregnant woman presents with congenital anomaly in the fetus, it is important to find out the cause in order to provide the prognosis and to determine the risk of recurrence.
- A thorough workup includes detailed history, examination, and investigations with the aim to identify the cause.
- The role of invasive testing in the form of CVS, amniocentesis, and cordocentesis is very useful.
- Conventional cytogenetic analysis karyotyping using in vitro culture of fetal nucleated cell takes 2–3 weeks.
- If there is suspicion of genetic disease, prenatal diagnosis is done by molecular techniques by obtaining the DNA sample from chorionic villi or amniotic fluid cells. The results take a week's time.
- FISH can be done on uncultured cells for rapid prenatal diagnosis and results can

be obtained in 24 hours, but the cost of the test is the limiting factor.
- CMA is replacing fetal karyotype as the investigation of choice for determining whether the anomaly is due to a chromosomal abnormality.
- Fetal autopsy can further add to the diagnosis in a significant number of cases.

REFERENCES

1. Queisser-Luft A, Stolz G, Wiesel A, Schlaefer K, Spranger J. Malformations in newborn: results based on 30,940 infants and fetuses from the Mainz congenital birth defect monitoring system (1990-1998). Arch Gynecol Obstet. 2002;266(3):163-77.
2. Bhat BV, Ravikumara M. Perinatal mortality in India: Need for introspection. Indian J Matern Child Health. 1996;7(2):31-3.
3. Phadke SR. Congenital malformation in Genetics for clinicians, 1st edition. Prism book Pvt Ltd; 2007. p. 140.
4. Mueller RF, Young ID. Genetics and congenital anomalies in Emery's elements of medical genetics, 11th edition. Churchill Livingstone: Harcourt Publications; 2001. p. 230.
5. James DK, Steer PJ, Weiner CP, Gonik B, et al. High Risk Pregnancy: Management Options, 3rd edition. India: Elsevier; 2006. pp. 325-471.
6. Gagnon A, Genetics Committee.. Evaluation of prenatally diagnosed structural congenital anomalies. J Obstet Gynaecol Can. 2009;31(9): 875-81, 882-9.
7. Drury S, Williams H, Trump N, Boustred C, GOSGene, Lench N, et al. Exome sequencing for prenatal diagnosis of fetuses with sonographic abnormalities. Prenat Diagn. 2015; 35(10):1010-7.
8. Wapner RJ, Driscoll DA, Simpson JL. Integration of microarray technology into prenatal diagnosis: Counselling issues generated during the NICHD clinical trial. Prenat Diagn. 2012;32(4):396-400.
9. Vimercati A, Grasso S, Abruzzese M, Chincoli A, de Genarro A, Miccolis A, et al. Correlation between ultrasound diagnosis and autopsy findings of fetal malformations. J Prenat Med. 2012;6(2):13-7.

SUGGESTED READING

1. American College of Obstetricians and Gynecologists' Committee on Practice Bulletins—Obstetrics; Committee on Genetics; Society for Maternal–Fetal Medicine. ACOG Practice Bulletin Number 162: Prenatal Diagnostic Testing for Genetic Disorders. 2016;127(5):e108-22.
2. Committee on Genetics and the Society for Maternal-Fetal Medicine. Committee Opinion No.682: Microarrays and Next-Generation Sequencing Technology: The Use of Advanced Genetic Diagnostic Tools in Obstetrics and Gynecology. Obstet Gynecol. 2016;128(6):e262-8.
3. Wilson RD; SOGC Genetics Committee. Prenatal screening, diagnosis, and pregnancy management of fetal neural tube defects. J Obstet Gynaecol Can. 2014;36(10):927-39.

16. Approach to a Pregnant Woman Presenting with Jaundice

Sharda Patra

INTRODUCTION

Jaundice refers to yellow discoloration of the conjunctiva, mucous membrane, skin, other tissues, and body fluids resulting from deposition of excess bilirubin. Jaundice is clinically detectable when the serum bilirubin level ≥ 2 mg/dL (normal range 0.2–0.9 mg/dL, 4–16 µmol/L).

The incidence of jaundice in pregnancy in India is estimated to vary from 0.4 to 0.9/1,000 deliveries.[1] It is one of the major indirect causes of maternal death responsible for 5–30% of all maternal deaths.[1] Jaundice in pregnancy encompasses a diverse range of liver diseases, some of which occur exclusively during pregnancy, some incidentally during pregnancy and still others due to preexisting liver diseases, which get unmasked or are worsened by pregnancy (Flowchart 1).

Flowchart 1: Algorithm of clinical approach to a pregnant women presenting with jaundice.

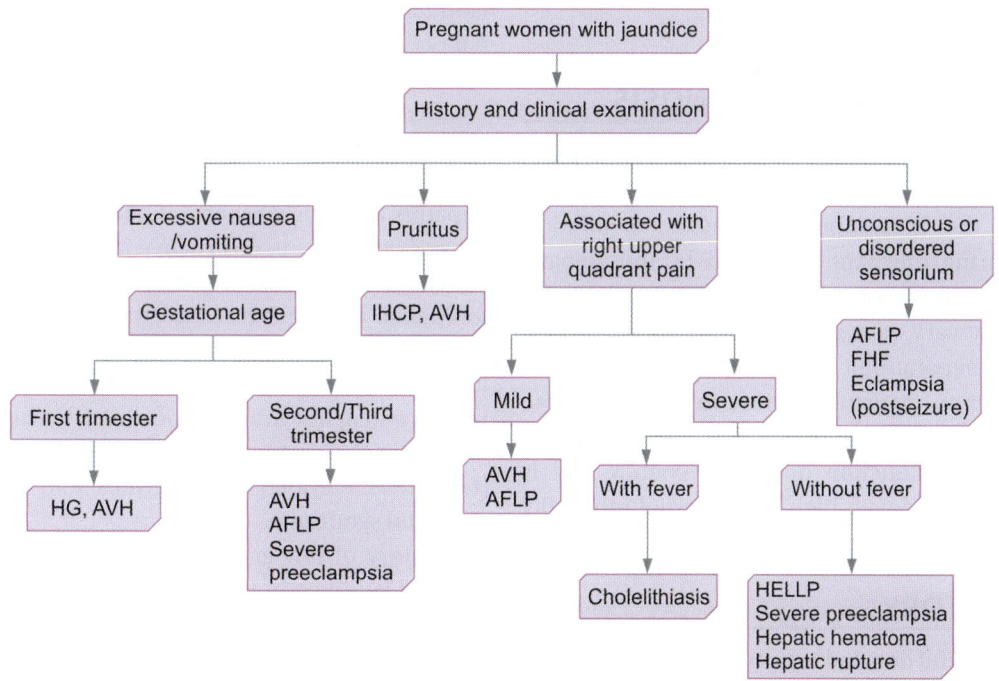

(AFLP: acute fatty liver of pregnancy; AVH: active viral hepatitis; FHF: fulminant hepatic failure; HELLP: hemolysis, elevated liver enzyme and low platelet; HG: hyperemesis gravidarum; IHCP: intrahepatic cholestasis of pregnancy)

Table 1: Differential diagnosis of jaundice in pregnancy.

Liver disease induced by pregnancy	Preexisting liver disease that worsens during pregnancy	Liver diseases incidental to pregnancy
First trimester Hyperemesis gravidarum	Cholelithiasis Primary biliary cirrhosis Dubin–Johnson syndrome	AVH DIH
Late second and third trimesters IHCP Preeclampsia and eclampsia HELLP syndrome Hepatic rupture AFLP	Wilson's disease Cirrhosis with PH Budd–Chiari syndrome Autoimmune hepatitis Hepatic adenoma Hepatocellular carcinoma	

(AFLP: acute fatty liver of pregnancy; AVH: acute viral hepatitis; DIH: drug-induced hepatitis; HELLP: hemolysis, elevated liver enzymes and low platelets; IHCP: intrahepatic cholestasis of pregnancy; PH: portal hypertension)

DIFFERENTIAL DIAGNOSIS

The differential diagnosis of jaundice in pregnancy is as given in Table 1. Viral hepatitis is the most common cause of jaundice during pregnancy followed by intrahepatic cholestasis of pregnancy (IHCP), but this may vary with geographic location. Though all hepatotropic viruses can affect pregnant women, hepatitis E virus infection is more common during pregnancy. It causes severe liver dysfunction during pregnancy and is associated with high fetomaternal morbidity and mortality.[1]

HISTORY

A careful detailed history is very important in finding out the cause of jaundice in pregnancy (Table 2). Many symptoms of liver disorders mimic normal symptoms of pregnancy; hence a high index of suspicion is required to make an early diagnosis during pregnancy.

History of Present Illness

The onset of jaundice, whether acute or insidious, and the duration of jaundice should be noted. The time of onset of jaundice in relation to the period of gestation provides an important clue to the etiology of jaundice (see Table 1). Liver diseases induced by pregnancy or incidental to pregnancy are usually acute in onset and of short duration (days), whereas jaundice due to preexisting liver diseases is insidious in onset and of long duration (months). One must enquire about the color of urine, whether it is yellowish and turns dark on standing or it is colorless. Appearance of dark-colored urine and pale stools followed by scleral icterus is characteristic of conjugated hyperbilirubinemia seen in obstructive jaundice, whereas scleral icterus with pale-colored urine suggests unconjugated hyperbilirubinemia due to hemolysis.

The history of altered bowel habits should be sought. The patient may complain of diarrhea in the prodromal phase of viral hepatitis A and E. Absence of bile acids may cause steatorrhea in obstructive jaundice.

Other associated constitutional symptoms such as fatigue, malaise, nausea, vomiting, and loss of appetite should be asked for as these symptoms precede the onset of jaundice in acute viral hepatitis (AVH), acute fatty liver of pregnancy (AFLP), and HELLP (hemolysis, elevated liver enzymes, and low platelets) syndrome.

History of low-grade fever precedes the onset of jaundice in viral hepatitis; however, high-grade fever in AVH is an ominous sign, indicative of fulminant hepatic failure (FHF). Fever is also present in jaundice due to infections such as malaria, leptospirosis,

Table 2: Pathognomonic clinical features of various causes of jaundice in pregnancy.

Condition	Clinical features
Hyperemesis gravidarum	Usually in first trimester, presents with intractable vomiting, dehydration, and mild jaundice (10%)
IHCP	Usually in second and third trimester, presents with pruritus often starts in the palms and soles and spreads to other parts of the body, more severe during night, mild jaundice in 20% of cases
AFLP	Usually in second and third trimester, presents with nausea, vomiting (70%), epigastric pain (65%), anorexia, mild jaundice, headache, altered sensorium (encephalopathy), deranged coagulation, 50% have high blood pressure, proteinuria, and edema
Preeclampsia with severe features	Usually in second and third trimester, presents with hypertension with or without proteinuria, epigastric pain radiating to hypochondrium, nausea, vomiting, tenderness on palpating the liver
HELLP syndrome	Usually in second and third trimester, presents with epigastric/right upper quadrant pain (50%), fatigue/malaise (90%), nausea, vomiting, headache (50%), 85% have preeclampsia
Preeclampsia with severe features and hepatic rupture	Severe right upper quadrant pain sudden in onset, nausea, vomiting, and hypotension
AVH	Fatigue, malaise, loss of appetite, diarrhea, mild fever, mild epigastric pain, mild pruritus, and mild-to-severe jaundice
FHF	Severe jaundice, encephalopathy, deranged coagulation, and renal dysfunction
Cholelithiasis	Fever, intermittent right upper quadrant pain, vomiting, and jaundice
Drug-induced hepatitis	History of drug intake
Budd–Chiari syndrome	Right upper quadrant pain, hepatomegaly with ascites, and mild jaundice

(AFLP: acute fatty liver of pregnancy; AVH: acute viral hepatitis; HELLP: hemolysis, elevated liver enzyme and low platelets; FHF: fulminant hepatic failure; IHCP: intrahepatic cholestasis of pregnancy)

disseminated tuberculosis (TB), and typhoid. Fever associated with chills or upper abdominal pain and/or a history of prior biliary surgery, is suggestive of acute cholangitis or cholecystitis.

Upper abdominal pain is a significant symptom, which is present late in pregnancy and could be due to HELLP, preeclampsia with severe features, AFLP, cholecystitis, or AVH. Severe upper abdominal pain, particularly in the epigastric area, occurs due to hepatic subcapsular hematoma or hemorrhage. Colicky pain with or without fever indicates biliary colic and/or acute cholangitis or cholecystitis.

Pruritus is the main complaint in patients with IHCP, biliary obstruction, or alcoholic hepatitis. Pruritus in IHCP characteristically starts in palms and soles and spreads to trunk and other parts of the body and is more severe during night. Jaundice follows pruritus in 20% cases of IHCP. Mild pruritus may be present in the cholestatic phase of viral hepatitis. Pruritus may be present in normal pregnancy but is generally limited to the abdomen and usually does not occur during night.

Altered sleep pattern and generalized slowing are early symptoms of encephalopathy. Loss of consciousness in a jaundiced patient is suggestive of hepatic encephalopathy and FHF. It may be present in AVH and AFLP. If the patient is unconscious, one should enquire about the duration of unconsciousness and symptoms preceding it like altered sleep pattern, convulsions, and severe headache. History of convulsions followed by unconsciousness could be due to eclampsia. Other important symptoms that should be elicited include headache, peripheral edema, foamy urine due to proteinuria, and decreased urine output suggestive of preeclampsia.

Past History

History should include history of hepatitis, pancreatic disorders, anemia, any inherited hemoglobinopathy such as thalassemia or sickle cell disease, and history of biliary disease or surgery. Ask about intake of hepatotoxic drugs such as acetaminophen, antitubercular drugs, antiepileptic, or antipsychotic drugs in recent past. One must also enquire about history of transfusion of blood or blood products and any intravenous drug abuse. History of contact with any person suffering from jaundice, especially within the household or travel to areas where hepatitis is endemic and intake of contaminated drinking water in areas with suspected food or waterborne outbreak should be elicited. History of multiple sexual partners, sexual contact with hepatitis B surface antigen (HBsAg)-positive person, and of chronic alcohol intake is important.

Occupational History

Healthcare workers, such as paramedical and medical staff handling blood and body fluids, are at an increased risk of contracting hepatitis.

Family History

Any history suggestive of inherited anemia, hemoglobinopathies, and liver disorders should be elicited. A family history of preeclampsia or IHCP is important. IHCP has a genetic predisposition and a positive family history is present in half of women with IHCP. Genetic predisposition of IHCP is due to an altered membrane composition of bile ducts and hepatocytes with resultant to increased sensitivity to sex steroids.

Obstetric History

History of jaundice and pruritus in the past pregnancies, its time of onset, and any associated complications should be elicited. This gives a clue to the diagnosis of IHCP. History of oral contraceptives in the past and occurrence of jaundice and or pruritus with intake of oral contraceptives are helpful in the diagnosis of IHCP.

EXAMINATION

The evaluation of a patient presenting with jaundice begins with a careful examination; it may not aid in narrowing the differential diagnosis but helps in determining the urgency of intervention.

General Physical Examination

The general condition of the patient on presentation should be assessed. In case of hyperemesis, HELLP, and AVH, the patient is likely to appear very ill and dehydrated. The level of consciousness, response to verbal commands, orientation to time, place, and person, and presence of irritability should be noted. The degree of jaundice and level of consciousness are important findings in assessing the severity of disease. Presence of severe jaundice with altered sensorium indicates FHF due to AVH. The AFLP should be suspected, if the patient has mild jaundice with altered sensorium. Mild jaundice with altered sensorium and significant peripheral edema may be present in eclampsia. In pregnancy, AVH and AFLP are two conditions where a patient deteriorates very fast and might present in FHF. Termination of pregnancy may be lifesaving in AFLP whereas AVH is managed conservatively; hence, an early diagnosis is very crucial.

Other findings that should be noted in the general physical examination are pallor, icterus, peripheral edema, generalized edema, and vital signs such as pulse, blood pressure, respiratory rate and temperature. High temperature with tachycardia and grunting respiration in a severely jaundiced unconscious patient are ominous signs indicating FHF either due to AVH or AFLP. Hepatic rupture should be suspected, if a conscious patient presents with severe epigastric pain, jaundice, tachycardia, and hypotension (signs of shock).

Mild jaundice with severe pallor could be due to hemolysis as in chronic anemia due to hemoglobinopathies. The presence of hypertension and edema points toward preeclampsia and AFLP.

Look for any rash, purpuric spots, or mucosal bleed; presence of these indicates disseminated intravascular coagulopathy with associated thrombocytopenia, which are present in AFLP, HELLP, and FHF following AVH. Look for scratch marks over abdomen, trunk, hands, and legs; it is indicative of severe itching as in IHCP. Spider angiomas and palmar erythema, which represent liver disease in nonpregnant women may be present in normal pregnancy.

Systemic Examination

Routine breast examination, respiratory and cardiovascular system examination should be done.

Per Abdomen Examination

Observe for any evidence of hepatosplenomegaly. It may not be possible to appreciate hepatosplenomegaly in advanced pregnancy due to the enlarged gravid uterus. Presence of hepatomegaly suggests either an acute or chronic liver disease. If the liver is not palpable, the liver dullness should be checked on percussion. The liver dullness is normally appreciated starting from fifth to seventh intercostal space till the right lower costal margin in the midclavicular line. If it is reduced, it indicates FHF as in AVH or AFLP. Splenomegaly may be present whenever there is hemolysis or if the patient is suffering from malaria or *Salmonella* infection.

Presence of shifting dullness due to ascites indicates chronic liver disease or Budd–Chiari syndrome. Rapid onset of hepatomegaly with ascites occurs in Budd–Chiari syndrome. The liver is tender to palpate in AVH and preeclampsia.

Neurological Examination

Neurological examination is done to assess the mental status of the woman including the level of consciousness and orientation for grading of hepatic encephalopathy (Table 3).

Table 3: Grades of hepatic encephalopathy (West Haven index)[2]

Grade	Clinical features
Minimal	No clinical abnormalities
I	Patient feels sleepy, may be irritable
II	Patient is drowsy, becomes disoriented intermittently
III	Patient is disoriented and confused
IVa	Patient is comatose, but responds to painful stimuli
IVb	Patient is comatose and does not respond to painful stimuli

Table 4: Differential diagnosis of jaundice in pregnancy based on laboratory investigations.

Condition	Bilirubin (mg/dL)	Transaminases (IU/mL)	Alkaline phosphatase (IU/mL)	Bile acids (µmol/mL)	Platelet count (1 × 10⁹/L)	PT/INR	Urine albumin	LDH
Hyperemesis gravidarum (HG)	<5	<200	<500	N	N	N	N	N
IHCP	<5	<200	<500	↑30–100 times >40	N	N	N	N
AFLP	<10	<200	<500	N	<100,000	↑↑↑	absent	N
Preeclampsia/Eclampsia	<5	200–1,000	<500	N	N to low	↑	Significant proteinuria	N
HELLP	<5	200–1,000	<500	N	<100,000	↑	Absent/Present	600–1,000
Hepatic rupture	<5	>1,000	2,000	N	Low	↑↑↑	N	N
AVH/FHF	>15 >20	>2,000 <500	500	N	N	↑↑↑ Or ↑↑↑	N	N
Drug-induced hepatitis	10–20	200–1,000	1,000	N	N	N	N	N
Cholelithiasis	<5	<200	1,000–2,000	N	N	N	N	N
Non-alcoholic steatohepatitis	<5	<500	<500	N	N	N	N	N

(AFLP: acute fatty liver of pregnancy; AVH: active viral hepatitis; HELLP: hemolysis, elevated liver enzymes and low platelets; FHF: fulminant hepatic failure; IHCP: intrahepatic cholestasis of pregnancy; INR: international normalized ratio; LDH: lactate dehydrogenase; N: normal; PT: prothrombin time)

Obstetric Examination

Obstetric examination is performed to assess the number of fetuses, presentation and, viability of fetus and presence or absence of uterine contractions. In the presence of obstetrical complaints like discharge or bleeding per vaginam or labor pains, per speculum and per vaginam examination may be indicated.

INVESTIGATIONS

A properly elicited history along with complete general physical examination narrows the differential diagnosis. All patients are subjected to complete blood count (CBC) with peripheral smear and liver function tests and then followed by specific investigations as guided by the provisional working diagnosis (Table 4).

Routine Investigations

Complete Blood Count with Peripheral Smear

Hemoglobin (Hb) < 11 g% indicates anemia in pregnancy. Presence of leukocytosis is

Table 5: Normal values of liver function tests in pregnancy.[3,4]

Biochemical marker	Nonpregnant	Pregnant		
		First trimester	Second trimester	Third trimester
Serum bilirubin (mg/dL)	0–1	0.2–0.9	0.1–0.7	0.1–0.8
(μmol/L)	0–17	4–16	3–13	3–14
AST (U/L)	7–40	10–28	10–29	11–30
ALT (U/L)	0–40	0–40	6–32	6–32
Alkaline phosphatase (U/L)	30–130	32–100	43–135	133–418
Gamma-glutamyltransferase (U/L)	11–50	5–37	5–43	3–41
Albumin (mg/dL)	3.3–4.1	2.4–3.1		
Bile acid (μmol/L)	0–14	0–14		

(ALT: alanine transaminase; AST: aspartate transaminase)

suggestive of infection. In AVH and AFLP, total leukocyte count (TLC) may increase to 20,000–25,000/mm³. Platelet count of < 50,000 × 10⁹/L is seen in HELLP syndrome whereas in AFLP, it may be < 100,000 × 10⁹/L. Thrombocytopenia is also a feature of FHF with disseminated intravascular coagulation (DIC) in viral hepatitis. The peripheral smear shows the type of anemia and other abnormalities such as presence of sickle cells as in sickle cell anemia, malarial parasite, or hemolysis. In HELLP syndrome, peripheral smear shows schistocytes, echinocytes, and spherostomatocytes whereas in drug-induced hemolysis, it shows only spherocytes. Microcytic hypochromic picture is suggestive of thalassemia.

Liver Function Tests[3,4]

While interpreting the values of various liver function tests in pregnancy, it is important to know that the normal range of values is altered in normal pregnancy. The enzymes alanine aminotransferase, aspartate amino-transferase and albumin are lower and alkaline phosphatase (ALP) is increased up to two to four times the nonpregnant levels in a pregnant woman. The normal values of various liver function tests in pregnancy are given in Table 5.

Serum Bilirubin

Serum bilirubin tests the liver's ability to clear metabolic products. Bilirubin remains in circulation in conjugated and unconjugated forms, which are measured as direct and indirect bilirubin. Generally, the normal value of direct bilirubin is 0.1–0.4 mg/dL and indirect bilirubin is 0.2–0.9 mg/dL. The normal ratio of direct and indirect bilirubin is 1:4. Elevated indirect bilirubin results from overproduction of bilirubin as seen in hemolysis (hereditary spherocytosis and sickle cell disease), impaired red blood cell (RBC) synthesis (megaloblastic, sideroblastic, and iron deficiency anemia), impaired uptake of bilirubin (drugs) and impaired conjugation (advanced liver disease, congenital hyperbilirubinemia). Elevated direct bilirubin signifies impaired intrahepatic excretion or regurgitation of unconjugated or conjugated bilirubin from hepatocytes of bile ducts and is a more sensitive indicator of hepatic disease.

Levels of >25 mg/dL may be seen in severe liver disease due to viral hepatitis though fractionated bilirubin is not useful in differentiating hepatocellular injury from cholestasis. If there is high clinical suspicion of liver disease, the aminotransferases, ALP, albumin, and prothrombin time (PT) should be evaluated. If all these values are normal, consider hemolysis or inherited disorders as the cause for jaundice. Gilbert's syndrome or Crigler–Najjar syndrome causes isolated unconjugated hyperbilirubinemia, and the Dubin–Johnson and Rotor syndromes cause isolated conjugated hyperbilirubinemia. In IHCP and AFLP, bilirubin levels are <5 mg/dL.

Serum Transaminases

Elevation of serum transaminases is an indicator of hepatocellular necrosis. As alanine transaminase (ALT) is the predominant enzyme in liver hence it is more specific of liver disease than aspartate transaminase (AST). Mild AST or ALT elevations of up to 1.5 times the upper limits of normal do not necessarily indicate liver disease, but serum levels of AST and ALT increase to some extent in almost all liver diseases. Marked elevation of >20 times or 1,000 U/L is common with conditions such as viral hepatitis, drug toxicity, and acute ischemic injury to liver. In AVH, its level in the initial phase may go up to 2,000–3,000 U/L. Elevated enzyme levels may reflect the extent of hepatocellular damage, but they do not always correlate with severity of liver damage. A declining AST and ALT following a rise in AVH may indicate either recovery or FHF. The highest level (up to 10,000 U/L) has been found in acute hepatic toxicity due to acetaminophen or acute ischemic injury to liver. Moderate increase in AST and ALT that is 3–20 times or 200–1,000 U/L are seen in HELLP syndrome, severe preeclampsia, AVH, chronic hepatitis, autoimmune hepatitis, and drug-induced hepatitis.

Mild increase in liver enzymes, i.e., up to one to three times or <200 U/L, is seen in conditions such as hyperemesis gravidarum, ICHP, AFLP, cholelithiasis, and alcoholic hepatitis.

The ratio of AST to ALT is useful in differentiating Wilson's disease, chronic liver disease, and alcoholic liver disease from other liver diseases and a ratio of >2 is usually observed in the former conditions. In nonalcoholic steatohepatitis (NASH) and viral hepatitis, the ratio of AST/ALT is <1. The ratio invariably rises to >1 as hepatic fibrosis develops in cirrhosis with resultant reduction of plasma clearance of AST secondary to impaired function of sinusoidal cells.

Alkaline Phosphatase

Alkaline phosphatase is a marker of bile stasis and is seen in cholestatic jaundice. In normal pregnancy, it rises to two to four times the normal values due to placental alkaline phosphatase. Hence, a level of more than this is considered as pathological in pregnancy. Mild-to-moderate elevation in ALP (four to five times) is seen in acute fatty liver of pregnancy, preeclampsia, HELLP syndrome, cholestasis of pregnancy, and hyperemesis gravidarum. Markedly elevated ALP (greater than six times the normal) is seen in extrahepatic biliary obstruction, hepatic rupture, primary biliary cirrhosis, and drug-induced cholestasis.

Serum Albumin

The serum albumin levels reflect synthetic liver function. With progressive liver disease, serum albumin levels fall, reflecting decreased synthesis as in chronic liver disease. However, in acute hepatic conditions such as in AVH, serum albumin remains in the normal range as it has a long half-life of 21 days. Hence, a low albumin in AVH indicates an underlying chronic liver disease and should be investigated. Further, the level of serum albumin also depends on factors such as the nutritional status, urinary and gastrointestinal losses, and the state of catabolism. Low albumin levels should be interpreted keeping all these factors in mind.

Serum Bile Acids

Elevated serum bile acids such as cholic acid, chenodeoxycholic acid, and deoxycholic acid, along with raised serum transaminases and bilirubin are diagnostic of IHCP. Serum bile acids level is a good predictor of fetal outcome in IHCP. Raised levels of serum bile acids correlate with adverse fetal outcome. The risk is low when serum bile acid level is <40 µmol/L, with an increase of each µmol/L thereafter the probability of the preterm delivery, birth asphyxia, and meconium staining increases by 1.5–2%.

Coagulation Profile

The presence of abnormal coagulation profile in the presence of liver disease reflects a poor synthetic function of liver and indicates an ongoing liver damage. The coagulation profile includes measurement of PT, partial thromboplastin time with kaolin (PTTK), international normalized ratio (INR), and fibrinogen degradation products (FDPs). An elevated PT and partial thromboplastin time (PTT) signify either a synthetic dysfunction due to liver damage or increased consumption secondary to DIC. Presence of FDPs indicates consumptive coagulopathy consequent to thromboplastins released by extensive liver damage.

Other investigations such as urine examination for albumin, sugar, bile salts and pigments, microscopy, serum cholesterol, blood sugar (random), kidney function test, and serum electrolytes should be done.

Specific Tests

Specific tests can be done based on the differential diagnosis by the history, physical examination, and liver functions tests.

If hemolysis is suspected (as in HELLP), serum lactic dehydrogenase (LDH) should be done. An elevated lactic dehydrogenase (LDH) and decreased haptoglobin levels can help to assess the severity of hemolysis.

In suspected cases of autoimmune hepatitis measurement of antinuclear, anti-smooth muscle and liver kidney microsomal (LKM) antibodies and for primary biliary cirrhosis, anti-mitochondrial antibodies (AMA) is indicated. In suspected cases of thalassemia, HPLC (high-performance liquid chromatography) for HbA2 for confirmation of diagnosis of thalassemia and serum levels of iron, transferrin, and ferritin are indicated to assess for body stores of iron. Serum levels of ceruloplasmin are done, if Wilson's disease is suspected. Measurement of alpha-1 antitrypsin activity is carried out for confirmation of the diagnosis of alpha-1 antitrypsin deficiency.

Viral Serology

Any patient with significant jaundice should be screened for viral hepatitis A, B, C, D, and E by viral serology. This includes immunoglobulin M (IgM) antibody to hepatitis A virus (anti-HAV IgM), hepatitis B core antigen (anti-HBc IgM), hepatitis C virus (anti-HCV IgM), hepatitis delta virus (anti-HDV IgM), hepatitis E virus (anti-HEV IgM), and HBsAg.

Other immunological tests for infections such as human immunodeficiency virus (HIV), herpes simplex virus (HSV), cytomegalovirus (CMV), and Epstein–Barr virus (EBV) should be done when indicated.

Imaging

Hepatic ultrasound can diagnose fatty liver, but liver may appear normal in AFLP as the fat is microvesicular. However, magnetic resonance imaging (MRI), computed tomography (CT) may help in identification of fat in liver. Presence of decreased attenuation on CT suggests fatty infiltration.

Ultrasound of liver with Doppler flow should be performed to identify evidence of portal hypertension, mass lesion or vascular obstruction such as portal vein or hepatic vein thrombosis. Ultrasound is safe and accurate in detecting gallstones.

Liver Biopsy[5]

Liver biopsy with special stains for fatty liver or electron microscopy is the gold standard for

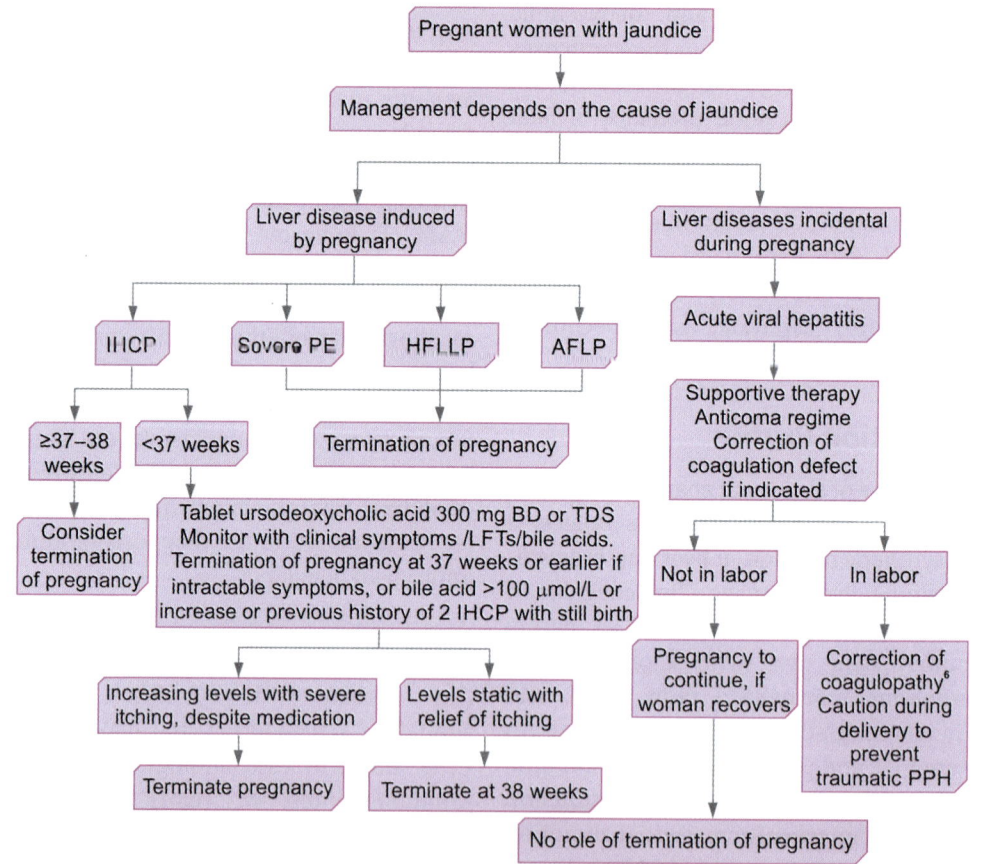

Flowchart 2A: Algorithm of management of a pregnant women presenting with jaundice.

(AFLP: acute fatty liver of pregnancy; IHCP: intrahepatic cholestasis of pregnancy; HELLP: hemolysis, elevated liver enzyme and low platelet; PE: pulmonary embolism; PPH: postpartum hemorrhage)

diagnosis of acute fatty liver of pregnancy. The microvesicular fatty infiltration of hepatocytes mainly in the central zone with periportal sparing is the typical histopathological lesion. There is mild or no inflammation or hepatocellular necrosis. Liver biopsy is not always essential and may not be practical in the presence of coagulopathy due to enlarged gravid uterus for the diagnosis of acute fatty liver of pregnancy. In fulminant failure due to hepatitis, the histopathological picture shows cholestasis and hepatocellular necrosis in the periportal area with inflammation.

MANAGEMENT

The management of jaundice without liver failure and with liver failure is given in Flowcharts 2A and B respectively.

Flowchart 2B: Algorithm of management of a pregnant woman presenting with severe jaundice with suspected liver failure—medical management.

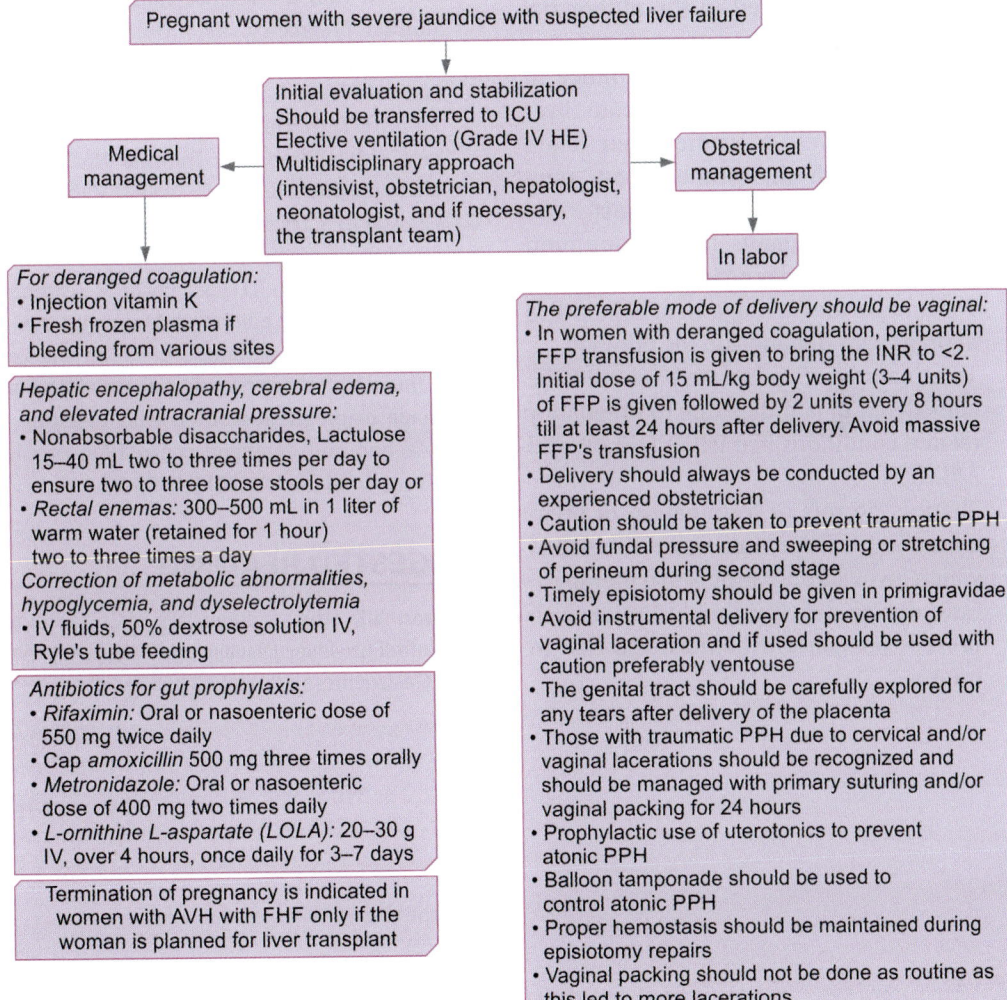

KEY POINTS

- Jaundice is one of the important causes of indirect maternal mortality in India.
- It can be due to causes related to pregnancy. A provisional diagnosis is formulated based on history and examination and further tests are performed to confirm the diagnosis.
- Any women with jaundice and elevated liver enzymes should first be screened for viral hepatitis.
- **If viral serology is negative, then other conditions more common in pregnancy should be considered in the differential diagnosis and managed accordingly.**
- The management of severe jaundice in pregnancy associated with acute liver failure involves a coordinated team approach with the primary care physician, obstetrician, hepatologist, and a transplant surgeon for an optimum maternal and fetal outcomes.
- The antepartum management of jaundice in pregnancy depends on the etiology.
- Termination of pregnancy should be considered in jaundice due to pregnancy related conditions like IHCP, HELLP, and AFLP.
- There is no role of termination of pregnancy in jaundice due to viral hepatitis which involves only supportive therapy.
- Care during delivery should be taken to prevent postpartum hemorrhage due to trauma.

REFERENCES

1. Chitra R, Aggarwal S. Jaundice in pregnancy. In: Trivedi SS, Puri M, Aggarwal S (Eds). Management of High-risk Pregnancy: A Practical Approach, 2nd edition. New Delhi: Jaypee Brothers Medical Publishers (P) Ltd; 2016. pp. 232-245.
2. Conn HO. The hepatic encephalopathies. In: Conn HO, Bircher J (Eds). Hepatic Encephalopathy: Syndromes and Therapies. Bloomington, IL: Medi-Ed Press; 1994. pp. 1-12.
3. Girling JC, Dow E, Smith JH. Liver function tests in pre-eclampsia: Importance of comparison with a reference range derived for normal pregnancy. Br J Obstet Gynaecol. 1997;104(2):246-50.
4. Nelson-Piercy C, Liver Disease. In: Nelson-Piercy C (Ed). Handbook of Obstetric Medicine, 4th edition. UK: Informa Healthcare; 2010. pp. 193-212.
5. Gimson AES. Liver and gastrointestinal diseases during pregnancy. In: Warrell DA, Cox TM, John D, Firth JD (Eds). Oxford's Textbook of Medicine, 5th edition; 2011. pp. 421-426.
6. Puri M, Patra S, Singh P, et al. Factors influencing occurrence of postpartum hemorrhage in pregnant women with hepatitis E infection and deranged coagulation profile. Obstetric Medicine. 2011;4:108-12.

SUGGESTED READING

1. Tran TT, Ahn J, Reau NS. ACG Clinical Guideline: Liver Disease and Pregnancy. Am J Gastroenterol. 2016;111(2):176-94.

17

Approach to a Pregnant Woman Presenting with Pallor

Indira Prasad

INTRODUCTION

Pallor or paleness is the waxy appearance or absence of coloration of the skin and mucous membrane.[1] "Pallor" and "anemia" are not interchangeable terms. Anemia is a pathological condition whereas pallor is a clinical entity. An anemic woman may not look pale as assessed from her palpebral conjunctiva or tongue in case she has conjunctivitis or glossitis and a person looking severely pale may not be grossly anemic as in Sheehan's syndrome.

Causes of pallor in pregnancy can be broadly grouped into those causing acute blood loss and/or shock, and those leading to chronic anemia. In acute shock, the body responds to the low circulating blood volume by increasing the heart rate and peripheral vasoconstriction to deliver adequate oxygen to the tissues and protect the vital organs such as brain, heart, and kidneys with resultant skin pallor. If left untreated, symptoms can worsen and may lead to low-volume pulse, hypotension, hypoxic ischemic encephalopathy, and loss of consciousness.

During the first 20 weeks of gestation, the most dangerous cause of acute blood loss and shock is ruptured ectopic pregnancy whereas the most common cause is spontaneous abortion, which can be inevitable, incomplete, complete, or septic. In 2–5% of antenatal women, acute blood loss occurs in late pregnancy (i.e., after 20 weeks of gestation) but before the birth of the baby, and is due to conditions such as placental abruption, placenta previa, and uterine rupture.[2] There can be a substantial blood loss either revealed or concealed, occasionally enough to cause hemorrhagic shock and severe pallor. However, acute shock can be nonhemorrhagic, as in cases with vasovagal attack, cerebrovascular accident, or neurogenic shock, where there is no blood loss, but shock and pallor are present.

Chronic anemia occurs in up to two third of women during pregnancy resulting in skin pallor. Causes leading to chronic anemia are same in both early and late pregnancy and are listed in Table 1. The most common cause is nutritional anemia.

DIFFERENTIAL DIAGNOSIS

For details of various conditions leading to pallor, refer Table 1. These are broadly divided into those resulting in pallor due to acute causes—hemorrhagic or nonhemorrhagic and those resulting in chronic anemia.

HISTORY

Pregnant women with chronic anemia are usually asymptomatic and pallor is noticed on general physical examination. Sometimes as the pregnancy advances, patient

Table 1: Differential diagnosis of pallor in pregnancy.

Acute causes		Chronic anemia
Hemorrhagic		
Early pregnancy	Late pregnancy	
Pregnancy-related causes: • Acute ruptured ectopic pregnancy • Abortion: Incomplete, inevitable or complete • Molar pregnancy in the process of expulsion • Ruptured corpus luteum cyst Pregnancy-unrelated causes: Traumatic hepatic or splenic rupture	Pregnancy-related causes: • Placental abruption • Placenta previa • Uterine rupture • Broad ligament hematoma • Hepatic rupture/hematoma Pregnancy-unrelated causes: • Traumatic hepatic or splenic rupture	Nutritional anemia: • Iron-deficiency anemia • Vitamin B_{12} deficiency anemia • Folic acid deficiency anemia • Combined anemia Hemoglobinopathies: • Hb C/S/E disease • Sickle cell disease • Thalassemias (β, β-δ, and α) Intrinsic RBC defects/membrane alterations: • PNH • Hereditary elliptocytosis • Hereditary spherocytosis Inherited enzyme deficiencies: • Embden–Meyerhof pathway defects • G6PD deficiency Infections: • Hookworm • Chronic malaria • Chronic kala-azar • Tuberculosis Chronic diseases: • Kidney diseases • Hypoproteinemia • Endocrine disorders Chronic blood loss: • Menorrhagia • Piles Malabsorption syndromes: Tropical sprue
Nonhemorrhagic shock		
• Septic shock: Septic abortion, pyelonephritis • Neurogenic shock: Ovarian torsion • Cardiogenic shock: Heart disease • Anaphylactic shock	• Septic shock: Chorioamnionitis, pyelonephritis • Neurogenic shock: Ovarian torsion • Cardiogenic shock: Heart disease • Anaphylactic shock	

(G6PD: glucose-6-phosphate dehydrogenase; Hb: hemoglobin; PNH: paroxysmal nocturnal hemoglobinuria; RBC: red blood cell)

decompensates and presents with symptoms such as increasing pallor, easy fatigability, breathlessness on exertion, progressively increasing weakness, lightheadedness, giddiness, anorexia, palpitations, angina, insomnia, tinnitus, and tingling sensation in extremities. There may be swelling of lower limbs or all over the body suggestive of hypoproteinemia or fluid retention due to associated preeclampsia.

The history in these women is directed to find out the likely cause of anemia such as poor diet, malabsorption, passage of worms in the stools, pica, and any chronic or recurrent infection such as urinary tract infection (UTI), tuberculosis, chronic blood loss consequent to menorrhagia, and piles.

It is important to know if the woman has been taking regular iron supplements in the current pregnancy or not. The color of the stools is black with iron intake. Many pregnant women have poor iron stores and increased demand during pregnancy resulting in iron deficiency anemia manifesting as increasing pallor.

Any history suggestive of hemoglobinopathy in the family such as need for repeated blood transfusions or episodes of acute pain suggestive of thalassemia, or sickle cell crisis is elicited. Any symptoms suggestive of hypothyroidism, which cause macrocytic anemia, should be asked for.

A pregnant woman brought to the emergency in shock or diagnosed as being in shock in the hospital, resuscitation should be done first followed by a systematic history from the attendants focused to find out the cause of shock whether it is hemorrhagic, hypovolemic, septic, cardiogenic, or neurogenic.

As the causes of acute shock in early and late pregnancy are different so is the history and examination. However, in pregnant woman with pallor due to chronic anemia, the causes are the same both in early and late pregnancy.

In a pregnant woman with acute shock in early pregnancy, it is important to find out any cause of severe blood loss as with abortions and molar pregnancy. The woman gives history of amenorrhea followed by profuse bleeding per vaginam with passage of products of conception or grape-like vesicles in incomplete abortion or molar pregnancy, respectively. In ectopic pregnancy, there is severe pain in the lower abdomen with or without syncope followed by mild bleeding per vaginam. Severe intermittent pain in lower abdomen with or without vomiting is the presenting complaint in women with twisted ovarian or paraovarian tumor or adnexal torsion.

In women presenting late in pregnancy, history of painless, causeless bleeding in bouts is suggestive of placenta previa. Bleeding associated with abdominal pain is suggestive of revealed placental abruption and severe abdominal pain with pallor is suggestive of concealed abruption. In a woman with a scarred uterus, severe suprapubic pain may be due to scar dehiscence. This is often associated with some urinary symptoms and fresh bleeding per vaginam.

Obstetrical History

It is important to find out if the woman has had repeated births or abortions in the past resulting in depletion of iron stores and anemia. In case there are repeated births, the interval between the successive births, compliance to antenatal and postnatal iron supplementation, and need for any blood transfusion are asked for.

Menstrual History

Menstrual history is important as the woman may be having heavy menstrual bleeding with resultant anemia.

Contraceptive History

Use of intrauterine copper devices can be associated with menorrhagia, anemia, and pallor.

Dietary History

A detailed dietary history should be elicited as nutritional anemia is the most common cause of anemia in pregnant women in developing countries.

Important points to be elicited in the history of a pregnant woman presenting with pallor are listed in Table 2.

EXAMINATION

General Physical Examination

Vitals are recorded including pulse rate, blood pressure, respiratory rate, and temperature. The degree of pallor is assessed as mild, moderate, or severe. This is assessed at multiple sites such as tongue, palpebral conjunctiva, nail beds, palmar creases, and soft palate (Figs. 1 to 3). This is a subjective assessment and may not always correlate with the hemoglobin levels. The hydration status is assessed. Jugular venous pressure may be raised in women with cardiac failure. Thyroid is looked for any enlargement. Any significant lymphadenopathy is noted. Any hematomas or petechiae are looked for on the body. Presence of edema on the legs, feet, or all over the body is checked for (Fig. 4).

Systemic Examination

A systematic examination of the cardiovascular, respiratory, and neurological

Table 2: Important points to be elicited in history.

Probable cause	Points elicited in history
Presence of infections (malaria, UTI, and TB)	Recurrent fever with chills and rigors, urinary complaints, prolonged productive cough
Chronic loss of blood	Bleeding gums, piles, or worm infestation
Malabsorption	Bulky stools and chronic diarrhea
Bleeding or coagulation disorder	Petechiae, bruises, and ecchymosis
Hemoglobinopathies	Repeated blood or blood component transfusion in self or family
Hemolysis	High-colored urine, yellow sclera, and drug intake
Dietary deficiency	Detailed dietary history, cooking habits, etc.
Menstrual history	Cycle length, duration, amount of bleeding, passage of clots, flooding, etc.
Obstetric history	Abortions, repeated childbirth, any complications such as APH, PPH, and blood transfusion in previous or current pregnancies
Contraceptive history	Use of IUCD with heavy menstrual cycles

(APH: antepartum hemorrhage; IUCD: intrauterine contraceptive device; TB: tuberculosis; PPH: postpartum hemorrhage; UTI: urinary tract infection)

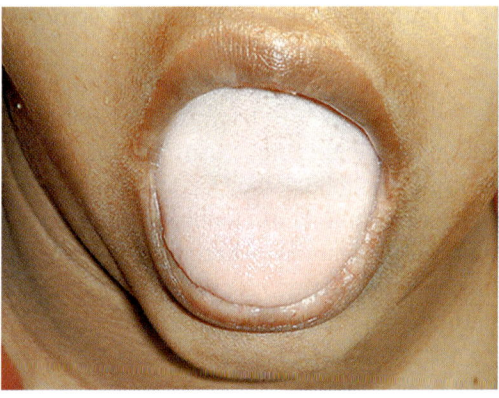

Fig. 1: Pale tongue.

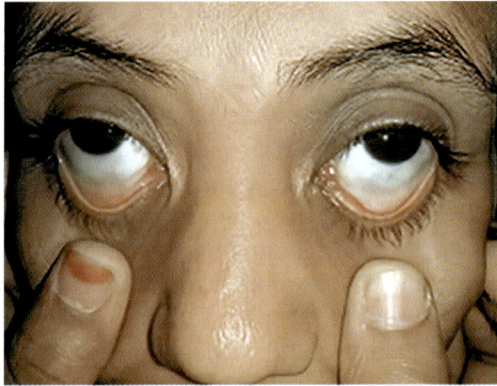

Fig. 2: Pale conjunctiva.

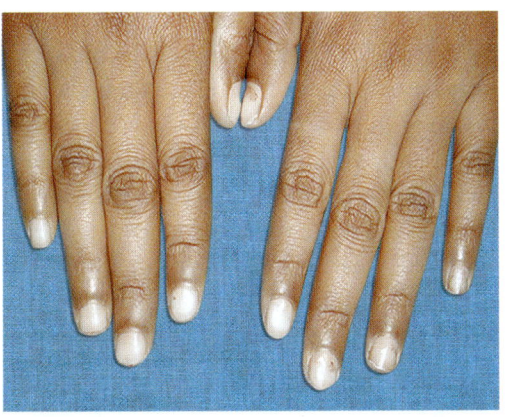
Fig. 3: Pale nails.

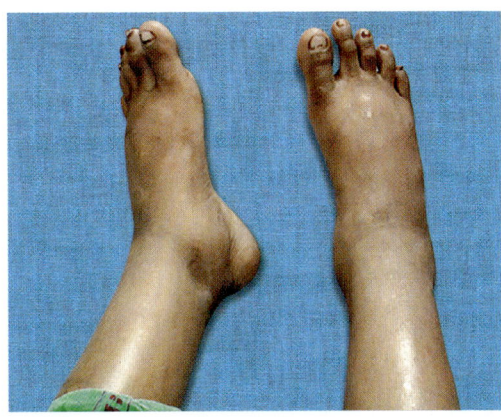
Fig. 4: Swollen feet and pitting edema.

systems is done. In respiratory system, any evidence of fine basal crepitation suggestive of cardiac failure, or any evidence of chest infection, or tuberculosis is looked for.

In cardiovascular system, hemic murmurs and hyperdynamic apex beat are often present in women with moderate or severe anemia.

A detailed abdominal examination is done to look for any organomegaly such as hepatomegaly and/or splenomegaly. Both spleen and liver are sites for extramedullary erythropoiesis and are firm, enlarged, and nontender in chronic anemia. Liver may be soft, enlarged, and tender in cases of cardiac failure. Significant splenomegaly is present in conditions associated with hemolysis such as sickle cell disease, and thalassemia. In advanced pregnancy, the palpation of liver and spleen may be difficult due to enlarged uterus.

Abdominal examination is carried out depending on the gestation whether it is early pregnancy or late pregnancy. In early pregnancy, look for any tenderness, peritoneal signs such as rebound tenderness, rigidity, guarding, and uterine size. Any evidence of free fluid in peritoneal cavity may be suggestive of intraperitoneal hemorrhage.

In late pregnancy, abdominal examination is done to assess the fundal height, contour of uterus, uterine tone, any uterine tenderness, ease with which fetal parts are palpable, amount of liquor amnii, any suprapubic, or scar tenderness. The contour of the uterus is lost, and fetal parts are felt superficially in cases of rupture uterus. The uterine height is more than the period of gestation, uterus is tense and tender, and fetal parts are felt with difficulty in concealed placental abruption. In placenta previa, the uterus is soft, relaxed, with an abnormal presentation or a free-floating head deviated on one side and normal feel of fetal parts.

The fetal heart sound (FHS) is heard and fetal heart rate (FHR) is noted. Fetal tachycardia may be present in decompensated cases of anemia, scar dehiscence, and mild abruption. Fetal bradycardia is noted in cases of impending uterine rupture and cases with severe abruption. FHS may be absent in women with scar rupture, uterine rupture, or severe abruption.

The signs to be observed in a pregnant woman with anemia are summarized in Table 3.

Table 3: Clinical examination in a pregnant woman with anemia.

General physical examination	Systemic examination
• Pulse rate, blood pressure, and respiratory rate • Skin and mucosa for pallor • Color of palmar creases • Petechiae, and ecchymosis	• Chest examination • Sternal tenderness • Any crepitation, fine basal or coarse apical
Eyes: • Pallor • Icterus	Cardiovascular (CVS) examination: • Murmurs
Oral cavity: • Glossitis • Stomatitis • Cheilosis	Per abdomen: • Edema of abdominal wall • Hepatosplenomegaly • Presence of free fluid
Nails: • Pallor • Platonychia or koilonychia • Clubbing	Obstetrical examination: • Height of uterus • Tone of uterus • Number of fetuses • Presentation of fetus • Amount of liquor • Fetal heart sound (FHS)
Neck: • Lymphadenopathy • Jugular venous pressure (JVP) • Thyroid enlargement	
Legs: • Edema • Ulcers • Peripheral neuropathy	

Examination of Genitalia

Inspection

The external genitalia are examined to assess for blood loss per vaginam.

Per Speculum Examination

Per speculum examination is done in all women with early pregnancy in shock. However, in those with late pregnancy, it may be deferred till the placenta is localized on ultrasonography and/or till 2–3 days after the bleeding stops.

In early pregnancy blood clots, products of conception or molar tissue may be seen on per speculum examination and the tissue so obtained may be sent for histopathological examination. The cervix and vagina are inspected for any purulent discharge, lesion, or tissue. In late pregnancy, it is done for ruling out any local cause of bleeding such as a cervical growth, erosion, or varices.

Per Vaginam Examination

Per vaginam examination should always be done in women presenting with pallor in early pregnancy to look for the size of uterus whether corresponding to the period of gestation or not, condition of internal os whether open or closed, and if open whether products of conception are felt in the uterine cavity or not. Presence of any tender adnexal mass, fullness, or bulge in pouch of Douglas, any induration, thickening or tenderness in fornices and cervical motion tenderness to diagnose conditions such as ectopic pregnancy, septic abortion, incomplete or inevitable abortion, and molar pregnancy in the process of expulsion. In late pregnancy, per vaginam examination is deferred till ultrasonography is done to rule out placenta previa.

INVESTIGATIONS

A pregnant woman presenting with pallor should be investigated for the severity of anemia, type of anemia, and causes of anemia. In women presenting in acute shock with pallor in addition to the investigations for assessing the severity and type of anemia, it is important to advice investigations to find out the cause of shock, whether hemorrhagic or nonhemorrhagic.

Complete Blood Count with Peripheral Smear

Complete blood count (CBC) gives information on the hemoglobin level, total and differential leukocyte, and platelet count. The peripheral smear helps in the diagnosis of the type of anemia whether it is microcytic (Fig. 5), macrocytic, or normocytic and whether it is hypochromic or normochromic (Table 4). The severity of anemia is classified as per the Indian Council of Medical Research ICMR (Table 5).

In iron deficiency anemia, the peripheral smear is microcytic hypochromic whereas in vitamin B_{12} and/or folic acid deficiency, it is macrocytic. Presence of target cells, schistocytes, and helmet cells are suggestive of hemolytic anemia (Fig. 6). Presence of malarial parasite, sickle cells, etc., can also be appreciated on peripheral smear (Figs. 7 and 8).

Reticulocyte Count

Reticulocyte count reflects the response of bone marrow to treatment and is the first to rise after treatment. The normal reticulocyte count is 0.5–2%. It is markedly raised in hemolytic anemia.

Investigations for the Cause of Anemia

Investigations include urine routine examination and culture sensitivity, liver function test (LFT) and kidney function test (KFT), serum electrolytes, high-performance liquid

Table 4: Differential diagnosis according to the type of anemia on peripheral smear.

Type of anemia	Cause of anemia
Microcytic	Iron deficiency, thalassemia, and chronic infections
Macrocytic	*Megaloblastic*: Folic acid deficiency, Vitamin B_{12} deficiency *Nonmegaloblastic*: Liver disease, hypothyroidism, and myelodysplasia
Normocytic	Post hemorrhagic, renal or hepatic disease, impaired marrow response, e.g., early iron deficiency, marrow hypoplasia, infiltrative disorder, and myelodysplasia
Dimorphic	Combined iron, folic acid, and vitamin B_{12} deficiency
Hemolytic	*Inherited*: Thalassemia, sickle cell disease, spherocytosis, glucose-6-phosphate dehydrogenase (G6PD) deficiency, and pyruvate kinase deficiency *Acquired*: Microangiopathic as in pregnancy-induced hypertension (PIH), cardiac hemolytic, autoimmune, pregnancy induced, infections, drugs
Pancytopenia	*Megaloblastic*: Folic acid and/or vitamin B_{12} deficiency *Aplastic*: Drugs, viral infections, exposure to toxic substances, etc.

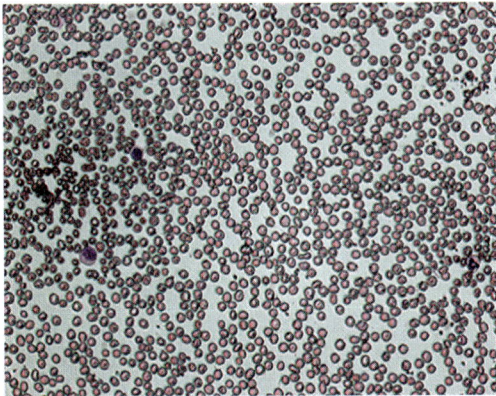

Fig. 5: Peripheral blood smear showing microcytic hypochromic red blood cells.

Table 5: ICMR classification of anemia according to severity.[3]

Severity	Hemoglobin levels (g/dL)
Mild	10.0–10.9
Moderate	7–9.9
Severe	<7
Very severe	<4

(ICMR: Indian Council of Medical Research)

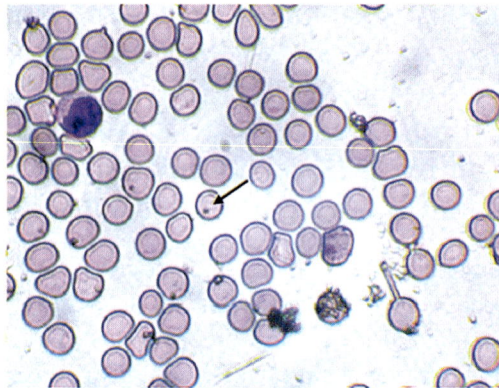

Fig. 7: Peripheral blood smear showing malarial parasite.

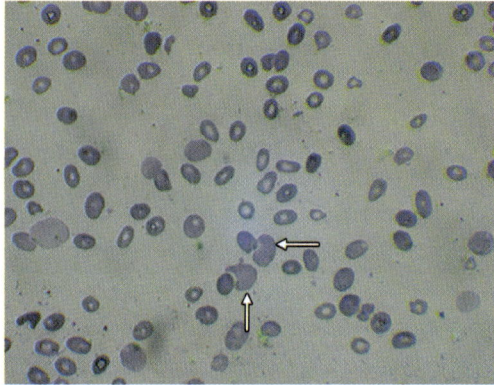

Fig. 6: Peripheral blood smear showing helmet cells.

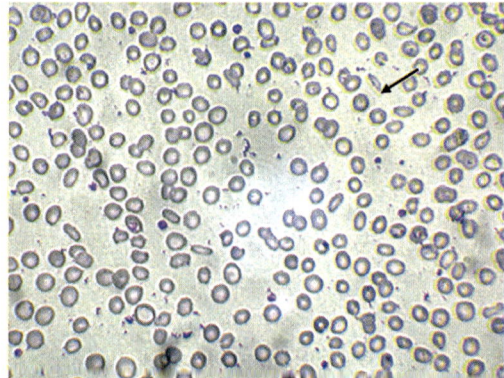

Fig. 8: Peripheral blood smear showing sickle cells.

chromatography (HPLC) for diagnosis of hemoglobinopathies such as thalassemia, blood group, X-ray chest after shielding the abdomen and electrocardiography (ECG) in women with cardiac failure. Echocardiography is done, if indicated. In women with swelling feet or generalized anasarca, serum proteins should be done to rule out hypoproteinemia. Coagulation profile and thyroid-stimulating hormone (TSH) may be advised in women with history of heavy menstrual bleeding.

An ultrasonography of abdomen is indicated to assess fetal well-being and rule out causes such as chronic ectopic in early pregnancy and retroplacental bleed in late pregnancy. In both these situations, the pregnant woman is pale, but stable.

In women who present in shock, in addition to the assessment of the degree and type of anemia, an assessment of function of vital organs such as liver, kidneys, heart, and lungs is done by carrying out LFT, KFT, ECG, and X-ray chest. Serum electrolytes and coagulation profile are done.

In early pregnancy, serum beta-human chorionic gonadotropin (β-hCG) along with transvaginal ultrasonography is helpful in the diagnosis of doubtful cases of ectopic pregnancy. Ultrasound is useful in diagnosing molar pregnancy and retained products of conception in incomplete abortion. Other than assessing the fetal maturity and well-being, ultrasonography is

Table 6: Investigations for finding out the cause of anemia.

Investigations	Cause of anemia
Peripheral smear	Malarial parasite, sickle cells, spherocytes, and evidence of hemolysis
Liver function tests	Liver disease and hemolysis
Renal function tests	Renal disease and renal insult
Serum proteins	Hypoproteinemia
Electrophoresis/high-performance liquid chromatography	Hemoglobinopathy
Urine examination	Urinary tract infection (UTI), occult hematuria, and schistosomiasis
Stool examination (3 consecutive days)	Ova and cyst, and occult blood
Bone marrow aspiration	Abnormal cells and iron stores
X-ray chest (after shielding abdomen)	Pulmonary tuberculosis

useful in the diagnosis of conditions such as placenta previa, placental abruption, hemoperitoneum, hepatic hematoma/rupture, and rectus sheath hematoma. Various investigations indicated for finding out the cause of anemia in pregnant woman are listed in Table 6.

The approach of a pregnant woman with pallor is summarized in Flowchart 1.

MANAGEMENT

The management of pallor depends upon the condition of the woman whether stable or unstable at the time of presentation and the cause of pallor whether hemorrhagic or non-hemorrhagic. Flowchart 2 summarizes the principles of management.

KEY POINTS

- Pallor in pregnancy can both be a symptom or a sign.
- Although pallor implies anemia, the terms are not interchangeable. Sometimes a woman may have a sallow complexion and look pale but is not anemic. On the other hand, an anemic woman may not have a pale tongue due to glossitis.
- The differential diagnosis of pallor depends essentially on the clinical presentation whether the woman presents in stable or unstable condition. The differential diagnosis, especially in acute unstable cases would also depend upon whether it is in early or late pregnancy. Stable cases with pallor are usually due to chronic anemia.
- The investigations are carried out to find out the severity, type, and cause of anemia. Function of vital organs must be assessed in women who present in shock.

REFERENCES

1. Kundu AK. Bedside Clinics in Medicine, 4th edition. Kolkata: Academic Publishers; 2005. p. 279.
2. McShane PM, Heye PS, Epstein MF. Maternal and perinatal mortality resulting from placenta previa. Obstet Gynecol. 1985;65(2): 176-82.
3. Federation of Obstetric and Gynecological Societies of India. Good clinical practice

Flowchart 1: Algorithm of clinical approach to a pregnant woman with pallor.

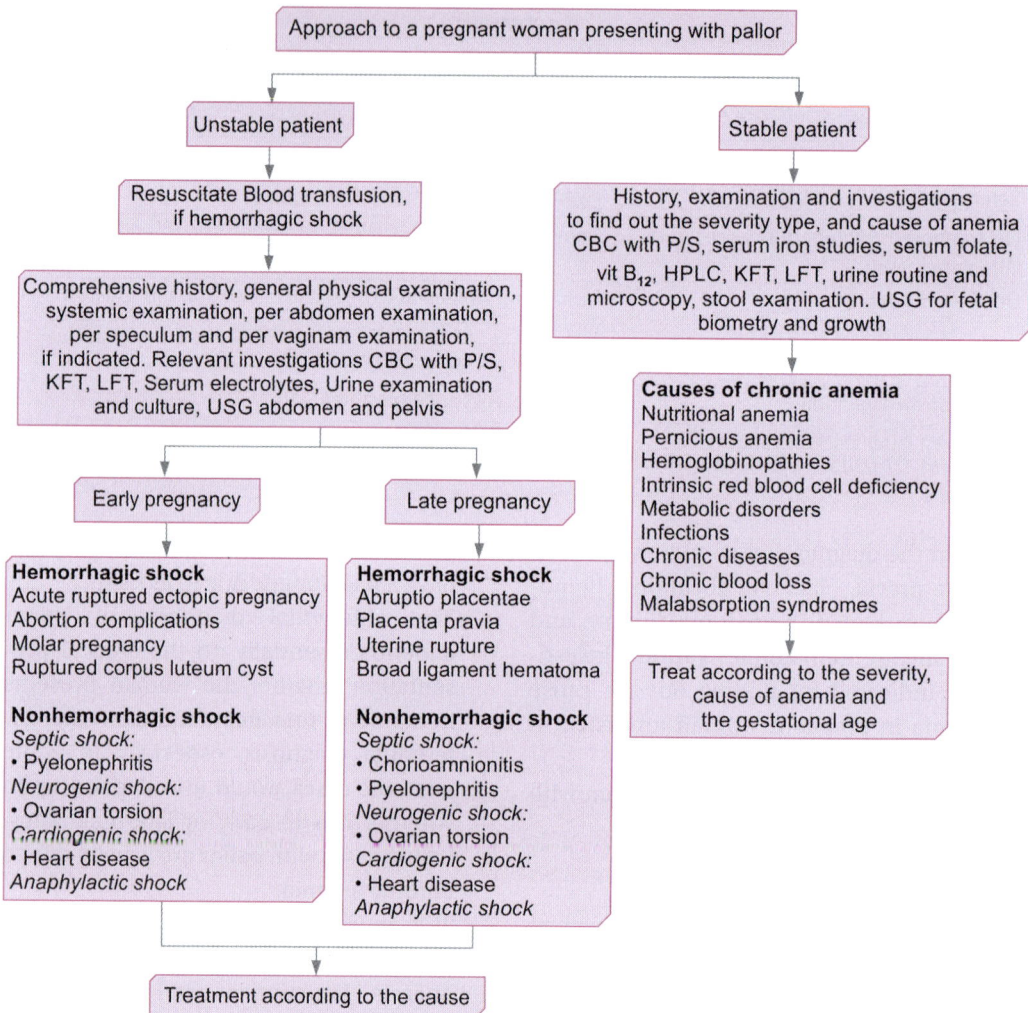

(CBC with P/S: complete blood count with peripheral smear; HPLC: high-performance liquid chromatography; LFT: liver function test; KFT: kidney function test; USG: ultrasonography)

recommendations for iron deficiency anemia (IDA) in pregnancy in India. J Obstet Gynecol India. 2011;61(5):569-71.

SUGGESTED READING

1. Federation of Obstetric and Gynecological Societies of India. (2016). FOGSI General Clinical Practice recommendations. Management of iron deficiency Anaemia in Pregnancy. [online] Available from: https://www.fogsi.org/wp-content/uploads/2017/07/gcpr-recommendation-ida.pdf. [Last accessed February, 2020].

2. Mane SV, Rani BSS. (2010). Antepartum haemorrhage. [online] Available from: https://www.fogsi.org/wp-content/uploads/fogsi-focus/antepartum_heamorrhage.pdf. [Last accessed February, 2020].

Flowchart 2: Algorithm of management of a pregnant woman with pallor.

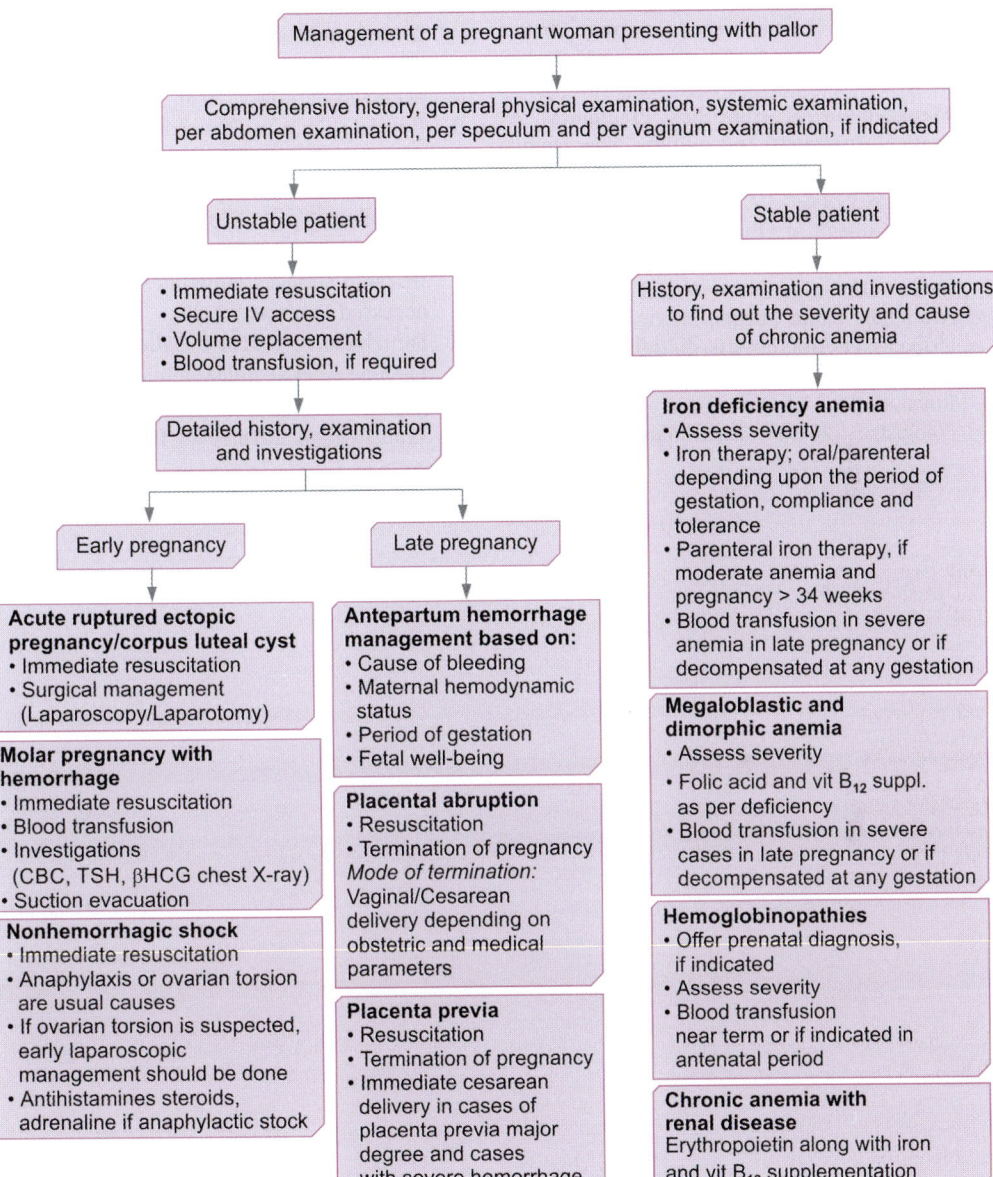

3. Morton MJ, Masterson M, Hoffmann B. Case report: Ovarian torsion in pregnancy-diagnosis and management. J Emerg Med. 2013;45(3):348-51.
4. National Institute for Health and Care Excellence. (2019). Ectopic pregnancy and miscarriage: diagnosis and initial management: NICE guidelines. [online] Available from: https://www.nice.org.uk/guidance/ng126/resources/ectopic-pregnancy-and-miscarriage-diagnosis-and-initial-management-pdf-66141662244037. [Last accessed February, 2020].
5. National Rural Health Mission. (2018). Annexure 1: Guidelines for prevention

of maternal Anaemia. [online] Available from: http://www.nrhmtn.gov.in/guideline/RGPMA.pdf. [Last accessed February, 2020].
6. Puri M, Malhotra N. Anemia in pregnancy. In: Trivedi SS, Puri M, Agarwal Swati (Eds). Management of High-Risk Pregnancy: A Pratical Approach, 2nd edition. New Delhi: Jaypee Brothers Medical Publishers (P) Ltd; 2015. pp. 273-5.
7. Royal College of Obstetricians and Gynaecologists. (2010). Antepartum Haemorrhage. (Green-Top guidelines No. 63). [online] Available from: https://www.rcog.org.uk/globalassets/documents/guidelines/gtg_63.pdf. [Last accessed February, 2020].
8. Royal College of Obstetricians and Gynaecologists. (2010). The management of gestational trophoblastic disease. (Green-Top Guideline No 38.). [online] Available from: https://www.rcog.org.uk/globalassets/documents/guidelines/gtg_38.pdf. [Last accessed February, 2020].
9. Royal College of Obstetricians and Gynaecologists. (2016). Diagnosis and management of ectopic pregnancy. (Green-Top Guideline No. 21) [online] Available from: https://www.rcog.org.uk/en/guidelines-research-services/guidelines/gtg21/. [Last accessed February, 2020].
10. Santaballa A, Garcia Y, Lainez N, Fuentes J, De Juan A, et al. SEOM clinical guidelines in gestational trophoblastic disease (2017). Clin Transl Oncol. 2018;20:38-46.

18
Approach to a Pregnant Woman Presenting with Hypertension

Shilpi Nain

INTRODUCTION

Hypertensive disorders of pregnancy account for approximately 5–10% of all pregnancies and contribute to significant maternal and perinatal morbidity and mortality.[1] Hypertension may antedate pregnancy or develop during pregnancy. The most common cause of hypertension developing during pregnancy is preeclampsia/eclampsia, which usually develops after 20 weeks of gestation. In women with hypertension antedating pregnancy or detected before 20 weeks gestation, 90% are essential hypertension and remaining 10% are secondary hypertension. These women are at increased risk of developing superimposed preeclampsia during pregnancy. Risk factors for superimposed preeclampsia in these patients include renal insufficiency, obesity, hypertension for at least 4 years and history of preeclampsia in prior pregnancy.[2,3]

Hypertensive pregnant women are at increased risk of developing adverse outcomes such as placental abruption, cerebral hemorrhage, disseminated intravascular coagulation, acute hepatic and renal failure, fetal growth restriction, and fetal death. The key to manage these patients is early detection, accurate disease classification, and timely termination of pregnancy.

HISTORY

History of time of onset of hypertension in relation to the pregnancy and the period of gestation is important. Hypertension with onset before pregnancy or prior to 20 weeks of gestation points toward chronic hypertension whereas that developing after 20 weeks of gestation is suggestive of pregnancy-related hypertension, i.e., gestational hypertension, preeclampsia, or eclampsia.

Enquire if the patient is taking any antihypertensive medication, its type, dose, and control achieved with the drug.

In pregnant woman developing hypertension after 20 weeks, ask for any history of severe features of preeclampsia such as headache, nausea, vomiting, epigastric pain, visual disturbances, and decreased urine output. Headache associated with preeclampsia/eclampsia is often bilateral, throbbing and is not relieved by salicylates. It may be associated with nausea and/or vomiting and is suggestive of severe disease or imminent eclampsia. Visual disturbances like blurred vision, scotoma, and diplopia are common with severe preeclampsia and eclampsia.[4,5] The underlying cause of headache and visual disturbances is cerebral ischemia from vasospasm. History of epigastric pain and right upper quadrant pain indicates worsening disease and is due to hepatocellular necrosis and ischemia. History of decreased urine output is suggestive of severe preeclampsia and is due to reduced renal perfusion and glomerular filtration (Table 1).

In pregnant woman with hypertension before pregnancy or detected before 20 weeks of gestation, symptoms of secondary disease like episodes of headache, sweating, and palpitations suggest pheochromocytoma. Symptoms like hematuria, dysuria, periorbital edema, or loin pain suggest renal disease. History of increased appetite with weight loss, diarrhea, heat intolerance, and nervousness is suggestive of hyperthyroidism. History of episodes of fever with arthralgia, myalgia, facial rash, photosensitivity, and anemia is common in patients with systemic lupus erythematosus (SLE). Presence of other risk factors such as smoking, diabetes, and dyslipidemia should be enquired.

Obstetric History

Ask for any history of high blood pressure (BP) in previous pregnancies, need for antihypertensive therapy, course and severity of disease, the gestational age at which the pregnancy was terminated, mode of termination of pregnancy; induction of labor or cesarean section, and pregnancy outcomes. History of complications like eclampsia, placental abruption, and PPH is important.

Past History

In patients with chronic hypertension, history of adverse events such as cerebrovascular accident, myocardial infarction, cardiac, or renal dysfunction in the past should be elicited, as these women are at increased risk of worsening or recurrence of such events during pregnancy. Any history of surgery for hyperthyroidism or pheochromocytoma should be asked for.

Family History

History of essential hypertension, myocardial infarction, stroke, and renal disease in both first- and second-degree relatives is important.

Table 1: Causes of hypertension in pregnancy.

Chronic hypertension (antedate pregnancy or develop before 20 weeks)	Pregnancy-related hypertension (manifests after 20 weeks of gestation)

• Idiopathic or essential hypertension
• Secondary hypertension:
  – Renal diseases:
    » Renal artery stenosis
    » Renal parenchymal disease
  – Endocrine diseases:
    » Pheochromocytoma
    » Primary hyperaldosteronism
    » Thyrotoxicosis
    » Cushing's syndrome
  – Vascular diseases:
    » Coarctation of aorta
  – Others:
    » Systemic lupus erythematosus (SLE)
    » Antiphospholipid antibody syndrome (APS)
	• Gestational hypertension:
	  – Blood pressure (BP) ≥ 140/90 mm Hg for first time in pregnancy without proteinuria or end organ dysfunction
	  – BP returns to normal in < 12 week postpartum
	• Preeclampsia:
	  – BP ≥ 140/90 mm Hg for first time in pregnancy
	  – With proteinuria ≥ 300 mg/24 h and or severe features
	• Eclampsia:
	  – Grand mal seizures in a woman with preeclampsia to which no other cause can be attributed
	• Preeclampsia syndrome superimposed on chronic hypertension:
	  – New-onset proteinuria ≥ 300 mg/24 h in hypertensive woman with no previous proteinuria
	  – Sudden worsening of hypertension or development of severe features in woman with hypertension before 20 weeks of gestation

EXAMINATION

General Physical Examination

A thorough general physical examination with special reference to some typical features that may point toward a specific disease—a moon-like face with buffalo hump is a sign of Cushing's disease, malar discoid or butterfly rash, painless oral ulcers, and/or alopecia are seen in SLE, a diffusely enlarged thyroid with a bruit may be present in Graves' disease. Proptosis with periorbital swelling is a sign of Graves' disease. Raised jugular venous pressure (JVP) is appreciated in a woman with congestive cardiac failure (CCF). Pedal edema, facial puffiness, and generalized anasarca indicate fluid retention and/or hypoproteinemia.

Pulse Rate

Pulse rate should be measured in both upper and lower limbs. Delayed and feeble femoral pulses are suggestive of coarctation of aorta.

Blood Pressure

Ideally, the patient should have rested for 5–10 minutes before recording the BP. The patient should be sitting with her feet rested on ground and legs uncrossed or semireclining with back supported or in a left lateral position with BP measured on the left arm. One should use a validated, calibrated device with appropriate cuff that is 1.5 times the circumference of the upper arm or bladder encircling more than 80% of the arm after supporting the arm on a desk. The cuff should be positioned in such a way that the middle of cuff is at the level of midpoint of sternum corresponding to right atrium level.

At first visit, the BP should be measured in both arms and if the difference in BP in both arms is 10 mm Hg or more, then the arm with a higher BP should be used for all future measurements. It is suggestive of unilateral arterial lesion or peripheral arterial disease. The first audible sound that is Korotkoff 1 is the systolic BP (SBP) and disappearance of sound that is Korotkoff 5 is used for recording diastolic BP (DPB). In case, the sounds are audible even with a deflated cuff Korotkoff 4 sound or muffling of sounds is recorded as the DBP. Repeat measurement should be at least after 1–2 minutes. Always note the time of recent BP medication taken before measurement. The BP should be measured in legs, if coarctation of aorta is suspected or if it cannot be measured in arms due to some surgery, vascular fistulae, etc.

Neurological System

Assessment of mental status with respect to level of consciousness should be done; as altered mental status ranging from confusion to coma may develop because of generalized cerebral edema in patients with severe preeclampsia or eclampsia. The deep tendon reflexes are brisk in women severe preeclampsia. Grand mal seizures suggest eclampsia.

Cardiovascular System

Points of special interest are palpation of forceful apical impulse, which is a sign of left ventricular hypertrophy due to chronic hypertension. On auscultation, a loud S2 and an audible S4 is also a sign of chronic hypertension. A prominent "to-and-fro" machinery murmur may be heard over the posterior chest in case of coarctation of aorta.

Respiratory System

Observe the respiratory rate and pattern of breathing. Auscultate the chest for any basal or diffused fine crackles suggestive of pulmonary edema or CCF.

Per Abdomen

In patients who present with hypertension early in pregnancy, the kidneys should be palpated to rule out any renal masses suggestive of adult onset polycystic kidney disease. Tenderness in the epigastrium or right hypochondrium is suggestive of hepatocellular ischemia and necrosis in patients with preeclampsia and indicates severe disease. The abdomen should be auscultated for bruit in the flanks suggestive of renal artery stenosis.

A detailed obstetrical examination is done to look for any features of uteroplacental insufficiency like fetal growth restriction or oligohydramnios.

Abdominal wall edema and ascites may be present in severe cases.

Local Examination

Vulvar edema may be present in preeclampsia/eclampsia suggesting fluid retention and possibly hypoproteinemia.

INVESTIGATIONS

Complete Blood Count

Hemoglobin

In patients with preeclampsia/eclampsia, because of diminished intravascular volume and hemoconcentration, hemoglobin values may be spuriously high, and anemia may be missed. Anemia secondary to hemolysis may be present in HELLP syndrome (characterized by hemolysis, elevated liver enzyme levels and a low platelet count). A sudden fall in hemoglobin may be suggestive of internal bleeding in the form of subcapsular hepatic hematoma, rupture of liver or placental abruption and needs to be correlated with clinical condition.

Platelets

Thrombocytopenia, platelet count of less than 100,000/μL, indicates severe disease and is an indication for termination of pregnancy in most cases. Other causes of thrombocytopenia like vitamin B_{12} and or folic acid deficiency, and antiphospholipid syndrome should be ruled out. A progressive fall in platelet count is more reliable than a single value. Thrombocytopenia should be confirmed by a peripheral smear test to rule out spurious thrombocytopenia due to clumping of platelets and correlated with clinical condition of the patient.

Peripheral Smear

In patients with preeclampsia/eclampsia syndromes, evidence of hemolysis on peripheral smear in the form of fragmented RBCs (schistocytes and burr cells) is suggestive of HELLP syndrome, which suggests severe disease. Similar blood smear may be found in case of hemolytic uremic syndrome (HUS) or thrombotic thrombocytopenic purpura (TTP).

Coagulation Profile

Coagulation profile is not indicated as a routine in all patients. It is indicated in patients who develop complications like placental abruption, deranged liver enzymes, or HELLP syndrome.

Liver Function Tests

Abnormalities in liver enzymes are due to reduced hepatic blood flow, potentially resulting in ischemia and periportal hemorrhage. Periportal and sinusoidal fibrin deposition and microvesicular fat deposition may affect hepatocyte function. Aspartate aminotransferase (AST) and alanine aminotransferase (ALT) are sensitive indicators of liver cell injury. Elevation of serum lactate dehydrogenase (LDH), ALT, and AST levels to more than two times the upper limit of normal is a marker of severe preeclampsia. In patients with chronic hypertension, marked elevations in serum AST and ALT indicate superimposed preeclampsia.

Renal Function Tests

Elevation in blood urea and serum creatinine may be present in preeclampsia/eclampsia and in secondary hypertension due to renal parenchymal disease. However, elevation in serum uric acid is typical of preeclampsia/eclampsia and hence can be used as a marker for distinguishing preeclampsia from chronic hypertension. Serum protein estimation is important in patients with significant proteinuria and anemia as hypoproteinemia and low albumin levels predispose the woman to pulmonary edema due to low oncotic pressure.

Serum Potassium

Hypokalemia in a hypertensive patient not on diuretics strongly suggests hyperaldosteronism. Hyperkalemia may be present in all forms of chronic kidney disease but is more prominent in patients with interstitial renal disease.

Urinalysis

Urinalysis is done for detection of hematuria, pyuria, proteinuria, and casts. A 24-hour urinary protein can be sent for protein excretion. Gross hematuria is characteristic of lower urinary tract disease and/or bleeding diathesis. Microscopic hematuria accompanied by proteinuria and urinary casts is most likely related to glomerulonephritis. Red cell casts are indicative of glomerulonephritis, white cell casts are suggestive of chronic interstitial nephritis, waxy and broad casts are seen in advanced renal disease. Proteinuria establishes the diagnosis of preeclampsia/eclampsia. It can be assessed by urine dipstick method from a fresh, clean voided midstream urine specimen (only if one of the quantitative methods is not available). Urine dipstick test is a semiquantitative method based on change in color of the dipstick and primarily detects albuminuria. An estimate of urine protein concentration as assessed by dipstick method is detailed in Table 2.

As dipstick test estimates protein concentration, it is influenced by the state of hydration of the woman. Therefore, *24-hours urinary protein excretion is considered gold standard for quantifying proteinuria.* Proteinuria of >300 mg/24 h in woman developing hypertension after 20 weeks of gestation is significant and confirms the diagnosis of preeclampsia.

The protein to creatinine ratio in a random urine sample can provide a rough estimate of protein excretion, a value of more than 0.3 mg urinary protein/mg urinary creatinine is suggestive of significant proteinuria that is equivalent to > 300 mg/24 h.

Fundus Examination

Retinopathy of preeclampsia is similar to hypertension associated retinopathy. Spasm of retinal arterioles, with decreased retinal artery-to-vein ratio correlates with severity

Table 2: Interpretation of urine dipstick test.

Dipstick grading	Urinary protein concentration
Negative/trace	10–20 mg/dL or 0.1 g/L
1+	30 mg/dL or 0.3 g/L
2+	100 mg/dL or 1 g/L
3+	300 mg/dL or 3 g/L
4+	1,000–2,000 mg/dL or 10 g/L

of hypertension. Hypertensive retinopathy (diffuse retinal edema, hemorrhages, exudates, and cotton-wool spots) may occur in case of severe hypertensive disorder. Other ocular abnormalities like papillophlebitis, Elschnig spots, macular edema, retinal pigment epithelial (RPE) lesions, retinal artery and vein occlusion, optic neuritis, optic atrophy, and ischemic optic neuropathy may be found in occlusive vascular disorders especially associated with antiphospholipid antibody (APLA).

Retinal detachment occurs in less than 1% of patients with preeclampsia and in 10% with eclampsia. It tends to be bilateral and resolves completely postpartum within few weeks.

Cortical blindness affects up to 15% of preeclamptic and eclamptic women and is often preceded or accompanied by headache or hyperreflexia. This visual loss often recovers over a period varying from 4 hours to 8 days.

Neuroimaging Studies

Noncontrast magnetic resonance imaging (MRI) findings consistent with vasogenic edema in the subcortical white matter and predominantly localized to the posterior cerebral (parieto-occipital) hemispheres are found in cases of posterior reversible encephalopathy syndrome (PRES). Computed tomography (CT)/MRI imaging shows involvement of cerebellum and brainstem commonly.

The PRES is characterized by headache, confusion, visual symptoms, and seizures in a patient of preeclampsia. It occurs as a result of endothelial dysfunction leading to disruption of blood-brain barrier and axonal swelling. Treatment of hypertension is the mainstay of treatment. Most patients recover within 2 weeks. A small number have residual neurologic deficits resulting from secondary cerebral infarction or hemorrhage; some patients may die as a result of increased intracranial pressure or as a complication of the underlying condition.

Obstetrical Ultrasound

Obstetrical ultrasound is indicated for assessing fetal well-being, amount of liquor amnii and to monitor fetal growth. Doppler flow studies are indicated if fetal growth restriction is suspected.

Tests for Ascertaining the Causes of Secondary Chronic Hypertension

Thyroid Function Tests

Thyroid-stimulating hormone (TSH) is a sensitive marker of thyrotoxicosis. Low TSH with high free thyroxine (T_4) is suggestive of primary thyrotoxicosis.

Screening for Adrenal Pathology

High levels of vanillylmandelic acid, catecholamines, and metanephrines in a 24-hour urine sample are diagnostic of pheochromocytoma. 24-hour urinary free cortisol measurement and overnight dexamethasone suppression test are helpful in establishing the diagnosis of Cushing's disease.

Lupus Anticoagulant and Anticardiolipin Antibody

Patients with early onset severe preeclampsia (before 34 weeks of gestation) should be screened for lupus anticoagulant and anticardiolipin antibodies. Immunoglobulin G (IgG) or IgM anticardiolipin or lupus anticoagulant antibodies in medium-to-high titers identified twice at least 12 weeks apart is diagnostic of APS. It should preferably be tested in nonpregnant state.

Antinuclear Antibody

Identification of antinuclear antibody (ANA) is the best screening test for SLE, but it is nonspecific. Antibodies to double-stranded DNA (dsDNA) and Smith (Sm) antigen are specific for SLE.

Ultrasound of Maternal Kidneys

The finding of bilateral small echogenic kidneys that are less than 9-10 cm depending on the body size on ultrasound, supports the diagnosis of chronic kidney disease. Doppler ultrasound of renal arteries gives a reliable estimate of renal blood flow velocity and hence helpful in the diagnosis of renal artery stenosis.

Magnetic Resonance Imaging

The imaging is useful for detection of adrenal tumors in patients with signs and symptoms of pheochromocytoma.

Tests for Ascertaining the Chronicity of Hypertension

The tests involve assessment of end organ damage that is eyes, heart, kidneys, and liver. Electrocardiography (ECG) is advised; evidence of left ventricular hypertrophy is suggestive of chronic hypertension. Two-dimensional (2D) echocardiography (ECHO) evaluates left ventricular function and diagnoses coarctation of aorta, if present (Flowchart 1).

Flowchart 1: Algorithm for clinical approach to a pregnant woman presenting with hypertension.

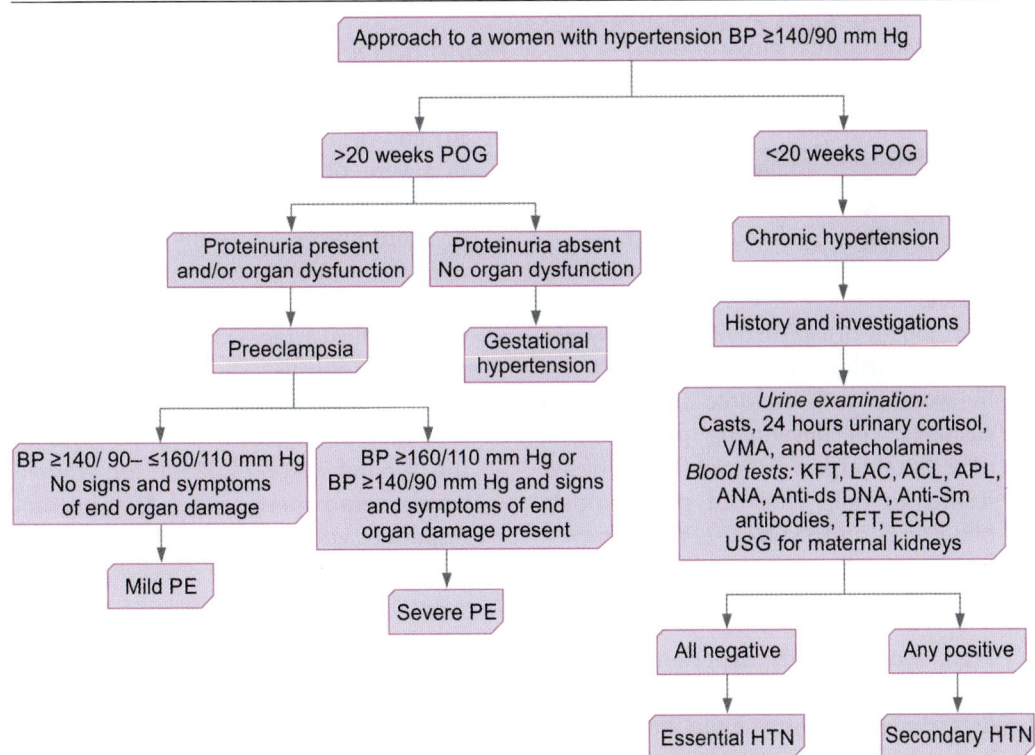

(ANA: antinuclear antibody; APS: antiphospholipid syndrome; dsDNA: double-stranded deoxyribonucleic; KFT: kidney function test; LAC: lupus anticoagulant; PE: pulmonary embolism; SLE: systemic lupus erythematosus; Sm: Smith; TFT: thyroid function test; USG: ultrasonography; VMA: vanillylmandelic acid)

CRITERIA TO DIAGNOSE SEVERE PE[6]

Preeclampsia with SBP ≥ 160 mm Hg or DBP ≥ 110 mm Hg or any of the following:
- New-onset cerebral or visual disturbance, such as photopsia, scotomata, cortical blindness, retinal vasospasm; severe headache that persists and progresses despite analgesic therapy and not accounted for by alternative diagnoses
- Platelet count < 100,000/dL
- Serum creatinine > 1.1 mg/dL or a doubling of the serum creatinine concentration in the absence of other renal disease)
- Severe persistent right upper quadrant or epigastric pain unresponsive to medication and not accounted for by an alternative diagnosis or serum transaminase concentration ≥2 times the upper limit of the normal range or both
- Pulmonary edema.

Management Principles

Prevention

- Identify patients at risk in antenatal period
- Start 150 mg of aspirin daily from 12 weeks until the birth of the baby
- In women with chronic hypertension suspected of developing preeclampsia offer placental growth factor (PlGF)-based testing to help rule out preeclampsia between 20 and 35 weeks of pregnancy.

Antihypertensive Agents

- Treat women with hypertension with one of the following: labetalol nifedipine, or hydralazine. Intravenous labetalol or hydralazine if BP ≥160/110 mm Hg oral labetalol, methyldopa or nifedipine if BP ≥ 150/100 mm Hg
- Start one antihypertensive drug and titrate till maximum dose. If hypertension is uncontrolled, add second drug. Target BP is systolic 130–150 mm Hg and diastolic 80–100 mm Hg
- Consider magnesium sulfate treatment, if one or more of the following features of severe preeclampsia is present—ongoing or recurring severe headaches, visual scotomata, nausea or vomiting, epigastric pain, oliguria, severe hypertension, and progressive deterioration in laboratory blood tests (such as rising creatinine or liver transaminases, or falling platelet count)
- If the woman has had an eclamptic fit, magnesium sulfate should be continued for 24 hours after the last fit. Recurrent fits should be treated with a further dose of 2–4 g given intravenously over 5–15 minutes.

Planning Delivery

- Thresholds include (but are not limited to) any of the following known features of severe preeclampsia or inability to control maternal BP despite using three or more classes of antihypertensives in appropriate doses, eclampsia, placental abruption, reversed end-diastolic flow in the umbilical artery Doppler velocimetry, a nonreassuring cardiotocograph, or intrauterine death
- Consider operative or assisted birth in the second stage of labor for women with severe hypertension which has not responded adequately to initial treatment.

Postdelivery Follow-up

- *Measure BP*: Two to four times daily for the first 2 days after birth, at least once between day 3 and day 5 after birth or as clinically indicated, if antihypertensive treatment is changed after birth.
- Aim to keep BP lower than 140/90 mm Hg.

Flowchart 2: Approach to monitor and manage a women presenting with hypertension.

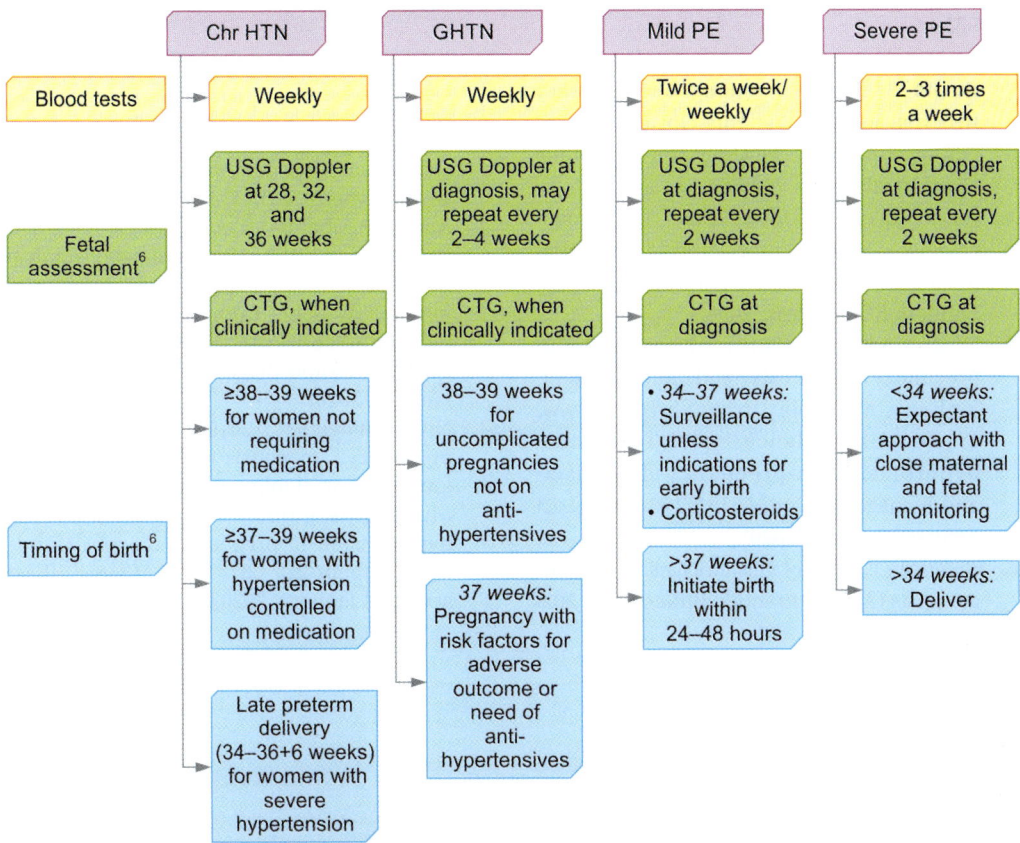

(CTG: cardiotocography; GHTN: gestational hypertension; HTN: hypertension; USG: ultrasonography)

- Review of antihypertensive treatment 2 weeks after the birth and a medical review 6–8 weeks thereafter.

KEY POINTS

- Preeclampsia/eclampsia is the most common cause of hypertension in pregnancy developing after 20 weeks of gestation.
- A systematic evaluation of all women presenting with hypertension is required.
- Home BP monitoring should be offered to women with gestational hypertension, chronic hypertension, and selected women with mild PE with a target BP of 135/85 mm Hg.
- Careful maternal and fetal monitoring (Flowchart 2) is indicated with timely termination of pregnancy to avoid adverse pregnancy outcomes.

REFERENCES

1. Borghi C, Esposti DD, Cassani AJ, Immordino V, Bovicelli L, Ambrosioni E. The treatment of hypertension in pregnancy. J Hypertens Suppl. 2002;20(2):S52-6.
2. Cunningham F, Leveno K, Bloom S, Hauth J, Rouse D, Spong C. Chronic hypertension. In:

Williams Obstetrics, 23rd edition. New York: McGraw Hill Publishing Division. 2010. pp. 983-95.
3. Cunningham FG, Leveno KJ, Hauth JC, Bloom S, Rouse D, Spong C. Pregnancy hypertension. In: Williams Obstetrics, 23rd edition. New York: McGraw Hill Publishing Division. 2010. pp. 706-56.
4. Royal College of Obstetricians and Gynaecologist. Severe preeclampsia/eclampsia management. Greentop guideline No. 10A. London: RCOG Press; 2006.
5. NICE guidelines. (2019). Hypertension in pregnancy: diagnosis and management. [online] Available from: https://www.nice.org.uk/guidance/ng133/resources/hypertension-in-pregnancy-diagnosis-and-management-pdf-66141717671365 [Last accessed January, 2020].
6. American College of Obstetricians and Gynecologists (ACOG) Practice Bulletin No. 202: Gestational Hypertension and Preeclampsia. Obstet Gynecol. 2019;133:e1-e25.

SUGGESTED READING

1. American College of Obstetricians and Gynecologists (ACOG) Practice Bulletin No. 202: Gestational Hypertension and Preeclampsia. Obstet Gynecol. 2019;133:e1-e25.
2. August P, Sibai BM, Lockwood CJ, Barss VA, UpToDate. (2019). "Preeclampsia: Clinical Features, Management and Prognosis". [online] Available from: https://www.uptodate.com/contents/preeclampsia-clinical-features-and-diagnosis [Last accessed January, 2020].
3. NICE guidelines. (2019). Hypertension in pregnancy: diagnosis and management. [online] Available from: https://www.nice.org.uk/guidance/ng133/resources/hypertension-in-pregnancy-diagnosis-and-management-pdf-66141717671365 [Last accessed January, 2020].

19. Approach to a Pregnant Woman Presenting with Heart Disease

Swati Agrawal

INTRODUCTION

Heart disease in pregnancy can be broadly classified into congenital and acquired heart disease with the latter comprising of rheumatic heart disease, ischemic heart disease, and cardiomyopathies. In the Western world, congenital heart disease is the most frequent type of cardiovascular disease presenting during pregnancy (75–82%), mainly with shunt lesions (20–65%). Rheumatic valvular disease dominates in developing countries comprising 56–89% of all women with cardiovascular disease in pregnancy.[1] Cardiomyopathies are rare, but serious form of cardiovascular disease complicating pregnancy.[2] Ischemic heart disease is becoming a rising concern amongst pregnant women consequent to pregnancies being planned at an older age and an increase in prevalence of cigarette smoking, obesity, and diabetes mellitus.[3]

DIAGNOSIS

The diagnosis of heart disease in a pregnant women is often challenging because of extensive pregnancy-induced physiological changes in the cardiovascular system, which influence the evaluation and interpretation of cardiac function in pregnancy.[4] During pregnancy, the plasma volume and cardiac output increase by 40–50%, heart rate by 10–20 beats/min, stroke volume by 30–50%, and the peripheral vascular resistance falls by about 20%. There is a fall in systemic arterial pressure and widening of pulse pressure as the fall in diastolic pressure is more as compared to systolic pressure. These changes mimic cardiac disease in the form of certain symptoms and signs in history, physical examination, and investigations in women with normal pregnancy (Table 1). Many asymptomatic pregnant women with heart disease can manifest for the first-time during pregnancy consequent to the pregnancy-induced physiological changes. Hence, cardiovascular system should be carefully examined in all pregnant women at their registration visit.

DIFFERENTIAL DIAGNOSIS

The differential diagnosis of a pregnant woman presenting with clinical features of heart disease as regard to the nature of heart disease is shown in Box 1.

Some pregnant woman may have undergone some surgery in the past for preexisting heart disease like closure of septal defects, balloon valvuloplasty or valve replacement, angioplasty for ischemic heart disease, or cardiac transplant for cardiac myopathies. It is important to know this as the woman may be on medications such as anticoagulants, aspirin, inotropes, etc.

Table 1: Signs and symptoms in normal pregnancy mimicking heart disease.

History	Examination	Investigations
Dyspnea Palpitations Fatigue Decreased exercise tolerance Swelling of lower limbs	Raised JVP with prominent pulsations Brisk and diffuse apex pulsation Loud heart sounds Widely split S_1, S_2 Occasional S_3 Aortic or pulmonary flow murmurs Mammary soufflé Venous hum	ECG changes: Sinus tachycardia Premature atrial and ventricular beats QRS axis deviation Small Q wave and inverted P wave in lead III CXR changes: Horizontal positioning of heart Straightening of left upper cardiac border Increased bronchovascular markings Echocardiography: Enlargement of ventricular dimensions Slight enlargement of left atrial size Functional tricuspid regurgitation Small pericardial effusion

(JVP: jugular venous pressure; ECG: electrocardiogram; CXR: chest X-ray)

Box 1: Differential diagnosis of heart disease in pregnancy.

Congenital heart disease:
- *Lesions with volume overload:* Atrial septal defect, ventricular septal defect, and patent ductus arteriosus
- *Lesions with obstruction:* Aortic stenosis, coarctation of aorta, pulmonary stenosis, and tetralogy of Fallot

Acquired heart disease:
- Rheumatic heart disease:
  - *Stenotic lesions:* Mitral stenosis and aortic stenosis
  - *Regurgitant lesions:* Mitral regurgitation and aortic regurgitation
  - Combination of lesions

Ischemic heart disease:
- Angina pectoris and myocardial infarction

Cardiomyopathies:
- Dilated and hypertrophic

HISTORY

A detailed history and examination are imperative in understanding the exact nature of heart disease, to prognosticate the maternal and fetal outcome, and decide upon the management of pregnancy.

Women who have congenital heart disease will have to be counseled regarding the increased risk of cardiac defect in the baby depending upon the nature of lesion in the woman. Those with acquired diseases can be reassured of no increase in risk of heart disease in the baby.

History of Present Illness

Women with heart disease usually present with breathlessness. An assessment of effort tolerance should be done to classify the heart disease as per New York Heart Association (NYHA) functional classification (Table 2).[5] Breathlessness, which is persistent, severe or progressive and presence of paroxysmal nocturnal dyspnea, or orthopnea are suggestive of increased severity of heart disease. History of nocturnal cough may suggest paroxysmal nocturnal dyspnea. History of hemoptysis is suggestive of heart failure in a patient with heart disease.

History of chest pain and/or syncope in relation to effort or exertion may be a

Table 2: New York Heart Association (NYHA) functional classification of heart disease in pregnancy.[5]

NYHA Class	Symptoms
I	Patient is asymptomatic and there is no limitation on ordinary physical activity like walking, climbing stairs, etc. despite diagnosed cardiac disease
II	Mild symptoms such as slight shortness of breath or angina on routine physical activity
III	Patient is comfortable only at rest, marked limitation of activity on less than ordinary activity such as walking short distance
IV	Severe limitation in activity due to the presence of symptoms even at rest; the patient is mostly bedridden

presenting symptom of ischemic heart disease in pregnancy.

Past History

History of Hospitalization

History of hospitalization in the past as regards the number, duration, and reason of admissions should be elicited to evaluate the severity of the heart disease. The previous records should be reviewed with respect to investigations, diagnosis, and treatment received.

History of Surgery

Any history of previous cardiac surgery, valvuloplasty, valve replacement, and angioplasty should be elicited, which may help in pointing towards the diagnosis. In those with valve replacement, it is important to find out if the replaced valve is synthetic or biological.

History of Drug Intake

It is important to know about the drugs, which the patient is currently taking, few drugs such as angiotensin-converting enzyme (ACE) inhibitors, amiodarone, and warfarin may be unsafe for the fetus and may need to be replaced. History of regular intramuscular injections every 3 weeks may suggest antibiotic prophylaxis in women with rheumatic heart disease to prevent subacute bacterial endocarditis.

History of Medical Disorders

Certain medical disorders such as diabetes and hypertension may further compromise the cardiovascular function in pregnant women with heart disease. The likelihood of ischemic heart disease is increased in pregnant women with comorbidities, especially if they are more than 35 years of age and obese.

History of Rheumatic Fever

History of fever with sore throat associated with fleeting pain and swelling of the joints or abnormal movements of limbs may be elicited in some patients with rheumatic heart disease.

Personal History

Personal history is essential to ask for any history of smoking for risk categorization in a patient with heart disease, especially in those with ischemic heart disease.

Obstetric History

In women with rheumatic heart disease, the timing of cardiac decompensation during previous pregnancy will provide information on the severity of lesion, cardiac reserve of the woman and her ability to tolerate the stress of pregnancy and labor. This is helpful in planning the management. History of any adverse event in the previous pregnancy such as cardiac failure in the last few months of pregnancy, or within 4–5 months after delivery in an otherwise healthy woman may point toward the diagnosis of peripartum cardiomyopathy.

Family History

History of sudden deaths in the family may suggest presence of congenital heart disease in the family. It is also important to elicit history of diabetes mellitus, hypertension and known congenital heart disease in the family.

EXAMINATION

The patient should be examined carefully from head to toe for any features suggestive of various types of cardiac diseases.

General Physical Examination

The degree of pallor should be noted as severe anemia may be responsible for the symptoms of the patient rather than her heart disease. Anemia needs to be aggressively treated in pregnant women with heart disease. Pitting edema in dependent parts may be suggestive of cardiac decompensation. Jugular venous pressure (JVP) may be raised significantly. One must look for features of Marfan's syndrome such as a tall, thin stature with long slender fingers, hyperextensibility of joints, and high-arched palate. Any thyroid enlargement should be looked for, as thyrotoxicosis can present with cardiac symptoms.

The pulse should be observed for rate, rhythm, volume, character, whether equal on both sides, condition of vessel wall, apex pulse deficit, radiofemoral delay, and carotid bruit. All the above qualities of the pulse help in pointing toward specific heart lesions and certain complications such as arrhythmias. Blood pressure (BP) should be measured in all four limbs as it may be unequal in two arms as in aortic stenosis and coarctation of aorta. There may be hypertension in upper limb and hypotension in lower limb in coarctation of aorta. The respiratory rate should be recorded as increased respiratory rate is an early sign of cardiac decompensation, normal respiratory rate in pregnancy is 12–18 breaths per min.

In respiratory system, bilateral lungs should be auscultated for the presence of crepts, especially at the lung bases. Both the lungs may be full of crepts in left heart failure or pulmonary edema. This may be associated with tender hepatomegaly on abdominal examination (Table 3).

Cardiovascular Examination

Inspection

The precordium should be observed for any bulge, which may be present in pleural or

Table 3: Clinical features of cardiac failure.

Symptoms	Signs
Dyspnea	Cachexia and muscle wasting
Orthopnea	Tachycardia
Reduced exercise tolerance, lethargy, and fatigue	Pulsus alternans
Nocturnal cough	Elevated jugular venous pressure
Wheeze	Crepitations in lungs
Ankle swelling	Third heart sound
Anorexia	Tender hepatomegaly
	Ascites
	Edema feet

pericardial effusion or mediastinal tumors. Look for any abnormal pulsations in the parasternal area, suggestive of right ventricular or left atrial enlargement, or aneurysm of aorta; in epigastrium suggestive of right ventricular hypertrophy, and a mass sitting on aorta; in suprasternal area as in aortic regurgitation and coarctation of aorta; in the neck suggestive of aortic regurgitation, carotid aneurysm or subclavian artery aneurysm; in the second left intercostal space as in dilated pulmonary artery, aneurysm of aorta, enlarged left atrium or hyperkinetic state and on the right side of the chest as in dextrocardia, right atrial enlargement. Presence of dilated veins over the chest wall may signify right-sided heart failure; or superior or inferior vena cava obstruction. Scars of previous cardiac surgery may be present and should be looked for and noted.

Palpation

Palpate the apex beat, which is normally shifted upward and outward in normal pregnancy. The apex beat may be tapping in patients with mitral stenosis and heaving in patients with left ventricular hypertrophy (LVH). Inability to palpate apex beat on the left side can be due to dextrocardia, pericardial effusion, thick chest wall, and obesity. A left parasternal heave may be palpated in patients with right ventricular enlargement. Presence of a thrill is a definite evidence of the presence of an organic disease of the heart and is usually present in stenotic lesions.

Percussion

Percussion is mainly done to determine the boundaries of the heart and is useful to detect pericardial effusion, and aortic aneurysm, rather than the size of the heart. The right, left, and upper borders are percussed. The lower border cannot be percussed as it cannot be distinguished from liver dullness. Normally, the left border is along the apex beat, the right border is retrosternal, and the upper border is in the third left intercostal space in the parasternal line.

Auscultation

The heart sounds are auscultated in all four areas of the chest, namely the mitral, tricuspid, pulmonary, and aortic. The intensity of S1 and S2 should be commented upon and the presence of any added sounds, and murmurs should be noted. Presence of any diastolic murmur or a systolic murmur of more than grade 3/6 is considered abnormal in pregnancy. The description of the grading of murmurs is as given in Table 4. As mitral stenosis is the most common lesion in women suffering from heart disease, mitral area should be auscultated to detect the presence of mid-diastolic murmur pathognomonic of mitral stenosis. It is best heard in the left lateral position with the bell of the stethoscope.

Obstetric Examination

Obstetric examination includes assessment of fundal height, amount of liquor amnii, and the number of fetuses. Uteroplacental insufficiency secondary to hypoxemia due to heart disease may lead to intrauterine growth restriction. Multiple pregnancy increases the morbidity associated with heart disease in a pregnant woman due to exaggerated hemodynamic changes and resultant increase in load on the heart.

INVESTIGATIONS

The various investigations that need to be offered in a pregnant woman with heart disease are as follows:

Table 4: Grading of heart murmurs.

Grade of murmur	Clinical character
I	The murmur is audible only on careful prolonged listening
II	The murmur becomes audible immediately upon putting the stethoscope on the chest
III	The murmur is loud and easily audible in the absence of palpable thrill
IV	The murmur is loud and is associated with a palpable thrill
V	The murmur is audible only with the rim of the stethoscope placed on the chest; palpable thrill is present
VI	The murmur is audible with the stethoscope placed close to the chest, but not in contact with it

Complete Hemogram

Complete hemogram is required to assess the degree and type of anemia, which may worsen the cardiovascular status. A raised leukocyte count may point toward subclinical infection and a search for a possible cause, and its treatment is indicated.

Coagulogram

Coagulogram is offered at regular intervals in patients on anticoagulants for monitoring and titrating the dose of anticoagulants.

Serum Electrolytes

Serum electrolytes are indicated in patients on diuretics that can result in hypokalemia and associated arrhythmias. It also sensitizes the heart to the effect of digoxin by competing with potassium ions for the same binding sites on the Na^+/K^+ ATPase pump.

Serum Markers for Ischemic Heart Disease

Serum markers are advised when there is a clinical suspicion of ischemic heart disease, such as occurrence of chest pain with sweating and syncope in pregnant women with unremarkable physical findings. These include troponin I, which is the marker of choice as its levels are not altered by normal pregnancy; and pregnancy-associated plasma protein-A (PAPP-A), a new marker of unstable angina and acute myocardial infarction (MI). A rising level of creatine kinase muscle brain (CK-MB) in the presence of signs and symptoms of MI is diagnostic although it is important to keep in mind that CK-MB level may be elevated in normal labor.

Urine Examination

Urine routine, microscopy, and culture are indicated to rule out asymptomatic bacteriuria.

Electrocardiography

A baseline electrocardiography (ECG) is required. It ensures a normal cardiac rhythm and may point toward a specific cardiac condition. Significant arrhythmias or heart block should be evaluated for underlying heart disease.

Holter Monitoring

Holter monitoring should be performed in patients with previous documented arrhythmias such as atrial fibrillation, atrial flutter, and in patients who complain of persistent palpitations.

Echocardiography

Echocardiography (ECHO) is the preferred screening method to assess cardiac function as well as to exclude, confirm, or monitor structural heart disease in pregnancy. Transesophageal echocardiography is safe, and can provide better visualization of left atrium and mitral valve. This measures the diameter of all the valves, size of the various chambers of the heart, and ejection fraction of the heart. Studies have shown that dimensions of cardiac chamber, left ventricular (LV) wall thickness, and mass may be higher in normal pregnancies than in nonpregnant women.[6] This knowledge is essential to pick up true abnormalities on ECHO in women with suspected cardiac disease.

Chest X-ray

Chest X-ray is useful in the assessment of the size of the heart and any evidence of pulmonary edema or pneumonitis. It is safe in pregnancy and should be carried out after shielding the abdomen.

Magnetic Resonance Imaging and Computed Tomography

Computed tomography (CT) is usually not indicated due to the radiation exposure involved except for ruling out pulmonary embolism. Magnetic Resonance Imaging (MRI) is safe and may be useful in the diagnosis of complex heart diseases, and those involving aorta, if other commonly used diagnostic procedures such as transthoracic and transesophageal echocardiography are inconclusive.

Fetal Surveillance

In addition to the routine antenatal surveillance of any high-risk pregnancy, women with family history of congenital heart disease should be offered screening for congenital cardiac malformations in the fetus. It can be initiated as early as 13 weeks of gestation along with Down screening by 11–14 weeks ultrasound.[7] Early detection of any major malformations allows parents to consider timely termination of pregnancy. Routine anomaly scan is done at 18–20 weeks gestation and is combined with a detailed fetal ECHO between 18 and 22 weeks of gestation to evaluate cardiac structure, function, rhythm, arterial, and venous flow.

Flowchart 1 summarizes the approach to a pregnant woman presenting with heart disease.

MANAGEMENT: PRINCIPLES

Preconception Risk Assessment and Counseling

- Preconception risk assessment and counseling is recommended in all women with suspected heart disease using the World Health Organization (WHO) classification of maternal risk with respect to the incidence of maternal cardiac events and maternal mortality and morbidity.[8]
- It includes a detailed history, assessment of functional status, information on prior interventions, thorough physical examination, a 12-lead electrocardiogram, and a transthoracic echocardiogram.
- Imaging of the aorta with either MRI or CT is recommended before pregnancy in patients with known aortic disease.
- Intervention is recommended before pregnancy in patients with severe aortic stenosis and severe mitral stenosis.

Antenatal Management

- Pregnancy in a patient with heart disease should be managed in a specialized

Flowchart 1: Algorithm for clinical approach to a pregnant woman with heart disease in pregnancy.

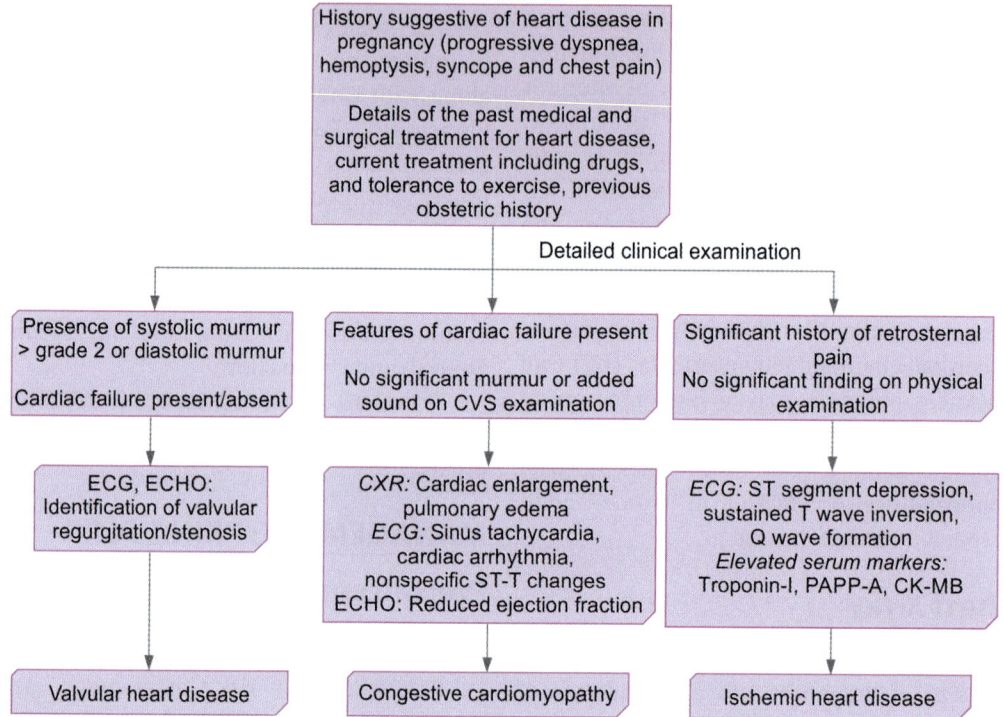

(CVS: cardiovascular examination; CXR: chest X-ray; CK-MB: creatine kinase muscle brain; ECG: electrocardiography; ECHO: echocardiography; LV: left ventricular; PAPP-A: pregnancy-associated plasma protein)

center by a multidisciplinary team consisting of an obstetrician, cardiologist, and anesthetist.

- Intervention in the form of percutaneous therapy or cardiac surgery should be avoided during pregnancy as far as possible but if the intervention is necessary, the best period is between the 13th and 28th week.
- Regular follow-up and close surveillance for cardiac decompensation is essential during pregnancy.
- The timing of admission depends on the severity of the cardiac lesion and the NYHA class.

Management during Delivery and Postpartum Period

- Vaginal delivery is recommended in most of the patients.
- Cesarean delivery is reserved for obstetrical indications or for patients with dilatation of the ascending aorta >45 mm, severe aortic stenosis, preterm labor while on oral anticoagulants, severe heart failure, or Eisenmenger's syndrome.
- Prophylactic antibiotic therapy during delivery for prevention of infective endocarditis is not recommended. However, antibiotic prophylaxis before vagi-

- nal delivery may be given at the time of membrane rupture in selected high-risk patients (e.g., unrepaired cyanotic congenital heart disease, repaired congenital heart disease with residual defects, or prosthetic heart valves).[9]
- Monitoring of maternal vitals and pulse oximetry is recommended during labor to detect early signs of decompensation.
- Regional anesthesia including epidural analgesia is usually preferred in these women but it should be carefully titrated especially in patients with obstructive valvular lesions or compromised ventricular function.
- Intravenous fluids, if required, should be administered cautiously to avoid fluid overload and heart failure.
- Assisted delivery with forceps or a ventouse should be considered to reduce maternal effort during the second stage of labor.
- Oxytocin and misoprostol may be used for the treatment for postpartum hemorrhage but ergometrine and prostaglandin F analogs should be avoided.
- Early ambulation is encouraged in postpartum period to reduce the risk of thromboembolism.
- Hemodynamic monitoring should be continued for at least 24–48 hours in these women as they are at high risk for heart failure in postpartum period due to significant hemodynamic changes and fluid shifts.

Contraception

- Estrogen-containing contraceptives are not advisable in women with cardiac disease due to the high risk of thrombosis and propensity to increase BP.
- Progestin-only contraceptives (implant or depot injection) have little or no (levonorgestrel-loaded intrauterine device or oral desogestrel) effect on coagulation factors, BP, and lipid levels and are preferred in these women.
- Barrier methods, Copper IUCD, and sterilization are safe. Vasectomy is preferred over tubectomy.

KEY POINTS

- The diagnosis of heart disease may be difficult in pregnancy because of profound physiological changes in the cardiovascular system during pregnancy.
- Heart disease in pregnancy can be broadly classified into congenital and acquired heart disease with the latter comprising of rheumatic heart disease, ischemic heart disease, and cardiomyopathies.
- Risk assessment and counseling on registration visit are important.
- A systematic cardiovascular examination may clinch the diagnosis, which can further be confirmed by investigations like chest X-ray, ECG, and ECHO.
- An assessment of effort tolerance should be done to classify the heart disease according to NYHA classification.
- Regular follow-up and careful evaluation of the pulse rate, respiratory rate, JVP, edema, and auscultation of the lungs is mandatory on each visit to exclude cardiac failure in all patients.
- Pregnancy should be managed in a specialized center by a multidisciplinary team consisting of an obstetrician, cardiologist, and anesthetist.
- The best time for any cardiac intervention during pregnancy is between 13th and 28th weeks of gestation.
- Vaginal delivery is recommended in most patients and cesarean delivery is reserved for obstetrical indications or select cardiac lesions.

- Careful monitoring of maternal vitals and pulse oximetry is recommended during labor to detect early signs of decompensation and should be continued for 24–48 hours postdelivery.
- Assisted delivery with forceps or a ventouse should be considered to reduce maternal effort during the second stage of labor.
- Postpartum contraceptive options include barrier contraceptives, male and female sterilization, intrauterine devices, and progesterone only contraceptives

REFERENCES

1. Regitz-Zagrosek V, Blomstrom Lundgvist C, Borghic C, Cifkova R, Ferreira R, Foidart JM, et al. ESC Guidelines on the management of cardiovascular diseases during pregnancy: the Task Force on the Management of Cardiovascular Diseases during Pregnancy of the European Society of Cardiology (ESC). Eur Heart J. 2011;32(24):3147-97.
2. Stergiopoulos K, Shiang E, Bench T. Pregnancy in patients with pre- existing cardiomyopathies. J Am Coll Cardiol. 2011;58(4):337-50.
3. Bondagji NS. Ischemic heart disease in pregnancy. J Saudi Heart Assoc. 2012;24(2): 89-97.
4. Vasu S, Stergiopoulos K. Valvular heart disease in pregnancy. Hellenic J Cardiol. 2009;50(6):498-510.
5. The Criteria Committee of the New York Heart Association. Nomenclature and Criteria for Diagnosis of Diseases of the Heart and Great Vessels, 9th edition. Boston: Little, Brown and Company; 1994. pp. 253-6.
6. Adeyeye VO Balogun MO, Adebayo RA, Makinde ON, Akinwusi PO, Ajayi EA, et al. Echocardiographic Assessment of Cardiac Changes During Normal Pregnancy Among Nigerians. Clin Med Insights Cardiol. 2016;10:157-62.
7. Rasiah SV, Publicover M, Ewer AK, Khan KS, Kilby MD, Zamora J. A systematic review of the accuracy of first-trimester ultrasound examination for detecting major congenital heart disease. Ultrasound Obstet Gynecol. 2006;28(1):110-6.
8. Regitz-Zagrosek V, Roos-Hesselink JW, Bauersachs J, Blomström-Lundqvist C, Cífková R, De Bonis M, et al. ESC Scientific Document Group, ESC Guidelines for the management of cardiovascular diseases during pregnancy. Euro Heart J. 2018;39(34):3165-241.
9. Warnes CA, Williams RG, Bashore TM, Child JS, Connolly HM, Dearani JA, et al. Guidelines for the management of adults with congenital heart disease: a report of the American College of Cardiology/American Heart Association Task Force on Practice Guidelines (writing committee to develop guidelines on the management of adults with congenital heart disease). Circulation. 2008;118(23):714.

SUGGESTED READING

1. ACOG Practice Bulletin No. 212: Pregnancy and Heart Disease. Obstetr Gynecol. 2019; 33(5):320-56.
2. Canobbio MM, Warnes CA, Aboulhosn J, Connolly HM, Khanna A, Koos BJ, et al. Management of pregnancy in patients with complex congenital heart disease: A scientific statement for healthcare professionals from the American Heart Association. Circulation. 2017;135(8):e50-e87.
3. RCOG. (2011). Cardiac disease and pregnancy (RCOG Good Practice No.13). [online] Available from: https://www.rcog.org.uk/en/guidelines-research-services/guidelines/good-practice-13/ [Last accessed January, 2020].
4. Stout KK, Daniels CJ, Aboulhosn JA, Bozkurt B, Broberg CS, Colman JM, et al. 2018 AHA/ACC Guideline for the Management of Adults With Congenital Heart Disease: Executive Summary: A Report of the American College of Cardiology/American Heart Association Task Force on Clinical Practice Guidelines. J Am Coll Cardiol. 2019;73(12):1494-563.

20
Approach to a Pregnant Woman with Suspected Fetal Growth Restriction

Sangeeta Gupta

INTRODUCTION

Fetal growth restriction (FGR) is among the most common complications of pregnancy. It is defined as failure of the fetus to achieve its biological growth potential and is associated with placental insufficiency and poor perinatal outcomes. Approximately, 4–8% of all infants born in developed countries and 6–30% of infants born in developing countries are classified as growth restricted.[1]

Diagnosis of FGR remains a challenge due to lack of uniformity in defining FGR. At present, there is no gold standard for the diagnosis of FGR. Other FGR-related dilemmas include lack of proper screening strategy, effective preventive interventions, recognition of variable phenotypes-early versus late onset, ideal monitoring protocols, optimal trigger for delivery, and choice of mode of delivery.

Fetal growth has been categorized in the following three groups based on percentiles of growth from a population-based reference growth charts for neonates:
- *Small for gestational age (SGA):* Neonates whose weights are lower than the 10th percentile.
- *Appropriate for gestational age (AGA):* Neonates whose birth weights were between the 10th and 90th percentiles.
- *Large for gestational age (LGA):* Neonates larger than the 90th percentile.

There are two concerns with the above classification. One, all SGA fetuses are not growth restricted and we need to differentiate between the constitutionally small and pathologically small. Two, all fetuses in AGA category may not be healthy some may have aberrant growth and at a higher risk of still birth. However, all fetuses below 3rd centile estimated fetal weight (EFW) are classified as pathological since the perinatal outcomes associated with this group are consistently poor. In AGA fetuses, if abdominal circumference (AC) or EFW cross centiles or growth curve plateaus or is associated with abnormal Doppler, FGR is the likely diagnosis. This category of AGA fetuses with abnormal growth contributes significantly to unexplained stillborns. Thus, an appropriate definition for FGR should include a fetal weight of less than the 3rd percentile and abnormal fetal growth velocity, umbilical artery Doppler, and cerebroplacental ratio (CPR). Fetuses with a normal growth velocity and umbilical flow, particularly greater than the 3rd percentile, are more likely constitutionally small normal fetuses. Considering the above observations, a panel of experts reached consensus on the definition of both early and late placental FGR through a Delphi procedure (Table 1).[2] The aim of the new criteria is to better identify fetuses at risk than done by criteria based solely on biometry. However, the new criteria needs further evaluation.

Table 1: Consensus-based definitions for early and late FGR in absence of congenital anomalies.[2]	
Early FGR: GA < 32 weeks	Late FGR: GA > 32 weeks
AC or EFW < p3 or UA AEDF or AC or EFW < p10 combined with one or both of the following: 1. PI in the uterine artery > p95 2. PI in the umbilical artery > p95	AC or EFW < p3 or At least 2 out of 3 of the following: 1. AC or EFW < p10 2. AC or EFW crossing centiles of more than two quartiles on growth centiles 3. CPR < p5 or UA > p95

(AC: abdominal circumference; AEDF: Absent end-diastolic blood flow; CPR: cerebroplacental ratio; EFW: estimated fetal weight; FGR: fetal growth restriction; GA: gestational age; UA: umbilical artery)

FETAL GROWTH CHARTS

The role of growth charts for detecting FGR cannot be overemphasized. Serial growth must be plotted on these charts whether monitoring is by symphysis-fundal height (SFH) or ultrasound biometry. The various charts available are World Health Organization (WHO) fetal growth charts and intergrowth-21. The WHO growth chart has been illustrated in Figures 1A to F.

Symmetrical and Asymmetrical Growth Restriction

In symmetrical FGR, both the fetal length and size are below normal percentiles for the gestational age. These fetuses account for 20–30% of fetuses affected by FGR. The cause of this phenotype is usually intrinsic where the impact of disease impedes cellular hyperplasia in early pregnancy like aneuploidy, anomalies, or fetal infections. While in asymmetrical FGR, the fetal length remains normal but size is reduced. The biparietal diameter, head circumference, and femur length (BPD, HC, and FL) remain normal but AC and EFW are reduced. This is usually the consequence of placental insufficiency or undernutrition.

Early versus Late-onset FGR

The discriminatory gestational age for the aforesaid categorization has been arbitrarily accepted as 32 weeks. The major differences between the two are listed in the Table 2. In early onset FGR, diagnosis is easier, but management is a challenge as iatrogenic prematurity is added to the existing severe fetal hypoxia. Whereas in late-onset FGR, management is easier as once diagnosed, delivery can be contemplated; however, diagnosis is often missed due to subtle presentation.

The cause of FGR may be maternal, fetal, or placental. The Box 1 enumerates various causes of FGR. It is important to diagnose the cause for purpose of counseling, appropriate referrals and planning management strategy.

DIFFERENTIAL DIAGNOSIS

The differential diagnosis of FGR is listed in Box 2.

Wrong Dates/Preterm

Poor recall of dates is common and hence, correct dating is most integral for the diagnosis of FGR. The best method to date is by ultrasound in first trimester. However, this

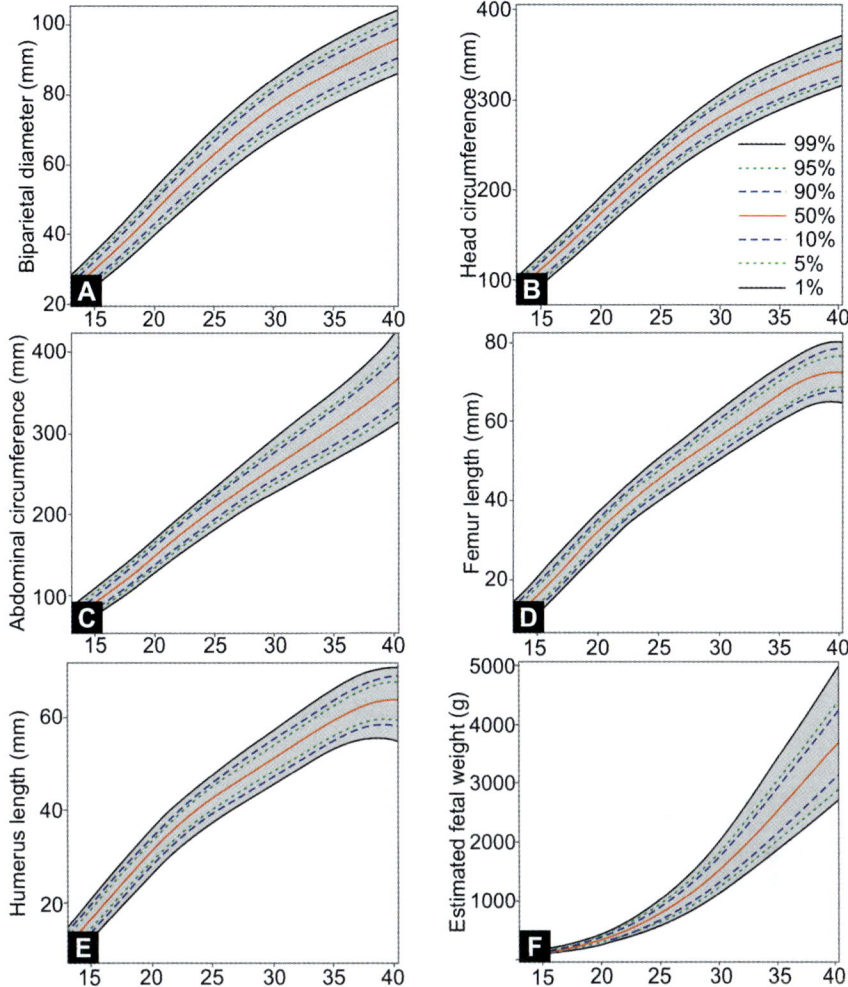

Figs. 1A to F: WHO growth charts with percentiles of BPD, HC, AC, FL, HL, and EFW from 14 to 40 weeks gestational age.[3]
(AC: abdominal circumference; BPD: biparietal diameter; EFW: estimated fetal weight; HC: head circumference; HL: humerus length; FL: femur length)

Table 2: Main differences between early versus late-onset FGR.[4,5]

Early-onset FGR	Late-onset FGR
Onset usually between 26 and 32 weeks	Onset usually after 32 weeks
Severe placental disease: Abnormal UA Doppler and high association with preeclampsia	*Mild placental disease:* Usually, normal UA Doppler, low association with preeclampsia
Severe hypoxia, abnormal DV Doppler	Mild hypoxia, abnormal CPR
High morbidity and mortality	Lower mortality but common cause of stillbirth as it goes unidentified.

(DV: ductus venosus; CPR: cerebroplacental ratio; FGR: fetal growth restriction; UA: umbilical artery)

> **Box 1:** Etiology of FGR.[6,7]
>
> *Maternal:*
> - Chronic hypertension or preeclampsia
> - Chronic medical disorders like antiphospholipid syndrome, SLE, chronic renal disease, cyanotic heart disease, COPD, malabsorption syndromes, and diabetes with vasculopathy
> - Sickle cell disease and beta-thalassemia
> - *Poor nutritional status:* Prepregnancy low BMI and poor weight gain during pregnancy
> - Smoking, alcohol, and drug abuse
> - Medications like anticonvulsant, antineoplastic agents, warfarin, and folic acid antagonists
> - Women residing in high altitude
>
> *Fetal:*
> - *Aneuploidy:* Trisomy 13, 18, 21, triploidy, and uniparental disomy
> - *Structural anomaly:* Gastroschisis, omphalocele, diaphragmatic hernia, and congenital heart defect
> - Fetal infections like TORCH and malaria
> - Multiple gestation
>
> *Placental:*
> - Placenta previa, morbidly adherent placenta, and abruption
> - Circumvallate placenta
> - Placental hemangioma
> - Confined placental mosaicism
> - Single umbilical artery
> - Velamentous cord insertion
> - Diffuse chronic villitis of unknown etiology
>
> (BMI: body mass index; COPD: chronic obstructive pulmonary disease; SLE: systemic lupus erythematosus)

> **Box 2:** Differential diagnosis of FGR.
> - Wrong dates
> - Prelabor rupture of membranes
> - Intrauterine death

Serial plotting of SFH or biometry will resolve the issue. A steady gain of SFH/AC/EFW will exclude the diagnosis of FGR. Doppler examination of umbilical artery and middle cerebral artery (MCA) will further facilitate clarifying the diagnosis.

Prelabor Rupture of Membranes

Leaking per vaginum leads to decrease in fundal height and oligohydramnios, both are features of FGR as well. However, a good history of vaginal leaking and per speculum examination usually clinches the diagnosis. In cases, where leaking is not demonstrable during per speculum examination, various tests like fern test or nitrazine test may be used to confirm the vaginal leaking.

Intrauterine Fetal Demise

History of loss of fetal movements, absence of cardiac activity on auscultation, and ultrasound confirm intrauterine fetal demise (IUD).

HISTORY

History gives insight into the cause of FGR and classifies women in high-risk group who are more likely to develop FGR during pregnancy. These women need closer surveillance during pregnancy for timely detection and management.

- *Present illness:* There is no specific complaint pertaining to FGR. She may have complaints of associated conditions like preeclampsia (headache and pedal edema).

remains a major challenge in many patients due to late bookings or complete lack of care or nonavailability in low resource settings. If dating is doubtful, following observations favor diagnosis of FGR:
- Presence of medical disorders like hypertension, chronic renal disease, or systemic lupus erythematosus (SLE)
- Associated oligohydramnios
- Size of head and its firmness relatively more for the period of amenorrhea.

- *Menstrual history:* The patient's menstrual history is considered adequate for the purpose of establishing the gestational age only if the last menstrual period was normal in duration and amount of flow, if the prior menstrual periods came at regular intervals and if the patient did not use oral contraceptives within 3 months of her last period.[8] However, the best method to date pregnancy is by ultrasound done in first trimester.
- *Obstetrical history:* History of FGR, stillbirth, and hypertension in previous pregnancies predisposes a woman to higher risk of FGR in current pregnancy.
- Poor socioeconomic status and undernourishment may also contribute to the impaired growth of fetus and hence it is important to enquire about prepregnancy weight and body mass index (BMI).
- *Personal history:* Smoking, alcohol abuse, and illicit drug abuse significantly impair fetal growth.
- *Medical history:* Chronic hypertension, chronic renal disease, antiphospholipid syndrome, SLE, and cyanotic heart disease are some medical disorders. In developing countries, chronic malaria is an important contributor to FGR.
- *Drug history:* Intake of drugs like antiepileptics (phenytoin and valproate), warfarin, and antineoplastic drugs.

EXAMINATION

Maternal Weight

It is an important determinant of fetal growth velocity. Low prepregnancy BMI as well as poor weight gain during pregnancy should be looked for. Measurement of blood pressure at every antenatal visit must be done. General examination may reveal features suggestive of severe undernutrition (pallor, cheilosis, and stomatitis) or hypertensive disorder of pregnancy (pedal edema).

Fundal Height Measurement

Discrepancy between period of amenorrhea and fundal height of more than 4 weeks should arouse suspicion of FGR. Fundal height is not a preferred method of monitoring as it lacks objectivity. Measurement of SFH in centimeters at every visit and plotting the same on growth charts is the first line tool to monitor fetal growth in *low-risk pregnancies*. Suboptimal growth is suspected when SFH falls below 10th centile or the growth velocity decreases or plateaus. Such cases need confirmation of diagnosis by ultrasound examination. In high-risk cases and multiple pregnancy, surveillance is primarily done by serial biometry. SFH measurement is influenced by maternal obesity, abnormal fetal lie, multiple gestations, polyhydramnios, large pelvic masses, e.g., fibroids, and fetal head engagement. There is considerable intra- and interobserver variability as well. The sensitivity for the detection of SGA has increased from 29 to 48% with the use of growth charts.

Oligohydramnios as assessed clinically is usually associated with FGR especially in those cases where cause is placental insufficiency.

INVESTIGATIONS

Serum Analytes

Abnormal serum screening [low pregnancy-associated plasma protein A (PAPP-A), raised β-human chorionic gonadotropin (β-hCG)] in first trimester predisposes the pregnancy to higher risk of FGR. These women are kept under closer surveillance. These serum analytes are routinely used for screening of aneuploidies but are not very robust for screening of FGR. Moreover, currently no preventive strategies are available for FGR.

Fetal Karyotype and Microarray

Amniocentesis or cordocentesis is indicated for collection of amniotic fluid or fetal blood for detection of chromosomal abnormalities using fetal karyotyping and or microarray.

Testing for Fetal Infections

This is done using maternal serology or polymerase chain reaction (PCR) DNA in amniotic fluid or fetal blood.

Ultrasound

Ultrasound is an indispensable tool for diagnosis, classification, detection of cause, monitoring, and management of FGR. It is the most reliable, preferred, and accepted modality.

It has following roles:
- Correct estimation of gestational age
- First-trimester uterine artery Doppler pulsatility index to assess placental invasion and screen patients at high risk of developing FGR
- Anomaly scan
- Serial biometry
- Arterial and venous Doppler
- Biophysical profile
- *Correct estimation of gestational age:* It remains an integral component of quality prenatal care and is the key to correct interpretation of fetal growth parameters. Dating by last menstrual period remains a challenge as discussed earlier. The gold standard for dating is by measuring crown-rump length between 7 and 13 weeks 6 days. In patients who have conceived by in vitro fertilization (IVF), dating will be done by embryo transfer and not CRL.
- *First trimester uterine artery Doppler pulsatility index (PI):* It has been used to assess placental invasion and screen patients at high risk of developing FGR. It may be combined with serum analytes to improve predictive values. However, like serum analytes the low prediction rates and lack of preventive strategy limit its utility in FGR.
- *Anomaly scan*: About a quarter of fetuses who have anomalies are growth restricted. Hence, a detailed anomaly scan is warranted in all pregnant women with FGR. The scan may also reveal soft markers of chromosomal abnormalities, which needs confirmation by invasive testing.
- *Biometry*: Measurement of various parameters like BPD, HC, AC, and FL gives vital information about EFW and whether FGR is symmetrical or asymmetrical. AC/EFW is the most sensitive parameter to monitor growth.

Plotting of AC/EFW on growth charts identifies fetuses below 10th centile. Serial biometry at intervals of 2–3 weeks is plotted on growth charts to observe the rate of growth. Following the rate of growth is of greater value than point estimates. This helps in distinguishing SGA from FGR. A growth curve below 10th centile but parallel to normal curve is representative of SGA which is not pathological (Fig. 2).

In symmetric growth restriction, all biometric parameters exhibit growth lag whereas in cases with placental insufficiency and nutritional deprivation, BPD and FL escape the insult and the AC lags causing asymmetrical growth restriction. The ratio of HC/AC differentiates between symmetrical and asymmetrical FGR, the ratio of more than one usually indicating asymmetrical growth. It is not uncommon to observe overlapping patterns. This categorization is important as it reflects the etiology of FGR. Symmetrical FGR is more often associated with intrinsic

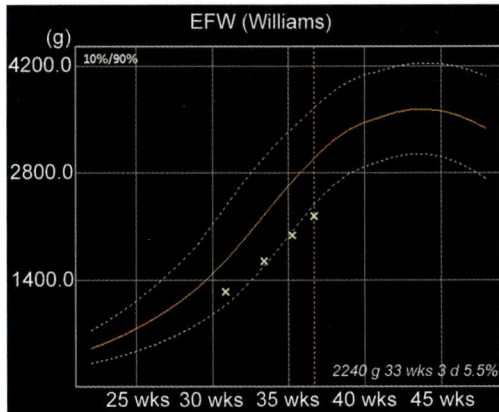

Fig. 2: Growth chart in small for gestational age.

Box 3: Indications of Doppler studies in FGR.

- Screening
- Differentiate SGA from FGR
- *Risk stratification:* Degree of placental disease (UA), level of redistribution (MCA and CPR), and degree of cardiac compromise (DV)
- Decide frequency of monitoring
- Decide the timing of delivery

(CPR: cerebroplacental ratio; DV: ductus venosus; FGR: fetal growth restriction; MCA: middle cerebral artery; SGA: small for gestational age)

causes like anomalies, aneuploidies, or fetal infections while asymmetric FGR with placental insufficiency and nutritional deprivation.

Arterial and venous Doppler: The indications of Doppler studies in FGR are listed in Box 3.

Umbilical artery Doppler (UAD):[9] It is the most accepted and widely used surveillance method in FGR. Placental pathology restricts the impedance to flow and this is reflected as increased UA PI (PI > 95th centile), absent or reversed diastolic flow in umbilical artery [absent end-diastolic velocity and reversed end-diastolic velocity (AEDV and REDV)]. An abnormal UA Doppler is associated with increased perinatal morbidity and mortality. Figures 3 and 4 illustrate normal UAD and UA REDV, respectively.

Middle cerebral artery:[9] PI decreases as an adaptive response to hypoxia-*brain sparing*. Currently, enough evidence is not available to use it as an isolated parameter to predict outcomes. Figures 5 and 6 depict normal MCA Doppler wave form and decreased MCA PI.

Cerebroplacental ratio[9,10] is ratio of MCA PI and UA PI. It is a more sensitive measure of cerebral redistribution. CPR is already decreased when its individual components suffer mild changes but are still within normal ranges. In growth restriction, CPR falls to less than 1 or below 5th centile. There is higher rate of intrapartum fetal distress, cesarean section, and adverse neonatal outcomes in these pregnancies.

Ductus venosus flow reflects atrial pressure-volume changes and is a sensitive marker of hypoxia and acidemia. It predicts short-term risk of fetal death in early onset FGR. It has a role in surveillance of preterm FGR fetuses with AREDV of UA and helps in deciding the time of delivery in preterm FGR. An absent or reversed "a" wave indicates severe cardiac decompensation and impending fetal death, hence calls for an urgent delivery with steroid cover. Figures 7 and 8 show normal DV waveform and reversed "a" wave in DV.

The Doppler studies play a vital role in deciding monitoring protocols of FGR fetuses and taking decisions of delivery. Tables 3 and 4 briefly describe the management protocols for early and late-onset FGR, respectively.[5,11]

When making decisions regarding termination of pregnancy in early onset FGR, following points should be considered:

- *Gestational age:* Each day gained intrauterine increases neonatal survival by about 1%
- Neonatal facilities available

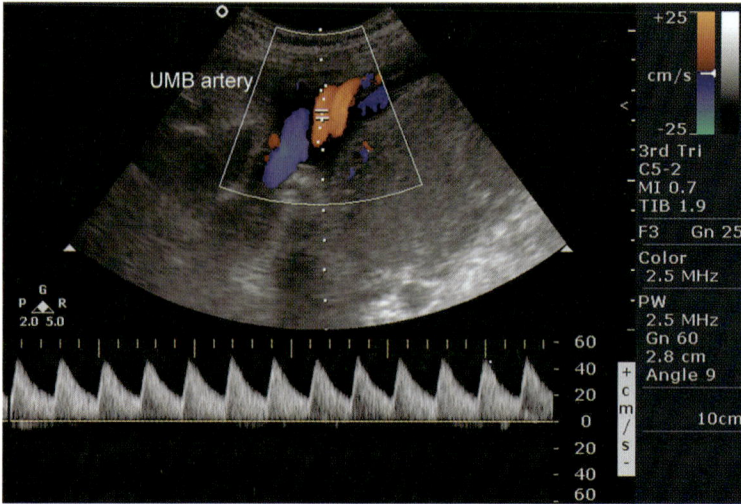

Fig. 3: Normal umbilical artery (UMB artery) Doppler wave form.

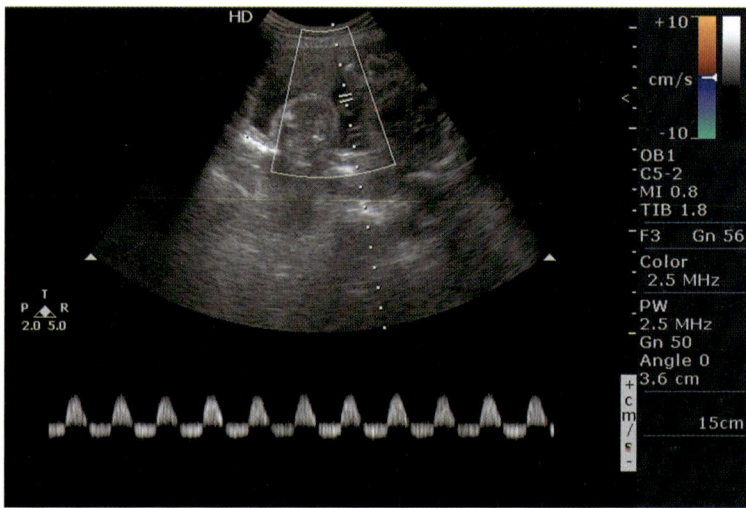

Fig. 4: Reversed end-diastolic flow in umbilical artery.

- Associated comorbidities in the mother especially severe preeclampsia or impending eclampsia
- *Parents' wish:* The parents should be counseled regarding possibility of IUD versus neonatal morbidity and mortality and long-term developmental outcomes.

Currently, the only fetal therapy available for FGR is delivery. There are inconsistencies in definitions of FGR and many diagnoses are missed in prenatal period. However, meticulous examination in low-risk population and serial plotting of growth charts holds the key to maximize improved outcomes.

Chapter 20: Approach to a Pregnant Woman with Suspected Fetal Growth Restriction

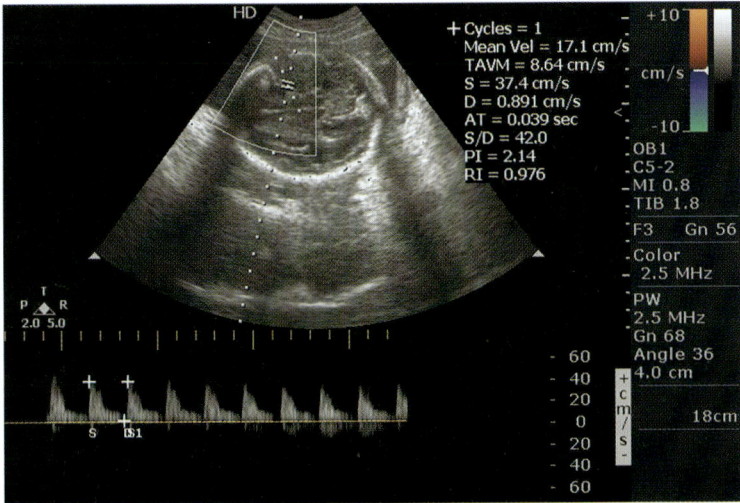

Fig. 5: Normal middle cerebral artery Doppler wave form.

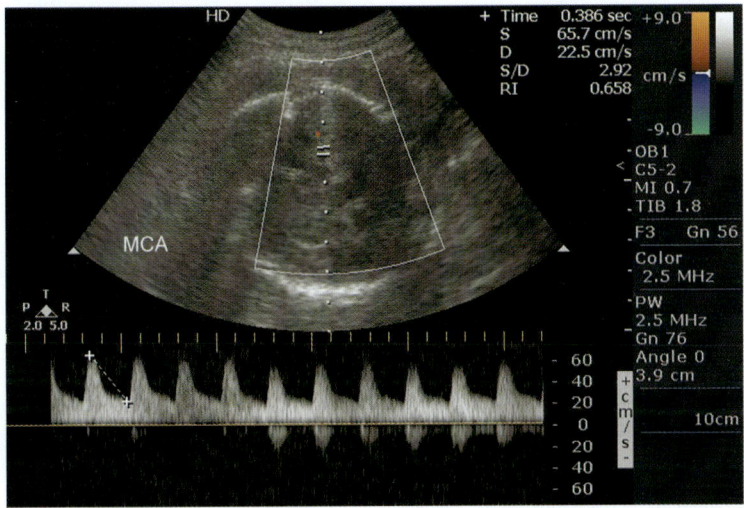

Fig. 6: Decreased middle cerebral artery (MCA) pulsatility index (PI).

KEYPOINTS

- Correct determination of gestational age is most elementary for diagnosis of FGR.
- Serial monitoring rather than point estimates are of greater value for assessing FGR, use of growth charts is mandatory for optimal prenatal care.
- Three important steps in FGR are identify SGA fetuses, distinguish SGA from FGR, and meticulously follow FGRs.

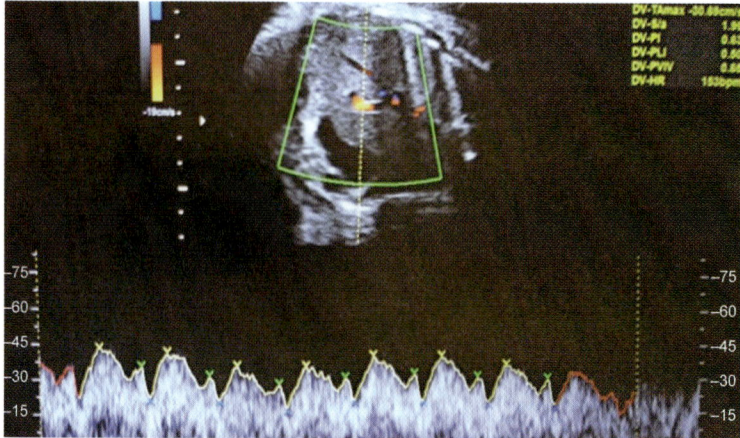

Fig. 7: Normal waveform of ductus venosus.

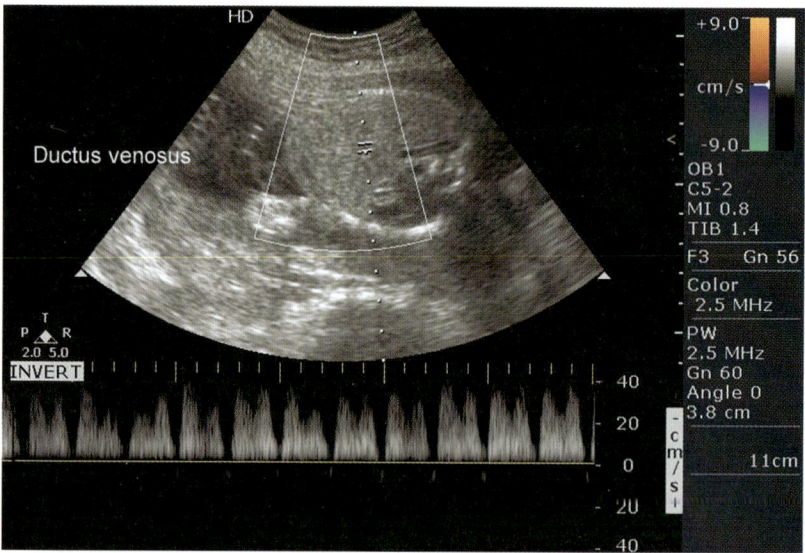

Fig. 8: Absent "a" wave in ductus venosus.

- Ultrasound and Doppler are the mainstay for the management of FGR.
- Monitoring intervals and timing of delivery are best achieved by an integrated protocol—serial measurements to assess growth velocity, combined with Doppler measurements to identify those fetuses with redistribution.
- Managing early FGRs is challenging due to associated prematurity—the trigger for delivery in early onset FGR should be based on late DV changes or abnormal CTG.
- Late FGR significantly contributes to unexplained SB—their diagnoses are a challenge and are identified when AC/EFW cross centiles or have abnormal CPR.

Table 3: Management protocol for early onset FGR (<32 weeks).

Fetal condition	Monitoring interval	Parameters	Termination of pregnancy
SGA: EFW <10th p, Doppler normal	2 weeks	Biometry + UA Doppler + BPP	40 weeks
FGR: EFW <3rd p/UA PI >95p/CPR <1	1 week	Biometry 2 weeks + UA Doppler + CPR + BPP/cCTG	37 weeks
UA AEDF	Admit, twice a week	UA Doppler + *DV Doppler* + BPP/cCTG	32–34 weeks
UA REDF or DV PI < 95th p	24–48 hours	UA Doppler + *DV Doppler* + BPP/cCTG	32 weeks, steroid cover
Absent reversed "a" wave on DV Spontaneous FHR decelerations cCTG reduced short-term variability (STV)	12–24 hours		Immediate delivery after administration of steroid and magnesium sulfate

(AEDF: absent end-diastolic blood flow; BPP: biophysical profile; cCTG: computerized cardiotocography; CPR: cerebroplacental ratio; DV: ductus venosus; EFW: estimated fetal weight; FGR: fetal growth restriction; FHR: fetal heart rate; PI: pulsatility index; SGA: small for gestational age; UA: umbilical artery)

Table 4: Management protocol for late onset FGR (>32 Weeks).

	Monitoring interval	Parameters	Termination of pregnancy
SGA: EFW < 10th p, Doppler normal	2 weeks	Biometry + UA Doppler + BPP	40 weeks
EFW < 3rd p/UA PI > 95 p/CPR < 1	Weekly	Biometry 2 weeks + UA Doppler + CPR + BPP	37 weeks
UA AEDF/REDF	Admit Twice weekly	UA Doppler + BPP	34 weeks

(AEDF: absent end-diastolic blood flow; BPP: biophysical profile; CPR: cerebroplacental ratio; EFW: estimated fetal weight; PI: pulsatility index; SGA: small for gestational age; UA: umbilical artery)

REFERENCES

1. Kramer MS. Determinants of low birth weight: methodological assessment and meta-analysis. Bull World Health Organ. 1987; 65:663-737.
2. Gordijn SJ, Beune IM, Thilaganathan B, Papageorghiou A, Baschat AA, Baker PN, et al. Consensus definition of fetal growth restriction: a Delphi procedure. Ultrasound Obstet Gynecol. 2016;48(3):333-9.
3. Kiserud T, Piaggio G, Carroli G, Widmer M, Carvalho J, Neerup Jensen L, et al. The World Health Organization Fetal Growth Charts: A Multinational Longitudinal Study of Ultrasound Biometric Measurements and Estimated Fetal Weight. PLoS Med. 2017; 14(1):e1002220.
4. Nawathe A, Lees C. Early onset fetal growth restriction. Best Pract Res Clin Obstet Gynaecol. 2017;38:24-37.

5. Figueras F, Gratacos E. An integrated approach to fetal growth restriction. Best Pract Res Clin Obstet Gynaecol. 2017;38:48-58.
6. Resnik R, Creasy RK. Intrauterine growth restriction, 7th edition. Philadelphia: Saunders; 2014. Maulik D. Fetal growth restriction: the etiology. Clin Obstet Gynecol. 2006;49(2): 228-35.
7. Arias F. Identification and surveillance of the high risk patient. In: Arias F (Ed). Practical Guide to High-risk Pregnancy and Delivery, 2nd ed. Missouri: Mosby Year Book; 1992. pp. 3-21.
8. Khalil A, Thilaganathan B. Role of uteroplacental and fetal Doppler in identifying fetal growth restriction at term. Best Pract Res Clin Obstet Gynaecol. 2017;38:38-47.
9. DeVore GR. The importance of the cerebroplacental ratio in the evaluation of fetal well-being in SGA and AGA fetuses. Am J Obstet Gynecol. 2015;213(1):5-15.
10. Figueras F, Gratacos E. Stage-based approach to the management of fetal growth restriction. Prenat Diagn. 2014;34(7):655-9.
11. Baschat AA. Planning management and delivery of the growth-restricted fetus. Best Pract Res Clin Obstet Gynaecol. 2018;49: 53-65.

SUGGESTED READING

1. McCowan LM, Figueras F, Anderson NH. Evidence-based national guidelines for the management of suspected fetal growth restriction: comparison, consensus, and controversy. Am J Obstet Gynecol. 2018; 218(2S):S855-68.
2. RCOG. The investigation and management of the small for gestational age fetus (Green-top31). London, England: RCOG; 2014.

21. Approach to a Pregnant Woman with Previous Cesarean Section

K Aparna Sharma

INTRODUCTION

The cesarean delivery rate worldwide is increasing contributing to an increasing population of pregnant women with previous caesarean scar. A pregnant woman with previous cesarean section (CS) can either undergo an elective repeat cesarean section (ERCS) or a trial of vaginal delivery. The ideal outcome would be a vaginal delivery with a healthy baby and mother.

Overall, the success rate of trial of labor after cesarean (TOLAC) ranges from 60 to 80% depending on various patient variables.[1] In properly selected women, a success rate of 72–75% can be given. In terms of absolute risk for the woman undergoing TOLAC, 1 in 1,000 trials of labor will result in neonatal death or significant neurological injury.[2] Specifically, 1 in 100 trials will result in scar rupture and 1 in 10 scar ruptures will result in neonatal death or neurological injury and 1 per 500 scar ruptures will result in a maternal death.[3]

The entire workup of the patient including a detailed history, general physical, abdominal, and vaginal examination can help in deciding whether the patient can undergo a trial of labor or needs a repeat CS delivery. It quantifies the chances of achieving a successful TOLAC, if a trial of labor is contemplated. The patient is counseled about the risks and benefits of the various options of delivery, i.e., TOLAC, elective repeat cesarean delivery (ERCD), and emergency cesarean after failed TOLAC.

The absolute contraindications to TOLAC are listed in Box 1.

Box 1: Absolute contraindications to trial of labor after cesarean (TOLAC).

- Previous classical or inverted "T" uterine scar
- Previous uterine rupture
- Presence of a contraindication to vaginal delivery such as placenta previa or malpresentation
- Woman declines a TOLAC and request elective repeat cesarean delivery (ERCD)
- Previous myomectomy with breach of uterine cavity

HISTORY

Patient Profile

Certain factors such as age, gravidity, and parity are important to determine the outcome of pregnancy in women undergoing trial of labor. Older women, >35 years of age, are less likely to opt for TOLAC and are also less likely to be successful if they opt for it.

History of Present Pregnancy

The period of gestation is important as studies have consistently shown that women who attempt TOLAC beyond 40 weeks of gestation are less likely to have a successful vaginal delivery.[4] Presenting complaints such as pain in lower abdomen, or bleeding per vaginum, or increased frequency of micturition may suggest scar dehiscence, especially in women presenting in labor.

Obstetric History

A detailed obstetric history should be elicited as described in Chapter 1 "Approach to a Pregnant Woman Attending Antenatal Clinic."

In women with previous cesarean section, certain specific points need to be asked in the obstetric history to assess the integrity of scar and the likelihood of the woman to have a successful TOLAC. These points are listed in Box 2.

The number of previous vaginal deliveries and number of vaginal births after CS (VBACs) are associated with higher chances of successful TOLAC.[5] The odds ratio (OR) for a successful TOLAC with prior vaginal delivery is 3.90, (95% CI 3.60–4.30); with prior VBAC is 4.76, (95% CI 4.35–5.26).[6] Previous successful TOLAC is the single best predictor of a successful TOLAC associated with a success rate of 85–90%.

History of interpregnancy interval is important as CS to conception interval of <6 months or an interdelivery interval of <18 months is an independent risk factor for both uterine rupture and maternal morbidity during TOLAC.[7] The number of previous CS is important as greater than two previous CS is a contraindication for TOLAC.

The rate of successful TOLAC depends on the indication for previous CS. Contracted pelvis is an indication for ERCS. Chances of successful TOLAC are low in case of previous section done for failure to progress in labor or cephalopelvic disproportion (54%), whereas chances of successful TOLAC are more, if previous CS was done for fetal distress (60%) or malpresentation such as breech (75%).[5] CS done in second stage of labor has low chances of successful TOLAC.

The gestation at which the previous CS was done is important, as TOLAC is less likely to be successful, if previous CS resulted in a preterm birth. At early gestation, lower uterine segment is poorly formed, so lower segment uterine scar may in fact result in a transverse incision in body of uterus.

History of puerperal infection or wound infection, or resuturing in postoperative period is associated with a weak scar. This is found by asking about any history of discharge from the stitch line, postoperative fever, or need for resuturing, the day on which the stitch removal was done, and the number of days of postoperative stay. History of blood transfusion, either pre- or postoperative, is suggestive of either the presence of anemia or excessive blood loss during surgery and likelihood of a weak scar. It is also important to know the type of anesthesia administered to the woman for CS.

If the old records are available, they should be reviewed for any complication or difficulty encountered during CS and the type of uterine incision given, whether it is horizontal, vertical, T or "J" shaped or was there any extension during surgery. The rate of scar rupture by incision type is as given in Table 1.[2]

Box 2: Specific points on obstetric history in a woman with previous cesarean section.

- Parity
- Number of previous vaginal deliveries
- Number of vaginal deliveries after cesarean section (CS)
- Interpregnancy interval or interdelivery interval
- Indication for CS
- Term or preterm CS
- Cervical dilatation at which CS was done
- Type of uterine scar
- Any extension of uterine scar
- Any postoperative infection, puerperal sepsis, or wound infection

Table 1: The rate of scar rupture by incision type.[2]

Type of scar	Risk of scar dehiscence/rupture
Low transverse	0.2–0.9%
Low vertical	1–7%
Prior classical/inverted T or J	2–9%
Multiple low transverse incisions	0.9–1.8%
Prior uterine rupture:	
• Lower segment	2–6%
• Upper segment	9–32%

EXAMINATION

In addition to the routine examination of a pregnant woman with a previous CS, it is important to establish scar integrity.

General Physical Examination

Height, Weight, and Body Mass Index

Shorter women and those with a body mass index (BMI) >30 kg/m² have a lesser likelihood of successful TOLAC.[5,8]

Vitals

The pulse, blood pressure (BP), temperature, and respiratory rate are recorded. Unexplained maternal tachycardia is an early sign of scar dehiscence. It is a trigger for careful abdominal examination to look for scar dehiscence, especially in women with previous CS in labor. Tachycardia with sudden fall in BP may occur following complete scar dehiscence or scar rupture.

Assessment of Pallor

In a woman with previous CS, it is important that anemia is diagnosed and corrected in antenatal period as the likelihood of repeat CS is more in these women. The complications of both surgery and anesthesia are higher in anemic women.

Systemic Examination

Examination of cardiovascular system (CVS) and respiratory system is done as described in Chapter 1 "Approach to Pregnant Woman Attending Antenatal Clinic."

Per Abdomen Examination

The woman is asked to empty her bladder and lie in a supine position with legs straight. On inspection, the contour of the uterus is observed along with the abdominal scar with respect to its position, length, width, any hyperpigmentation, hypertrophy, or keloid formation (Figs. 1 and 2). The scar is observed for whether it has healed by primary or secondary intention (Fig. 3). A puckered scar adherent to underlying structures is suggestive of surgical site infection in the previous surgery with healing of the wound by secondary intention. An abdominal scar, which extends above the umbilicus, is likely to be a classical CS and a pfannenstiel incision scar practically rules out classical CS.

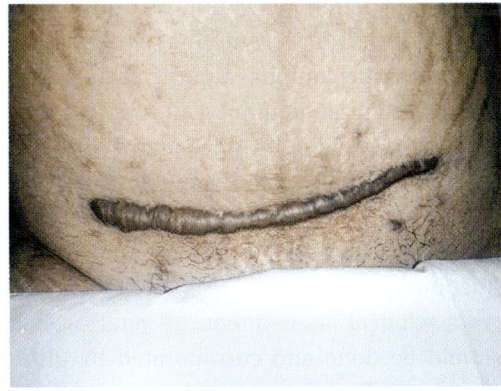

Fig. 1: Hyperpigmented hypertrophic scar.

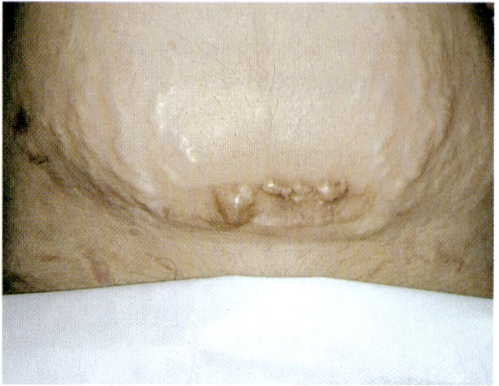

Fig. 2: Scar keloid.

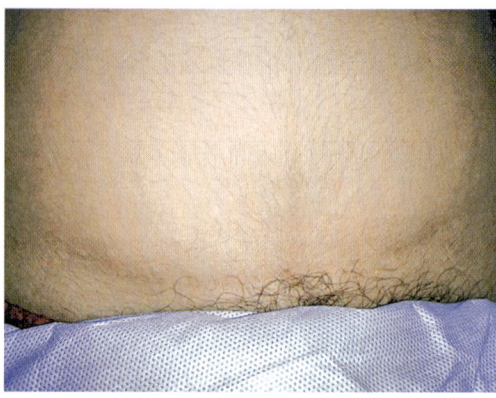

Fig. 3: Normal scar healed by primary intention.

The fundal height and girth are measured. The Leopold's maneuvers are done as described in Chapter No. 1. The uterine scar site is palpated for any scar tenderness in all women with previous CS during abdominal examination. Presence of scar tenderness is an early sign of scar dehiscence. To elicit scar tenderness, the obstetrician palpates the suprapubic area with the flat of fingers along the site of previous uterine scar, irrespective of the abdominal scar. The whole length of the uterine scar is palpated. All this while, the obstetrician keeps the woman engaged in conversation to divert her attention and continue to look at her face for any wincing (Fig. 4).

During labor, scar rupture presents as sudden cessation of uterine contractions, loss of uterine contour, superficially felt fetal parts through abdominal wall, uterus forming a firm swelling on one side of the fetus (complete rupture), and sometimes a bulge is felt on one side of the uterus due to retroperitoneal hematoma in the broad ligament (incomplete rupture).

A clinical assessment of fetal weight should be done and corroborated by ultrasound as fetal macrosomia, i.e., a fetus weighing >4,000 g reduces the likelihood of successful TOLAC. The odds ratio (OR) for successful TOLAC for birth weight >4,000 g is 0.55, 95% CI (0.49–0.61).[5]

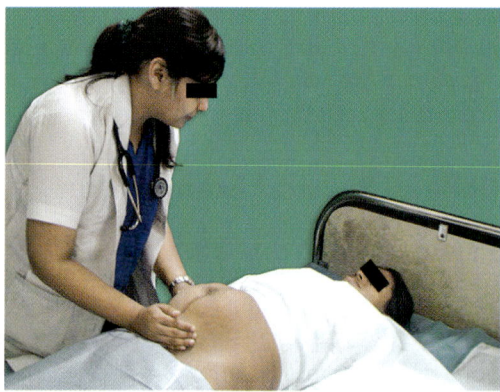

Fig. 4: Eliciting scar tenderness.

Fetal heart is auscultated for any fetal heart rate (FHR) abnormalities; mostly recurrent variable or late decelerations and prolonged bradycardia are suggestive of scar dehiscence.

Pelvic Examination

Per Speculum Examination

Look for any vaginal discharge, leaking, or bleeding. Slight fresh red vaginal bleeding during labor is sign of scar dehiscence.

Per Vaginal Examination

Per vaginal examination is done in the antenatal period near term to assess for the adequacy of the pelvis and decide the options of delivery to be offered to the woman and help her take an informed decision regarding mode of delivery.

In women, who report in early labor, the cervical findings and station of head are assessed in addition to the pelvic assessment. Women in spontaneous labor and those with favorable pelvic findings at admission are more likely to have a successful TOLAC compared to women who are being induced or who have unfavorable pelvic findings. In women in established labor, loss of presenting part from its former position in pelvis is suggestive of scar rupture.

INVESTIGATIONS

Routine antenatal investigations are carried out in pregnant women with previous CS. Hemoglobin (Hb) levels are carefully followed to ensure that the woman has a Hb level of >11 g%. Ultrasound is indicated for ruling out placenta previa accreta and is repeated near term to assess for the fetal weight as fetal macrosomia is associated with higher rates of unsuccessful TOLAC.

All the previous ultrasound reports should be reviewed and the period of gestation confirmed. This is important in women, who are planned for ERCS to prevent iatrogenic prematurity. Imaging techniques have been used to predict women at increased risk of uterine rupture with mixed results. The most common technique is ultrasound measurement of the thickness of the lower uterine segment in the third trimester. Full lower uterine segment thickness is the smallest measurement between the amniotic fluid and urine in the maternal bladder. A value of 2.1–4.0 mm provides a strong negative predictive value for occurrence of scar dehiscence during TOLAC and a value of 0.6–2.0 mm provides a strong positive predictive value for scar dehiscence in TOLAC. However, there is no clinically useful ideal ultrasonic measurement of the lower uterine segment in late pregnancy, i.e., 100% predictive or protective of catastrophic uterine disruption.[9]

Algorithm for approach to a pregnant woman with previous cesarean section is shown in Flowchart 1.

Flowchart 1: Algorithm for clinical approach to a pregnant woman with previous cesarean section (CS).

- Pregnant woman with previous CS
- **History**
  - Age of woman, period of gestation
  - Dating of pregnancy
  - Assessment of scar integrity by detailed obstetric history including parity, number of previous vaginal deliveries, number of vaginal deliveries after CS and interpregnancy interval
  - Reviewing previous operative records as regards indication for CS, i.e. term or preterm CS, cervical dilatation at which CS was done, nature of uterine scar, and any extension of uterine scar, any postoperative infection, and puerperal sepsis or wound infection
- **Examination**
  - Height, weight, body mass index (BMI), and pallor
  - *Per abdomen:* Uterine contour, fetal weight, scar tenderness and for any signs of scar rupture, especially in woman in labor
  - Per vaginum examination
  - Pelvic assessment near term
- **Investigations**
  - Routine investigations, ultrasonography (USG) for confirming the dates, estimation of fetal weight and fetal well-being are carried out
- Decision regarding mode of delivery; trial of labor after cesarean (TOLAC) or elective repeat cesarean section (ERCS)

MANAGEMENT

The management includes an assessment of the pregnant woman with previous CS and a discussion regarding the options for mode of delivery. This should include the advantages and disadvantages of both ERCS and TOLAC and of the emergency CS following failed TOLAC. The complications are maximum after emergency CS for failed TOLAC. The discussion needs to be done and documented in the antenatal records well before the expected date of delivery. ERCS should be planned after 39+0 weeks for optimal neonatal outcome and a plan in the event woman goes into spontaneous labor prior to planned ERCS should be documented. For those planned for TOLAC, an informed consent should be taken.

Table 2 summarizes the morbidities associated with both the options. This can be used for counseling the woman regarding mode of delivery.[10]

The evidence suggests that most women are candidates for TOLAC, except those who are at high risk of rupture (e.g., those who had a prior uterine rupture or a T-shaped incision on the uterus or in those who had extensive transfundal surgery) or those in whom vaginal delivery is otherwise contraindicated. Some studies have proposed a prediction model for success of TOLAC based on factors in history and examination. Maternal-Fetal Medicine Units website provides a free calculator for predicting the success of TOLAC based on the information available on first antenatal visit that includes factors such as maternal age, BMI, race, prior vaginal delivery, history of a VBAC, and indication for prior caesarean delivery.[10]

As regards special situations, Table 3 gives the evidence which can be used for antenatal counseling regarding mode of delivery.

Table 2: Comparison of maternal and neonatal morbidities with ERCD and VBAC.[11]

Risks	ERCD (one CD)	VBAC (previous one CS)
Scar rupture	0.7%	0.02%
Maternal death	4/100,000 (1–16/100,000)	13/100,000 (4–42/100,000)
Risk of transient respiratory morbidity	2–3% 6% if done before 38 weeks instead of 39 weeks	4–5%
Hypoxic ischemic encephalopathy (HIE)	0.01% (1 per 10,000)	0.08% (8 per 10,000)
Perinatal death	Nil	0.04% (4 per 10,000) Comparable to the risk for a nulliparous woman

Table 3: Evidence for TOLAC in special situations.[12]

Condition	Evidence
Previous two cesarean section (CS)	Limited data is available. Studies have reported a scar rupture rate of 0.9–1.9%
Twin gestation	Women with one previous CS with a low transverse incision, who are suitable for twin vaginal delivery, can be offered trial of labor after cesarean (TOLAC).
Induction of labor (IOL)	IOL increases the risk of uterine rupture when compared to spontaneous labor therefore, the risks and benefits of IOL should be considered by the clinician and discussed with the patient. Misoprostol is contraindicated. There are no definite recommendations regarding the use of prostaglandin E_2.

KEY POINTS

- A pregnant woman with previous CS is a high-risk pregnancy.
- The woman needs to be thoroughly evaluated in the antenatal period on history and examination to assess, if she can be offered TOLAC. Review of old records can provide some vital information that can influence the management.
- The benefits of successful TOLAC are derived from avoidance of risks associated with repeat cesarean delivery. Immediate benefits of TOLAC include shorter hospital stay, fewer postpartum complications, quicker return to normal activities, and lower maternal morbidity and mortality. Long-term potential complications that accrue with multiple cesarean deliveries can be avoided.
- The benefits of ERCD are scheduling convenience, ease of sterilization at the time of delivery, and avoidance of the risks associated with failed TOLAC.
- After counseling, the ultimate decision to undergo TOLAC or a repeat cesarean delivery should be made by the patient in consultation with her obstetrician or obstetric care provider.
- The potential risks and benefits of both TOLAC and elective repeat cesarean delivery should be discussed. Documentation of counseling and the management plan should be included in the medical record.
- Because of the risks associated with TOLAC, including uterine rupture and other unpredictable complications, it should be attempted in facilities that can provide cesarean delivery.

REFERENCES

1. Sabol B, Denman MA, Guise JM. Vaginal birth after cesarean: an effective method to reduce cesarean. Clin Obstet Gynecol. 2015;58(2):309-19.
2. Cunningham FG, Leveno KJ, Bloom SL, Corton MM. Williams Obstetrics, 24th edition. New York: Appleton-Century-Crofts; 2014.
3. Wen SW, Huang L, Liston R, Heaman M, Baskett T, Rusen ID, et al. Severe maternal morbidity in Canada, 1991-2001. CMAJ. 2005;173(7):759-64.
4. National Institutes of Health Consensus Development Conference Panel. National Institutes of Health Consensus Development conference statement: vaginal birth after cesarean: new insights, March 8-10, 2010. Obstet Gynecol. 2010;115(6):1279-95.
5. Landon MB, Leindecker S, Spong CY, Hauth JC, Bloom S, Varner MW, et al. The MFMU Cesarean Registry: factors affecting the success of trial of labor after previous cesarean delivery. Am J Obstet Gynecol. 2005;193(3):1016-23.
6. Van der Merwe AM, Thompson JM, Ekeroma AJ. Factors affecting vaginal birth after caesarean section at Middlemore Hospital, Auckland, New Zealand, N Z Med J. 2013; 126(1383):49-57.
7. Stamilio DM, DeFranco E, Paré E, Odibo AO, Peipert JF, Allsworth JE, et al. Short interpregnancy interval: risk of uterine rupture and complications of vaginal birth after cesarean delivery. Obstet Gynecol. 2007;110(5): 1075-82.
8. Hibbard JU, Gilbert S, Landon MB, Hauth JC, Leveno KJ, Spong CY, et al. Trial of labor or repeat cesarean delivery in women with morbid obesity and previous cesarean delivery, Obstet Gynecol. 2006;108(1):125-33.
9. Kok N, Wiersma IC, Opmeer BC, de Graaf IM, Mol BW, Pajkrt E. Sonographic measurement of lower uterine segment thickness to predict uterine rupture during a trial of labor in women with previous Cesarean section: a metaanalysis. Ultrasound Obstet Gynecol. 2013;42(2):132-9.
10. Maternal-Fetal Medicine Units Network. Vaginal birth after cesarean (calculator). [online] Available from https://

mfmunetwork.bsc.gwu.edu/PublicBSC/MFMU/VGBirthCalc/vagbirth.html. [Last accessed March, 2020].

11. Royal College of Obstetricians and Gynaecologists. (2015). Birth after previous caesarean birth (Green-top Guidelines No. 45). [online] Available from https://www.rcog.org.uk/globalassets/documents/guidelines/gtg_45.pdf. [Last accessed March, 2020].

12. National Institute of Child Health and Human Development. Maternal–Fetal Medicine Units (MFMU) Network. N Engl J Med. 2004;351:2581-9.

SUGGESTED READING

1. ACOG Practice Bulletin No. 205. Obstet Gynecol. 2019;133(2):e110-27.
2. The Royal Australian and New Zealand College of Obstetricians and Gynaecologists. (2019). Birth after previous caesarean section. [online] Available from https://ranzcog.edu.au/RANZCOG_SITE/media/RANZCOG-MEDIA/Women%27s%20Health/Statement%20and%20guidelines/Clinical-Obstetrics/Birth-after-previous-Caesarean-Section-(C-Obs-38)Review-March-2019.pdf?ext=.pdf. [Last accessed March, 2020].

22 Approach to a Pregnant Woman with Multiple Pregnancy

Shalini Warman, Neelam Jain

INTRODUCTION

Multiple pregnancy refers to a pregnancy with two or more fetuses. Delayed childbirth and the use of assisted reproductive techniques (ARTs) have increased the incidence of multiple pregnancies. Twins are the most common. Triplets are far less common than twins and higher orders even rarer.

The twins can be monozygotic (30%) or dizygotic (70%). The differences between the monozygotic and dizygotic twins are listed in Table 1. The prevalence of monozygotic twins (3–5/1,000 births) is constant throughout the world but the that of dizygotic twins varies markedly with maternal age, race, and geographical distribution.[1,2]

Multiple pregnancies are associated with a high risk of perinatal morbidity and mortality. Women with multiple pregnancies have an increased risk of miscarriage, preterm labor, hypertensive disorders, anemia, gestational diabetes mellitus (GDM), operative delivery and postpartum hemorrhage (PPH).

Risk to babies depends upon the chorionicity and amnionicity of the pregnancy. Chorionicity refers to placentation and amnionicity to the membranes separating the twins (Table 2). Depending on chorionicity and amnionicity there can be three types of twin pregnancies: (1) dichorionic diamniotic, (2) monochorionic diamniotic, and (3) monochorionic monoamniotic. Monochorionic pregnancies have a higher rate of perinatal loss and handicap compared to dichorionic pregnancies. Monochorionic pregnancies have a shared fetoplacental circulation with presence of vascular anastomoses. These anastomoses are bidirectional in 80% of cases and rarely lead to hemodynamic imbalance between the two fetal circulations. Sometimes there may be unbalanced blood flow in anastomotic vessels along the equatorial plate of the shared placenta leading to an increased risk of fetal death. Twin-to-twin transfusion syndrome (TTTS) and twin reversed arterial perfusion (TRAP) sequence complicate

Table 1: Monozygotic versus dizygotic twins.

	Identical twins (monozygotic)	Fraternal twins (Dizygotic)
Frequency	One-third (30%) of all twin pregnancies	Two-thirds (70%) of all twin pregnancies
Origin	Division of the fertilized oocyte into two	Fertilization of two oocytes with two spermatozoa
Genetics	Genetically identical and have same sex	Genetically different may be of same or different sex
Placenta	May be monochorionic or dichorionic	Always dichorionic separate or fused

Table 2: Monozygotic twins.[4]

Type of twinning	Description	Frequency	Timing of cleavage from fertilization
Diamniotic-dichorionic	Two placentae, two sacs	20–30%	First 3 days
Monochorionic-diamniotic	Single placenta, two sacs	70%	4th–7th day
Monochorionic-monoamniotic	Single placenta, single sac	1–5%	8th–12th day
Conjoined twins	Single placenta, single sac, conjoined	<0.1%	13th day onward

twins sharing a single placenta and account for approximately 20% of all stillbirths in multiple pregnancies.[3] Other complications associated with multiple pregnancies are selective fetal growth restriction (sFGR), cord entanglement, conjoined twins, single fetal demise, and congenital anomalies. Early diagnosis and careful monitoring of multiple pregnancies is important for optimizing the fetomaternal outcomes.

HISTORY

A detailed history should be taken from any patient with multifetal gestation.

Age: Maternal age is an important risk factor, maximum incidence being between 30 and 35 years. This may be related to increasing levels of follicle stimulating hormone with age.

Parity: Parity has a direct relationship with the incidence of multifetal gestation, especially for fifth gravida onwards. It is independent of maternal age. Moreover, older women are more likely to use fertility treatments.

Complaints: All common annoyances of pregnancy are more troublesome in multiple pregnancy. The symptoms of nausea, vomiting is more severe in the first trimester due to an increase in the level of circulating hormones [human chorionic gonadotropin (hCG)] as compared to a singleton pregnancy. Women are more predisposed to hyperemesis gravidarum.

The pressure effects come earlier and are more severe. These include pressure in the pelvis, backache, varicosities, constipation, hemorrhoids, abdominal distension, and cardiorespiratory embarrassment. Due to increased weight of the uterus, there is an early onset of pedal edema and the woman may present with swelling feet.

Multiple pregnancy worsens the medical disorders of pregnancy. A woman with multiple pregnancy is at an increased risk of anemia due to an increase in the requirement of iron and folate. A history of increasing pallor, easy fatiguability, breathlessness, palpitations, and anorexia should be elicited.

The incidence of cholestasis increases from 1% in singleton pregnancies to 21% in multiple pregnancies.[5] The increased incidence is probably due to increased levels of estrogen in multiple pregnancies. Hence a history of itching in palms and soles, worsening at night and not associated with skin lesions should be asked for. It usually starts in the third trimester.

Metabolic disorders such as GDM are common with multiple pregnancy due to an increase in anti-insulin hormones. These patients may give a history of discharge and pruritis per vaginum suggestive of vaginal candidiasis; dysuria and increased frequency of micturition suggestive of urinary tract infection which may be recurrent. The pregnant woman may complain of overdistension of the abdomen due to multiple fetuses or hydramnios associated with GDM or TTTS in monochorionic twin pregnancy.

Multifetal gestation carries a nearly fourfold risk of pre-eclampsia and this is independent of race and parity. It is due to an abundance of chorionic villi. Significant history related to pre-eclampsia such as swelling of feet, facial puffiness, tightening of rings, headache, blurring of vision, epigastric, and upper abdominal pain should be asked. Early onset pre-eclampsia (<20 weeks) can present with multiple pregnancy.

Low lying placenta may occur due to an increase in placental area, therefore any history of bleeding per vaginum should be asked. Bleeding with pain abdomen may be a symptom of placental abruption complicating such pregnancies.

Multigravidas may complain of increased fetal movements compared to their previous singleton pregnancy. Monitoring fetal well-being by keeping a fetal kick count may not be an effective method in multiple pregnancies.

Menstrual history: Presence of irregular delayed cycles with history of infertility may suggest anovulatory infertility and use of ovulation induction drugs. Date of last menstrual period (LMP) is important for calculating the exact gestational age. However, in induced and ART treated cycles, date of intrauterine insemination or embryo transfer should be considered.

Obstetrical history: Duration of active married life that is history of conjugal years after marriage is to be enquired. If there is a history of infertility, the reason of infertility should be asked. Ovulation induction and ovarian stimulation contribute significantly to multiple births. Improvement in ART protocols limiting embryo transfers to only one or two can result in fewer multiple births from ART.

Family history: Enquire about a history of twinning on the maternal or paternal side of the pregnant woman. The association is stronger with maternal family history. A positive family history of the biologic father does not have any effect on his partner's risk of having twins, but the trait may be passed on to the daughter. The propensity for dizygotic or heterozygous twins seems to be driven by genetics as the tendency to release multiple ova is probably inherited. This does not hold true for monozygotic twins.

EXAMINATION

General Physical Examination

A thorough general physical examination should be done with emphasis on the following points:
- Height and weight are recorded at the first registration visit. Taller and heavier women have a higher incidence of twinning than short and malnourished ones.
- Pallor is noted in lower palpebral conjunctiva and the other mucosal surfaces as anemia complicates most of these pregnancies. Blood pressure is recorded at each visit for early diagnosis of pre-eclampsia. The respiratory rate may be increased if the abdomen is overdistended causing cardiorespiratory embarrassment. Pedal edema may be present due to compression of the iliac veins by the large gravid uterus. It may also be a feature of pre-eclampsia or hypoproteinemia.

Systemic Examination

Done in the usual way as described in Chapter 1.

Per Abdominal Examination

Inspection

There is overdistension of the abdomen due to excessive enlargement of the uterus. The overlying skin is stretched and umbilicus is everted.

Palpation

Fundal height is more than the period of gestation. Other causes of fundal height more than the period of gestation should be ruled out (Box 1). Leopold's grips are done as described in Chapter 1. Multiple fetal parts are palpable. Palpation of at least three fetal poles that is, two cephalic poles and one podalic pole confirms twin gestation. The presentation of the lower or presenting twin decides the mode of delivery. There may be difficulty in feeling fetal parts if hydramnios is present. Serial assessment of fundal height is not useful in monitoring fetal growth in multiple pregnancy, serial biometry by ultrasound is indicated.

Auscultation

Two distinct fetal hearts can be auscultated simultaneously. These are not synchronous with each other and with the maternal pulse and there is a variation of at least 10 beats/min. The distance between the two heart sounds should be measured and is approximately 10 cm. *Arnaux sign* is the occasional superimposition of two heart sounds which produces a galloping rhythm.[6]

INVESTIGATIONS

Routine antenatal (ANC) investigations include hemoglobin, blood group and Rh typing, urine routine and culture sensitivity, oral glucose tolerance test (OGTT), human immunodeficiency virus (HIV), hepatitis B surface antigen (HBsAg), venereal disease research laboratory test (VDRL), and thyroid stimulating hormone (TSH). For details refer to Chapter 1.

The other biochemical investigations are advised depending on the coexisting medical conditions such as pre-eclampsia, GDM, and intrahepatic cholestasis of pregnancy. The hemoglobin, OGTT, and urine examination are repeated at 28 weeks of gestation.

Screening for Aneuploidy

First Trimester Serum Screening

A combined screening that is a combination of biochemical markers β-hCG and pregnancy-associated plasma protein A (PAPP-A) and ultrasonic marker nuchal translucency (NT) is recommended between 11 and 13^{+6} weeks of pregnancy in multiple pregnancy to provide a fetus specific risk of Down syndrome. Biochemical markers alone are not reliable as both fetuses contribute to these and the values are double than that with singleton pregnancy. Moreover, an early pregnancy loss of one fetus may affect the levels and interpretation. NT is more reliable but false positive rates are common with monochorionic pregnancies as it is an early marker for development of TTTS. NT is also

---

Box 1: Causes of fundal height more than period of gestation.

- Multiple fetuses
- Distended bladder
- Wrong date of last periods
- Excessive liquor
- Hydatidiform mole
- Uterine fibroids and other uterine masses
- Adnexal mass
- Fetal macrosomia

raised in other aneuploidies and congenital malformations.

Second Trimester Serum Screening

Maternal free β-hCG, unconjugated estriol, inhibin-A, and α-feto protein (AFP) are measured in quadruple test. In multiple pregnancy it is not reliable as it has a high false positive rate of 10%.[7] This method of screening in multiple pregnancies is used only if first trimester screening is not done and is more sensitive than screening by maternal age alone. No biochemical tests should be done in cases of spontaneous fetal death, selective fetal reduction, and vanishing twins.

In a monozygotic pregnancy the risk of Down syndrome is same for both the fetuses whereas in a dizygotic pregnancy risk of one affected fetus is assumed to be twice that of an age-matched woman with singleton pregnancy, e.g., at the maternal age of 40 years, compared to a risk of 1/85 (0.01) in a singleton pregnancy the risk is 1/85 × 2 (0.023) at delivery for one affected fetus whereas the risk of both affected fetuses will be 1/85 × 1/85 (0.0006).[8]

Risk of trisomy 21 in monochorionic twins is calculated per pregnancy based on average risk of the both fetuses (as the fetuses have the same karyotype). In dichorionic twins, the risk is calculated per fetus as 90% have different karyotype.

Noninvasive prenatal testing (NIPT) is a reliable screening test based on sequencing of fetal cell free DNA for Down syndrome screening.

Ultrasonography

Ultrasound is the most important tool for diagnosis, follow-up, and to identify and monitor the risk of adverse outcomes. Ultrasound should be done frequently for all pregnant women carrying multiple fetuses. We should see for the following during a scan in the pregnant women.

Dating of Pregnancy

Ideal dating done between 11+0 and 13+6 weeks when crown rump length (CRL) is between 45 and 84 mm (Fig. 1). In cases where there is a disparity in the CRL of fetuses, consider the largest CRL for calculation of gestational age as the other fetus/es may be growth restricted. After 14 weeks, we should consider the larger head circumference for gestational age calculation.

Nuchal Translucency

It refers to an ultrasonographic sonolucency in the posterior aspect of fetal neck (Fig. 2). It depends on gestational age and increases 15-20% per week. It is also done at the CRL measurements of 45-84 mm. Down syndrome detection rate with NT is same as for singletons and we should offer it to all patients with multiple pregnancy. In monochorionic twins each fetus has the same risk of being affected with Down syndrome. Whereas in dichorionic twins it is considered separately and has an independent risk.

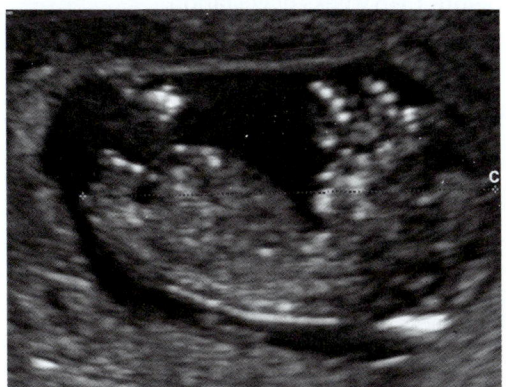

Fig. 1: Crown rump length (CRL) measurement.

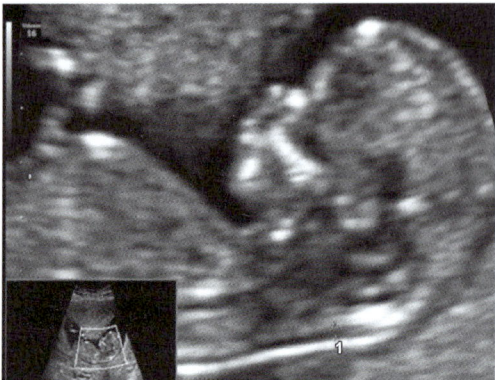

Fig. 2: Nuchal translucency.

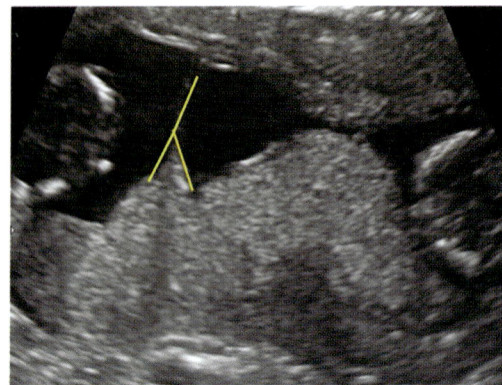

Fig. 3: Lambda sign.

Thus, chorionicity has a major impact on the interpretation of NT results. In multifetal pregnancy screening with NT and maternal age is an acceptable option.

Determining Chorionicity and Amnionicity

Determination of chorionicity is the most important part of management of twin pregnancy as monochorionic pregnancies are at a much higher risk than dichorionic pregnancies. Management of twin pregnancy depends upon the chorionicity and not zygosity. An ultrasound to determine chorionicity should be offered to all women before 13+6 weeks of gestation.

The earliest time to determine is 6–8 weeks however it is the most accurate between 10 and 13 weeks of gestation. It depends upon the presence of λ (lambda) or T sign at the site of insertion of the amniotic membrane into the placenta. Presence of a λ sign or twin peak sign (Figs. 3 and 4) evident by presence of a small portion of placental tissue in-between the two amniotic sacs is diagnostic of dichorionic pregnancy. There is a thick layer of fused chorionic membranes with two thin amniotic layers, one on each side, which separates the two

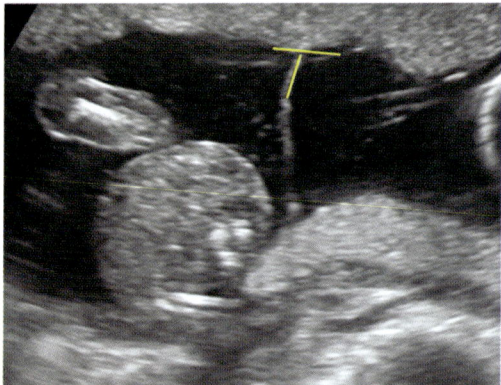

Fig. 4: T sign.

fetuses. Diagnosis of a dichorionic diamniotic (DADC) pregnancy is also made by two separate placentae. However, presence of a T sign with papery thin separating membrane is diagnostic of monochorionic diamniotic pregnancy (MCDA).

After 14 weeks, discordant fetal sex also points toward dizygotic twins. Cord entanglement on using pulsed-wave Doppler USG is suggestive of monoamniotic twins.

Labeling of Twins Fetus

The twins are labeled as right or left, upper or lower to follow the growth of each fetus on subsequent scans (Fig. 5).

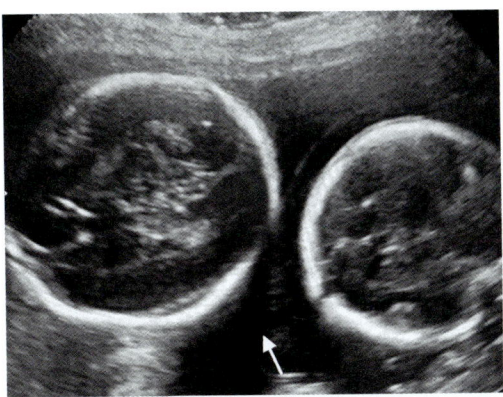

Fig. 5: Twins both cephalic (right and left).

Anomaly Scan (Targeted Imaging Fetal Anomalies—TIFFA)

The risk of congenital malformations is three- to fivefold higher in monozygotic twins as compared to dizygotic twins or singleton pregnancies. An anatomic survey for fetal anomalies is indicated for all patients between 18 and 20 weeks and an echocardiography to rule out congenital heart disease (CHD) at 18–22 weeks in all monochorionic twins. CHD is diagnosed in 5–7.5% of at least one twin on routine echocardiography in monochorionic pregnancies.[9]

In monochorionic twins, middle cerebral artery-peak systolic velocity (MCA-PSV) should be recorded from 20 weeks to screen for TRAP sequence (Figs. 6A to C).

Monitoring of Fetal Growth and Discordant Growth

In uncomplicated dichorionic twins growth scan is advised every 4 weeks after a detailed anomaly scan at 18–20 weeks. In complicated dichorionic twins scan can be offered more frequently.

In uncomplicated monochorionic twins growth scan is advised every 2 weeks from 16 weeks till 24 weeks for early diagnosis of TTTS and then every 2–3 weeks for diagnosis of sFGR and TTTS. For complicated monochorionic twins, scanning should be done more frequently.

For screening of TTTS, serial assessment of maximum vertical pocket of amniotic fluid in both sacs, presence and size of fetal bladders, Doppler measurement of MCA-PSV, Doppler measurement of umbilical artery (UA) end-diastolic flow velocity and placental discordant echogenicity should be done every 2 weeks for an early diagnosis. Presumptive diagnosis of TTTS is made when there is oligohydramnios MVP < 2 cm in one sac and polyhydramnios > 8 cm in other sac in a monochorionic twin pregnancy. As the condition progresses the bladder of the donor twin is not visible followed by abnormal Doppler flow studies on umbilical artery in either twin. Finally, one or both twins may become hydropic and finally die. Table 3 describes the various stages of TTTS Quintero classification.

Growth abnormalities can manifest as selective growth restriction when one twin is smaller (sFGR) or there can be a discordance in the sizes of twins of ≥20% difference in estimated weights with none being small for gestational age or both twins may be small for gestational age. Selective growth restriction may be due to some chromosomal anomaly, genetic syndrome, congenital anomaly, and placental abnormality.

MANAGEMENT

Principles of Management

- Management of twin pregnancy must be by a multidisciplinary team comprising an obstetrician, a fetal medicine specialist, and a pediatrician.
- Women with multiple pregnancy of higher order than twins should be counseled

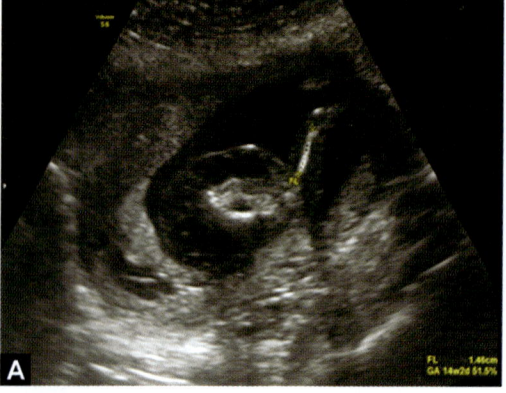
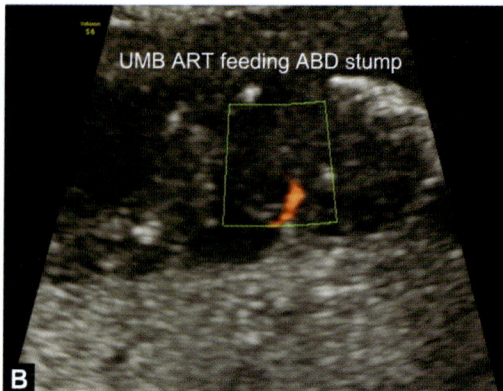
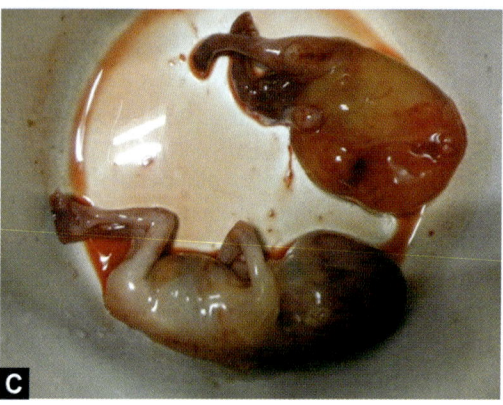

Figs. 6A to C: Acardiac twinning twin reversed arterial perfusion (TRAP). (A) Acardiac twin with femur bone; (B) Doppler showing umbilical artery feeding abdominal stump; and (C) Abortus showing an acardiac twin.

Table 3: Stages of twin-to-twin transfusion syndrome (TTTS) (Quintero classification).[10]	
Stage	Ultrasonic features
I	• Oligohydramnios and polyhydramnios • Bladder of both fetuses' present • Normal Doppler flow studies (UA, UV, DV)
II	• Oligohydramnios and polyhydramnios • Bladder of donor fetus absent • Normal Doppler flow studies (UA, UV, DV)
III	• Oligohydramnios and polyhydramnios • Bladder of donor fetus absent • Abnormal Doppler flow studies (UA, UV, DV) • *One of the following*: absent or reversed end-diastolic velocity in the UA, reversed flow in a-wave of the DV, or pulsatile flow in the UV
IV	• Oligohydramnios and polyhydramnios • One or both fetuses' hydropic
V	One or both fetuses' dead

and offered fetal reduction preferably after aneuploidy screening to optimize the outcome of pregnancy.

- Determination of chorionicity is the most important step in the management of twin pregnancy and should be advised in the first trimester.
- Aneuploidy screening should be offered by either NT or a combined test between 11 and 13 + 6 weeks gestation.
- Frequency of antenatal visits in a dichorionic pregnancy is every 4 weeks from 20 weeks with serial ultrasounds for monitoring growth of the fetuses. Whereas in monochorionic pregnancies it is every 2 weeks from 16 weeks to 24 weeks for early detection of TTTS and then every 2–3 weeks for any discordant growth.

- Women are carefully screened for anemia, pre-eclampsia, GDM, and intrahepatic cholestasis of pregnancy during antenatal period.
- Early diagnosis of complications and timely referral to appropriate center should be done.
- The delivery is planned at 37–38 weeks in uncomplicated dichorionic twins, 36–37 weeks in uncomplicated monochorionic twins, and 32–34 weeks in monoamniotic monochorionic twins.
- Preferred mode of delivery depends upon the presenting twin. It is vaginal if the presenting twin is cephalic. Cesarean section is recommended for monoamniotic monochorionic twins. Preparedness for management of PPH is important as it is a common complication with multiple pregnancy.

KEY POINTS

- Incidence of multiple pregnancy is on the rise mainly due to women delaying pregnancy and increase in use of ovulation induction agents and ART procedures.
- Multiple pregnancy is a high-risk pregnancy.
- There is an increase in maternal risk due to a higher incidence of anemia, hypertensive disorders, gestational diabetes, cesarean delivery and PPH.
- Premature births, low birth weight, small for gestational age, congenital malformations, TTTS, and TRAP add to the higher incidence of neonatal morbidity and mortality in such pregnancies.
- Dichorionic pregnancies have a lower perinatal risk compared to the monochorionic ones.
- Women with multiple pregnancy need to have more frequent antenatal check-ups compared to singleton pregnancy and carefully screened for maternal complications.
- Early determination of chorionicity in the first trimester is paramount for the antenatal care of multiple pregnancies because of the inherent and treatable risks associated with monochorionic twins.
- When screening is done by NT and maternal age, a pregnancy-specific risk should be calculated in monochorionic twins. In dichorionic twins, a fetus-specific risk should be calculated.
- With apparently high positive predictive value and low false positive rate, NIPT has the potential to be used as a good test for screening in these pregnancies.
- Serial ultrasounds with Doppler are recommended in these pregnancies for early detection of complications such as TTTS and discordant growth for timely management.
- A collaboration between a neonatologist and an obstetrician is important to manage the pregnancies as majority of them would require preterm terminations.
- The risk of maternal morbidity and perinatal morbidity and mortality increase with the presence of each additional fetus therefore, selective reduction offers a cure to reduce the number of fetuses to a safe number.

REFERENCES

1. Iyiola OA, Oyeyemi FB, Raheem UA, Mark FO. Frequency of twining in Kwara State, North-Central Nigeria. Egyptian J Med Hum Genet. 2013;14(1):23-5.
2. Akinboro A, Azeez MA, Bakare AA. Frequency of twinning in southwest Nigeria. Indian J Hum Genet. 2008;14(2):41-7.
3. American College of Obstetricians and Gynecologists; Society for Maternal-Fetal

Medicine. ACOG Practice Bulleitin No. 144: Mulifetal gestations: twin, triplet, and higher-order multifetal pregnancies. Obstet Gynecol. 2014;123(5):1118-32.
4. Mark C. (2005-11-02). "Twinning". Focus Information Technology. Retrieved 2008-10-10.
5. Gonzalez MC, Reyes H, Arrese M, Figueroa D, Lorca B, Andresen M, et al. Intrahepatic cholestasis in twin pregnancies. J Hepatol. 1989;9:84-90.
6. GFMER (Geneva Foundation for Medical Education and Research). Obstetrics Simplified, Diaa M. El-Mowafi, Multiple Pregnancy.
7. Garchet-Beaudron A, Dreux S, Leporrier N, Oury JF, Muller F; ABA Study Group, et al. Second-trimester Down syndrome maternal serum marker screening: a prospective study of 11040 twin pregnancies. Prenat Diagn. 2008;28:1105-9.
8. Boyle B, Morris JK, McConkey R, Garne E, Loane M, Addor MC, et al. Prevalence and risk of Down syndrome in monozygotic and dizygotic multiple pregnancies in Europe: implications for prenatal screening. BJOG. 2014;121(7):809-20.
9. Best KE, Rankin J. Increased risk of congenital heart disease in twins in the North of England between 1998 and 2010. Heart. 2015;101:1807-12.
10. Quintero RA, Dickinson JE, Morales WJ, Bornick PW, Bermúdez C, Cincotta R, et al. Stage-based treatment of twin-twin transfusion syndrome. Am J Obstet Gynecol. 2003;188:1333-40.

SUGGESTED READING

1. ACOG: Committee Opinion No. 719 multifetal pregnancy reduction. Obstet Gynecol. 2017;130(3):670-1.
2. American College of Obstetricians and Gynecologists (ACOG). (2016, reaffirmed 2019). Practice bulletin on multifetal gestations—Twin, triplet, and higher-order multifetal pregnancies. [online] Available from https://www.acog.org/clinical/clinical-guidance/practice-bulletin/articles/2016/10/twin-triplet-and-higher-order-multifetal-pregnancies [Last accessed March, 2020].
3. Chitayat D, Langlois S, Douglas Wilson R. Society of Obstetricians and Gynaecologists of Canada (SOGC): Prenatal screening for and diagnosis of aneuploidy in twin pregnancies. J Obstet Gynaecol Can. 2017;39(9):e380-e394.
4. National Institute for Health and Care Excellence (NICE). (2019). Guideline on twin and triplet pregnancy [online] Available from https://www.nice.org.uk/guidance/ng137/documents/draft-guideline [Last accessed March, 2020].
5. RCOG. (2016). Green-top guideline for the management of monochorionic twin pregnancy. [online] Available from https://www.rcog.org.uk/en/guidelines-research-services/guidelines/gtg51/ [Last accessed March, 2020].
6. Royal Australian and New Zealand College of Obstetricians and Gynaecologists (RANZCOG). (2017). Management of monochorionic twin pregnancy. [online] Available from https://ranzcog.edu.au/RANZCOG_SITE/media/RANZCOG-MEDIA/Women%27s%20Health/Statement%20and%20guidelines/Clinical-Obstetrics/Management-of-Monochorionic-Twins-(C-Obs-42)-review-July-2017.pdf?ext=.pdf [Last accessed March, 2020].
7. SOGC. (2017). Ultrasound in twin pregnancies (reaffirmed 2017) No. 260-Ultrasound in Twin Pregnancies. [online] Available from https://www.jogc.com/article/S1701-2163(17)30823-X/pdf [Last accessed March, 2020].

23 Approach to a Pregnant Woman Presenting with Rh-negative Pregnancy

Sumita Agarwal

INTRODUCTION

Rhesus (Rh) alloimmunization leading to hemolytic disease of fetus and newborn (HDFN) or hydrops fetalis was once a major contributor to perinatal morbidity and mortality. The introduction of Rh-immune globulin has substantially reduced the incidence of this disease. Proper and timely management can result in a favorable outcome in >90% of cases.

The Rh blood group system consists of five antigens (C, c, D, E, and e) present on the surface of red cell membrane. These antigens are coded by two genes which are located on the short arm of chromosome 1. There is no evidence of an isoform for the major antigen D, so the notation "d" is used to indicate an absence of the D antigen. The D antigen is the most potent among various Rh antigens expressed early in gestation and hence clinically most important. The presence or absence of D antigen determines whether an individual is Rh-positive or negative. The Rh genotype of an individual may be either homozygous or heterozygous for each antigen inheriting one set from each parent. Rh-negative individuals are homozygous for complete absence of RhD antigen. The genotype of the male partner is important. If a Rh-negative woman has a homozygous Rh-positive partner, then all their offspring will be Rh-positive but if he is heterozygous Rh-positive, only 50% of their children will be Rh-positive.

The incidence of Rh negativity has racial and ethnic variations. It is primarily a Caucasian trait. Its incidence is around 15% in whites, 35% in Basques, 4–8% in blacks, and 1% in Asians.[1]

Almost three fourths of women have evidence of fetal transplacental hemorrhage (TPH) at some time during pregnancy or at delivery, the size of which is usually small, around 5 mL in 1% and 30 mL or more in 0.25%. The various sensitizing events are mentioned in Box 1.

> **Box 1:** Sensitizing events.
>
> - *Pregnancy related (fetomaternal transplacental bleed):*
>   - *Delivery*: Vaginal and cesarean section
>   - Miscarriage (threatened, incomplete)
>   - Medical termination of pregnancy (MTP)
>   - Ectopic pregnancy
>   - Partial molar pregnancy
>   - *Antepartum hemorrhage*: Abruption
>   - Maternal blunt abdominal trauma
>   - Intrauterine death
>   - *Procedures*: External cephalic version and manual removal of placenta
>   - *Prenatal invasive diagnostic procedures*: CVS, amniocentesis, cordocentesis, and fetoscopy
> - *Pregnancy unrelated*: Transfusion of Rh-positive blood or platelets

(CVS: chorionic villus sampling; Rh: rhesus)

Table 1: Differential diagnosis.

Disease/condition	Differentiating features
Nonimmune fetal hydrops	• Maternal serum anti-D antibodies are negative • Features such as FGR, placental calcifications, and oligohydramnios may be present • Chromosomal abnormalities may be present
Congenital infections such as parvovirus	• Virus-specific IgM antibodies may be present • Amniotic fluid PCR is diagnostic for fetal affliction
Non RhD hemolytic disease, e.g., Kell alloimmunization	• Usually transfusion related • Prior obstetric history does not reliably predict occurrence in subsequent pregnancy • Maternal antibody titer does not correlate with severity
Placental chorioangioma	• Large masses >5 cm may lead to fetal anemia, hydrops, polyhydramnios, and poor perinatal outcome • Can be detected by USG and color Doppler • Maternal serum alpha-fetoprotein levels may be raised
Twin–twin transfusion syndrome	• Develops in monochorionic twin pregnancies • USG finding progresses from poly-oligo sequence to discordant growth to Doppler changes and finally hydrops and death
Thalassemia and autoimmune hemolytic anemia	• HPLC • DNA testing • Detection of specific antibodies helps in diagnosis

(DNA: deoxyribonucleic acid; FGR: fetal growth restriction; HPLC: high-performance liquid chromatography; PCR: polymerase chain reaction; Rh: Rhesus; USG: ultrasonography)

DIFFERENTIAL DIAGNOSIS

Other conditions to be suspected in case of HDFN or a hydropic fetus are summarized in Table 1.

HISTORY

The important points to be noted in the history of a woman with Rh-negative pregnancy with a Rh-positive partner include any bleeding per vaginum, abdominal trauma, invasive procedures such as amniocentesis, chorionic villus sampling, or cordocentesis in current pregnancy. All these events are associated with an increased risk of fetomaternal hemorrhage (FMH). Per vaginal bleeding with pain abdomen is suggestive of placental abruption and an increased risk of FMH.

Any history of anti-D prophylaxis in pregnancy is recorded. Antepartum prophylaxis is indicated to cover any of the sensitizing events during pregnancy and prophylactically at 28 weeks of gestation. Any history of blood transfusion in the past should be elicited.

Obstetrical History

Previous obstetric history must be recorded in detail for each of the previous pregnancies, irrespective of the outcome for the following:
- Any sensitizing event in the past pregnancies (see Box 1)
- Any antenatal or postnatal anti-D prophylaxis received in each pregnancy
- Whether there is any history suggestive of birth of an afflicted baby.

This is evident if a previous baby developed jaundice within 24 hours of birth, needed phototherapy or exchange transfusion, or was born hydropic. In women with previous alloimmunized pregnancy, it is important to know if any intrauterine transfusions (IUTs) were needed and at what period of gestation. This is important because if previous baby was affected, then the severity of the affliction in subsequent pregnancy is likely to be more severe and at an earlier gestational age. If a woman has previously had a hydropic baby, there is an almost 90% chance

Chapter 23: Approach to a Pregnant Woman Presenting with Rh-negative Pregnancy

of the fetus being hydropic in the subsequent pregnancy if it is Rh-positive.

All previous records should be reviewed.

EXAMINATION

Detailed general physical and systemic examination should be carried out (Refer to Chapter 1). Per abdominal examination is done to determine the presentation of the fetus, growth, and assessment of liquor and per vaginal examination is done when indicated. Development of hypertension, features of polyhydramnios (overdistended abdomen, fundal height more than the period of gestation, tense abdomen with shiny skin, fetal parts not easily felt, and fetal heart sound not heard easily) may indicate development of hydrops fetalis.

INVESTIGATIONS

Routine antenatal investigations must be done. Specific investigations related to Rh disease are as mentioned in Table 2.

Table 2: Specific investigations.

Indirect Coombs test	If positive, a titer should be obtained. A "critical titer" is one at which there is significant risk of fetal hydrops. It is typically between 1:8 and 1:32 dilutions, which varies in different laboratories.[2] Most labs consider 1:16 as the critical titer.
Anti-D antibody levels	Levels between 4 and 15 IU/mL correlate with a moderate risk of developing hemolysis whereas levels >15 IU/mL are associated with severe HDFN and mandate intervention
Ultrasound	• Features of hydrops such as ascites, pleural effusion, pericardial effusion, scalp edema, cardiomegaly, placentomegaly, and polyhydramnios may be present • Doppler studies for measurement of middle cerebral artery peak systolic velocity (MCA PSV) help in predicting fetal anemia and can be started as early as 18 weeks of gestation
Tests to quantify fetomaternal hemorrhage (FMH)	• *Kleihauer–Betke acid elution test*: Smear prepared from maternal blood is treated with citric acid phosphate buffer which elutes adult hemoglobin causing maternal RBCs to appear colorless or ghost-like whereas fetal RBCs retain their pink color as fetal hemoglobin is acid resistant. The smear is fixed and stained. The number of mean RBC count per high power field (HPF) is calculated. Next fetal RBCs in 30 HPF are estimated and their percentage is calculated. The percentage is expressed as decimal, e.g., 1% = 0.01. Volume of fetal blood is calculated by the formula (decimal fraction of fetal cells × maternal blood volume assumed as 5,000 mL). Fetal cell count of 1% is equivalent to $0.01 \times 5,000 = 50$ mL fetal blood • Other tests for estimating FMH are Rosette test and flow cytometry
Cell-free fetal DNA in maternal plasma	Noninvasive technique to assess fetal RhD status
Invasive tests	• Amniocentesis to assess degree of fetal anemia indirectly by using Liley's charts for determining bilirubin levels in the amniotic fluid reflected by change in optical density at 450 nm wavelength (ΔOD450) by spectrophotometric analysis is no longer preferred due to availability of noninvasive Doppler USG • Cordocentesis for fetal blood sampling to assess the degree of anemia and to perform intrauterine blood transfusion

(HDFN: hemolytic disease of fetus and newborn; USG: ultrasonography; DNA: deoxyribonucleic acid)

MANAGEMENT

Management of a Rh-negative mother depends upon whether the pregnancy is Rh nonimmunized or Rh-isoimmunized pregnancy (Flowchart 1).

Management of a Rh-negative Nonimmunized Pregnancy

The main goal of management in a nonimmunized Rh-negative mother is to prevent isoimmunization by administration of prophylactic Rh-immune globulin to cover for spontaneous FMH and additional sensitizing events.

In the absence of any prophylaxis, it is estimated that around 1% of Rh-negative women will develop antibodies by the end of first Rh-positive pregnancy. Additional 7–9% would become sensitized at the time of delivery and another 7–9% would develop antibodies within 6 months postpartum. So, by the end of second pregnancy almost 17% Rh-negative mothers would become sensitized. The risk of alloimmunization is only 2% if postnatal prophylaxis is given and around 0.02% if both antenatal and postnatal prophylaxes are administered.[3,4]

A routine antenatal anti-D prophylaxis is recommended at 28 weeks (dose of 300 µg deep intramuscular in deltoid muscle) which is to be repeated after delivery within 72 hours (can be given up to 4 weeks) if the baby's blood group is positive and the direct Coombs test (DCT) is negative. 1 µg is equal to 5 IU of anti-D. It should also be given after every sensitizing event before delivery, after miscarriage, and after any invasive antenatal procedure. A dose of 300 µg neutralizes FMH of 15 mL fetal red cells or 30 mL fetal whole blood. Half-life of anti-D is around 21–30 days and it provides protection for 12 weeks. Indirect Coombs test (ICT) may become positive after anti-D but titers do not exceed 1:4.

Various guidelines recommend a dose of 50–150 µg for events <12 weeks (threatened miscarriage, induced miscarriage, ectopic pregnancy, partial molar pregnancy, and chorionic villus sampling). After 12 weeks, a full dose of 300 µg is recommended. Events such as second-trimester miscarriage, amniocentesis, cordocentesis, antepartum hemorrhage, external cephalic version, retained placenta, and blunt trauma over abdomen require a dose of 300 µg. In cases where excessive FMH is suspected, Kleihauer–Betke test should be done to assess the amount of fetal bleed and additional dose of anti-D is given. Additional 10 µg of anti-D should be given for every additional 0.5 mL of fetal RBCs in maternal circulation.

First-trimester spontaneous complete miscarriage without any instrumentation does not require anti-D. Complete mole does not require anti-D as RBCs are not formed. Threatened miscarriage with persistent bleeding may require anti-D every 6 weeks.

During labor stripping of membranes, oxytocin for induction should be avoided. Cord should not be clamped from the maternal side. Placenta should be allowed to deliver spontaneously and manual removal should be avoided. Vaginal and perineal wounds and lacerations should be protected from being exposed to fetal blood spilled from cord. During cesarean section, abdominal packs should be used before opening the lower segment to prevent blood spilled from placenta to enter the peritoneal cavity.

At birth, cord blood sample should be obtained for baby blood group, DCT, hemoglobin (Hb), hematocrit (Hct), and bilirubin levels. Postnatal anti-D prophylaxis given as discussed previously.

Chapter 23: Approach to a Pregnant Woman Presenting with Rh-negative Pregnancy

Flowchart 1: Approach to management of Rh-negative pregnancy.

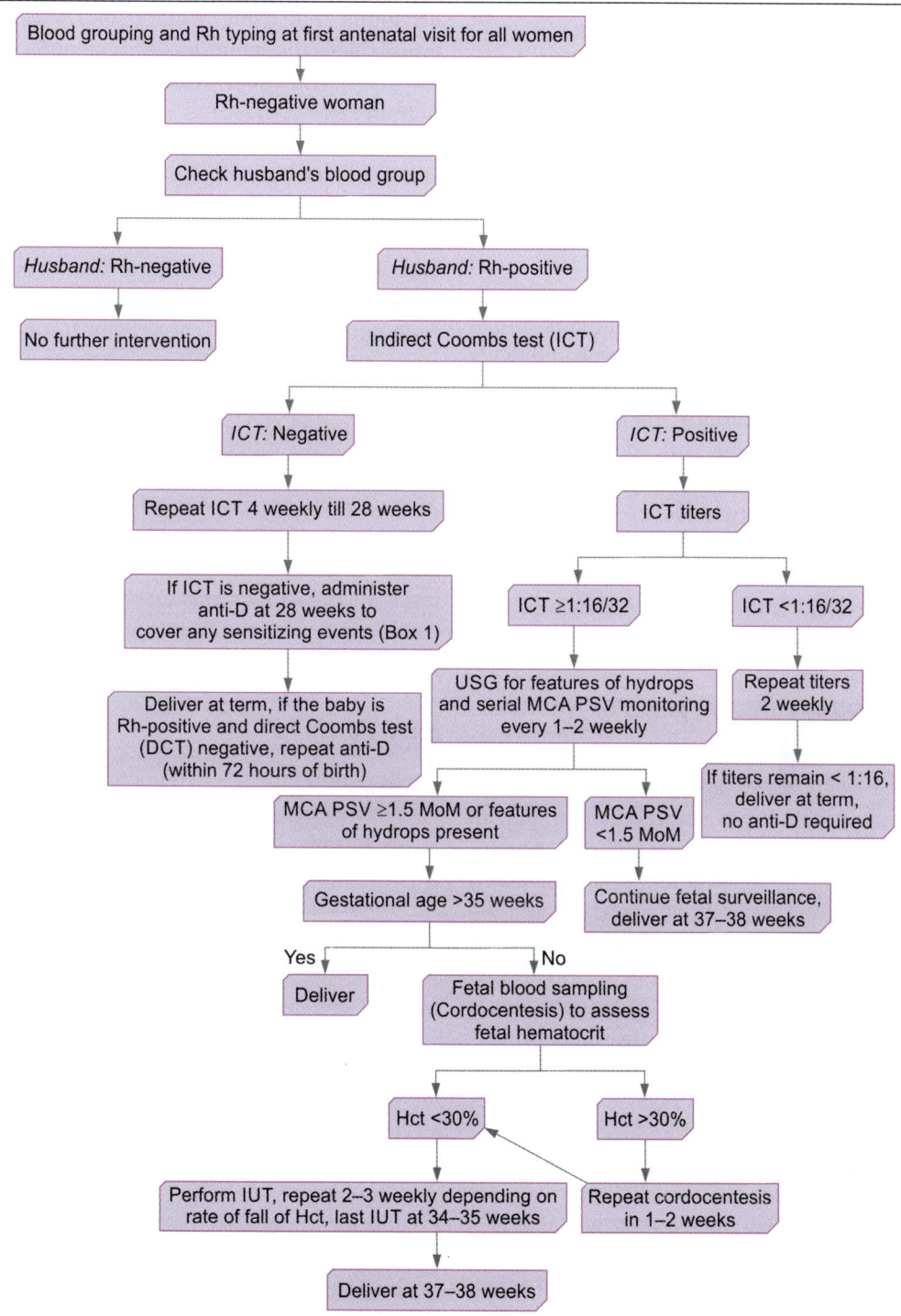

(Hct: hematocrit; IUT: intrauterine transfusion; MCA PSV: middle cerebral artery peak systolic velocity; MoM: multiples of median; Rh: rhesus; USG: ultrasonography)

Management of Rh-negative Isoimmunized Pregnancy

The goal of management is early detection of fetal anemia and therapeutic intervention in the form of IUT to prevent development of fetal hydrops.

First Affected Pregnancy

Once sensitization is detected by a positive ICT, it is repeated in dilutions and if below the critical levels, it is repeated every 2 weeks. The pregnancy can be carried to term. When the critical titer is reached, a detailed ultrasound with middle cerebral artery peak systolic velocity (MCA PSV) is done to look for any evidence of fetal anemia and hydrops and repeated every 1–2 weeks. Delivery should be planned at approximately 38–39 weeks if there is no evidence of fetal anemia.

Previously Affected Fetus or Neonate

These patients should be managed at a perinatal center with adequate experience in the management of severely isoimmunized pregnancies. Zygosity of paternal phenotype should be determined if possible and if heterozygous, fetal RhD status should be determined from the cell-free fetal DNA circulating in maternal plasma or amniocentesis performed at 15 weeks' gestation to determine the fetal genotype. Further monitoring is required only if the fetus is Rh-positive.

More commonly, however, serial MCA Doppler measurements are used to monitor pregnancies for development of fetal anemia. Testing is initiated at 18 weeks and repeated every 1–2 weekly. Once the MCA PSV is >1.5 MoM (multiples of median), fetal blood sampling is performed with availability of blood for IUT and if the Hct is found to be <30%, then IUT is done. A meta-analysis of 12 studies found that using a cutoff of 1.5 MoM, fetuses with moderate-to-severe anemia are identified with a sensitivity of 86% and specificity of 71%.[5]

Intrauterine transfusion is the cornerstone of management of severely anemic fetuses of Rh-isoimmunized mothers. The routes of IUT can be intraperitoneal, intravascular, combined, or intracardiac. Freshly collected adult blood of O-Rh-negative group from which white cell component has been removed and which has been packed to Hct of 80–85% and sterilized by double irradiation and tested for hepatitis B and C, HIV and cytomegalovirus is used.

Management of neonate: After delivery of the baby, cord blood samples are obtained for blood group, DCT, Hb, Hct, and bilirubin levels. Baby may require exchange transfusion if either Hct <30% or bilirubin >5 g/dL or both. Additional phototherapy may be required.

KEY POINTS

- Rh-isoimmunization is not uncommon in our country.
- Maternal Rh-isoimmunization occurs when immune system of Rh-negative mother is exposed to Rh-positive RBCs during pregnancy, delivery or blood transfusion.
- Administration of anti-D antenatally and postnatally can prevent alloimmunization effectively and should be used in appropriate dosages after all sensitizing events.
- Diagnosis of isoimmunization is based on detection of anti-D antibody in maternal circulation.
- It is recommended that Rh typing should be offered to all pregnant women at their booking visit. If negative, her partner's Rh typing is done. If he is positive, maternal

anti-D testing is done and repeated at 28 weeks and near term.
- Rh-isoimmunized pregnancies can be monitored with titers of anti-D initially and once the critical titer is crossed (usually 1:16–32), further monitoring is done with serial ultrasound for MCA PSV every 1–2 weeks.
- IUT is considered when MCA PSV is >1.5 MoM. Repeated IUT can assure excellent outcomes in both hydropic and nonhydropic babies.

REFERENCES

1. Zipursky A, Paul VK. The global burden of Rh disease. Arch Dis Child Fetal Neonatal Ed. 2011;96(2):F84-5.
2. Nicolaides KH, Rodeck CH. Maternal serum anti-D antibody concentration and assessment of rhesus isoimmunization. BMJ. 1992; 304(6835):1155-6.
3. Bowman JM. Controversies in Rh prophylaxis. Who needs Rh immune globulin and when should it be given? Am J Obstet Gynecol. 1985;151(3):289-94.
4. Bowman JM. The prevention of Rh immunization. Transfus Med Rev. 1988;2(3):129-50.
5. Martinez-Portilla RJ, Lopez-Felix J, Hawkins-Villareal A, Villafan-Bernal JR, Paz Y Miño F, Figueras F, et al. Performance of fetal middle cerebral artery peak systolic velocity for prediction of anemia in untransfused and transfused fetuses: systematic review and meta-analysis. Ultrasound Obstet Gynecol. 2019;54(6):722-31.

SUGGESTED READING

1. Committee on Practice Bulletins-Obstetrics. Practice Bulletin No. 181: Prevention of Rh D alloimmunization. Obstet Gynecol. 2017; 130(2):e57-70.
2. Fung KFK, Eason E. No. 133-prevention of Rh alloimmunization. J Obstet Gynaecol Can. 2018;40(1):e1-10.
3. Royal Australian and New Zealand College of Obstetricians and Gynaecologists (RANZCOG) (2019). Guidelines for the use of Rh(D) immunoglobulin (anti-D) in obstetrics. [online] Available from https://ranzcog.edu.au/RANZCOG_SITE/media/RANZCOG-MEDIA/Women%27s%20Health/Statement%20and%20guidelines/Clinical-Obstetrics/Use-of-Rh(D)-Isoimmunisation-(C-Obs-6).pdf?ext=.pdf. [Last accessed March, 2020].
4. Royal College of Obstetricians and Gynaecologists (2014). The management of women with red cell antibodies during pregnancy (Green-top Guideline No. 65). [online] Available from https://www.rcog.org.uk/globalassets/documents/guidelines/rbc_gtg65.pdf. [Last accessed March, 2020].
5. World Health Organization (2016). WHO recommendation on antenatal anti-D immunoglobulin prophylaxis. [online] Available from https://extranet.who.int/rhl/topics/preconception-pregnancy-childbirth-and-postpartum-care/antenatal-care/who-recommendation-antenatal-anti-d-immunoglobulin-prophylaxis. [Last accessed March, 2020].

24. Approach to a Pregnant Woman with Trauma

Prabha Lal

INTRODUCTION

In recent years, trauma has been considered as the leading cause of nonobstetric death during pregnancy, accounting for up to 36% of nonobstetric deaths and even higher number of fetal deaths.[1,2] Trauma affects 6–7% of all pregnant women in United States of America (USA), mostly in the last trimester with 0.3–0.4% of these requiring hospitalization.[3] As a rule, pregnancy must always be suspected in any female trauma patient of reproductive age group until proved otherwise. This is particularly pertinent in women who are unconscious or have altered sensorium consequent to head injury, intoxication, hypoxia or profound shock, and unable to give history.

Trauma during pregnancy may be unintentional or intentional. Unintentional causes include motor vehicle accidents, falls, poisoning, and burns. Whereas intentional causes are assault, intimate partner violence, suicide, homicide, etc.[4] Intimate partner violence should be suspected in pregnant women presenting with vague or inconsistent symptoms repeatedly to the hospital.[5]

PHYSIOLOGICAL CHANGES DURING PREGNANCY AFFECTING TRAUMA MANAGEMENT

Significant anatomical and physiological changes take place during pregnancy. This results in variations in the pathophysiology and site of trauma-related injuries in pregnant women as compared to nonpregnant women.[6] Most trauma-related deaths in pregnancy are due to head injuries, respiratory failure, and hypovolemic shock. Traumatic injuries can be classified as blunt, penetrating, burns, and electrical injuries. Blunt trauma is the most common form of injury most often caused by motor vehicle accidents. Maternal shock accounts for majority of fetal deaths. Hence, fetal condition is assessed only after initial maternal resuscitation. Direct fetal injury is relatively uncommon as the uterus, placenta, and amniotic fluid diminish the force of trauma on the fetus.

The initial assessment and resuscitation of pregnant woman with trauma is the same as that of a nonpregnant woman. However, in view of the unique pregnancy induced anatomical and physiological changes the resuscitation process needs to be modified (Box 1). Hence, it is essential for the attending obstetrician to understand all the changes that occur during pregnancy to provide appropriate care to both mother and fetus.

Maternal Changes

Cardiovascular System

There is a 30–50% increase in blood volume during pregnancy consequent to a 40–50%

> **Box 1:** Steps in the management of a pregnant patient with severe trauma.
>
> *Primary survey:*
> A: Airway maintenance with cervical spine protection
> B: Breathing and ventilation
> C: Circulation with hemorrhage control
> D: Disability (neurological evaluation)
> E: Exposure/environmental control

increase in plasma volume and 15–20% increase in red cell mass. The resultant hemodilution in pregnancy allows the pregnant woman to tolerate blood loss better during parturition.[5,6]

Due to the pressure of enlarged uterus on inferior vena cava, pregnant woman is susceptible to supine hypotension, which can reduce cardiac output by 30%. Therefore it is essential that pregnant woman should be transported and resuscitated in lateral position so as to keep the uterus displaced.

Respiratory System

The most important respiratory change that occurs during pregnancy is reduction in functional residual capacity (FRC) by 25%. This is coupled with 20% increase in oxygen consumption. Hence, oxygen supplementation should be done, while doing resuscitation.

Gastrointestinal System

Increased hormonal levels in pregnancy predispose to aspiration due to decreased competency of gastroesophageal sphincter. During pregnancy uterine enlargement displaces the intestines laterally and upwards and stretches the peritoneum making abdominal examination findings unreliable.

Renal System

Renal blood flow increases by 25–40% during pregnancy. Blood urea and serum creatinine are reduced due to increased glomerular filtration rate and urinary excretion.

Central Nervous System

The pregnancy induced neurological changes reduce anesthetic requirement by 25–40%, indicating loss of consciousness even at a sedation dose.

FETAL PHYSIOLOGY

The blood flow to uterus is directly related to maternal systemic blood pressure. The effect of trauma on fetal survival depends on the gestational age (GA), type and severity of trauma and the extent of disruption of normal uterine and fetal circulation. Fetal response to trauma where oxygenation or perfusion is affected includes bradycardia or tachycardia, decrease in the baseline variability, absence of heart rate acceleration, or presence of recurrent decelerations.[7]

GENERAL APPROACH TO A PREGNANT TRAUMA PATIENT

Care of pregnant trauma patients with severe injuries often requires a multidisciplinary team approach, involving an emergency clinician, trauma surgeon, obstetrician, and neonatologist.

Prehospital Care

As in any trauma patient, the airway, breathing, and circulation (ABC) of trauma resuscitation must be followed. The mother should always receive supplemental oxygen. Patients beyond first trimester should be tilted 25–30° to the left to prevent supine hypotension syndrome from the gravid uterus compressing the inferior vena cava. Fetal heart sound is auscultated if the pregnancy is advanced for assessment of fetal well-being and to reassure the mother. If military antishock trousers (MAST) are used, care is taken to inflate only the leg compartments.

Emergency Department Care

It is important to focus on initial assessment and resuscitation of the mother rather than getting distracted by the presence of obviously gravid uterus. Priority of treatment of an injured pregnant woman is same as that for a nonpregnant woman. Once the mother is assessed, fetal assessment should follow. Patients with minor injuries should receive routine medical treatment and fetal assessment. Patients with severe injury should be managed as per recommendations of advanced trauma life support system (ATLS).

The management of such patients is divided into primary survey and secondary survey (see Box 1).

Primary Survey

The initial period is used to assess severity of trauma and initiation of resuscitative measures. During the primary survey, a basic neurological assessment is made to see if the woman is conscious and alert, drowsy or unconscious. A more detailed neurological assessment is performed after the primary survey to establish the patient's level of consciousness, size and reaction of pupils, lateralizing signs, and level of spinal cord injury, if any. In view of the physiological changes in pregnancy the modifications of resuscitative measures in pregnancy are listed in Box 2.

Secondary Survey

Secondary survey begins after maternal condition stabilizes following adequate resuscitative efforts. It is evaluation of the trauma patient from head to toe. This includes complete history including obstetric history and a systematic physical examination to identify injuries to both mother and fetus. At the same time, evaluation and monitoring the fetus is initiated. Previous history of preterm labor or placental abruption increases the risk of recurrence of the same.

Box 2: Modification of resuscitative measures in pregnancy.

Modification of resuscitative measures in pregnancy:
- Perform manual left lateral tilt by 25–30° to reduce aortocaval compression
- Increased chest wall compression force to overcome the decreased chest wall compliance due breast hypertrophy and elevated diaphragm
- Use cricoid pressure if assistance is available to prevent gastric aspiration
- Perform compression higher on sternum slightly above center of sternum
- Remove fetal and uterine monitors before defibrillation else it may reduce cardiac shock dose or produce skin burns at monitor site
- Heimlich maneuver; a first aid procedure for dislodging an obstruction from a person's windpipe in which a sudden strong pressure is applied on their abdomen, between the navel and the ribcage. Use chest thrust if unable to encircle the gravid uterus

Advanced cardiac life support:
- Early tracheal intubation using smaller endotracheal tube and laryngoscope to overcome difficult intubation due to pharyngeal edema, breast hypertrophy, and elevated diaphragm
- After 4 minutes perform emergency hysterotomy, if required, as life-saving measure to facilitate resuscitation if pregnancy > 20 weeks

HISTORY

The patient's history should include the following points:

The mechanism of trauma whether the trauma was a direct abdominal trauma or trauma related to some weapon, sharp object or use of seat belt. The date of last menstrual period (LMP) and estimated date of delivery

(EDOD) is recorded. Any history of complications such as premature labor, premature rupture of membranes, and vaginal bleeding should be elicited. It is important to find out if the woman is perceiving normal fetal movements or not. Any history of depression, substance abuse or previous visits to emergency is elicited as these factors may suggest attempt to suicide or domestic violence.

EXAMINATION

General Physical Examination

Physical examination is mostly done as a part of primary survey, but can be repeated to look for any obvious injuries. In cases of domestic violence, ecchymoses of the breasts, abdomen, and upper extremities may be present and the observed injuries are in varying stages of healing.[8]

Systemic Examination

Systemic examination involves a careful examination of the chest, cardiovascular system (CVS), and neurological system.

Per Abdomen Examination

Examination of abdomen is especially relevant compared to nonpregnant women. Pregnant women have higher incidence of serious abdominal injuries, but a lower incidence of chest and head injury due to the presence of protruding gravid uterus.

Abdomen is inspected for any bruises especially across the lower abdomen, which is seen with seat belt injury. The uterus is palpated for its contour, any uterine tenderness or contractions. Gestational age can be estimated by the fundal height and abdominal girth.

Uterine tenderness and height of the uterus more than the period of gestation may occur in placental abruption. Loss of uterine contour and superficial palpation of fetal parts is suggestive of uterine rupture.

Fetal heart rate is assessed with stethoscope, Doppler fetal monitor or ultrasonography (USG). In advanced pregnancy, rebound tenderness and guarding may be less evident due to decreased concentration of pain fibers in peritoneum due to its stretching. Thus, the peritoneal signs are often veiled and hemoperitoneum may be missed. The flanks must be percussed for dullness suggestive of blood or fluid collection. The percussion note is normally resonant due to displaced bowel loops.

Evaluation of Perineum and Genital Tract

The area is inspected for any injury in a patient suffering from polytrauma. Pelvic, vaginal, and rectal examination should be done except in women with unstable spine and fracture of pelvis and femur, because positioning may risk further injury. This is carried out only after orthopedic clearance. Maternal pelvic fractures are associated with injury to the maternal bladder and urethra, retroperitoneal bleeding, and fetal skull fracture. The bladder may be catheterized if trauma to urethra or bladder is suspected. Mostly in woman with pelvic trauma an examination under anesthesia is required.

Per Speculum Examination

Per speculum examination is done for observing any discharge, bleeding, leaking, and lacerations in the vagina. Presence of bone fragments in vagina indicates an open pelvic fracture. The vaginal discharge should be tested for pH and ferning. The vaginal pH in normal pregnancy is acidic, around

3.8–4.2 whereas in women with ruptured membranes it is 7 due to presence of amniotic fluid. Presence of ferning is suggestive of liquor amnii.

Per Vaginum Examination

Per vaginum examination is done when indicated usually in operation theater.

INVESTIGATIONS

A complete laboratory evaluation must be done in all cases of pregnant trauma patients (Box 3). Additional tests should be dictated by the patient's condition and clinical situation.

It is important to understand that the clinical evaluation of trauma patients has limitations. Large studies reveal 5–10% of abdominal injuries during pregnancy are missed if diagnosis is made based only on clinical findings. Hence the importance of other diagnostic modalities such as imaging studies can not be overlooked.[7,8] Choice for appropriate imaging modality causes anxiety to the obstetrician due to their concern for radiation exposure to the fetus. Computed tomography (CT) scan has radiation concerns whereas USG and magnetic resonance imaging (MRI) have no fear of ionizing radiation exposure. The concerns about radiation exposure to the fetus should not influence the decision to use a radiographic imaging modality in a pregnant trauma patient, injury detection always takes priority.[8]

X-rays

The treating physician should interpret the X-rays in the background of pregnancy-related anatomical changes. These include an increase in anteroposterior (AP) diameter, mild pulmonary vascular cephalization, cardiomegaly and a slight widening of mediastinum on X-ray chest and widening of the sacroiliac joints and symphysis pubis on X-ray pelvis.

Ultrasonography and Focused Assessment with Sonography for Trauma

Ultrasound is done to assess fetal age, number, position, viability, amount of liquor amnii, and any evidence of placental abruption. It also evaluates for free fluid or hemorrhage in the peritoneal cavity. Ultrasound has low sensitivity (24%) but high specificity (96%), for diagnosing placental abruption. It has a positive predictive value of 88% and a negative predictive value of 53%.[9,10]

Focused assessment with sonography for trauma (FAST) is a routine in many trauma centers. It is a noninvasive bedside test that can be repeated easily if required. It is highly specific. Focus is directed in locating fluid in the pericardium, pleural cavity, pararenal, retroperitoneal space, paracolic gutters, and peritoneal cavity. FAST reduces the need for CT.

Box 3: Laboratory evaluation.

Investigations:
- Complete blood count (CBC) with platelet count
- Blood grouping and crossmatching
- Coagulation profile including D-dimer levels
- Serum electrolytes
- Liver function tests (LFTs)
- Renal function tests (RFTs)
- Serum amylase
- Arterial blood gas (ABG) analysis
- Urine analysis
- Urine pregnancy testing, if status is unknown in a young female
- Urine and blood toxicology studies
- Kleihauer-Betke (KB) test*

*This test is used to detect fetal-to-maternal hemorrhage.

Computed Tomography

Computed tomography scans for abdomen should be pursued without hesitation using the lowest possible dose to achieve necessary information where USG has been inconclusive. Head and chest CT may be used when indicated as the amount of radiation exposure to the fetus is not significant.

Magnetic Resonance Imaging

Not usually indicated.

Continuous Electronic Fetal Monitoring

Recently, continuous electronic fetal monitoring (CEFM) is considered as a standard of care for a viable fetus following trauma. Monitoring should be started as soon as maternal condition is stabilized, because most placental abruptions occur shortly after trauma. Fetal distress is manifested by fetal heart rate variations like bradycardia, tachycardia, loss of beat-to-beat variability, and late decelerations. Fetal monitoring can be useful for both fetal and maternal assessment as fetal distress is an early marker of impending maternal hemodynamic compromise. Hence, fetal heart rate is considered the fifth vital sign in addition to pulse, blood pressure, respiratory rate, and temperature in an injured pregnant woman. Ideal duration for fetal monitoring is unclear; however, it can range from 4 to 24 hours depending upon the severity of injury.[11,12]

ROLE OF PERIMORTEM CESAREAN DELIVERY

It may save the life of the fetus when done after a period of viability. It leads to a survival benefit for the mother as delivery increases venous return and cardiac output by 25–30%.[13] The American Heart Association recommends considering perimortem cesarean delivery if advanced cardiovascular life support (ACLS) has not returned spontaneous circulation within 4–5 minutes of cardiac arrest.

ROLE OF EMERGENCY HYSTEROTOMY

- Gestational age less than 20 weeks with singleton pregnancy emergency hysterotomy is not recommended unless it is a multiple pregnancy.
- Gestational age 20–23 weeks emergency hysterotomy is indicated for successful resuscitation, but not for survival of fetus.
- Gestational age more than 23 weeks emergency hysterotomy is indicated to save life of both mother and fetus.
- Emergency hysterotomy should not be delayed while attempting to listen to fetal heart sound (FHS) and do USG to document gestational age.
- Omission of a timely emergency hysterotomy or delay may lead to unnecessary loss of two lives although the decision is multidimensional.
- Skilled obstetrician should perform the procedure quickly.

KEY POINTS

- Trauma is an important cause of non-obstetric maternal death, especially in developed countries.
- The initial assessment and resuscitation of pregnant woman with severe injury are the same as that of nonpregnant traumatized patient.
- Modifications of resuscitative measures are required in view of explicit anatomic

Flowchart 1: Algorithm for clinical approach to a pregnant woman with trauma.

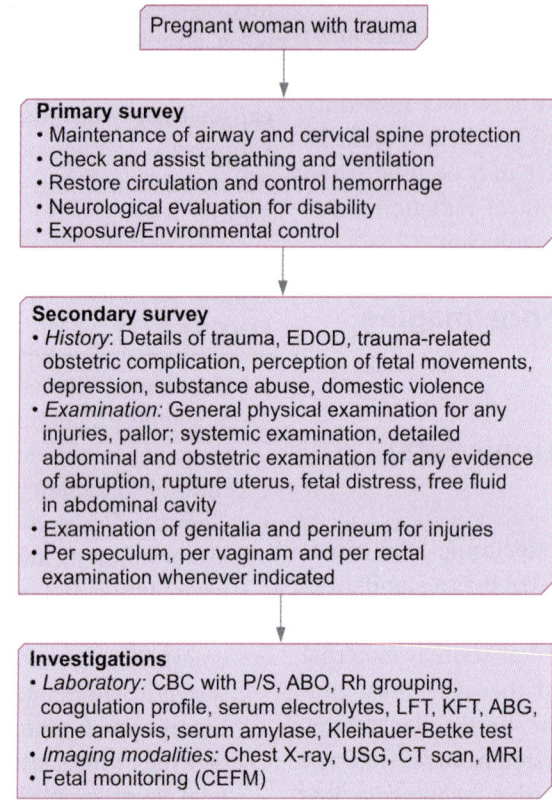

(ABG: arterial blood gas; CBC: complete blood count; CEFM: continuous electronic fetal monitoring; CT: computed tomography; EDOD: estimated date of delivery; KFT: kidney function test; LFT: liver function test; MRI: magnetic resonance imaging; P/S: peripheral smear; Rh: rhesus; USG: ultrasonography)

and physiologic changes that occur during pregnancy.
- A detailed history and thorough examination are done to look for injuries after initial stabilization.
- A careful obstetric examination is done for any trauma-related pregnancy complication and fetal well-being.
- The accuracy of symptoms and signs in diagnosing various injuries is not very high, so aid of imaging modalities like X-ray, USG, CT scan and MRI, is useful.
- The concerns about radiation exposure to the fetus should not influence the decision to use a radiographic imaging modality in a pregnant trauma patient.
- Fetal distress is an early marker of impending maternal hemodynamic compromise, so CEFM should be done.

REFERENCES

1. Jacob S, Bloebaum L, Shah G, Varner MW. Maternal mortality in Utah. Obstet Gynecol. 1998;91(2):187-91.
2. Connolly AM, Katz VL, Bash KL, McMahon MJ, Hansen WF. Trauma and pregnancy. Am J Perinatol. 1997;14(6):331-6.
3. Shah KH, Simons RK, Holbrook T, Fortlage D, Winchell RJ, Hoyt DB. Trauma in pregnancy:

maternal and fetal outcomes. J Trauma. 1998;45(1):83-6.
4. Mendez-Figueroa H, Dahlke JD, Vrees RA, Rause DJ. Trauma in pregnancy: an updated systematic review. Am J obstet gynecol. 2013; 209(1):1-10.
5. American College of Surgeons. Trauma in pregnancy and intimate partner violence. Advanced Trauma Life Support Student Mannual, 9th edition. Chicago: American college of Surgeons; 2012.
6. Harvey MG. Physiology change of pregnancy. In: Clark SL (Ed). Critical Care Obstetrical Nursing. Gaithersburg: Aspen Co; 1991.
7. Goodwin TM, Breen MT. Pregnancy outcome and fetomaternal hemorrhage after non-catastrophic trauma. Am J Obstet Gynecol. 1990;162(3):665-71.
8. Schurink GW, Bode PJ, van Luijt PA, van Vugt AB. The value of physical examination in the diagnosis of patients with blunt abdominal trauma: a retrospective study. Injury. 1997;28(4):261-5.
9. Glantz C, Purnell L. Clinical utility of sonography in the diagnosis and treatment of placental abruption. J Ultrasound Med. 2002; 21(8):837-40.
10. ACOG Committee on obstetric practice. ACOG Committee Opinion. Number 299, September 2004 (replaces No. 158, September 1991). Guidelines for diagnostic imaging during pregnancy. Obstet Gynecol. 2004;104:647-51.
11. Diercks DB, Mehrotra A, Nazarian DJ, Promes SB, Decker WW, Fesmire FM. Clinical policy: Critical issues in the evaluation of adult patients presenting to the emergency department with acute blunt abdominal trauma. Ann Emerg Med. 2004;43:278-90.
12. Curet MJ, Schermer CR, Demarest GB, Bieneik EJ 3rd, Curet LB. Predictors of outcome in trauma during pregnancy: identification of patients who can be monitored for less than 6 hours. J Trauma. 2000;49:18-25.
13. Katz VL, Dotters DJ, Droejemueller W. Perimortem caesarean delivery. Obstet gynecol. 1986;68(4):571-6.

SUGGESTED READING

1. Dennis Henlon. Current Concepts in Management of the Pregnancy Trauma Patient. AP of Emergency Medicine Residency and Director of Emergency Medicine, Stanford University.
2. Trauma in Pregnancy: Assessment and Treatment: SAGE Journal by P-Petrone 2006.
3. Trauma in Pregnancy: Family Practice Notebook.

25
Approach to a Pregnant Woman Brought in a Collapsed State

Aimee Teong Chuin Ai, Kazila Bhutia

INTRODUCTION[1-3]

Maternal collapse is defined as acute events resulting in partial or complete loss of consciousness involving cardiorespiratory system and/or brain at any stage in pregnancy and up to 6 weeks postpartum. Data from the US Nationwide Inpatient Sample suggest that cardiac arrest occurs in 1:12,000 admissions for delivery. Though it is a rare event, outcome can be catastrophic. The first few minutes of resuscitation are vital to reduce morbidity and mortality.

It is essential that all healthcare professionals including paramedics involved in resuscitation of pregnant woman should be aware of anatomical and physiological changes pertinent to pregnancy, which make the resuscitation less effective.

After 20 weeks' gestation, the gravid uterus in supine position can cause aortocaval compression resulting in decrease cardiac stroke volume. This can be minimized by tilting the woman in left lateral position using wedge, pillows or even rescuer's knee. Pregnant women at term have increase in oxygen consumption by 20% and decrease in pulmonary function residual capacity by 25%, hence have a tendency to become hypoxic more rapidly than nonpregnant women. The enlarged uterus together with diaphragmatic splinting and decreased lung compliance make ventilation during cardiac arrest difficult. Increased weight gain and large breast size in later part of pregnancy contribute to difficulty in providing effective ventilation during cardiopulmonary resuscitation (CPR) as well as difficult intubation due to laryngeal edema.

DIFFERENTIAL DIAGNOSIS[1,3-5]

There are multiple causes of collapse, which may be either related to pregnancy or pre-existing conditions not related to pregnancy. Detailed discussion of all causes is outside the scope of this chapter. The most common causes of maternal collapse are vasovagal syncope and postural hypotension. The most common reversible causes of collapse can be ascertain using the 5T's, the 4H's and E as employed by the Resuscitation Council (UK) (Table 1).

RISK REDUCTION[1,6]

Antenatal Care

Thorough assessment of women during antenatal visit must be done. All high risks group with pre-existing significant medical issues should be referred to concerned specialist to optimize their care involving multidisciplinary team. Local protocols should be in place to manage the symptoms such as chest pain, breathlessness, and calf tenderness.

Chapter 25: Approach to a Pregnant Woman Brought in a Collapsed State

Table 1: Differential diagnosis of maternal collapse—4H's and 4T's + E.[1,4,5]

Reversible causes		Causes in pregnancy
4H's	Hypovolemia	• *Most common cause*: Hemorrhagic shock from ante- or postpartum hemorrhage • High epidural/Dense spinal block; Neurogenic shock
	Hypoxia	• Pregnant mothers can become hypoxic quickly • *Cardiac events*: Cardiomyopathy, myocardial infarction, aortic dissection, aneurysm
	Hypo/hyperkalemia or other electrolyte abnormalities	No more likely
	Hypothermia	No more likely
4T's	Thromboembolism	• *Venous thromboembolism (VTE)*: Incidence of venous thrombosis is same antenatal and postnatal, but pulmonary embolism is much higher postnatally • *Amniotic fluid embolism*: Anaphylactic type of reaction to fetal skin squames and amniotic fluid entering maternal circulation • Air emboli • Myocardial infarct
	Toxicity	• Local anesthetic-induced arrhythmias • Hypermagnesemia • Illicit drugs • *Anaphylaxis*: Food, drugs, animal and plant products etc.
	Tension pneumothorax	Following trauma, suicide attempt
	Tamponade (cardiac)	Following trauma, suicide attempt
E	Pre-eclampsia and eclampsia	• Includes intracranial hemorrhage • It can cause ante-, intra- or postpartum collapse; need to exclude epilepsy

Source: Reproduced with the permission of the Royal College of Obstetricians and Gynaecologists. Royal College of Obstetricians and Gynaecologists. (2011). Green-top Guideline no.56: Maternal collapse in Pregnancy and the Puerperium (Figure 1 of page 4 of 24). [online] Available from: https://www.rcog.org.uk/globalassets/documents/guidelines/gtg_56.pdf [Last accessed March, 2020].

Inpatient Care

The use of an early warning score chart should be part of routine care. Important parameters should be observed:
- Pulse rate
- SBP
- DBP
- Respiratory rate
- Oxygen saturation
- Temperature
- Consciousness.

This allows prompt escalation to senior staffs as well as early recognition and timely management of the deteriorating patient.

MANAGEMENT[1,3,5-9]

Successful management of maternal collapse depends on early communication and teamwork. Prompt resuscitation is paramount while considering the differential diagnosis. All maternity units should have well-established local protocols, including basic life support (BLS) in pregnancy and advanced cardiovascular life support (ACLS) in pregnancy. Early involvement of senior experienced staff where possible, including obstetrician, anesthetist, midwife, neonatologist, and intensivist, is essential to optimize outcome.

Flowchart 1: Algorithm for maternal collapse.[1,6-9]

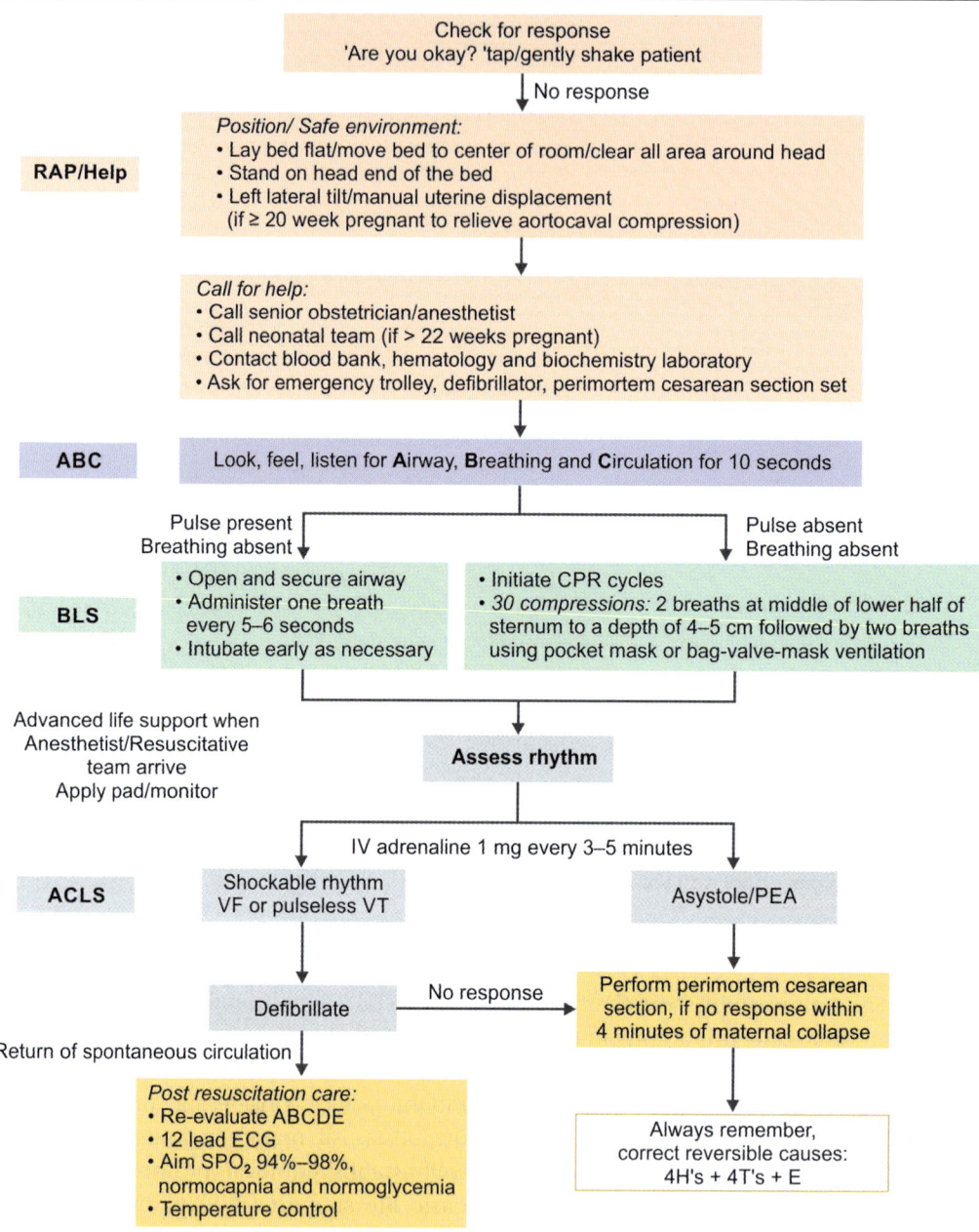

(ACLS: advanced cardiovascular life support; BLS: basic life support; PEA: pulseless electrical activity VF: ventricular fibrillation; VT: ventricular tachycardia)

The resuscitation should follow the commonly used airway, breathing, and circulation (ABC) pattern as in all medical emergencies. Brief history should be taken from the family members, paramedics or hospital staff along with simultaneous assessment of ABC (Flowchart 1).

Airway

Airway patency should be assured, check for any foreign body or vomitus obstructing airway. In unconscious woman, a head tilt/chin lift or thrust may be required to keep the airway patent. Consider intubating as soon as skilled person is available. Intubation not only helps in effective ventilation but also protects the airway from regurgitation and aspiration. This is due to progesterone effect relaxing the lower esophageal sphincter and delayed gastric emptying. One should always be aware of head and spinal cord injury. Various factors such as pregnancy-related weight gain, laryngeal edema, and large breasts could contribute to challenging intubation, hence early involvement of senior anesthetist is paramount.

Breathing

As pregnant women have low threshold to withstand hypoxia, 100% high-flow oxygen should be administered as soon as possible either by face mask or intubation. If breaths do not go in, retilt head and give two more breaths. Suspect choking if breath does not go in.

Circulation

Two large bore cannulas should be sited immediately, and blood should be sent for crossmatch, full blood count, coagulation profile, baseline liver and kidney function tests, and arterial blood gas analysis. There should be aggressive approach to fluid replacement in the presence of hemorrhagic shock.

Basic Life Support

Absence of breathing movement or gasping breathing is a common feature of absence of circulation and cardiac arrest and should not be taken as sign of life, time should not be wasted on palpation for pulse. The CPR should be commenced immediately in the form of standard rate and ratio of chest compression and ventilation (30:2). The United Kingdom Resuscitation Council Guidelines recommend starting CPR using airway and defibrillation within 3 minutes of collapse due to cardiac arrest. The circulation status should be reassessed after every 10 ventilation/chest compression cycles (approximately 2 minutes) taking not more than 10 seconds. Change rescuer every 2 minutes, if possible, to prevent ineffective compressions due to exhaustion.

Advanced Cardiac Life Support

Defibrillation according to cardiac rhythm should be initiated as soon as possible, if there is no sign of circulation even after effective CPR. The team leader should decide on defibrillation and use of drugs sequence based on shockable or nonshockable rhythm. When indicated, defibrillation should be performed in the pregnant patient without hesitation or delay. The risk to the mother in delaying appropriate defibrillation would outweigh any potential concern about defibrillation in the setting of fetal monitors. Compressions should then immediately resume after defibrillation. It is recommended that ACLS drugs should be administered at recommended doses without modifications.

For the following emergencies:
- *Cardiac arrest*: IV adrenaline (epinephrine) 1 mg for shockable rhythms (to give after second shock then every second cycle) and for nonshockable rhythms (to give immediately and then every 3–5 minutes)
- *VF/VT*: Amiodarone IV 300 mg after 3rd shock

- *Opiate overdose*: IV Naloxone 400–800 μg
- *Magnesium toxicity*: IV Calcium gluconate 10 mL of 10% slowly
- *Local anesthetic toxicity*: 1.5 mL/kg 20% lipid emulsion (e.g. intralipid 20%).

In immediate postpartum woman, hemorrhagic shock is the most common cause of postpartum collapse, aggressive approach to fluid replacement should be there till blood and blood products are available. Vasopressors are administered as necessary.

Perimortem Cesarean Section (Resuscitative Hysterotomy)

Pregnant woman tends to develop anoxia faster than the nonpregnant woman and can suffer irreversible brain damage within 4–6 minutes after cardiac arrest. If there is no response after effectively performed CPR in pregnant woman after 20 weeks of gestation, inform the operation theater team and neonatologists, cesarean section delivery should be initiated within 4 minutes and the baby should be delivered by 5 minutes of cardiac arrest. Delivery of fetus allows resuscitation to carry out easily, reduces maternal oxygen consumption, increases venous return, and alleviates aortocaval compression. Maternal indication is paramount as compared to prognosis of fetus due to prematurity. No time should be wasted by moving patient to an operating theater for perimortem cesarean and it should be performed as same area where resuscitation is taking place. CPR should be continued during the entire process.

While continuing resuscitation process, simultaneous assessment should be carried out to rule out cause of collapse including a detailed systemic and vaginal examination. Once stabilized, the woman is transferred to intensive care unit for further monitoring. Continuing care should be directed to specific etiology to optimize the outcome.

CLINICAL GOVERNANCE[1,8,10]

Documentation

Clear documentation of the entire process in a stepwise manner is important whether resuscitation is successful or not. Timeline of cardiac arrest, staff attendance, drug/fluid/blood products administration, defibrillation, and delivery should be documented clearly and legibly retrospectively as soon as possible after the event.

Debriefing

It is a good practice to ensure the partner/relatives are kept informed about regular updates of ongoing events during resuscitation. The woman should be debriefed about the entire events once she recovers, about the possible outcome or recurrence in future pregnancy. Involvement of professional counselor reduces the chances of post-traumatic stress disorder and postnatal depression. Arrange for further follow-up appointment.

Incident Reporting

All the maternal collapse cases should be reported in clinical incident reporting system and thorough review of the care given to the woman should be reviewed through the local clinical governance committee.

Training

All maternity staff should have annual formal training in generic life support and the management of maternal collapse, with regular appraisal.

KEY POINTS

- Maternal collapse is an uncommon event but requires prompt action.
- Effective communication and teamwork are paramount for optimum outcome.
- Lateral tilt to 15°, if more than 20 weeks period of gestation is followed by management of cardiac arrest using basic and advanced life support.
- If the resuscitation is successful, the woman is transferred to intensive care unit (ICU) and further management is etiology specific along with continued intensive monitoring.
- Conversely, if resuscitation is unsuccessful, cesarean delivery should be initiated within 4 minutes of resuscitation.
- Clear documentation of the entire sequence of events is mandatory.

REFERENCES

1. Royal College of Obstetricians and Gynaecologists. (2011). Green-top Guideline no.56: Maternal collapse in pregnancy and the puerperium. [online] Available from https://www.rcog.org.uk/globalassets/documents/guidelines/gtg_56.pdf [Last accessed March, 2020].
2. Mhyre JM, Tsen LC, Einav S, Kuklina EV, Leffert LR, Bateman BT. Cardiac arrest during hospitalization for delivery in the United States, 1998-2011. Anesthesiology. 2014;120(4):810-8.
3. Lombard H, Pillay PS. Managing acute collapse in pregnant women. Best Pract Res Clini Obstet Gynaecol. 2009;23(3):339-55.
4. Resuscitation Council (UK). Guidelines 2005. [online] Available from https://www.resus.org.uk/archive/guidelines-2005/ [Last accessed March, 2020].
5. Bhatti S, Penna L. Maternal collapse. Obstetrics, Gynaecology & Reproductive Medicine. 2012;22(7):191-8.
6. Jeejeebhoy FM, Zelop CM, Lipman S, Carvalho B, Joglar J, Mhyre JM, et al. Cardiac Arrest in Pregnancy: A Scientific Statement From the American Heart Association. Circulation. 2015;132(18):1747-73.
7. Resuscitation Council (UK). Guidelines 2010. [online] Available from: https://www.resus.org.uk/resuscitation-guidelines/ [Last accessed March, 2020].
8. SA Maternal, Neonatal & Gynaecology Clinical Community of Practice. (2017). Perinatal Practice Guideline. Collapse (Maternal). [online] Available from: https://www.sahealth.sa.gov.au/wps/wcm/connect/32d24804ee4fc8297449fd150ce4f37/Collapse+%28Maternal%29_PPG_v2.0.pdf?MOD=AJPERES&CACHEID=ROOTWORKSPACE-32d2e4804ee4fc8297449fd150ce4f37-n1mkzns [Last accessed March, 2020].
9. Ching CK, Leong SH, Chua SJ, Lim SH, Heng K, Pothiawala S, et al. Advanced cardiac life support: 2016 Singapore Guidelines. Singapore Med J. 2017;58(7):360-72.
10. Black RS, Brocklehurst P. A systemic review of training in acute obstetrics emergencies. BJOG. 2003;110(9):837-41.

SUGGESTED READING

1. Katz VL, Dotters DJ, Droegemueller W. Perimortem cesarean delivery. Obstet Gynecol. 1986;68(4):571-6.
2. Knight M, Bunch K, Tuffnell D, Jayakody H, Shakespeare J, Kotnis R, Kenyon S, Kurinczuk JJ (Eds) on behalf of MBRRACE-UK. Saving Lives, Improving Mothers' Care - Lessons learned to inform maternity care from the UK and Ireland Confidential Enquiries into Maternal Deaths and Morbidity 2014-16. Oxford: National Perinatal Epidemiology Unit, University of Oxford; 2018.
3. Lee A, Sheen JJ, Richards S. Intrapartum maternal cardiac arrest: A simulation case for multidisciplinary providers. MedEdPORTAL. 2018;14:10768.
4. Lipman S, Cohen S, Einav S, Jeejeebhoy F, Mhyre JM, Morrison LJ, et al. The Society for Obstetric Anesthesia and Perinatology consensus statement on the management of cardiac arrest in pregnancy. Anesth Analg. 2014;118(5):1003-16.
5. Zelop CM, Einav S, Mhyre JM, Martin S. Cardiac arrest during pregnancy: ongoing clinical conundrum. Am J Obstet Gynecol. 2018;219(1):52-61.

26

Approach to a Postnatal Woman

Sumi P Thampi, Anu Handa

INTRODUCTION

Puerperium, the period between delivery and complete physiologic involution, has been referred to as the fourth trimester of pregnancy. The duration of this period is between 4 and 6 weeks after childbirth; however, some authors consider it till 12 weeks. In both developing and developed countries, more than 60% of maternal deaths occur in the postpartum period. Of these, 45% of postpartum deaths occur in the first 24 hours, more than 65% within 1 week, and more than 80% within 2 weeks;[1] hence, the postpartum period is a very critical time.

HISTORY-TAKING

Detailed history plays an important role in the management of a postnatal woman. After the general details such as name, age, date of delivery, condition of the baby, the woman is asked about any specific complaint. In case there is none, then a detailed history of the delivery including questions related to the labor and newborn are asked. In case there is any specific complaint, then relevant history pertaining to that complaint is elicited followed by a detailed history of delivery. This includes questions related to the delivery and the newborn.

History of Delivery

It is important to know whether the delivery was vaginal or abdominal, term or preterm, and spontaneous or induced. In case it was induced, then the indication of induction, method of induction, and induction to delivery interval are asked.

Any history suggestive of ruptured membranes before delivery is important. Prolonged leaking of more than 18 hours may be associated with chorioamnionitis and resultant puerperal sepsis. The total duration of labor is noted.

For vaginal deliveries, it is important to know if the delivery was spontaneous or assisted with instruments such as forceps or ventouse. Instrumental deliveries are more likely to be associated with complications such as injuries to the genital tract and newborn. The woman is asked if any episiotomy was done or postplacental intrauterine contraceptive device (IUCD) was inserted.

History of any complications such as excessive blood loss, blood transfusion, repair of any perineal, vaginal or cervical tears, or vulvovaginal hematoma is asked for.

For cesarean delivery, it is important to know the indication of cesarean section, whether it was an elective or emergency procedure, and the type of anesthesia received whether, general anesthesia or regional block. All this information influences the postoperative management of the woman.

Any significant perioperative surgical or anesthetic event such as difficulty during surgery or anesthesia, any injury to bladder or bowel, excessive blood loss, and blood transfusion is asked for. It is important to know if the woman has had tubal ligation or post placental IUCD insertion during cesarean section.

Depending upon the postoperative day of the woman, she is asked for the duration for which the urinary catheter was retained and if she is passing urine normally after the removal of catheter.

For those operated more than a week back, one can ask if the sutures have been removed or not and is the incision line healthy or is there any discharge from it.

As regards the newborn, it is important to know about the number of babies, baby weight, sex of the baby, whether the baby cried immediately after birth or not, when was the baby roomed in, when was the breastfeeding initiated, and how is the baby doing.

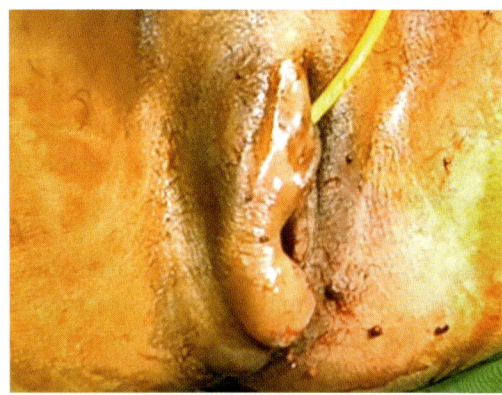

Fig. 1: Bleeding or discharge per vaginum.

remember that severe perineal, vaginal, or rectal pain, or urinary retention always warrants careful inspection and palpation of perineal area and episiotomy site to rule out any vulvovaginal or episiotomy hematoma (Fig. 1).

History of Specific Complaints

In puerperium, the woman can complain of pain in lower abdomen, pain in perineal or abdominal stitch line, bleeding or discharge, problems related to breastfeeding, fever, urinary or bowel complaints, and swelling or pain in the leg. She should be asked for detailed history pertaining to the specific problem.

Pain

A postpartum woman can have pain due to several reasons such as intermittent pain lower abdomen (after pains), pain in perineum due to episiotomy or perineal trauma or in abdominal wound in case of abdominal delivery, breast pain if engorged, and headache consequent to leakage of cerebrospinal fluid through postdural puncture in neuraxial anesthesia or analgesia. It is important to

Bleeding or Discharge Per Vaginum

In puerperium, the woman has bleeding for first few days which becomes progressively pale and is replaced by yellowish white discharge. This postpartum vaginal discharge or lochia continues for 4–6 weeks and is consequent to sloughing and shedding of decidua after delivery. It contains serous exudate, erythrocytes, leukocytes, fragments of decidua, bacteria, and epithelial cells. For the first 24 hours, there is bleeding which is followed by lochia rubra for a few days, then lochia serosa for 2–3 weeks, and finally lochia alba for another 2 weeks.[2]

Any history of excessive bleeding in first few days of puerperium is important. The assessment is subjective. The woman can be asked about the number of pads she is soaking every day and if there is passage of clots. Soakage of more than one pad in an hour, or more than five pads per day, or passage of clots is suggestive of excessive bleeding.

Ask for the amount, color, and odor of the vaginal discharge. Foul smelling discharge may be suggestive of either poor hygiene or puerperal sepsis.

Normal menses usually return in 6–8 weeks if the woman is not breastfeeding. Lactating women may start menstruating as early as the 2nd or as late as 18th month after delivery.[3]

Fever

Low-grade fever in the first 24 hours after delivery can be due to exertion or exhaustion and resolves spontaneously and is not diagnosed as puerperal pyrexia. Any fever of ≥38.0°C (≥100.4°F) on any 2 of the first 10 days postpartum may be suggestive of some puerperal complication and needs to be investigated. A detailed history and examination to look for any focus of infection is indicated.

Bowel and Bladder Function

Bladder and bowel problems are common in puerperium. It is important to ask whether the woman is passing urine and stools normally. Urinary retention with overdistended bladder is common after neuraxial analgesia or anesthesia, instrumental delivery, cesarean section, episiotomy, or perineal trauma following delivery. Vulvovaginal hematoma should be ruled out in women with urinary retention following vaginal delivery. Urinary frequency and dysuria may be present following urinary catheterization during delivery or cesarean section and urinary tract infection should be ruled out.

Constipation is common in puerperium due to change in eating pattern during labor and after cesarean section and sometimes due to perineal trauma-related pain. However, some women may complain of increase in frequency of passing motion consequent to altered bowel flora because of intake of broad-spectrum antibiotics prescribed to them.

Breastfeeding

After delivery, the breasts begin to secrete colostrum. The secretion persists for approximately 5 days with gradual conversion to mature milk during the ensuing 4 weeks.

It is important to ask if the woman is breastfeeding her baby and if she is facing any problems regarding the same.

There can be breastfeeding-related problems such as no or inadequate milk secretion, painful feeding, inability to latch on the baby, engorged breasts, cracked or fissured nipples which need to be addressed by a lactation consultant.

All postpartum women are encouraged to breastfeed their newborn within 1 hour of childbirth and encourage skin-to-skin contact. Initially, breastfeeding is attempted at least every 2 hours and then builds up to 8–12 times in 24 hours.

Ambulation

Women are encouraged for early ambulation within a few hours after vaginal delivery and by the day after surgery following cesarean section. Woman should initially be assisted, especially after cesarean section. Early ambulation lowers the risk for venous thrombosis and pulmonary embolism. It also lowers complications such as urinary retention and constipation.

Drug History

Detailed history of intake of any drug for chronic disease states such as thyroid disorders, hypertension, diabetes mellitus, or seizure disorders is important as the dosages of many medications may require adjustment in puerperium.

Women who develop hypertension and diabetes during pregnancy need to be monitored postnatally to taper the medications.

Contraceptive History

It is important to discuss contraception with the postnatal woman. Her contraceptive need and knowledge are assessed. Spacing of 2–3 years is optimum for women wishing for another pregnancy. The discussion can be initiated by asking her if she has used any contraceptive in the past. If yes, then whether she wishes to continue that method. In case she wishes to continue, then method-specific counseling can be reinforced; otherwise she is counseled about other options available to her.

Dietary History

It is important to ask about the dietary intake of the postnatal woman. The dietary requirement is increased by 500 kcal in breastfeeding mothers. After normal vaginal delivery, the postnatal woman is advised to have full meals and plenty of fluids whereas after cesarean section, the woman is kept nil orally till bowel sounds return, usually for 6 hours, and then she is started on clear fluids. Full diet is gradually introduced by next day. Myths about restriction of certain foods and water in postnatal women should be allayed.

EXAMINATION OF A POSTNATAL WOMAN

Careful and frequent monitoring (every 15–30 minutes) should be done in the first 1 hour following vaginal delivery, then once at 6 hours, followed by once or twice a day till discharge. Women after cesarean section need to be monitored frequently for the first 2 hours and then every 4–6 hours for next 24 hours and once or twice a day till discharge.

The woman is assessed for her pulse, temperature, blood pressure, uterus well contracted or not, fundal height, abdominal incision line in postcesarean women, perineum for any vaginal bleeding or any abnormal discharge, any perineal swelling, or discoloration.

Following low risk vaginal delivery, BP is checked once and then again after 6 hours. Urine void is documented in 6 hours for all vaginal deliveries.[2]

General Physical Examination

The vitals including pulse rate, blood pressure, respiratory rate, and temperature are recorded. Increased pulse rate, fever, and increased respiratory rate are suggestive of sepsis and need further evaluation. For details of general physical examination, refer to Chapter 1.

The hydration status is assessed. Any pallor is looked for and noted.

Breast Examination

Examine both the breasts. Whether nipples are normal or poorly formed (Fig. 2) or retracted or are there any cracks or fissures on

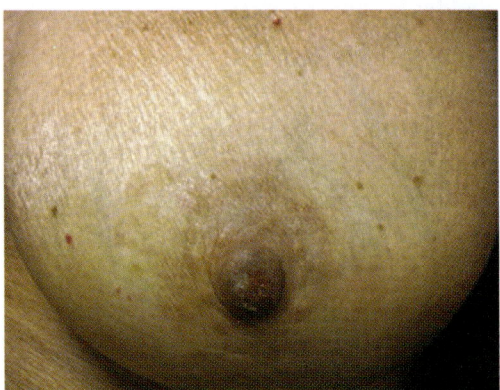

Fig. 2: Poorly formed flat nipple.

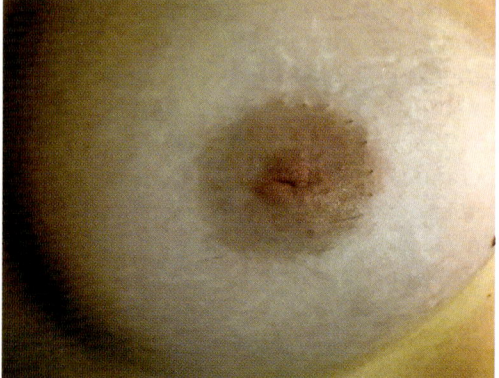
Fig. 3: Cracked nipple.

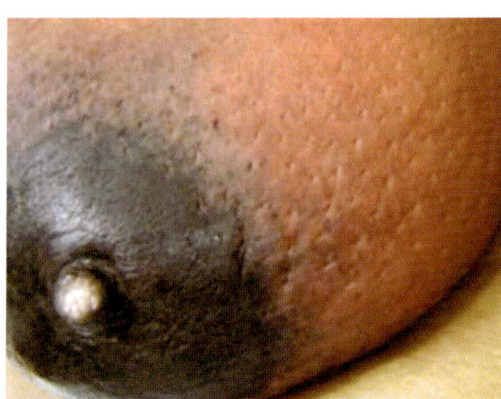
Fig. 4: Engorged breast.

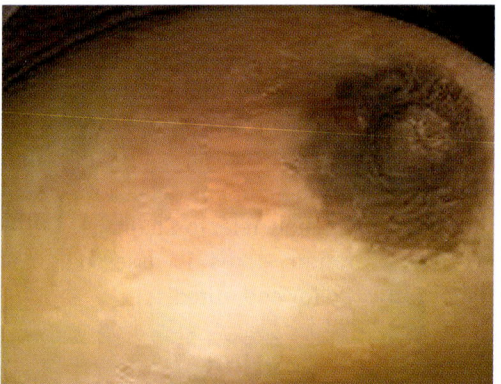
Fig. 5: Lactational breast abscess.

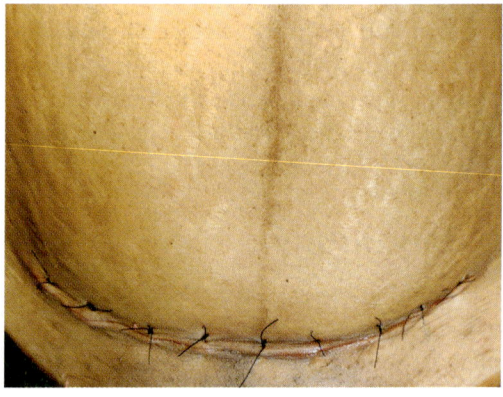
Fig. 6: Inspection of cesarean section (CS) wound—normal stitch line.

the nipples (Fig. 3)? Whether breasts are soft or engorged (Fig. 4)? Whether there is any palpable mass or an area which is firm, red, and tender? Is the inflamed area fluctuant? Whether milk or colostrum can be expressed from the breasts? Identification of abnormal findings (Fig. 5) can facilitate timely intervention for establishment of successful breastfeeding.

Systemic Examination

The cardiovascular, respiratory, and central nervous systems are systematically examined for any abnormality. For details of systemic examination, refer to Chapter 1.

Per Abdomen Examination

Inspection

Look for any obvious swelling or distension of abdomen. In case of cesarean section check whether the dressing is dry or soaked? In case there is no dressing the incision line is inspected for any redness, swelling, or discharge (Figs. 6 and 7).

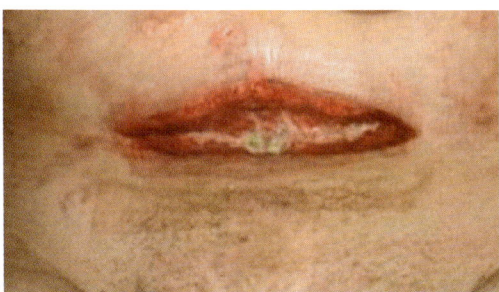

Fig. 7: Inspection of cesarean section (CS) wound—infected stitch line.

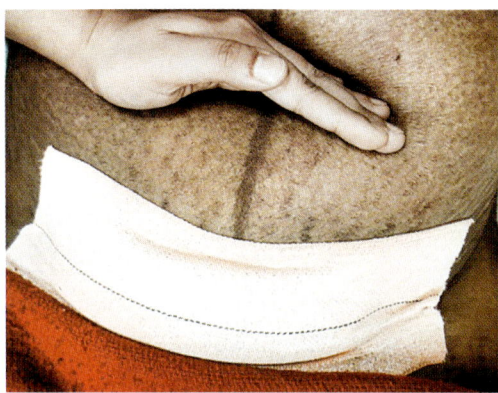

Fig. 8: Palpating postpartum uterus for involution.

Palpation

The abdomen is palpated for the uterus; its fundal height, consistency, and any tenderness.

Immediately after placental expulsion, the fundus of the contracted uterus is central and usually lies midway between umbilicus and pubic symphysis (Fig. 8). It rises to just below or above the umbilicus in next 12 hours. Then decreases at the rate of 1 cm per day and becomes a pelvic organ by 2 weeks postpartum due to involution. There is no involution of the uterus in the first 24 hours; it is contracted and retracted and should be described as that. Thereafter, it can be described as well involuted or subinvoluted. The uterus may appear larger in women with hydramnios and multiple pregnancy and smaller in women with fetal growth restriction, preterm birth, and lactating mothers.

The uterus is usually central but may be deviated on one side in the presence of a full bladder or a broad ligament hematoma. The uterus may be tender on palpation in women with cesarean section in the early postoperative period but tenderness later may suggest infection.

In women with abdominal distension, a distended bladder is ruled out and abdomen is systematically palpated for any tenderness, guarding, rigidity, or mass.

In women with an abdominal incision, the incision site is palpated for any induration or tenderness.

Percussion

Percussion is very useful to detect any fluid collection in abdominal cavity. In a postpartum woman, moderate amount of blood or fluid collection in abdomen may be missed on palpation due to laxity of abdomen following delivery of the baby. Careful percussion of the flanks for any dullness and eliciting shifting dullness is helpful in diagnosing free fluid in abdomen.

Auscultation

Abdomen is auscultated for the bowel sound for their presence or absence and their character. The bowel sounds are hypotonic in paralytic ileus and hyperdynamic in bowel obstruction.

Local Pelvic Examination

The vulva is examined for any swelling, discoloration, episiotomy site, and any purulent discharge. Routinely, no per speculum, per

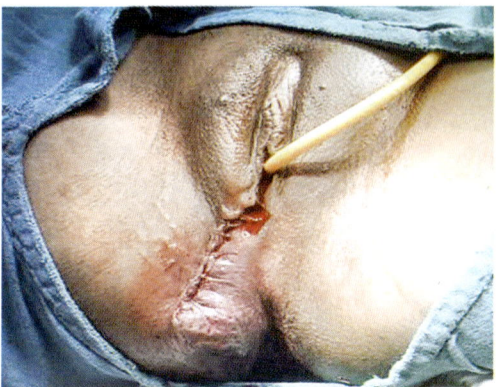

Fig. 9: Vulval hematoma.

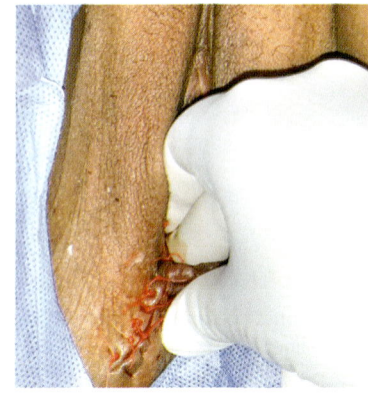

Fig. 10: Palpating episiotomy for induration.

vaginum, or per rectal examination is done. Per vaginal and per rectal examinations are done if a postnatal woman complains of retention of urine or extreme perineal pain or if there is a swelling or discoloration on the perineum or episiotomy site to exclude any vulvovaginal hematoma (Fig. 9). Per vaginal examination is also done to check for induration along the episiotomy site—if there is suspicion of infection later in puerperium (Fig. 10).

The perineal pad of the woman should be inspected for the color and odor of lochia.

INVESTIGATIONS

Usually, no investigations are required following normal vaginal delivery, but are indicated if any complication arises. Generally, following cesarean section, hemoglobin level, total and differential leukocyte count and urine examination are done as a routine on the third operative or second postoperative day.

EXAMINATION OF BABY

A detailed examination of the baby must be done by a neonatologist within 24 hours of birth (Box 1). The range of normal measure-

Box 1: Examination of newborn.[4]

- *Newborn's general appearance*: Whether looking well or ill
- *Observe the newborn's state of alertness*: The normal term newborn is alert and responsive
- Newborn's *gestational age* is verified
- *Head-to-toe examination*:
  - *Appearance*: Color, posture, activity, breathing behavior
  - *Skin*: Color and texture, birthmarks, rashes
  - *Head*: Size, shape, any swellings, and the cranial sutures are palpated
  - *Growth*: Record head circumference, weight, and length
  - *Face, nose, and eyes*: Observe for appearance and symmetry
  - *Mouth*: Check palate and tongue
  - *Ears*: Check for placement, shape, and symmetry
  - *Neck and clavicles*: Check for masses in the neck
  - *Heart*: Check color of mucus membranes and murmers
  - *Lungs*: Observe breathing
  - *Abdomen*: Check umbilical cord. Note for any abnormalities
  - *Genitalia*: Ask if there were any concerns raised about male infant's testes. Inspect female genitalia
  - *Spine*: Check for sacral dimple. Check skin integrity
  - *Upper and lower limbs*: Check for length, proportion, and symmetry; check for extra digits
  - *Hips*: Check tone and mobility of joint
  - *Central nervous system*: Check tone, behavior, movements, posture, and reflexes
  - *Cry*: Note the sound of baby's cry

Table 1: Variable range of normal values for neonates.[4]	
Heart rate	100–160 bpm
Respiratory rate	30–60 breath per min
Temperature	36.5–37.5°C
Length	48–53 cm
Head circumference	32–38 cm

Box 2: Signs of good attachment.
- Mother is sitting comfortably with her back straight and the back of the baby is straight
- Baby's mouth is wide open
- Areola is more visible above the baby's mouth than below
- Baby's lower lip is turned outward
- Baby's chin is touching mother's breast

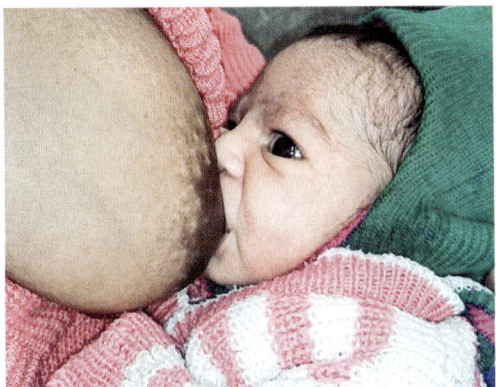

Fig. 11: Good attachment.

Box 3: Postnatal advice.
- Take enough rest and sleep
- Avoid heavy work for 6 weeks*
- Take extra and nutritious food
- Do exclusive breastfeeding for 6 months
- Take oral calcium and iron regularly for 6 months
- *Importance of washing for prevention of infection*:
  - Wash hands before handling baby
  - Wash perineum daily and after excretion
  - Change perineal pads every 4–6 hours and dispose them properly
  - Wash body daily
- Contraceptive advice
- Immunization advice
- Avoid sexual intercourse till perineal wound heals or 4 weeks, if no wound
- Follow-up after 6 weeks or earlier for any danger signal

*For postoperative cesarean section, women should avoid heavy work, especially lifting heavy weight for at least 3 months.

ments of a newborn are as given in Table 1. On daily rounds, the obstetrician or neonatologist should ask if the baby is feeding and sleeping well and passing urine and stools normally. The latching of the baby is observed for signs of good latching (Fig. 11 and Box 2).

The baby is checked for its hydration status, jaundice, and state of umbilical cord stump. Ask for any other complaints regarding baby such as fever or discharge from the eyes.

MANAGEMENT

Before discharge, the patient should be given proper advice regarding the care she should take of herself and her newborn (Box 3). She is told about the danger signs that should trigger a visit to health facility (Box 4). The World Health Organization (WHO) recommends at least three postnatal contacts for all mothers and newborns, on day 3 (48–72 hours), between days 7 and 14 after birth, and 6 weeks after birth.[5]

KEY POINTS

- The postnatal period is a time of rapid physiological adjustment for the mother to the return to the nonpregnant state, and for the newborn adapting to life outside the uterus.
- After an uncomplicated vaginal birth in a health facility, healthy mothers and

Flowchart 1: Algorithm for clinical approach to a postnatal woman.

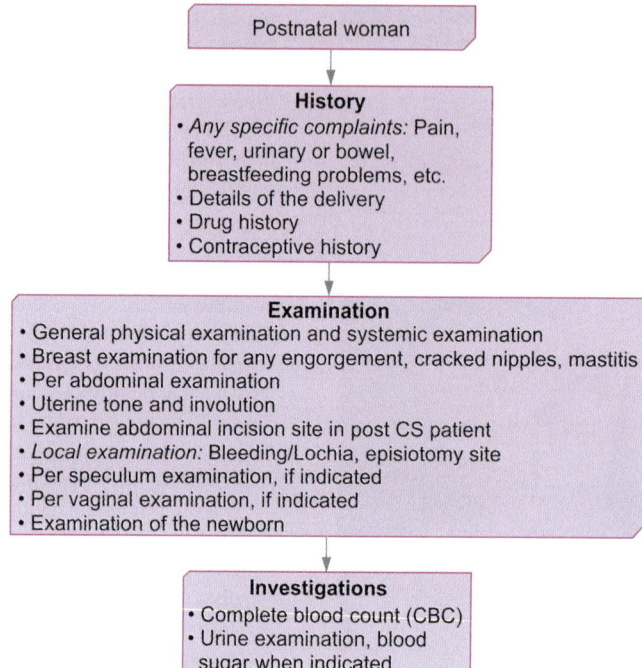

Box 4: Danger signals.

Red flag (Report to health facility immediately):
- Excessive vaginal bleeding
- Convulsions
- Headache with blurred vision
- Fast or difficult breathing
- Fever and too weak to get out of bed
- Severe abdominal pain
- Calf pain, redness, or swelling
- Shortness of breath or chest pain

Others (Go to health center as soon as possible):
- Fever
- Abdominal pain
- Feels ill
- Breasts swollen, red or tender breasts, or sore nipple
- Urine dribbling or pain on micturition
- Pain in the perineum or draining pus
- Foul-smelling lochia
- Severe depression or suicidal behavior (ideas or attempts)

newborns should receive care in the facility for at least 24 hours after birth.
- Starting from the first hour after birth, all postpartum women should have regular assessment of pulse, uterine tone, temperature, fundal height, and vaginal bleeding.
- Blood pressure should be measured shortly after birth. If normal, the second blood pressure measurement should be taken within 6 hours.
- Urine void should be documented within 6 hours.
- Health assessment of the well mother and baby should occur within 2–4 days of leaving the hospital and then at 7–10 days of delivery.
- Breastfeeding progress should be assessed at each postnatal contact and exclusive breastfeeding should be encouraged.

- Postnatal women and their newborns should be screened for any danger signs.
- Mother and family should be encouraged to seek healthcare early if they identify any of the danger signs in between postnatal care visits.
- Women should be counseled on nutrition, hygiene, birth spacing, and family planning. Contraceptive options should be discussed, and contraceptive methods should be provided if requested.

REFERENCES

1. Li XF, Fortney JA, Kotelchuck M. The postpartum period: the key to maternal mortality. Int J Gynaecol Obstet. 1996;54(1):1-10.
2. Campbell OMR, Gray RH. Characteristics and determinants of postpartum ovarian function in women in the United States. Am J Obstet Gynecol. 1993;169(1):55-60.
3. Oppenheimer LW, Sherriff EA, Goodman JD, Shah D, James CE.. The duration of lochia. Br J Obstet Gynaecol. 1986;93(7):754-7.
4. Public Health England. (2018). Service Specification No. 21: Newborn and Infant Physical Examination Screening Programme. [online] Available from https://www.england.nhs.uk/wp-content/uploads/2017/04/Gateway-ref-07842-180913-Service-specification-No.-21-NHS-Newborn-and-Infant-Physical-Examination.pdf. [Last accessed January, 2020].
5. World Health Organization (2013). WHO recommendations on postnatal care of the mother and newborn. [online] Available from https://www.who.int/maternal_child_adolescent/documents/postnatal-care-recommendations/en/. [Last accessed January, 2020].

SUGGESTED READING

1. ACOG Committee Opinion No. 736: Optimizing Postpartum Care. Obstet Gynecol. 2018;131(15):e140-50.
2. American College of Obstetricians and Gynecologists. (2018). ACOG Postpartum Toolkit. [online] Available from https://www.acog.org/-/media/Departments/Toolkits-for-Health-Care-Providers/Postpartum-Toolkit/2018-Postpartum-Toolkit.ashx. [[Last accessed January, 2020].
3. Berens P. (2019). Overview of the postpartum period: Physiology, complications, and maternal care. [online] Available from https://www.uptodate.com/contents/overview-of-the-postpartum-period-physiology-complications-and-maternal-care. [Last accessed January, 2020].
4. Haran C, van Driel M, Mitchell BL, Brodribb WE. Clinical guidelines for postpartum women and infants in primary care–a systematic review. BMC Pregnancy Childbirth. 2014;14:51.
5. National Institute for Health and Clinical Excellence. (2006). Postnatal care up to 8 weeks after birth NICE guideline. [online] Available from https://www.nice.org.uk/guidance/cg37. [Last accessed January, 2020].
6. World Health Organization. (2012). WHO recommendations for the prevention and treatment of postpartum haemorrhage. [online] Available from https://www.who.int/reproductivehealth/publications/maternal_perinatal_health/9789241548502/en/. [Last accessed January, 2020].

27. Approach to a Woman with Specific Problems in Puerperium

Priyanka Arora, Isha Khurana Vashisht

INTRODUCTION

Puerperium is often referred to as the fourth trimester of pregnancy, a period between delivery and complete physiological involution. This period tests the true resilience of the postnatal woman to adapt both physically as well as mentally from being a woman to a mother. This phase does not get as much attention as it should. The role of the obstetrician does not just end with delivering the baby; he/she needs to take the woman through this demanding phase of reproductive process. This chapter focuses on the approach to various common problems of puerperium, which are often perplexing as well as challenging. These include:
- Fever
- Pain in lower abdomen
- Malodorous discharge per vaginum
- Breast complaints
- Swelling of the leg
- Urinary complaints
- Bowel complaints.

The history of a woman presenting with some complaint in postnatal period would essentially be guided by the presenting complaint. The knowledge of the differential diagnosis for each complaint is important to elicit a good history. The relevant details for various complaints listed above are given below along with the relevant history, examination, and investigations for each complaint.

FEVER

Low-grade fever in the first 24 hours of postnatal period is normal, especially following normal vaginal delivery. Presence of fever up to or >100.4°F (38°C) on at least two occasions 24 hours apart within first 10 days following delivery excluding the first 24 hours is defined as postpartum febrile morbidity or puerperal pyrexia. Postpartum shivering is common and is observed in 25–50% women. It starts within 1–30 minutes after delivery and lasts for 2–60 minutes. The exact cause is not known but is probably a response to fall in body temperature due to bleeding during delivery, placental separation, oxytocic agents, or bacteremia.[1]

History of Presenting Complaint

A detailed history of the presenting complaint is elicited as regards its onset, duration, severity, and pattern. Fever occurring within 24 hours may be due to stress of labor or due to antepartum causes such as urinary tract infection (UTI), premature rupture of membranes (PROM) and chorioamnionitis, or causes unrelated to pregnancy such as COVID, malaria and chest infection.

Duration is important to correlate it with any antecedent event. The severity and pattern of fever gives a clue regarding the underlying pathology. It is low grade and associated with dry cough, myalgias or breathlessness in COVID. The fever is intermittent with rigors and chills in malaria, UTI, septicemia, abscess, etc. It is without rigors and chills in endometritis, breast engorgement, thrombophlebitis, and wound infection. It is high grade in genitourinary infections, pneumonia, septicemia and usually low grade in tuberculosis and endometritis.

History of High-risk Factors

An important aspect of history in postnatal women with fever is to look for any high-risk factors by taking a detailed history of any contact with COVID positive person or if she is from containment area. The details of delivery as regards the place where it was conducted and the person who conducted the delivery, whether the birth attendant observed aseptic precautions such as washing hands and wearing sterile gloves. It is important to know if there was any history of prolonged leaking per vaginum (>18 hours), duration of labor, number of prevaginal examinations done, mode of delivery; vaginal or abdominal, whether any episiotomy was given, was it an instrumental delivery. Was there any third-stage complication such as postpartum hemorrhage (PPH), retained placenta, manual removal of placenta (MRP), repair of any genital tract trauma, or any history of blood transfusion or any comorbid condition such as anemia, diabetes mellitus, HIV, or any chronic illness during pregnancy?

History of Localizing Features

The woman should be asked for any associated complaints for localization of the source of fever. Table 1 gives the various causes of fever with the relevant history and examination findings.

Table 1: Differential diagnosis of fever.

Cause	Specific history points	Specific findings on examination	Specific investigations
Surgical site infection	Throbbing pain along incision in abdomen/perineum, purulent discharge, and gaping of wound	The area is red swollen indurated and purulent discharge may be seen	Wound swab for culture sensitivity (CS)
Breast complications (Breast engorgement and mastitis)	Pain, redness, hardness, and cracking of nipples difficulty and pain in feeding (Fig. 1)	Cracked nipples, any area of redness, engorgement, induration, or presence of a fluctuant swelling suggestive of breast abscess	• Pus for CS • Ultrasound of breast to detect an abscess
Urinary tract infection	Frequency of micturition, dysuria, pain in lower abdomen and lumbar region	Suprapubic tenderness and costovertebral angle tenderness	Urine for complete examination and CS
Endometritis	• Mild lower abdominal pain or there may be no symptoms, except fever • *Risk factors*: History of prolonged leaking per vaginum > 18 hours, multiple prevaginal examinations, home delivery by unskilled attendant without aseptic precautions	• Purulent discharge on per speculum examination • A subinvoluted tender uterus on per abdomen or per vaginal examination is indicative of endometritis • Retained products of conception or placental bits may be felt in uterine cavity	• High vaginal or cervical swab for CS • USG of abdomen or pelvis for any retained products in uterus, collection in pelvis or abdomen

Contd...

Contd...

Cause	Specific history points	Specific findings on examination	Specific investigations
Septic thrombophlebitis (ovarian vein or pelvic veins)	Swelling and or pain in leg/s or iliac fossa or lower abdomen	Leg swelling and tenderness are important signs of deep vein thrombosis. Presence of calf muscle tenderness is elicited by Homan's sign (Fig. 2)	Compressive ultrasound and venous Doppler studies
Infusion site thrombophlebitis	Pain at infusion site	Swelling, redness, and tenderness along the vein (Fig. 3)	
Injection site abscess (gluteal or upper arm)	Pain and hardness at injection site	Redness in the area, indurated tender mass with or without fluctuations (Fig. 4)	
Retained pack/swab in vagina or abdomen	• History of surgical intervention episiotomy, CS • Abdominal pain and distension in retained abdominal pack • Foul-smelling discharge per vaginum in case of retained vaginal swab	• A swab may be seen in vagina on per speculum examination • Purulent discharge from the wound, ill-defined mass may be palpable per abdomen	CT scan for any foreign body in abdomen or pelvis
Respiratory complications (after GA)	Cough, breathlessness, and difficulty in breathing	Tachypnea and use of accessory respiratory muscles	X-ray chest ABG
Incidental causes: • Malaria • TB • Gastroenteritis COVID 19	• Intermittent fever with chill and rigors • Productive cough • Abdominal pain, vomiting, and/or diarrhea • History of contact, fever with dry cough breathlessness	• No specific findings • Crepts and rhonchi in chest • Abdominal tenderness • No signs • ↓ oxygen saturation • Crepts and rhonchi in chest	• Peripheral smear for malarial parasite • X-ray chest, sputum for AFB • Throat swab RT PCT SARS-CoV-2 • X-ray chest

(AFB: acid-fast bacilli; CS: culture and susceptibility; CT: computed tomography; GA: general anesthesia; USG: ultrasonography; TB: tuberculosis; ABG: arterial blood gases)

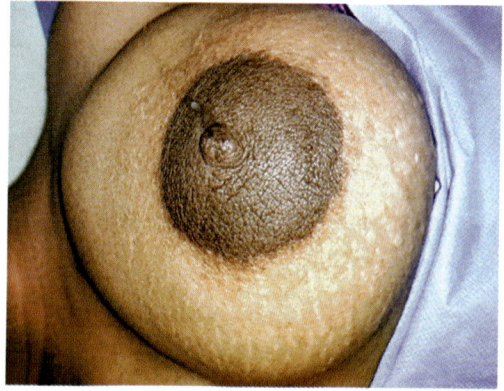

Fig. 1: Engorged breast.

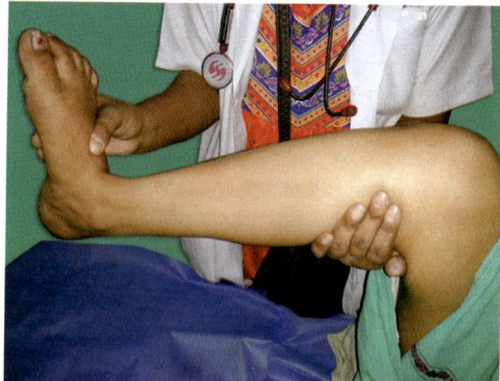

Fig. 2: Eliciting Homan's sign.

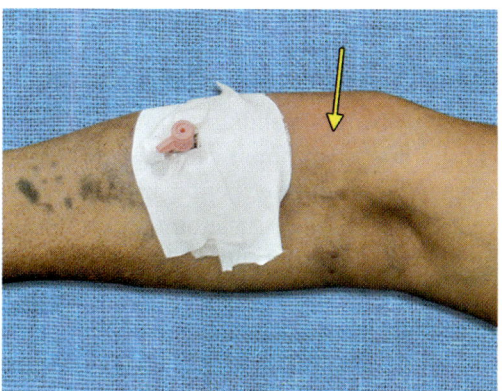

Fig. 3: Superficial thrombophlebitis.

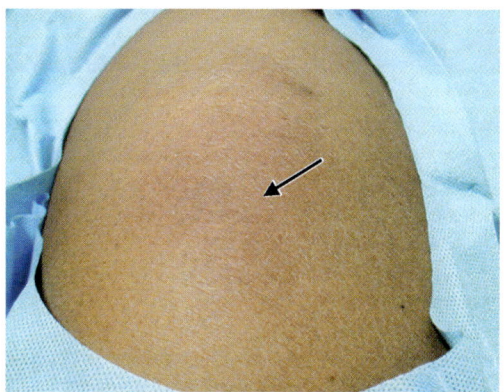

Fig. 4: Injection site abscess.

PAIN IN LOWER ABDOMEN

Pain is a common symptom in the immediate postpartum period. It is usually related to common puerperium-related conditions such as afterpains, incision site pain, and constipation. It may be due to serious gynecological or nongynecological conditions unrelated to puerperium needing immediate attention.

The approach is the same as in nonpregnant women with the initial aim to identify those with a serious cause requiring urgent intervention (Refer to Chapter 35, Approach to a woman with pain lower abdomen).

Afterpains are hypertonic uterine contractions for the first 36–48 hours after birth causing spasmodic central, intermittent lower abdominal pain, which usually improve by the end of 1st week of postpartum period. Typically, it gets exacerbated by breastfeeding and is worse in multiparous women.

In a woman who has undergone lower segment cesarean section (LSCS), incision site pain is usually severe, steady, and worsens with movement or deep breathing. However, it diminishes markedly after the first 12 or 24 hours. In addition, the woman may experience afterpains and pain due to constipation and failure to pass flatus following LSCS. These are usually relieved by second to third postoperative day, once the patient becomes ambulatory and starts taking full diet. Persistence of gas pains strongly suggests the onset of subacute intestinal obstruction.

Onset of a new pain or increase in pain at incision line in the postoperative patient demands urgent attention and meticulous search for cause. Rapidly increasing pain which is out of proportion to signs is suggestive of necrotizing fasciitis.

Differential Diagnosis

The causes of abdominal pain in puerperium can be puerperium related or nonpuerperium related. The causes unrelated to puerperium can be gynecological or nongynecological, as in nonpregnant women (Refer to Chapter 35, Approach to a woman with pain lower abdomen). The puerperium-related causes of pain abdomen are listed in Table 2.

History

The history and physical examination are vital in making the differential diagnosis of abdominal pain and steer the assessment.

Table 2: Puerperium-related causes of lower abdominal pain in puerperium.

Common	Uncommon

• Afterpains (uterine involution)
• UTI/acute urinary retention
• Incisional complications (hematoma, seroma, infection, and dehiscence)
• Endometritis
• Postoperative ileus
	• Life-threatening causes:
	  – Necrotizing soft-tissue infection (postcesarean section and episiotomy)
	  – Group A streptococcal infection (endomyometritis and wound infection)
	• Other serious causes:
	  – Hemorrhage/uterine scar dehiscence
	  – Unrecognized injury to viscera
	  – Foreign body left in abdomen during cesarean section
	  – Intra-abdominal or pelvic abscess
	  – Pregnancy-related liver disease (HELLP)
	  – Ovarian vein thrombophlebitis
	  – Myocardial infarction
	  – *Clostridioides difficile*
	  – Acute colonic Pseudo-obstruction

(HELLP: hemolysis, elevated liver enzymes, low platelet count; UTI: urinary tract infection)

History of Present Illness

The location of abdominal pain is important in making the diagnosis. Midline, intermittent, lower abdominal, and back pain are generally due to uterine involution. Pain associated with incisional complications in cesarean section such as hematoma is more diffuse and over the stitch line. Unexplained pain over stitch line, which increases rapidly over time may be the first manifestation of necrotizing fasciitis. Suprapubic and abdominal pain with difficulty or inability to pass urine may point toward UTI or acute urinary retention. Pain associated with rare postpartum condition—ovarian vein thrombophlebitis is localized to the side of affected vein in the flank or back.

Pain in upper abdomen in puerperium can be due to common causes such as gastroesophageal reflux, peptic ulcer disease, gallbladder disease, skeletomuscular injury, or due to uncommon and serious causes such as rectal sheath hematoma, bowel obstruction, perforation, hepatitis, aneurysmal rupture, hiatus hernia, and HELLP (hemolysis, elevated liver enzymes, low platelet count).

Appendicitis often produces pain in the periumbilical area and right lower quadrant; diverticulitis usually gives rise to lower abdominal pain in the midline or left lower quadrant. Pain due to ovarian torsion or rupture is unilateral and may be associated with a rounded swelling near the uterus but separate from it. It is almost always associated with vomiting at the onset of pain. However, in appendicitis the vomiting usually presents late. In postpartum endometritis and degeneration in a leiomyoma, the pain is over the uterus, which may be soft and subinvoluted on palpation.

Onset of pain helps in determining the underlying pathology. Acute intermittent pain in lower abdomen not persisting beyond first week postpartum suggests afterpains. Pain due to constipation can be both insidious and acute. It generally relieves with passage of flatus. Pain due to stitch line complications is generally insidious in onset and slowly progressing. Acute onset lower abdominal pain may also be due to appendicitis, biliary or renal colic, mesenteric infarction, cystitis, and gastroenteritis.

Character of the pain is important for understanding the origin of pain. Visceral pain is usually dull aching in character. Parietal pain is sharp and well-localized. Referred pain is aching in character and perceived to be near the surface of the body. Intermittent colicky pain abdomen can be due to afterpains, gas pains, colitis, renal or biliary colic. Constant pain in abdomen can be due to stitch line complications, urinary retention, hemoperitoneum, and constipation.

The onset, frequency, and duration of the pain are helpful features. The pain associated with postpartum endometritis usually develops within the first postpartum week.

It is important to ask the patient for factors that aggravate or alleviate the pain. Pain of peritonitis is minimized or relieved if the woman lies straight and motionless on her back. Pain in twisted ovarian cysts is also related to position as some postures may relieve the tension on the twisted pedicle.

Symptoms such as nausea, vomiting, fever, chills, weight loss, diarrhea or constipation, happening in relation to abdominal pain may give important clues to the diagnosis and help in differential diagnosis. Vomiting with constipation occurs in cases of bowel obstruction. Vomiting usually precedes pain in gastroenteritis. In appendicitis, vomiting usually occurs a few hours after the onset of pain. Vomiting also occurs almost always with the pain due to adnexal torsion or rupture of ovarian cysts due to peritoneal irritation.

Fever is usually present in cases of torsion of ovarian cyst, postpartum endometritis, degeneration of fibroids, ovarian vein thrombosis, and incision site complications. Associated urinary symptoms such as frequency or dysuria or inability to pass adequate volume of urine may point toward a UTI or acute urinary retention.

Past Medical and Surgical History

Past medical and surgical history is important, including details of any abdominal surgery. Any history of abdominal surgery increases the risk of bowel obstruction. History of adnexal pathology such as ovarian or paratubal cyst and hydrosalpinx is a risk factor for adnexal torsion. History of similar episodes of pain points toward inflammatory bowel disease.

Examination

General Physical Examination

The general appearance and level of comfort or discomfort should be noted. A patient of ovarian torsion would be writhing in pain, whereas in peritonitis, the patient lies still to avoid any movement which incites pain. Pallor of skin is noted. Hydration status is checked for by looking at the tongue. Dehydration will be marked in cases of bowel obstruction, gastroenteritis, or ovarian cyst rupture.

Vital signs are recorded. Tachycardia can occur due to pain or dehydration. Women with internal bleed or severe sepsis as with group A *Streptococcus* (GAS) may be hemodynamically unstable. There is tachycardia and low blood pressure and it calls for immediate resuscitation and urgent intervention. Pallor is an accompanying sign in a woman with internal bleed.

Low-grade fever can be present in a variety of conditions such as torsion of ovarian cysts, degeneration of a fibroid, septic thrombophlebitis, and ovarian vein thrombophlebitis.

The eyes should be examined for scleral icterus and the skin for jaundice.

Chest and Cardiovascular Examination

The lungs need to be examined for signs of consolidation and the heart for murmurs and rubs.

Per Abdomen Examination

In postcesarean women with rapidly increasing severe pain at surgical site, look for erythema, skin necrosis, induration, crepitus, and anesthesia which is suggestive of necrotizing fasciitis.

Palpation of the abdomen must be performed gently. It is important to keep the patient distracted, to rule out psychogenic pain. It is best to begin the palpation at an area away from the site of pain. Rigidity and muscle guarding are important and early signs of peritonitis. They can be localized as in a patient with a focal inflammatory mass, such as a diverticular abscess or diffuse as in peritonitis. Guarding is typically absent with deeper sources of pain such as renal colic. In cases of appendicitis and pelvic peritonitis with endometritis, there may be rebound tenderness due to peritonitis.

Palpation also may detect enlarged organs or masses. A full bladder may be palpable in cases of urinary retention. Subinvoluted and tender uterus may be palpable in cases of endometritis. Tenderness over the fibroid or the uterus may be present in cases of a degenerating leiomyoma. Tenderness may be present in the pelvis in cases of torsion or rupture of ovarian cysts and ovarian vein thrombophlebitis. Pelvic tenderness is typically absent in cases of septic pelvic thrombophlebitis.

Auscultation of the abdomen may be helpful in the evaluation of abdominal pain. Bowel sounds are absent in advanced peritonitis or adynamic ileus, whereas they are exaggerated in early bowel obstruction. Ileus may be present in peritonitis, injury to viscera during cesarean section and sometimes in ovarian vein thrombophlebitis.

Pelvic Examination

A pelvic examination is generally indicated in all women with acute lower abdominal pain. The pelvic examination is critical for determining whether abdominal pain is due to uterus and adnexa or due to nongynecological causes. A per speculum examination may reveal purulent cervical/vaginal discharge in endomyometritis. Per vaginum and per rectal examination is done to confirm the size of uterus, whether tender or not, and for any collection or mass in the pouch of Douglas. Fullness in fornices is present in cases of collection in pelvis.

Investigations

The investigations are advised depending on the working diagnosis based on history and examination. The initial aim is to rule out life threatening and serious conditions such as intraperitoneal hemorrhage, acute obstruction, ovarian torsion, or peritonitis. After an acute surgical emergency is excluded, search for other causes of abdominal pain is done. Patients are kept nil per oral till acute surgical emergency is ruled out.

Ultrasound examination is a useful tool to rule out intraperitoneal bleed or collection in abdomen and pelvis, rectus muscle, or liver hematoma, any ovarian cyst, fibroid uterus, to mass, appendicitis, etc.

Abdominal radiographs including an upright radiograph are important for finding the cause of acute abdomen. Proximally dilated bowel loops are characteristic of intestinal obstruction and air under the diaphragm confirms the suspicion of intestinal perforation. However, if computed tomography (CT) is available, it is preferable for the diagnosis of suspected partial or complete intestinal obstruction.

Abdominal CT is helpful as an alternative to ultrasound or for resolving the equivocal ultrasound findings.

The following laboratory tests should be done:
- Complete blood count (CBC) with differential leukocyte count
- Serum amylase and serum lipase
- *Serum electrolytes*: Serum sodium, potassium, and calcium
- Liver function test (LFT), kidney function test (KFT), and blood glucose
- Prothrombin time and partial thromboplastin time
- Urine routine, microscopy, and culture.

Sometimes, when proper diagnosis is not possible with radiological modalities, then diagnostic laparoscopy may be required.

MALODOROUS DISCHARGE PER VAGINUM

Postnatal woman may present with the complaint of foul-smelling discharge per vaginal. It is important to understand the evolution of normal lochia, i.e., normal shedding of decidua and blood for the initial few days. It is dark red or brown for a few days (lochia rubra), then progressively becomes watery and pinkish brown for 2–3 weeks (lochia serosa), and then turns yellowish white (lochia alba). It usually lasts for 4 weeks and is not accompanied with any foul smell. Concern usually arises, if there is heavy bleeding per vaginum with passage of clots or if there is foul-smelling discharge per vaginum. Foul-smelling discharge suggests underlying infection.

Differential Diagnosis

Foul-smelling vaginal discharge can be due to a spectrum of causes (Box 1).

History

Details regarding the nature of discharge should be inquired as regards its onset, duration, and any recent change in the nature.

Box 1: Causes of foul-smelling vaginal discharge.
- Infection (endometritis or local episiotomy site)
- Foreign body (forgotten packs and/or swabs)
- Fistulae (urinary or fecal)
- Malignancy (undiagnosed)
- Others

The color of discharge is asked whether it is white, yellow, greenish, bloody, or clear like urine. It is yellowish in women with rectovaginal fistula or anal incontinence due to soiling with fecal matter. Its consistency is noted whether watery, mucoid, frothy, or thick. Its smell is noted whether it is uriniferous or fecal, or foul smelling. The amount is important, whether scanty or copious. Presence of any associated features such as fever, itching, burning, and dysuria are noted. Any problem related to episiotomy is asked pain, discharge or dehiscence.

History of presence of risk factors for endometritis such as prolonged labor, prolonged rupture of membranes, multiple vaginal examinations, compromised hygiene and nutrition, place of delivery, and any internal monitoring are asked for.

History of any medical disorder likely to lower immunity such as diabetes mellitus, human immunodeficiency virus (HIV) infection, anemia, or any chronic disease is elicited. Any history suggestive of genital tract malignancy should be elicited.

Examination

General Physical Examination

Signs of infection such as tachycardia and pyrexia should be looked for. Assessment of general nutrition, anemia, and other diseases should be done.

Abdominal Examination

Localizing signs such as lower abdominal tenderness, bulky subinvoluted tender uterus, or abdominal mass is suggestive of endometritis, parametritis and/or pelvic peritonitis.

Speculum Examination

Appearance of vulva and vagina, any discharge, and presence of forgotten vaginal packs are looked for. The vaginal discharge is inspected for its nature, amount, color, smell, and whether blood-stained or not, and whether it is coming out through the cervix. Vagina and cervix should be visualized for the presence of erosions, tears, growth or any defect (vesicovaginal fistula or rectovaginal fistula).

Per Vaginal Examination

Bimanual examination should be done to assess for uterine involution, any retained products and tenderness. Presence of any mass in fornices, especially pouch of Douglas may suggest tubo-ovarian (TO) masses or pelvic abscess. Pelvic collection can be confirmed on per rectal examination. The episiotomy is palpated for any induration or any communication with rectum, which can be further confirmed on per rectal examination.

Investigations

Complete blood count is done to detect neutrophilia, which suggests bacterial infection. Swabs for culture sensitivity from vagina, cervix, or infected episiotomy helps in identifying causative organism as well as its sensitivity to specific antibiotics.

Imaging techniques such as pelvic ultrasound helps to detect retained products, TO mass and detection of intra- and extrauterine collections. Cystoscopy, CT pyelography, proctosigmoidoscopy, and barium enema are indicated to diagnose genital fistulae.

BREAST COMPLICATIONS

One of the most important events in puerperium is establishment of lactation or breastfeeding. Even though it is a natural eventuality, it is often be sought with numerous problems, which need to be handled promptly or else lead to tremendous stress and anxiety often resulting in failure of lactation. The aim of the management is to carefully evaluate the symptom complex, reach a diagnosis, and plan treatment so that the lactation can be resumed.

History

Presenting Complaint

The main complaint with which the patient presents to the physician should be asked in detail. The spectrum of breast-related complaints includes no milk or less milk production or severe pain while breastfeeding.

Problems related to milk production: Most often the postnatal women complain of inadequate milk production. Only <1% women are physiologically incapable of lactation. Patient should be asked about the nature of secretion that can be expressed from the breast. Initially for first few days after delivery scanty thick yellowish colostrum can be expressed, proper flow of milk gets established after 2–3 days. This normal physiological pattern should be explained to the woman. It is prudent to ask for the breastfeeding practices being followed.

Engorgement: It is usual for the breasts to become distended and firm usually 1 or 2 days after delivery, due to let down reflex. Any prolonged engorgement should be addressed as it can ultimately lead to mastitis and fever.

Pain: Women may present with pain during breastfeeding. It is mostly due to breast

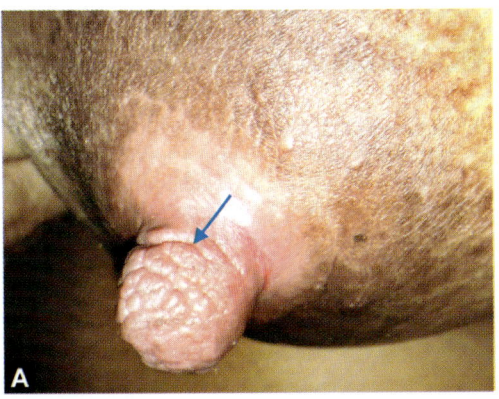 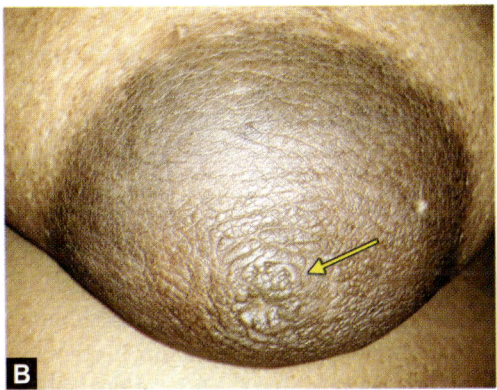

Figs. 5A and B: Breast conditions. (A) Cracked nipple; (B) Poorly formed flat nipple.

engorgement or cracked nipples rarely it may be due to mastitis and breast abscess. It can range from dull ache to severe pain. The woman may complain of hardening of breasts.

Nipple problems: This includes both sore and/or cracked nipples and retracted or poorly formed nipples (Figs. 5A and B). The associated pain with sore/cracked nipples can pose problems in breastfeeding.

Retracted nipples may also lead to poor attachment and inadequate milk flow with related problems such as engorged breasts and mastitis.

Associated Symptoms

The woman is asked about presence of fever, generalized body ache, malaise, and flu-like symptoms.

Breastfeeding Practice

It is extremely important to ask about breastfeeding practice, i.e., how the mother feeds her baby. Most common cause of puerperal breast problems is wrong breastfeeding practices. Details regarding the positioning, attachment, adequacy of feeding on alternate breast, frequency of feeding should be asked for.

Many times, proper counseling, and education is enough to resolve breast-related problems.

Baby Details

While evaluating the mother for breast problems, always remember to evaluate the baby. Feeding inadequacy may arise due to poor sucking in preterm, growth-restricted, and sick babies. Also babies with tongue-tied or cleft palate may have feeding difficulties, ultimately resulting in poor let-down reflex in the mother.

Unfortunately, all pregnancy outcomes are not happy. Mothers suffering from early perinatal loss face a different set of breast problems, which include engorged breasts, mastitis, etc., that needs to be handled differently as compared to mothers with live babies.

Examination

General Physical Examination

The general condition may vary from a stable to an extremely distressing state. The woman may be febrile and have tachycardia in conditions such as breast engorgement, mastitis, and breast abscess. A note of general nutrition and hydration should be made as these factors may cause inadequate lactation.

Breast Examination

The nipples may be cracked, retracted, or normal; bilateral breasts appear distended with prominent dilated veins on inspection and feel firm to hard and tender when engorged. In the presence of mastitis, the affected area looks red and it is warm, tender, and indurated on palpation. Sometimes mastitis progresses to an abscess which is fluctuant in the center.

A note of other breast conditions such breast mass, fibroadenoma, Paget's disease, or breast malignancy should be sought for as a part of opportunistic screening.

Investigations

Though clinical diagnosis is enough to identify the specific breast problem, some investigations may aid the diagnosis and provide useful information.

Complete blood counts for neutrophilia, ultrasonography of the breast for the diagnosis of breast abscess, and sometimes milk or pus for culture sensitivity are indicated. However, milk for culture sensitivity may not provide useful information due to contamination by maternal skin commensals.

SWELLING OF LEG

Swelling of leg/s is not a common problem and may be unilateral or bilateral (Table 3). The common causes of swelling of leg/s in postnatal women are deep vein thrombosis and hypoproteinemia. The risk of thrombosis is 2–5 times more common in postnatal period compared to antenatal period. The risk is highest in the first 6 weeks returning to that of a nonpregnant woman by 18 weeks' postpartum.[2] It is usually left sided due to venous stasis due to compression of left iliac vein by right iliac artery and of inferior vena cava by pregnant uterus. It is mostly femoral or iliac vein thrombosis.

The differential diagnosis of swelling of leg in a postnatal woman is listed in Table 3.

Careful clinical assessment of this symptom is necessary to detect underlying cause which can sometimes be life threatening.

Table 3: Differential diagnosis of a postnatal woman presenting with swelling of leg(s).

Unilateral	Bilateral
• Deep vein thrombosis (leg veins)	• Deep vein thrombosis (pelvic veins)
• Infection: Cellulitis	• Nutritional: Anemia, hypoproteinemia
• Trauma (calf muscle pull/tear)	• Medical disorders: Cardiac, hepatic, renal
• Surgery	
• Lymphatic: Filariasis	• Endocrine: Myxedema
• Malignancy: Compression, metastasis, and radiation	• Drug induced: Calcium channel blockers, steroids, etc.

History

The following points should be asked in case of leg swelling in puerperium: Whether it was pre-existing or developed in postpartum period; was the onset sudden or gradual; whether only one leg is involved or both legs are involved; is it confined to the foot or leg or is involving the whole limb; and whether there is any swelling of other parts of the body.

Any associated features such as pain, erythema, and tenderness may be suggestive of features of deep venous thrombosis (DVT). Pain in buttock, pelvis, or leg is suggestive of DVT. History of any preceding event such as trauma, surgery and immobilization, and exposure to some drug is elicited. Any aggravating factors such as increase on walking and/or squatting and any relieving factors such as rest, leg elevation, medication, etc. is inquired. Predisposing factors such as history of prolonged immobilization, cesarean section, thrombotic disorders and puerperal infection are looked for. Any history suggestive of medical diseases such as cardiac, renal, and hepatic disease is important.

Examination

On general physical examination in women with anemia and hypoproteinemia, pallor and other features of malnutrition such as cheilosis and glossitis may be present. The woman may be febrile if thrombophlebitis or puerperal sepsis is present. A detailed cardiovascular and respiratory examination for any valvular lesion or any sign of cardiac failure is done. Signs of pulmonary embolism, such as unexplained tachycardia, tachypnea, chest pain, fainting, and collapse, may be present. On per abdomen examination, any palpable mass in the iliac region or lower abdomen likely to be pressing on the iliac veins should be looked for, followed by a pelvic examination for any pathology causing pressure.

Most important tool for diagnosing deep vein thrombosis is clinical suspicion. It usually causes asymmetrical swelling in one limb, which is >2 cm greater in diameter than the other limb. The affected limb is red and warm. Pain in the calf during passive dorsiflexion of foot (Homan's sign) is positive in a third of women with DVT and is not a very reliable sign.

Investigations

These are noninvasive or invasive. Compressive ultrasound (CUS) is the preferred first-line investigation for diagnosis of proximal DVT. A positive CUS triggers treatment whereas a negative CUS in the presence of a strong clinical suspicion triggers alternate imaging modality Doppler ultrasound of iliac veins or a CT or MR venography. If the clinical suspicion is low, CUS can be repeated after 3 and 7 days.[3]

Advanced noninvasive imaging includes CT venography and magnetic resonance venography. It involves injection of intravenous contrast followed by imaging. It forms the gold standard for judging imaging methods. It is diagnostic for obstruction to blood supply from the affected vessel. Cost, invasiveness, availability restricts its use.

Invasive diagnostic technique includes conventional venography. With advent of CT and MR venography, its use is limited to complicated cases.

Blood investigations include CBC, coagulation profile, and D-dimer. CBC gives an overview of hemoglobin levels, leukocytosis, and thrombocytopenia. Coagulation profile detects the presence of any coagulation defect. D-dimer is a fibrinogen degradation product and an elevated level can result from plasmin dissolving a clot.

Allied investigations such as tests of pulmonary embolism include chest X-ray, electrocardiography (ECG), CT pulmonary angiography, ventilation perfusion scan. These may be indicated in some cases.

URINARY COMPLAINTS

Urinary problems are common in the immediate postpartum period. The common urinary problems are voiding difficulties, urinary retention, postpartum urinary incontinence mainly stress incontinence, or true incontinence and other problems such as urinary frequency, dysuria, and urgency suggestive of UTI. These are due to the impact of labor and delivery on the bladder and urethra. Both these organs are near the cervix and vagina and undergo stretching during labor and delivery. Timely diagnosis and correct management of these conditions is essential for restoration of normal bladder function.

Postpartum Urinary Retention

The exact incidence of the postpartum urinary retention (PPUR) is uncertain; it ranges from 0.05 to 37% in different studies.[4] The large variation in the incidence is because of difference in the focused symptoms ranging from overt and covert urinary retention to persistent urinary retention. Overt PUR is absence of spontaneous micturition after 6 hours of vaginal delivery or 6 hours of removal of catheter. Covert PUR is postvoid residual urinary volume >150 cc.

Postpartum Urinary Incontinence

Involuntary passage of urine with sudden increase in the intra-abdominal pressure is a common complaint during pregnancy and postpartum period. Prevalence of postpartum stress urinary incontinence (PPSUI) ranges from 7 to 40% according to different studies.[5]

The other type of incontinence is true incontinence or continuous dribbling of the urine, which generally occurs soon after cesarean section or cesarean hysterectomy due to surgical injury to the urinary bladder or ureter and following obstructed labor due to pressure necrosis of bladder neck. The vesicovaginal fistula due to surgical trauma presents in early postoperative period, but that due to obstructed labor-related pressure necrosis presents late, after 7–10 days of delivery or cesarean section.

The other common urinary problem is increased urinary frequency, which is mostly related to covert urinary retention and resolves with time. However, it may be an early symptom of UTI. Dysuria or painful micturition is generally related to infections of urinary tract, episiotomy, and peripartum catheterization.

Differential Diagnosis

The differential diagnosis of urinary problems is essentially related to the nature of urinary complaint (Table 4).

History

History of Present Illness

The history of present illness should include a detailed description of the nature of problem, its duration, timing of onset in relation to

Table 4: Postnatal urinary complaints and differential diagnosis.

Nature of urinary problem	Clinical presentation	Cause
Urinary retention overt or covert	• Inability to pass urine or passage of small amounts of urine. Full bladder palpable on per abdomen examination • Overt postpartum urinary retention (PPUR) is absence of spontaneous micturition after 6 hours of vaginal delivery or 6 hours of removal of catheter. Covert PPUR is postvoid residual urinary volume >150 cc	• Vaginal delivery, painful episiotomy, perineal tears, vulvar hematoma • Prolonged labor • Instrumental delivery • Epidural or spinal block • Postcesarean section • Intake of drugs like antidepressants, anticholinergic

Contd...

Contd...

Nature of urinary problem	Clinical presentation	Cause
Urinary incontinence: • Stress urinary incontinence	• Involuntary passage of urine on raising intra-abdominal pressure • Demonstration of escape of urine per urethra on coughing in a woman with full bladder	• Due to vaginal delivery, big baby, prolonged labor and instrumental delivery • Caused by stretching of pelvic tissues, and leading to disruption of integrity of urethral sphincter, and innervation of urethral sphincter and bladder neck
• True incontinence	• Continuous dribbling of urine	• Due to vesicovaginal or ureterovaginal fistula following cesarean section or cesarean hysterectomy or obstructed labor due to pressure necrosis
• Overflow incontinence	• Frequency or continuous dribbling of urine • Urinary bladder is distended and palpable per abdomen	• Covert retention urine
Dysuria	Painful micturition or burning during micturition	Urinary tract infection (UTI), episiotomy or perineal tear, and peripartum catheterization

delivery of baby, whether it was present in prepregnant state or during antenatal period, and any treatment received. Any history suggestive of diabetes mellitus needs to be recorded. Any history of fever, pain in lower abdomen, lumbar region, or perineum should be asked for. Fever with rigors and chills is suggestive of UTI. Any history of drug intake such as antidepressants with anticholinergic action such as imipramine should be elicited.

Obstetrical History

Obstetrical history includes the parity, mode of delivery whether spontaneous vaginal delivery, instrumental vaginal delivery, or cesarean section. The details recorded are:
- Duration of both first stage and second stages of labor
- Whether the labor was prolonged?
- Was the delivery difficult?
- Was there any instrumentation?
- Number of pelvic examinations done during labor
- What was the indication of cesarean section?
- If a cesarean birth, when was the woman catheterized for how long?
- What was the weight of the baby?

It is important to know, if the woman has an episiotomy or perineal tear and is it painful. History of any associated symptoms such as fever, pain in lower abdomen, or lumbar region is suggestive of UTI.

Examination

A general physical examination is carried out as in any other postnatal woman. The mental status of the woman is assessed, whether she is well oriented to time, place, and person. Her mood is assessed it may be low or sad as in postpartum depression or blues. A complete neurological examination is done to see the integrity of sensory and motor nerve fibers of S2, S3, and S4 (Refer to Chapter 42, Approach to a Woman Presenting with Urinary Incontinence).

Per Abdomen Examination

Assess whether the bladder is full. Palpate for any tenderness in lower abdomen and in renal angles, which is suggestive of cystitis or pyelonephritis, respectively. The uterus is assessed for its size and whether it is central, lifted, or deviated to one side as with full bladder.

Local Examination of Perineum

The woman is first examined with a full bladder in dorsal position with legs flexed at the hip and knee joints, and buttocks at the edge of the table. The labia are separated, and she is asked to cough—any demonstrable leak of urine is observed? She is then asked to pass urine for further examination with empty bladder. The episiotomy site is inspected for any swelling, redness, and tenderness. Presence of any vulvar, periurethral, vaginal, or perineal bruising, hematoma or lacerations is looked for.

Per Speculum Examination

Per speculum examination includes visualization of any vaginal hematoma, laceration, fistula, mass and any uterovaginal prolapse or inversion of the uterus.

Per Vaginal Examination

Per vaginal examination is done to detect any mass in the vagina such as fibroid polyp, uterine inversion, cervical fibroid, cervical descent, or any mass in pouch of Douglas.

Investigations

Investigations include a CBC with peripheral smear, kidney function tests, blood urea, and serum creatinine. The urine is subjected to routine microscopic examination, urine culture and sensitivity. Ultrasound abdomen and pelvis for kidneys, bladder, amount of residual urine, back pressure changes in urinary tract, bladder stones, and any pelvic hematomas.

Imaging of the pelvic floor is indicated to assess for the degree of trauma to levator ani muscle by three-dimensional (3D) translabial ultrasound and magnetic resonance imaging (MRI) in patients with postpartum urinary dysfunction.

Woman who is not relieved of the symptoms should be referred to an urogynecologist for a proper urodynamic evaluation and management. Patients with fistula are investigated and managed according to the site of fistula. The surgical intervention is indicated after 3 months once the tissues become healthy.

BOWEL COMPLAINTS

Bowel complaints are not uncommon in puerperium. The usual bowel complaints are constipation, diarrhea, and anal incontinence. These are mainly due to the trauma sustained by the perineal body during vaginal delivery, changes in diet during labor, and effect of drugs in postoperative or postnatal period. There is proximity of the anal canal to the vagina and perineal body and all are subjected to considerable stretch during labor with resultant neuromuscular damage such as pudendal neuropathy, fascial tears, and decreased muscular tone. It is more marked in prolonged labor.

Differential Diagnosis

The differential diagnosis of various bowel problems in postpartum period is detailed in Table 5.

History

History of Presenting Complaint

Postpartum anal incontinence:
In women presenting with complaints of anal incontinence, it is important to find

Table 5: Differential diagnosis of bowel problems in postpartum period.

Bowel complaints	Causes
Anal incontinence	Episiotomy, third- or fourth-degree perineal tears
Postpartum diarrhea	• *Drug induced*: Prostaglandins, broad-spectrum antibiotics, and iron supplements • Puerperal sepsis with pelvic abscess • Gastroenteritis • Pre-existing conditions such as: 　– Inflammatory bowel disease 　– Irritable bowel syndrome 　– Malabsorption syndrome
Postpartum constipation	• Decreased colonic motility due to vasodilatory prostaglandin and vascular endothelial substances • Change in diet and decreased intake of fluid and fibers • Postpartum stress and depression • Postponement of bowel movement due to painful tears or episiotomy • Reduced physical activity in postpartum • Other uncommon conditions such as hypothyroidism, drugs such as codeine, morphine, and anticholinergic drugs, postpartum depression

out the nature and severity of incontinence, whether it is involuntary and recognized passage of flatus, liquid, or solid stool, i.e., urge incontinence, or unrecognized anal leakage, i.e., passive incontinence or fecal soiling of clothes. The duration of symptom and its relation to delivery is asked, whether it was present in antenatal period or before pregnancy. It is important to take a detailed obstetric history including the parity, duration of labor, mode of delivery vaginal, or cesarean section, whether any instrumentation was done or not, epidural analgesia received or not, episiotomy given or not, any tears sustained during delivery and the weight of the baby. All these are risk factors for anal incontinence. It is also important to know, if there was any infection of the episiotomy site or repaired tear.

It is important to assess the impact of anal incontinence on the quality of life of the woman by enquiring about any alteration in lifestyle, need to wear a perineal pad and inability to socialize due to incontinence.

Postpartum diarrhea:
The details of the nature and severity of symptom are asked as regards frequency of stools, consistency, passage of blood and mucus, and any associated nausea and vomiting. This is suggestive of infection of the gastrointestinal tract. History of urgency of defecation is associated with injury to external anal sphincter or may sometimes be drug induced. Pain in lower abdomen, fever, and unhealthy vaginal discharge along with passage of loose stools are suggestive of puerperal sepsis with pelvic abscess.

It is important to find out any history of administration of drugs such as any broad-spectrum antibiotics or any oral iron preparation or prostaglandins specially PGF2α, which contracts smooth muscles, and causes vomiting and diarrhea.

Sometimes, the problem may have been existing even before pregnancy or in antenatal period and gets aggravated in the postpartum period as with conditions such as malabsorption syndrome, inflammatory bowel disease, and irritable bowel syndrome. Any treatment received for the same in the past should be recorded.

Postpartum constipation:
Postpartum constipation is a common problem often encountered in the postpartum period. The history should be directed

toward the onset, duration, and severity of problem. Whether the woman had constipation before or during pregnancy? What treatment did she take? She should be asked about her dietary intake. Is she taking adequate amount of liquids and fibers; does she have an episiotomy and is it painful? Is the defecation painful and is there any bleeding per rectum? This is suggestive of anal fissure and piles, respectively.

History of drug intake is important. Iron preparations sometimes cause constipation although most often they cause diarrhea. Anticholinergic drugs such as antidepressants, and antiallergics cause constipation.

The woman should be interviewed for any symptoms of depression such as low or sad mood, tearfulness, lack of drive, easy fatigability, and loss of appetite. Constipation is an important symptom of depression and depression per se is common in postpartum period.

Whether the woman is ambulatory or not also has an impact on her bowel function. In women who are not ambulatory, especially in postcesarean women ambulation improves the general well-being and helps restore the bowel activity.

Examination

In women presenting with anal incontinence, there may be an unrepaired third-or fourth-degree perineal tear present on local examination of the perineum. Local scarring and gaping of anal orifice and perianal soiling may be observed. There may be absence of cutaneous anal reflex on local examination of perineum.

On per speculum examination, a rectovaginal fistula may be appreciated. On per rectal examination, there may be absence of tone of external anal sphincter.

In women with diarrhea due to gastroenteritis, fever, tachycardia, and dehydration may be present on general examination. On abdominal examination, abdomen may be distended with generalized tenderness and the bowel sounds may be tinkling suggestive of paralytic ileus. In Crohn's disease, perineal examination may show presence of fistula and scarring, and postperineal repair sepsis.

Patients with pelvic abscess or peritonitis may also complaint of diarrhea with fever among other findings as discussed before.

In women with postpartum constipation abdomen may be distended with exaggerated bowel sounds suggestive of obstruction. On per rectal examination, the rectum is loaded lumpy, and firm to hard pieces of stools are felt. A loaded rectum can also be appreciated on per vaginal examination, can be digitally evacuated. Sometimes, the fecaliths felt in the sigmoid colon or rectum can be confused with a pelvic mass. Successful indentation of fecaliths and per rectal examination confirms the diagnosis. Anal spasm and tenderness due to external hemorrhoids or anal fissure may be present.

Investigations

Anal Incontinence

Anal manometry is indicated to assess the tone and contractile function of the anal sphincter. Endoanal ultrasound is done to assess anatomic integrity of the internal and external anal sphincters. Detailed neurophysiological assessment should be done in women presenting for secondary anal sphincter repair.

Diarrhea

No specific investigations are indicated in most women. Serum electrolytes and kidney function tests are done in all women. Stool examination for ova, cyst, pus cells, and culture sensitivity may be carried out. In women with fever, total and differential counts and ultrasound of abdomen and pelvis for any collection in pelvis is done. However, in Crohn's disease and inflammatory bowel disease sigmoidoscopy or colonoscopy may be indicated to confirm mucosal inflammation.

Constipation

Proctoscopic examination may show internal hemorrhoids.

MANAGEMENT

The management of each complication is according to the cause identified. It is important to identify life-threatening complications such as headache, new hypertension, seizures, excessive bleeding, chest pain, dyspnea, and severe pain in abdomen or perineum at the earliest and institute immediate treatment to prevent maternal mortality and morbidity. Refer to the section on suggested reading for the management of various complications in the postnatal period.

KEY POINTS

- Postpartum period is the 6–8 weeks period from delivery of the baby during which the various organs of the woman revert to their nonpregnant state.
- This period should be carefully supervised for early diagnosis and treatment of life-threatening complications such as hemorrhage, severe pre-eclampsia, eclampsia, pulmonary embolism, necrotizing fasciitis, and GAS infection.
- The common non-life-threatening problems in puerperium include fever, pain in lower abdomen, malodorous vaginal discharge, breast problems, swelling of the leg, urinary and bowel problems, and perinatal depression.
- The knowledge of the various causes of these symptoms is important to systematically identify and confirm the diagnosis and institute-specific treatment.

REFERENCES

1. Benson MD, Haney E, Dinsmoor M, Beaumont JL. Shaking rigors in parturients. J Reprod Med. 2008;53(9):685-90.
2. Kamel H, Navi BB, Sriram N, Hovsepian DA, Devereux RB, Elkind MS. Risk of a thrombotic event after the 6-week postpartum period. N Engl J Med. 2014;370(14):1307-15.
3. Bates SM, Jaeschke R, Stevens SM, Goodacre S, Wells PS, Stevenson MD, et al. Diagnosis of DVT: Antithrombotic Therapy and Prevention of Thrombosis, 9th ed: American College of Chest Physicians Evidence-Based Clinical Practice Guidelines. Chest. 2012;141(2 Suppl.):e351S-418S.
4. Lim JL. Post-partum voiding dysfunction and urinary retention. Aust N Z J Obstet Gynaecol. 2010;50(6):502-5.
5. Reilly ET, Freeman RM, Waterfield MR, Waterfield AE, Steggles P, Pedlar F. Prevention of postpartum stress incontinence in primigravidae with increased bladder neck mobility: a randomised controlled trial of antenatal pelvic floor exercises. BJOG. 2002;109(1):68-76.

SUGGESTED READING

1. ACOG Committee Opinion No. 736: Optimizing Postpartum Care. Obstet Gynecol. 2018;131(5):e140-50.
2. ACOG Committee Opinion No. 742: Postpartum Pain Management. Obstet Gynecol. 2018;132(1):e35-43.
3. Committee on Practice Bulletins--Gynecology, American College of Obstetricians and Gynecologists. ACOG Practice Bulletin No. 84: Prevention of deep vein thrombosis and pulmonary embolism. Obstet Gynecol. 2007;110(2 Pt 1):429-40.

4. Royal College of Obstetricians and Gynaecologists (RCOG). (2012). Bacterial sepsis following pregnancy (Green-top Guideline No. 64b). [online] Available from https://www.rcog.org.uk/globalassets/documents/guidelines/gtg_64b.pdf. [Last accessed April, 2020].
5. Royal College of Obstetricians and Gynaecologists (RCOG). (2015). Reducing the risk of venous thromboembolism during pregnancy and the puerperium. [online] Available from https://www.rcog.org.uk/globalassets/documents/guidelines/gtg-37a.pdf. [Last accessed April, 2020].
6. Royal College of Obstetricians and Gynaecologists (RCOG). (2015). Thromboembolic Disease in Pregnancy and the Puerperium: Acute Management (Green-top Guideline No. 37b). [online] Available from https://www.rcog.org.uk/globalassets/documents/guidelines/gtg-37b.pdf. [Last accessed April, 2020].
7. World Health Organization (WHO). (2015). WHO recommendations for prevention and treatment of maternal peripartum infections. [online] Available from https://apps.who.int/iris/bitstream/handle/10665/186171/9789241549363_eng.pdf;jsessionid=C5E5698214C1C62D17321A3D7FBC2793?sequence=1. [Last accessed April, 2020].

28 Approach to a Woman with Abnormal Behavior in Puerperium

Jasmeet K Monga

INTRODUCTION

An abnormal behavior of a woman during puerperium can be due to an organic cause or a psychiatric disorder. Those due to psychiatric disorders are a common cause of maternal morbidity that often goes unrecognized and untreated, until and unless the woman is violent or completely withdrawn. It is important for the obstetrician to be aware of all the possible differential diagnosis of abnormal behavior and systematically rule out an organic cause and treat it, if identified.

Postnatal affective disorders are not rare. Depending on the severity, they are of three types: Postpartum blues, postpartum depression, and postpartum psychosis.

Postpartum blues is the term used to describe the essentially normal emotional and behavioral changes that occur after childbirth. This affects >50% of all the new mothers.[1] The onset is typically within two to three days of delivery, usually after initial few days of being happy. The blues are characterized by emotional lability with spells of tearfulness, distress, agitation, anxiety, and feelings of incompetence. This condition is usually self-limiting. It peaks over a few days and resolves within two weeks of onset.

Postpartum depression, a depressive illness of varying severity develops in about 10–15% of all recently delivered women.[2] The onset occurs before or during pregnancy in about 50% of women. The symptoms of postnatal depression develop gradually and manifest within first few months usually first six weeks[3] after childbirth. There is no consensus on the time frame in which the symptoms should develop. The severity may vary from mild-to-severe with symptoms ranging from anxiety and irritability to early morning awakenings, mood swings, mental slowing, lack of concentration and feelings of incompetence, guilt, difficulty in coping with everyday tasks, and loss of appetite and weight. It is differentiated from postpartum blues as they are self-limiting and resolve within 2 weeks of onset.

Postpartum psychosis is relatively rare; the incidence of a psychotic illness arising in a previously well woman following childbirth is 1–2 per 1,000 births.[4] Postpartum psychosis is characterized by acute onset, usually after the third postpartum day and rapid deterioration. The woman is agitated, confused, distressed, frightened, and suspicious of those around her. Emotional lability, delusions of paranoia, guilt, and incompetence are common as are disinhibition, and urinary and fecal incontinence. The woman neglects self-care and infant care. Delusional ideas lead to a risk of suicide and occasionally, infanticide.

These illnesses occur around a time when happiness and contentment are the expected feelings. The new mother is coming to terms with her revised personal and social responsibilities, and adjusting to the various physical and psychological changes. The challenge for the care givers and the healthcare providers lies in being able to recognize symptoms of serious illness, while at the same time, helping the woman understand, and rationalize the normal changes associated with childbirth and motherhood.

This chapter discusses the diagnostic approach of a woman presenting with abnormal behavior during the postpartum period.

DIFFERENTIAL DIAGNOSIS

The differential diagnosis of an abnormal behavior in a woman in the puerperium includes a wide variety of conditions as listed in Box 1.

Box 1: Differential diagnosis of abnormal behavior in a woman in puerperium.

Causes of abnormal behavior
- Organic causes:
  - *Metabolic conditions*:
    » Electrolyte disturbances
    » Hypoglycemia and hyperglycemia
    » Blood loss, anemia, and hypoxia
    » Hyperthermia and hypothermia
    » Hepatic encephalopathy
    » Preeclampsia and eclampsia
    » Dehydration
    » Renal failure and uremia
  - *Drugs and toxins*: Prescription medicines, drugs of abuse, and poisons
  - *Central nervous system infections*: Meningitis, encephalitis, brain abscess, tuberculoma, and cerebral malaria
  - *Systemic infections*: Urinary tract infection (UTI), puerperal sepsis, and pneumonia
  - *Endocrinological conditions*: Hypothyroidism manifesting with nonpsychotic depressive illness in postpartum period
  - *Cerebrovascular conditions*: Hemorrhage and stroke
  - *Seizure*: Postictal state
- Nonorganic causes:
  - Postpartum blues
  - Postpartum depression
  - Postpartum psychosis

EVALUATION OF THE PATIENT

History

In the history of present illness, it is important to find out the nature of abnormality in behavior, its onset, and duration. History of any such episode in the past, especially following previous childbirth is asked for. In case it is present, then old records are reviewed for the diagnosis and the treatment received. Any past history of psychiatric illness such as bipolar disorder in self or the family is asked for. Any adverse event such as a traumatic delivery or birth of a stillborn baby or a neonatal death is asked for.

History of any medication is important. Administration of some drugs such as metoclopramide for vomiting, can make the woman restless due to extrapyramidal symptoms. The woman may be a known case of psychiatric disorder on medications, in these women drug compliance should be assessed. Any history of drug abuse should be elicited, as use of and more so sudden withdrawal of such drugs can give rise to abnormal behavior.

Any history suggestive of jaundice, such as yellow discoloration of urine, sclera, passage of clay-colored stools, loss of appetite, nausea, and vomiting, is elicited as hepatic encephalopathy can result in abnormal behavior. Any history of vomiting and or diarrhea leading to dehydration is suggestive of electrolyte imbalance. Any history suggestive of any endocrinopathy, such as diabetes mellitus and hypothyroidism, should be elicited. Any history of significant blood loss leading to severe anemia and hypoxia is important. Any history suggestive of preeclampsia, hypertension, severe headache, and convulsions should be taken. History of some preexisting or current renal disease is elicited to rule out uremia as a cause of abnormal behavior. History suggestive of tuberculosis may be suggestive of intracranial lesion in the form of tuberculoma. History of severe headache, projectile vomiting, and convulsion with abnormal behavior suggests an intracranial pathology. History of fever points toward infection as a cause of abnormal behavior as with malaria, viral and bacterial infections, etc.

EXAMINATION

Examination including a detailed general physical, neurological, and gynecological examination is indicated. Fundus examination is advised, whenever any intracranial pathology is suspected.

INVESTIGATIONS

Investigations includes a complete blood count with peripheral smear to rule out infections, malaria, and anemia.

Serum electrolytes including sodium, potassium, calcium, magnesium, and phosphorus to rule out electrolyte imbalance, liver function tests including serum albumin to diagnose liver dysfunction and related hepatic encephalopathy.

Kidney function tests to rule out uremia; infection screen including urine culture, blood culture, and chest X-ray is done.

Thyroid function tests and blood sugar levels should be assessed. Arterial blood gas analysis is done, in women with tachypnea where hypoxia is suspected as a cause of abnormal behavior.

Lumbar puncture is indicated to send the cerebrospinal fluid (CSF) for examination to rule out meningitis.

Electrocardiogram (ECG) is done whenever any cardiac pathology is suspected.

Brain imaging is advised, when there is any neurological symptom or sign and electroencephalography (EEG) is indicated, when seizure-related etiology is suspected.

The algorithm for clinical approach to a postnatal woman presenting with abnormal behavior is shown in Flowchart 1.

MANAGEMENT

The management of various mild and major mood disorders and psychiatric illnesses in postpartum period has special considerations. These include the physical safety issues of the neonate, breastfeeding and transmission of drugs through milk to the baby, sleep deprivation and general hygiene of the postpartum woman. Table 1 outlines the principles of management of various mental illnesses in the postpartum period.

KEY POINTS

- Abnormal behavior in a woman in puerperium can either be due to an organic pathology or due to some psychiatric disorder.
- Knowledge of the differential diagnosis and systematic evaluation of such women is important.
- Organic causes resulting in abnormal behavior need to be addressed on emergency basis, because if left untreated it can result in serious complications.
- The psychiatric disorders can be minor like postpartum blues or major like postpartum depression or postpartum psychosis.
- Minor problems such as postpartum blues pass off without much problem,

Section 1: Obstetrics

Flowchart 1: Algorithm for clinical approach to a postnatal woman presenting with abnormal behavior in puerperium.

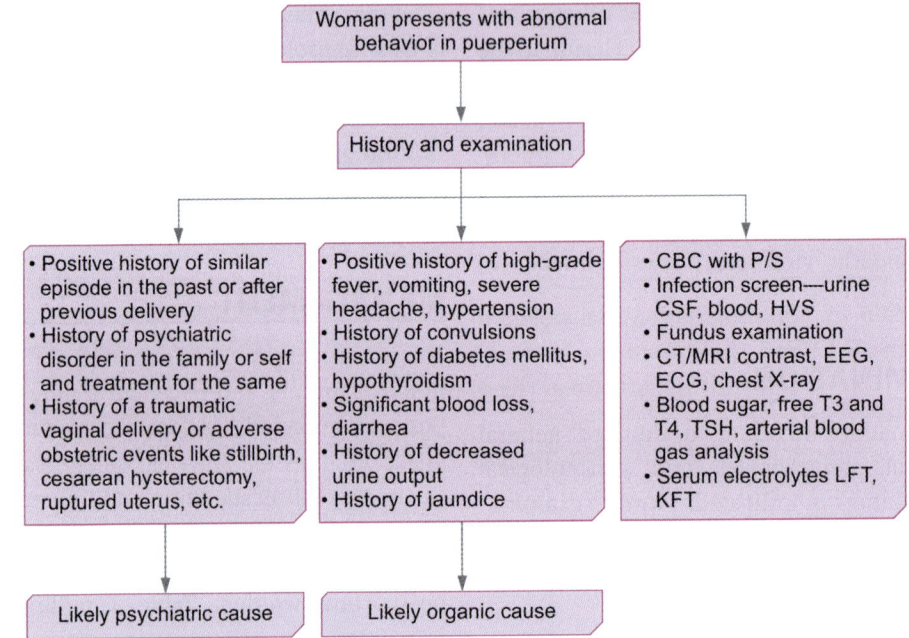

(CBC: complete blood count; CSF: cerebrospinal fluid; CT: computed tomography; ECG: electrocardiogram; EEG: electroencephalogram; HVS: high-vaginal swab; KFT: kidney function test; LFT: liver function test; MRI: magnetic resonance imaging; P/S: peripheral smear; TSH: thyroid-stimulating hormone; T3: triiodothyronine; T4: thyroxine)

Table 1: The principles of management of various mental illnesses in postpartum period.

Diagnosis	Principles of treatment
Postpartum blues	• Conservative • Watchful expectancy • Reassurance and support to woman and her family • Adequate rest and sleep • Cognitive behavioral therapy/pharmacotherapy or both • If symptoms worsen and persist beyond 2 weeks or suicidal ideation, assess for depression
Postpartum depression	• Psychotherapy • Pharmacotherapy • Combined psychotherapy and pharmacotherapy • *Adjunctive treatments*: Exercise, parenting education, and couple/family therapy
Postpartum psychosis	• Medical emergency • Hospitalization • Organic causes need to be ruled out • Second-generation antipsychotics preferred (quetiapine, risperidone, and olanzapine) • Benzodiazepines, mood stabilizer, or antidepressant may be added as per presentation • Treated till remission and 1 year thereafter

but major disorders such as postpartum depression and psychosis can result in serious consequences like suicide and infanticide, if left untreated.

REFERENCES

1. Howard LM, Molyneaux E, Dennis CL, Rochat T, Stein A, Milgrom J. Non-psychotic mental disorders in the perinatal period. Lancet. 2014;384(9956):1775-88.
2. Gaillard A, Le Strat Y, Mandelbrot L, Keïta H, Dubertret C. Predictors of postpartum depression: prospective study of 264 women followed during pregnancy and postpartum. Psychiatry Res. 2014;215(2):341-6.
3. World Health Organization. International Classification of Diseases (ICD) ICD-10 online version: 2016 http://www.who.int/classifications/icd/en.
4. VanderKruik R, Barreix M, Chou D, Allen T, Say L, Cohen LS. The global prevalence of postpartum psychosis: a systematic review. BMC Psychiatry. 2017;17(1):272.

SUGGESTED READING

1. Hasan A, Falkai P, Wobrock T, Lieberman J, Glenthøj B, Gattaz WF, et al. World Federation of Societies of Biological Psychiatry (WFSBP): Guidelines for biological treatment of schizophrenia. Part 3: 2015 Update Management of special circumstances: Depression, suicidality, substance use disorders and pregnancy and lactation. 2015;16(3):142-70.
2. McAllister-Williams RH1, Baldwin DS3, Cantwell R, Easter A, Gilvarry E, Glover V, et al. British Association for Psychopharmacology (BAP): Consensus guidance on the use of psychotropic medication preconception, in pregnancy and postpartum 2017. 2017;31(5): 519-52.
3. Molenaar NM, Kamperman AM, Boyce P, Bergink V. Guidelines on treatment of perinatal depression with antidepressants: An international review. Aust N Z J Psychiatry. 2018;52(4):320-7.

Section 2

Gynecology

- History Taking and Clinical Examination of a Woman Presenting with Gynecological Complaints
- Approach to a Woman Presenting with Vaginal Discharge
- Approach to a Woman Presenting with Abnormal Uterine Bleeding
- Approach to a Woman Presenting with Infertility
- Approach to a Woman Presenting with Dysmenorrhea
- Approach to a Woman Presenting with Dyspareunia
- Approach to a Woman Presenting with Lower Abdominal Pain
- Approach to a Woman Presenting with Abdominal Lump
- Approach to a Woman Presenting with Pelvic Organ Prolapse
- Approach to a Woman Presenting with Urinary Incontinence
- Approach to a Woman Presenting with Anal Incontinence
- Approach to a Woman Presenting with Pruritus Vulvae
- Approach to a Woman Presenting with Vulvar Lesion
- Approach to a Woman Presenting with Amenorrhea
- Approach to a Woman Presenting with Hirsutism
- Approach to a Girl Presenting with Precocious Puberty
- Approach to a Girl Presenting with Delayed Puberty
- Approach to a Woman Presenting with Breast Lump
- Approach to a Woman Presenting with Nipple Discharge
- Approach to a Survivor of Sexual Assault

29 History Taking and Clinical Examination of a Woman Presenting with Gynecological Complaints

Shalini Singh

INTRODUCTION

History-taking and clinical examination are the basic steps in the workup and the management of any patient presenting to the outpatient department or in emergency. These are the stepping stones in making the provisional diagnosis and differential diagnosis. These skills are imperative to decide on the investigations and their sequence to reach or confirm the final diagnosis on the basis of which the patient is counseled as regards the treatment options and prognosis. These skills are not only about how to take history or how to examine the patient but also about comprehending the facts intelligently and placing them in a meaningful sequence to reach a provisional diagnosis. This is an art, which every student needs to master to become a fine clinician.

HISTORY-TAKING

History-taking forms a vital part in approaching patient's problem and arriving at a diagnosis. Giving proper attention to the complaints of the patient and allowing her to explain her problem in her own words makes the patient comfortable and cooperative, and allows the physician to get maximum information from the patient.

In order to establish a rapport with the patient, her demographic data in the form of name, age, address, marital status, parity, and occupation must be documented. The common complaints with which women usually present to the outpatient department of gynecology are menstrual abnormalities, abdominal pain, inability to conceive, discharge per vaginum, dysmenorrhea, abdominal lump, mass coming out per vaginum, pruritus vulva, urinary complaints, and urinary or anal incontinence.

The various components of history-taking are listed in Box 1.

History of Present Illness

History of present illness should be recorded in a chronological order. It should include the duration, evolution, and progress of the problem, any aggravating or relieving factors and their relation to menstrual cycles. For example, a woman presenting with complaint of discharge per vaginum should be asked about its duration, amount, need for use of pads, its

Box 1: Components of history-taking.
- History of present illness
- Past history
- Family history
- Menstrual history
- Obstetric history
- Marital and sexual history
- Socioeconomic history
- Personal history

color, smell, associated itching or rash, its relationship to the menstrual cycle, and any symptoms in the partner.

Past History

History of previous illness should include all important medical and surgical illnesses, both for its association with present complaint and for the purpose of fitness of the patient for anesthesia, in case surgical management is required. For example, a girl with history of tuberculosis (TB) in childhood may present with hypomenorrhea and infertility, and patients with diabetes mellitus (DM) may present with pruritus vulvae. Previous history of abdominal or pelvic surgery can subsequently result in infertility and previous conservative surgery for fibroid uterus or ovarian cyst may be followed by recurrence.

Family History

Purpose of family history is to find out any disease in the family, which might be relevant to the present illness of the patient. Some gynecological problems such as premature menopause, polycystic ovarian syndrome and certain malignancies, e.g., breast cancer, ovarian cancer, endometrial cancer, and carcinoma in colon, run in families due to environmental or genetic factors. TB, thalassemia, DM, and hypertension may affect more than one member of the family.

Menstrual History

Menstrual history should be sought in detail including age at menarche, date of last normal menstrual period, cycle length and duration, any recent change in pattern and amount of bleeding, and number of pads/tampons used per day.

Dysmenorrhea, whether primary or secondary, as secondary dysmenorrhea is usually pathological. The time of onset of pain in relation to menstrual cycle and its duration are often helpful in pointing toward a specific pathology. Pelvic pain and discomfort occurring a few days before menstruation suggests pelvic congestion possibly due to pelvic inflammatory disease (PID), fibroid, or endometriosis.

Any history of intermenstrual or post-coital bleeding must be given special attention.

Age of menopause, perimenopausal period, and any episode of postmenopausal bleeding should be recorded.

Marital and Sexual History

Marital and sexual history includes details regarding the relationship of the woman with her partner. Wherever relevant, history of problems such as vaginismus, decreased libido, difficulty in coitus, frequency of coitus, dyspareunia, and inability to achieve orgasm, should be sought. The number of partners and history of partner's occupation are important in cases of suspected sexually transmitted disease, such as genital ulcer, recurrent PID, or discharge per vaginum. History of sexual dysfunction like impotence, premature ejaculation, and hypospadias, and of any surgical or medical illnesses such as mumps, hernia, hydrocele, and varicocele is important in the male partners of women presenting with infertility.

Obstetric History

Obstetric history includes recording any difficulty in conception, details of all pregnancies, their outcome including medical termination of pregnancies (MTPs), spontaneous abortions, and ectopic pregnancies.

The number of children, details of ante-, intra- and postnatal periods, any obstetrical complications, e.g. postpartum hemorrhage (PPH), perineal tears, postabortal or puerperal sepsis, or postnatal depression should be elicited, as they may have a bearing on the present illness of the woman.

Age of youngest child, milestones of children, their immunization status, and details of any contraceptive method used are recorded.

Socioeconomic and Personal History

Socioeconomic and personal history including level of education, occupation, income, environment at home and workplace, lifestyle, any addictions, smoking or alcohol intake, sleeping patterns, her decision-making power, etc. should be enquired; it helps in guiding management options for patient's problem.

EXAMINATION

Examination should be done with the verbal consent of the patient, maintaining privacy and after explaining the procedure to the patient. It is mandatory for the male physicians to have a female attendant present at the time of examination. Patient should be made comfortable and provided with a clean sheet to cover her. A complete examination includes general physical examination, systemic examination, and gynecological examination.

General Physical Examination

General physical examination is a careful examination of the patient as a whole. Appearance of the patient, gait, height, and weight are to be recorded.

Body Mass Index

Body mass index (BMI) is calculated as weight in kilograms by height in meters square, i.e., kg/m^2. The current World Health Organization (WHO) BMI and Asian BMI criteria cutoffs are given in Table 1.[1,2]

For public health action, especially in reference to Asian population who have a higher percentage of body fat than whites, Asian cutoffs are used.[2]

Women with high BMI are at risk of polycystic ovary syndrome (PCOS), infertility, breast cancer, endometrial cancer, and anesthetic complications. Women with anorexia nervosa, thyrotoxicosis, and malignancy have a low BMI.

Height has got both obstetrical and gynecological significance. Women with height <2 standard deviation of mean for that chronological age are considered short stature. Short stature is associated with chromosomal anomalies, e.g., Down syndrome and Turner's syndrome.

A note is made of secondary sexual characters, hair distribution, signs of hyperandrogenism such as acne, hirsutism, alopecia, and presence of acanthosis nigricans.

Table 1: Body mass index criteria cutoffs.

Category	WHO standard	Asian standard
Underweight	< 18.5 kg/m²	< 18.5 kg/m²
Normal range	18.5–24.9 kg/m²	18.5–22.9 kg/m²
Overweight	25–29.9 kg/m² (pre-obese)	23–24.9 kg/m² (pre-obese)
Obese	≥ 30 kg/m²	≥ 25 kg/m²

Pallor

Pallor is looked for in lower palpebral conjunctiva, tip and dorsum of tongue, nail beds, soft palate, palmer creases, and soles (Figs. 1A to C).

Most women attending gynecological clinics in our country have nutritional deficiency anemia. Any signs of nutritional deficiencies such as glossitis, cheilosis, and angular stomatitis, should be recorded (Fig. 2A). Presence of icterus or cyanosis should be looked for (Fig. 2B). Thyroid should be inspected and palpated for any enlargement or nodule. Cervical, supraclavicular, axillary, epitrochlear, and inguinal lymph nodes are palpated; these may be enlarged in diseases such as TB, syphilis, malignancy, and human immunodeficiency virus (HIV) (Fig. 2C).

Edema

Edema is demonstrated by applying firm pressure over medial malleolus and lower end of tibia for at least 5 seconds and to look for depression (Figs. 3A and B). In a bedridden patient, edema is demonstrable on sacrum, which is the most dependent part. In cases of anasarca, there is generalized swelling of face, hands, abdomen, thighs, vulva, and legs. Edema may be present in cases of hypoproteinemia, chronic anemia, myxedema, ovarian malignancy, large abdominal tumors, or with use of certain drugs such as amlodipine.

Breast Examination

Breast examination should be done as a routine in all women presenting to the gynecology outpatient department. Breasts are inspected for any asymmetry and skin changes such as puckering. This is followed by palpation for any lump or any discharge from the nipple (Refer to chapter on breast). Care should be taken not to omit the axillary tail of the breast during palpation.

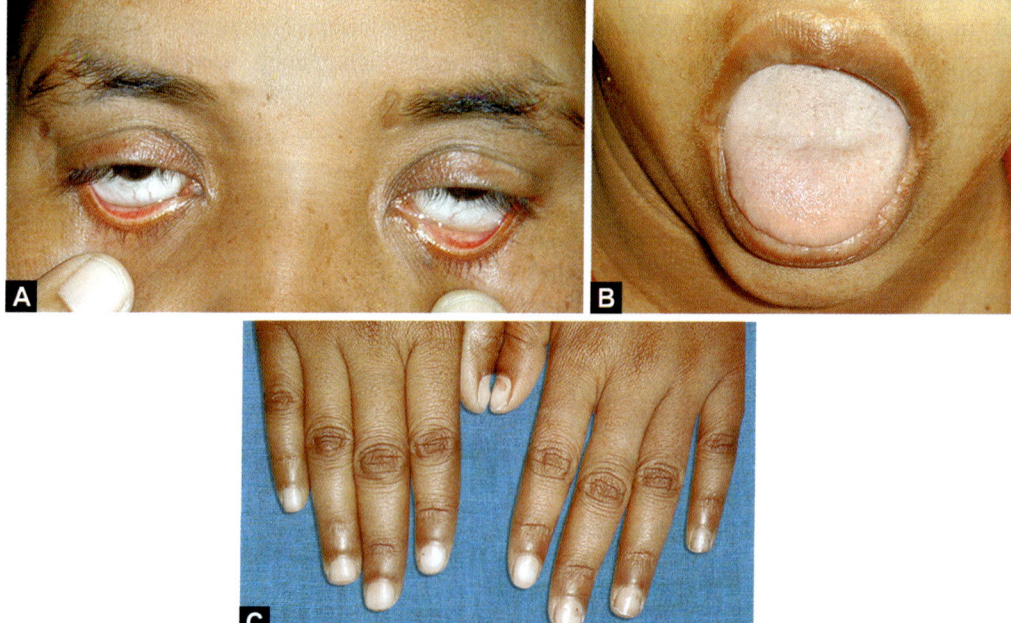

Figs. 1A to C: Demonstration of pallor. (A) Normal conjunctiva; (B) Pale tongue; (C) Pale nails.

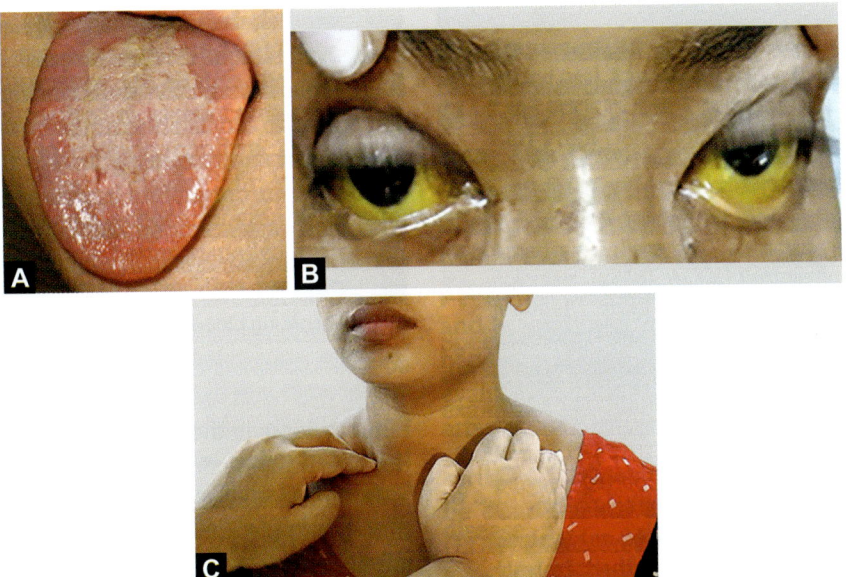

Figs. 2A to C: (A) Glossitis; (B) Presence of icterus; (C) Palpation of supraclavicular lymph nodes.

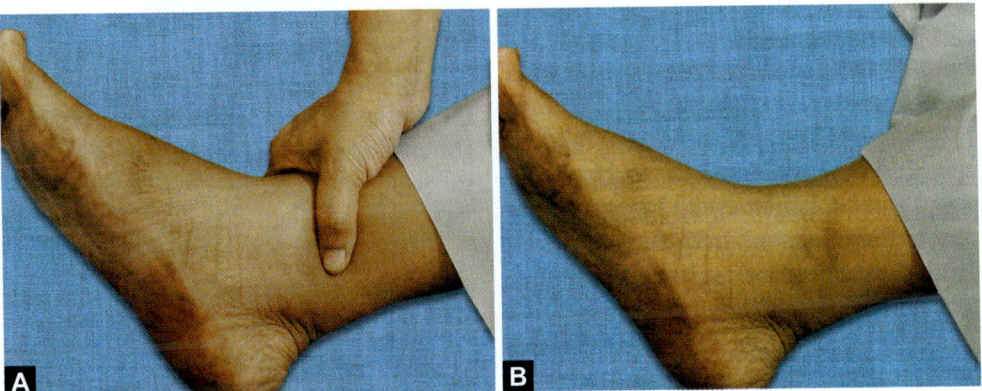

Figs. 3A and B: Demonstration of edema. (A) Application of firm pressure over a bony surface (medial malleolus); (B) Visualization of area of depression.

Vital Parameters

Vital parameters such as pulse, blood pressure, temperature, and respiratory rate are recorded. Temperature is recorded for at least 1 minute with a thermometer in the mouth or axilla. Temperature of mouth and rectum is half a degree higher than at groin and axilla. Normal temperature ranges from 36.6 to 37.2°C (98–99°F). Pulse rate is counted in radial artery with forearm semi-pronated and wrist slightly flexed against radial bone for at least 1 minute and any variation in rate, rhythm, volume, and character should be recorded (Fig. 4).

Sinus tachycardia is pulse rate or heart rate of >100 beats per minute, while sinus bradycardia is pulse rate or heart rate of <60

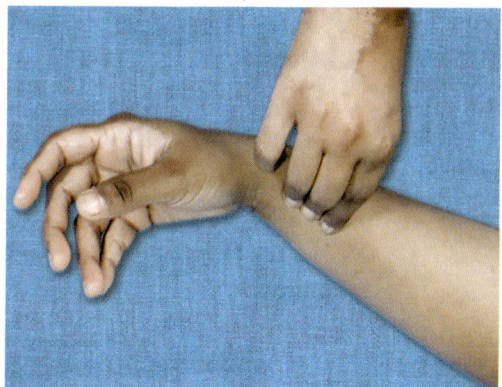

Fig. 4: Recording pulse rate.

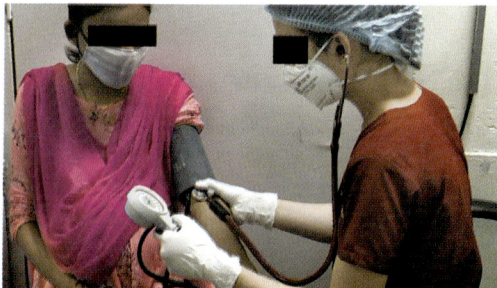

Fig. 5: Recording blood pressure.

beats per minute in the absence of any irregularity of the rhythm. In cases of hypovolemia and shock, brachial and radial pulses may not be palpable due to low-pulse pressure, so carotid and/or femoral artery pulsations are palpated.

Respiratory rate is measured by counting the number of rise and fall of the chest wall in 1 minute. While recording respiratory rate, an effort should be made to deviate attention of the patient by pretending to record pulse rate and looking at the watch. Respiratory rate is recorded by keeping the other hand over shoulders to appreciate chest movements, as it is not possible to see the chest movements and time simultaneously. Normal respiratory rate is 14–18 breaths per minute. Any difficulty in breathing and irregularity should be noted.

Blood pressure is measured in right brachial artery in supine, sitting, or standing position after ensuring that the level of arm is at the level of heart, i.e., at fourth intercostal space (Fig. 5). The patient should be seated for at least 5 minutes and relaxed to prevent white coat hypertension. The cuff of sphygmomanometer should be snugly fitted; a lose cuff gives false higher values, while a tight cuff gives lower measurements. The center of the bladder lies over the brachial artery. The bladder should encircle at least 80% of the arm and not more than 100%. The appearance of first Korotkoff sound and disappearance of fifth Korotkoff sound marks the systolic and diastolic pressure, respectively.

Systemic Examination

Cardiovascular System

Precordium is inspected for any obvious abnormality in shape and contour. Any scars, sinuses, or dilated veins should be noted. Apical impulse is normally palpated in fifth intercostal space just medial to midclavicular line. Precordium is palpated for any thrill or palpable heart sounds. All the areas of precordium, namely tricuspid, mitral, pulmonary, and aortic, should be auscultated for murmurs, opening snaps, ejection clicks, or splitting of heart sounds. Patients with known or suspected heart disease must have complete cardiac workup before they are planned for any surgery to avoid intra- or postoperative complications.

Respiratory System

Rate and rhythm of breathing is noted. Any spinal deformity in the form of scoliosis or kyphosis is recorded. Normally both sides of chest wall move uniformly during respiration without any bulge or flattening. Any deviation from normal is recorded. Accessory muscles of respiration are not required in the normal act of breathing. On percussion, any change in the normal resonant note of the chest is observed; it may be dull or hyperresonant in different respiratory disorders.

The normal low-pitched vesicular breath sounds have a rustling character due to passage of air into alveoli, which becomes blowing and hollow (bronchial) in character in cases of lung diseases. Presence or absence of added sounds should be noted. Rales, crepitations, or crackles are nonmusical interrupted added sounds, which may be fine or coarse according to origin of production. Fine end-inspiratory crepitations over both lung bases are an early sign of left ventricular failure. Rhonchi or wheeze are musical continuous added sounds heard on auscultation in asthma and emphysema.

Gynecological Examination

Abdominal Examination

Inspection: Shape of the abdomen, position, and direction of umbilicus, presence of prominent veins, and divarication of recti, flanks, and hernia sites should be inspected. The hernial sites include epigastric, umbilical, paraumbilical, inguinal, femoral, and incisional hernias. Condition of skin for striae, pigmentation, scars, ulcers, and any other lesion is noted. The details of the scar as regards its location, size (length and width), any puckering, hypertrophy, keloid formation, hyperpigmentation, healing by primary or secondary intention, and whether adherent to underlying tissues or not are noted. Movement of all quadrants of abdomen with respiration is observed.

Palpation: Abdomen is palpated to feel for temperature of overlying skin, tenderness, any guarding or rigidity, its consistency, presence of any lump, and fluid thrill. Deep palpation is done to appreciate any enlargement of liver and/or spleen, any lump in abdomen, and presence of rebound tenderness. In cases of peritonitis, there is restricted movement of the abdomen and extreme tenderness on palpation. Surgical causes of abdominal pain should be ruled out by examining McBurney's point, epigastric region, and renal angle for any tenderness.

While examining a lump in the abdomen, its site, size, shape, surface, margins, consistency, and mobility are noted. On palpation, it is important to trace the lower margin of the mass as it is usually made out in ovarian masses and not made out in uterine masses such as fibroids. Smooth, round, mobile, and cystic swellings are usually benign, while solid, irregular, hard, and fixed lumps may be malignant in nature.

In women with advanced pregnancy and ovarian tumor, it may be difficult to appreciate two separate swellings. Abdominal examination in Trendelenburg position (Head end down) displaces the ovarian tumor upward and a groove between the two swellings can be appreciated (Hingorani sign).

Percussion: Uterine myomas and ovarian cysts are dull on percussion but the flanks are resonant. Dullness in the flanks and shifting dullness indicate presence of free fluid in the peritoneal cavity. Ascitis may be associated with tuberculosis, peritonitis, malignancy, or pseudo-Meigs syndrome.

Auscultation: It is done for appreciating bowel sounds, whether normal, hypokinetic, or hyperkinetic, and for presence of any bruit.

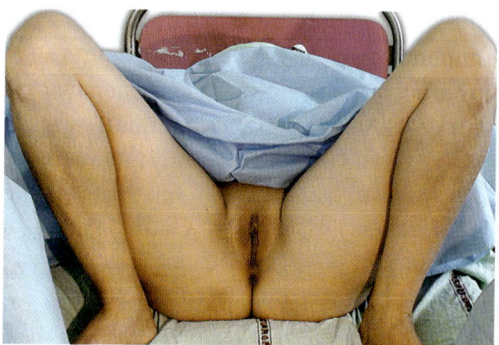

Fig. 6: Dorsal position.

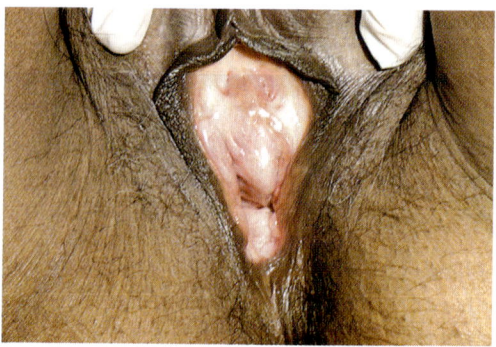

Fig. 7: Local examination of genitalia.

Pelvic Examination

Patient is asked to empty her bladder, except if she is presenting with complaints suggestive of stress urinary incontinence (SUI) where the initial examination is done with full bladder. Pelvic examination is usually performed with the patient in dorsal position with the buttocks at the edge of the table (Fig. 6). Examination is done under good light and with aseptic precautions.

Distribution of pubic hair is noted. Vulval, urethral, perineal, and perianal areas should be inspected for any lesion, growth, swelling, pigmentation, discharge, blood, or any signs of trauma. Labia are separated by thumb and index finger and mucosal characteristics of labia minora, clitoris, urethral orifice, introitus, hymen, perineal body, and anus are inspected (Fig. 7). Fourchette is examined for its intactness and presence of any old healed perineal tears.

Patient is asked to strain and presence of any polyp, vaginal, uterine, or rectal prolapse, is noted. SUI can be demonstrated by asking the patient to cough with a full bladder with labia separated to expose the urethral meatus and observe for any leakage of urine per urethra (Fig. 8). Bonney's test can be performed by placing two fingers in the

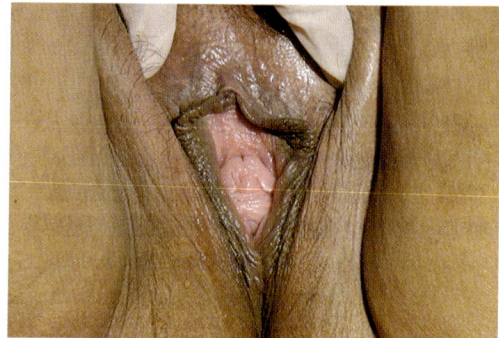

Fig. 8: Demonstration of stress urinary incontinence (SUI).

vagina at the urethrovesical junction on either side of urethra and bladder neck region and elevating the bladder neck (Fig. 9). On repeat straining or coughing, absence of leakage of urine indicates a positive Bonney's test and suggests that correction of incontinence by surgical procedures is likely to be effective. Bartholin's gland is palpated by keeping index finger in the vagina and thumb on posterior part of labia majora above the fourchette (Fig. 10). Normally, it is not palpable.

Per Speculum Examination

Appropriate size of speculum should be selected and inserted with blades oblique and gently rotated along the posterior

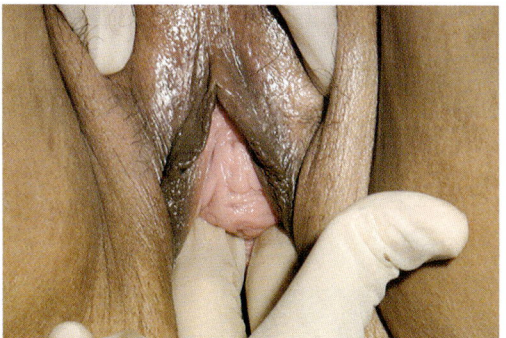

Fig. 9: Bonney's test.

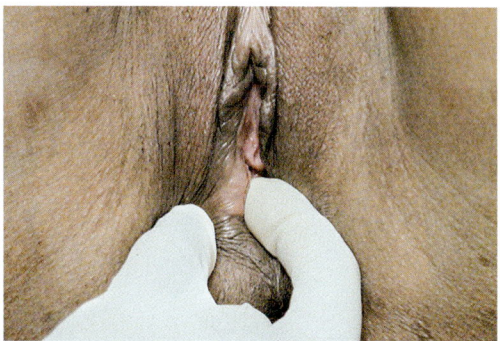

Fig. 10: Palpation of Bartholin's gland.

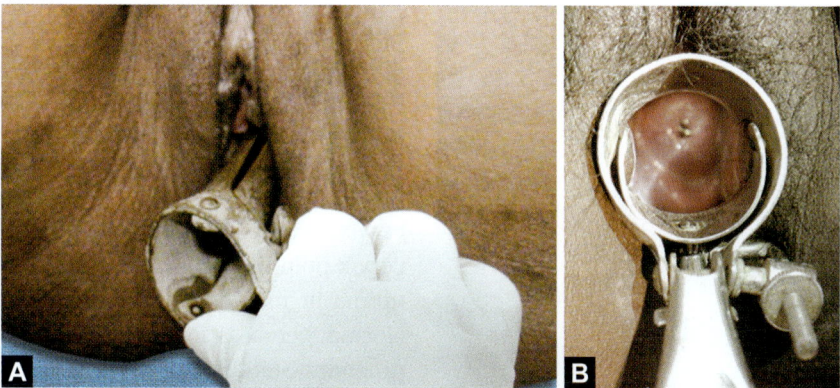

Figs. 11A and B: Per speculum examination using Cusco's speculum. (A) Introduction of speculum in oblique position; (B) Cusco's speculum in position.

vaginal wall avoiding contact with urethra as it is a very sensitive area (Figs. 11A and B). Vagina and cervix are inspected for rugosities, color, scarring, pigmentation, any bleeding, discharge, growth, ulcer, and descent.

Per speculum examination is done. Cusco's speculum is ideal for taking Pap smear, collecting vaginal discharge, and colposcopic examination (Figs. 12A to C). However, Sim's speculum with anterior vaginal wall retractor allows better assessment of uterine and vaginal wall prolapse, but it requires the help of an assistant in case any minor procedure such as Pap smear or cervical swab for culture sensitivity is to be collected. (Figs. 13A

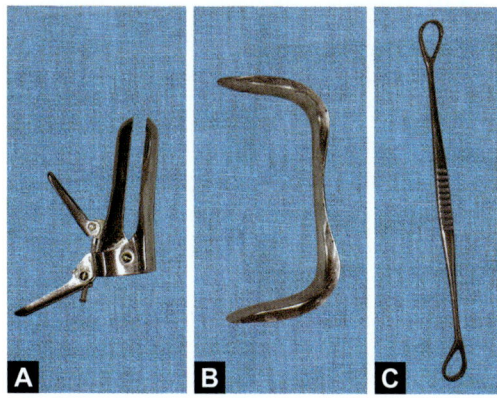

Figs. 12A to C: (A) Cusco's bivalve self-retaining vaginal speculum; (B) Sim's double bladed vaginal speculum; (C) Anterior vaginal wall retractor.

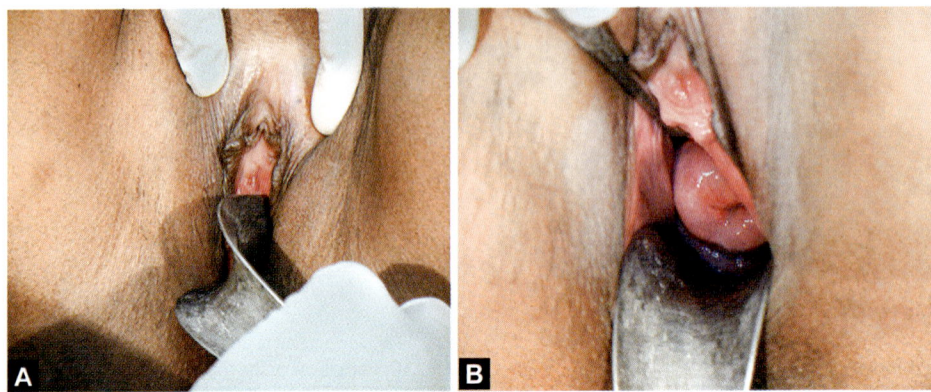

Figs. 13A and B: Per speculum examination using Sim's speculum. (A) Introduction of Sims speculum; (B) Visualization of cervix and vagina with Sim's speculum and anterior vaginal wall retractor.

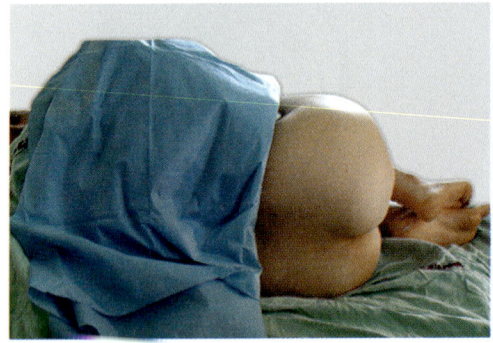

Fig. 14: Sim's lateral position.

and B). Patients with vesicovaginal fistula or anterior wall lesions can be examined with Sim's speculum in the Sim's lateral position for better visualization of anterior vaginal wall (Fig. 14). Pap smear should be offered to all women undergoing per speculum examination using Ayer's spatula and endocervical brush (Figs. 15A and B).

Per Vaginum Examination

The woman is asked to empty her bladder. The labia are separated by the index finger and thumb of nondominant hand and lubricated middle and index fingers of the dominant hand are gradually introduced into the vagina until cervix is reached. Position, consistency, and tenderness and mobility of cervix are noted. If anterior lip of cervix is touched first, it is suggestive of a cervix pointing backward and an anteverted uterus in majority of cases and vice versa. Normal cervix is firm in feel; it feels soft in pregnant state and firm to hard in carcinoma cervix. Cervical motion tenderness is demonstrable in ectopic pregnancy and acute salpingo-oophoritis.

Uterus is evaluated with bimanual pelvic examination in which vaginal fingers lift the cervix and are coordinated with nondominant hand kept over suprapubic region or lower abdomen (Figs. 16A and B). Position, size, shape, symmetry, consistency, tenderness and mobility of uterus should be noted. This is followed by bimanual palpation of the lateral fornices starting from the lateral wall of the uterus to the lateral pelvic wall on either side, to feel for any adnexal pathology (Fig. 17).

Adnexal structures are normally not palpable. Ovary, if palpable, is tender, firm, and freely mobile. If an adnexal mass is found, its location in relation to uterus and

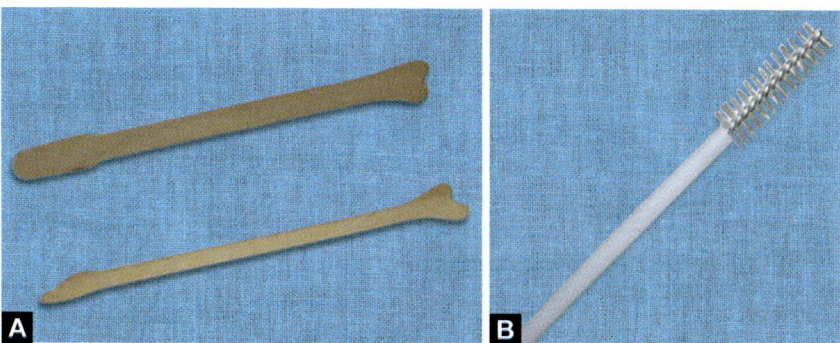

Figs. 15A and B: Pap smear collection. (A) Ayers spatula; (B) Endocervical brush.

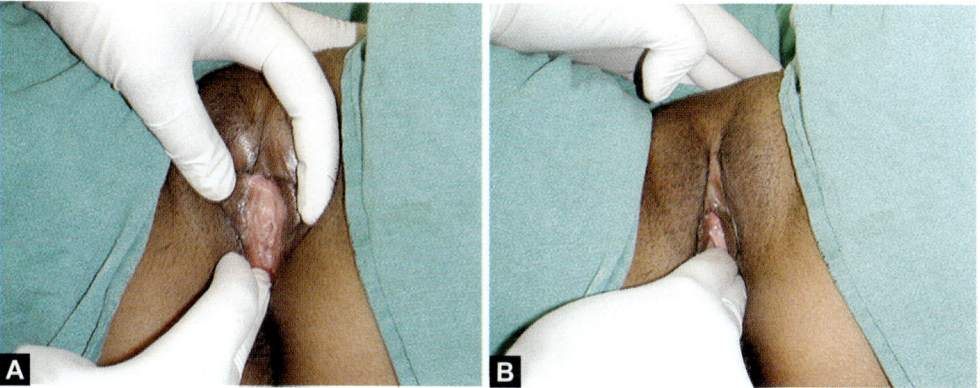

Figs. 16A and B: Per vaginum examination. (A) Introducing middle finger of dominant hand making space for index finger with labia retracted by nondominant hand; (B) Introducing both index and middle fingers of dominant hand in vagina with other hand on lower abdomen.

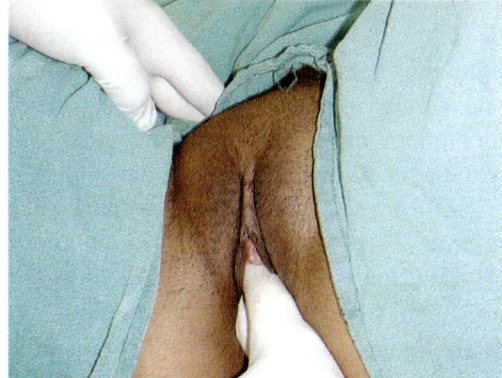

Fig. 17: Assessment of fornices by per vaginum examination.

cervix, its consistency, tenderness, and mobility is assessed. Movement of cervix is transmitted to the masses arising from the uterus but not to adnexal masses. This finding helps in differentiating a uterine mass from an ovarian mass. Posterior fornix is palpated for any thickening, tenderness, scarring or nodularity, which is present in endometriosis and PID. The uterosacral ligaments can be assessed through pouch of Douglas (POD). They are thick and tender in PID. Nodularity in POD is also felt in malignant ovarian tumors and is suggestive of peritoneal deposits.

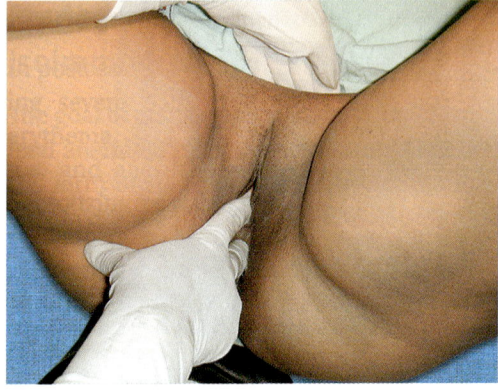

Fig. 18: Rectovaginal examination.

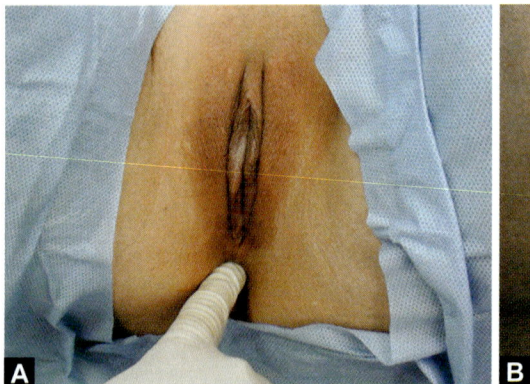 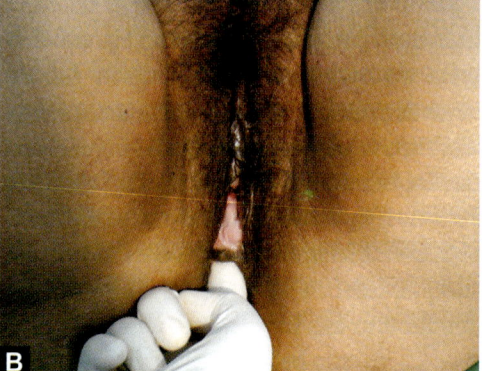

Figs. 19A and B: Per rectal examination. (A) Introducing finger; (B) Turning the finger around.

Tone and bulk of levator ani muscle is assessed in patients of genital prolapse by keeping middle and index finger toward lateral vaginal wall and thumb over the perineum by the side of anus and asking the patient to contract her pelvic muscles.

Per vaginal examination is followed by rectovaginal examination. It is done by placing index finger in posterior fornix and middle finger in rectum, and both directed toward abdominal hand. It is helpful in diagnosing lesions in the rectovaginal space (Fig. 18).

A digital rectal examination is done in virgin women, in women suspected to be suffering from endometriosis, cervical cancer, or ovarian tumor. It is helpful in assessing any collection or mass in the POD. A well-lubricated, gloved index finger of dominant hand is introduced into the anus and cervix, uterus, and POD are palpated bimanually through the anterior rectal wall with the nondominant hand on the abdomen (Figs. 19A and B). This examination is also important for the assessment of parametrium (Mackenrodt's ligaments) which are felt on either side of the cervix extending up to the lateral pelvic wall (Fig. 20). In PID, Mackenrodt's ligaments may be thick, indurated, and tender. In carcinoma cervix, parametrial involvement is appreciated by its

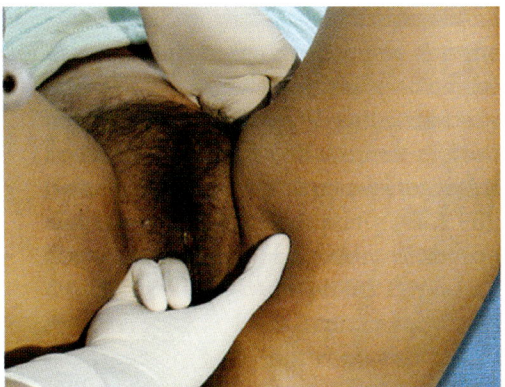

Fig. 20: Palpating parametrium on bimanual per rectal examination.

irregularity and induration. It helps in staging of carcinoma cervix. Tone of anal sphincter is assessed by asking the woman to contract her perianal area with finger in the anus.

Per rectal examination also helps in differentiating between enterocele and rectocele in women with pelvic organ prolapse.

KEY POINTS

- History taking is an art and an essential part of training as a medical student.
- The patient should be allowed to describe her complaints in her own words with very few interruptions from the physician.
- It is followed by relevant leading questions by the physician to extract relevant information from the patient to make a differential diagnosis.
- Detailed history is followed by a systematic examination to fine tune the differential diagnosis considering the findings on examination.

REFERENCES

1. Obesity: preventing and managing the global epidemic. Report on a WHO Consultation. World Health Organ Tech Res Ser. 2000;894:i-xii, 1-253.
2. WHO Expert Consultation. Appropriate body-mass index for Asian populations and its implications for policy and intervention strategies. Lancet. 2004;363(9403):157-63.

SUGGESTED READING

1. Dewhurst's Textbook of Obstetrics and Gynaecology, 9th edition 2019 by Keith Edmonds and Christoph Lees, Wiley Blackwell.
2. Oxford Textbook of Obstetrics and Gynaecology, Edited by Sabaratnam Arulkumaran, William Ledger, Lynette Denny.
3. Shaw's Textbook of Gynaecology, 17th edition 2018 by VG Padubidri.
4. Williams Gynecology, 3rd edition by Barbara L Hoffman, John O Schorge.

30. Approach to a Woman Presenting with Vaginal Discharge

Seema Singhal, Namita Jain

INTRODUCTION

Vaginal discharge is the most common complaint of women in the reproductive age group presenting to the gynecology outpatient department.[1] Vagina near its opening carries glands which produce mucus to keep the vagina moist. Most of the time vaginal discharge is physiological. It is thick, sticky, and nonfoul smelling, but becomes clearer, watery, and stretchy for a short period around the time of ovulation. These changes do not occur in women using oral contraceptives. Vaginal discharge contains vaginal squamous epithelial cells in a serous transudate and secretions from sebaceous, sweat, and Bartholin glands, and from the cervix. The predominant organisms are lactobacilli, which are large gram-positive rods. The vaginal pH is between 3.8 and 4.2 usually below 4.5. The quantity of normal discharge varies from woman to woman and with the different phases of menstrual cycle. The physiological increase in the amount of discharge is seen during ovulation, sexual arousal, and pregnancy. Normal discharge does not have any offensive odor and is not associated with vaginal irritation, itching, or burning.[2]

Pathological vaginal discharge is caused by a variety of infectious and noninfectious (less common) causes. It is characterized by a change in color, consistency, volume, and/or odor, and may be associated with symptoms such as itch, soreness, dysuria, pelvic pain, or intermenstrual or postcoital bleeding. With the availability of various over-the-counter medications for vaginal discharge, many symptomatic women seek these products before evaluation by a healthcare professional.

A careful history and physical examination help in differentiating pathological from physiological discharge and provide clues to the possible cause of discharge.

DIFFERENTIAL DIAGNOSIS

Differential diagnosis of vaginal discharge is listed in Table 1.

Table 1: Differential diagnosis of vaginal discharge.

Physiological	
• Puberty • Sexual stimulation • Pregnancy	
Pathological	
Infective	Noninfective
Vaginal: • Trichomonas vaginitis • Candida vaginitis • Bacterial vaginosis • Primary syphilis • Viral warts	• Cervical erosion • Cervical ectropion • Cervical polyp • Surgery on cervix or vagina

Contd...

Infective	Noninfective
Cervical: • Gonococcal • *Chlamydia trachomatis* • Herpes simplex virus • Primary syphilis • Viral warts • Tuberculosis *Pelvic infection*: • Postoperative infections • Postabortal infections • Puerperal pelvic infections • Chronic pelvic infection	*Trauma*: • Iatrogenic • Allergic • Foreign body *Malignancy*: • Vaginal cancer • Cervical cancer • Uterine cancer *Fistulae*: • Rectovaginal • Vesicovaginal

History alone has been shown to be insufficient for accurate diagnosis and prescribing medication for vaginitis. Therefore, a careful history, examination, and laboratory testing to determine the etiology of vaginal symptoms is warranted. The three diseases most frequently associated with vaginal discharge are bacterial vaginosis, *Trichomonas vaginalis*, and candidiasis.

HISTORY

The onset and duration of symptoms should be elicited. The color, odor, consistency of vaginal discharge and its relationship to the menstrual cycle, whether bloodstained or not, and presence or absence of any associated symptoms should be asked. Relationship with menstrual cycle is important as physiological discharge follows a typical pattern. It is observed in the mid-cycle and is usually not noticed for a few days just before and after the periods.

If character of discharge is thin or mucoid, it is usually suggestive of physiological discharge, but sometimes after minor surgical procedures on cervix such as cervical conization, cryotherapy, or electrocautery, there is profuse thin mucoid discharge; hence, the importance of eliciting history of any surgical procedure done on the cervix in the recent past. If the character of discharge is thick and curdy white, then it is suggestive of *Candida* infection; yellowish frothy vaginal discharge is usually present in women with trichomoniasis.

The discharge in vaginal infection such as candidiasis is usually odorless; however, it is malodorous in bacterial vaginosis and trichomoniasis. The malodor associated with bacterial vaginosis is worse after sexual intercourse and during menstruation due to increase in release of amines by the anaerobic bacteria consequent to increase in vaginal pH due to presence of semen or blood. Foul-smelling discharge is associated with malignancies or retained foreign body such as tampons and condoms.

Blood-stained vaginal discharge is seen in women with polypoidal growths such as endocervical or fibroid polyps, malignancies, and atrophic vaginitis. Associated symptoms such as pruritus vulvae, lower abdominal pain, urinary complaints, postcoital bleeding, intermenstrual bleeding, and constitutional symptoms provide clues to the nature of the cause of vaginal discharge. Constitutional symptoms such as fever and lower abdominal pain are present in pelvic inflammatory disease (PID). These symptoms are common with infection due to *Chlamydia trachomatis* and *Neisseria gonorrhoeae*.

Pruritus is an important symptom of vaginal trichomoniasis and candidiasis. Urinary symptoms such as frequency and dysuria are present in women with candidiasis and trichomoniasis. It is important to differentiate between true dysuria and vulval dysuria or splash dysuria, as vulval dysuria is due to urine coming in contact with raw or sore area of the vulva and is suggestive of vulvovaginal candidiasis. Superficial dyspareunia may also point toward vulvovaginitis. Postcoital bleeding is common with malignancies of cervix and vagina.

History of drug intake in the form of immunosuppressive agents such as corticosteroids, and broad-spectrum antibiotics such as ampicillin, and cephalosporins, is important as they predispose the woman to vaginal candidiasis.

Contraceptive History

Contraceptive history is important as the use of combined oral contraceptive pills can predispose a woman to vaginal candidiasis.

Personal History

Personal hygiene such as use of soaps and douching, may be associated with increased chances of chemical irritation of vagina.

Sexual History

All women presenting with vaginal discharge should be screened for any sexually transmitted infections (STIs). It is important to elicit history of multiple sexual partners, frequent change of partner, or a new partner in the last 3 months. Symptoms such as dysuria or any genital lesion in the partner or any previous history of STI should be asked for.

Menstrual History

Menstrual history is important as any intermenstrual or postcoital bleeding may be suggestive of a cervical or vaginal growth. Any recent change in pattern of menstrual cycle and amount of flow is suggestive of pelvic infection. Date of last menstrual period is important to know if the woman is pregnant or not.

History of Past Illness

Any history of diseases such as diabetes mellitus or human immunodeficiency virus (HIV) infection should be inquired as recurrent vulvovaginal candidiasis may be a manifestation of these diseases. Patients with renal transplant, who are taking immunosuppressive drugs may develop recurrent genital warts and discharge per vaginum. History of any treatment taken for this problem in the past should be elicited.

Family History

History of diabetes mellitus in the family should be enquired, especially in patients with recurrent candidiasis.

EXAMINATION

General Physical Examination

The general built, body mass index (BMI), nutrition, and presence or absence of anemia are important. In obese patients, there are increased chances of excoriation and rashes in the vulval region due to increased vaginal discharge.

Per Abdomen Examination

Presence of tenderness in lower abdomen or a mass may be suggestive of PID. Inguinal lymph nodes should be palpated. These may be normally palpable, but if they have enlarged recently and are tender, it may be suggestive of some acute infection.

Examination of Genitalia

Inspection of vulva and perineal region should include labia majora, labia minora, and clitoral region. Vulval erythema with edema is suggestive of vulvovaginal candidiasis and it may be associated with fissures. Trichomoniasis also causes vulval erythema, usually in conjunction with a profuse frothy discharge, which may cause maceration of the upper thighs.

Vulva and perineum should be inspected for presence of warts or ulcers. The lesions of genital herpes range from clusters of small erythematous patches, vesicles, or ulcers of variable size on the labia.

Per Speculum Examination

The cervix and vagina are inspected. Presence of hyperemia, ectropion, ulcer, erosion, growth, or warts on the cervix should be noted. The vaginal walls are inspected for any evidence of hyperemia, atrophy, ulcers, warts, or growth. Any discharge if present, is observed for its character, color, and odor. In vaginal candidiasis, the discharge is curdy white and in lumps (Fig. 1). This is often adherent to vaginal walls and has an erythematous base. Bacterial vaginosis does not cause vaginal inflammation, but results in a homogeneous white or gray discharge that may have a fishy odor. In *Trichomonas* vaginitis, the discharge is usually profuse, frothy, and yellow, and is associated with inflammation of the cervix and vagina. There may be submucosal punctate hemorrhages on the cervix and vagina (strawberry cervix). Lubricating jelly may be used to facilitate the introduction of the speculum, if the patient feels pain during per speculum examination (Table 2).

Per Vaginum Examination

Bimanual examination should be performed. Size and consistency of the uterus should be noted. An enlarged, soft uterus is suggestive of pregnancy. Cervical excitation pain and tenderness in the fornices is suggestive of PID. Adnexal mass may be palpable in PID. The pelvic examination can be deferred in cases, where there is severe vaginitis to avoid extreme discomfort to the patient.

INVESTIGATIONS

Routine microscopy and culture form the standard of care for the purpose of distinguishing between the common causes of vaginal discharge (Table 3). Cervicitis may be suspected if the cervix is inflamed on examination or if there are numerous WBCs on microscopic examination, especially in the absence of Trichomonas infection.

Wet Smear

Wet Smear with Saline

The discharge collected on the blade of vaginal speculum or collected with a swab stick can be used to a make a wet smear. A drop of discharge is placed on a clean slide along with a drop of saline, covered with a cover slip, and examined under microscope for *T. vaginalis*, clue cells and hyphae.

T. vaginalis are motile organisms of the size of a WBC (Fig. 2). They have a characteristic

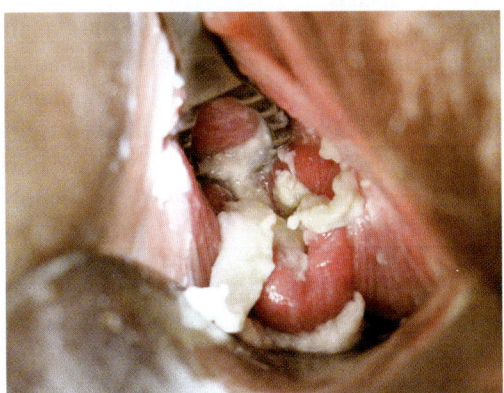

Fig. 1: Candidal discharge.

Table 2: Clinical features associated with common causes of vaginal discharge in women in reproductive age group.[3-5]

Feature	Vulvovaginal candidiasis	Bacterial vaginosis	Trichomoniasis	Neisseria gonorrhoeae	Chlamydia
Symptoms	Thick white discharge	Thin discharge	Scanty-to-profuse or frothy yellow discharge	Increased or altered vaginal discharge	Profuse vaginal discharge
	• Vulval itch • Superficial dyspareunia • Dysuria	No discomfort, soreness, or itch	• Vulval itch or soreness • Dysuria • Lower abdominal pain • Dyspareunia	Rarely menorrhagia and intermenstrual bleeding	Postcoital bleeding, dysuria, lower abdominal pain, and deep dyspareunia
Signs	Vulval erythema, edema, fissuring, satellite lesions	• Discharge coating vagina and vestibule • No inflammation of vulva	Vulvitis and vaginitis "Strawberry" cervix	Mucopurulent discharge, contact bleeding, and pelvic tenderness	Mucopurulent discharge ± contact bleeding, pelvic tenderness, and cervical motion tenderness

Table 3: Site/specimen and test offered to diagnose common causes of vaginal discharge.[3-5]

Infection	Site/specimen	Test
Vulvovaginal candidiasis	High vaginal swab (anterior fornix) or self-collected vaginal swab	• *Microscopy*: Wet smear with KOH and Gram staining of smear • Culture
Bacterial vaginosis	Vaginal swab	• *Microscopy*: Wet smear with saline and Gram stain of smear (Amsel and Hay/Ison criteria) • Whiff test
Trichomoniasis	High vaginal swab (posterior fornix) or self-collected vaginal swab or first pass urine	• *Microscopy*: Wet smear with saline and Gram stain of smear • Culture • Nucleic acid amplification test (NAAT)
Neisseria gonorrhoeae	• Endocervical swab • Urethral swab	• *Microscopy*: After Gram staining • Culture • Nucleic acid amplification test
Chlamydia trachomatis	• Vulvovaginal swab • Endocervical swab • First-catch urine • Urethral swab	Nucleic acid amplification test

twisting motion. Clue cells are vaginal epithelial cells with irregular indistinct margins due to adherent bacteria. Yeast is seen as hyphae or budding cells and are better visualized in smear prepared with potassium hydroxide (KOH). Presence of a few WBCs or leukocytes may be normal, but presence of >10 per high-power field (HPF) is abnormal.

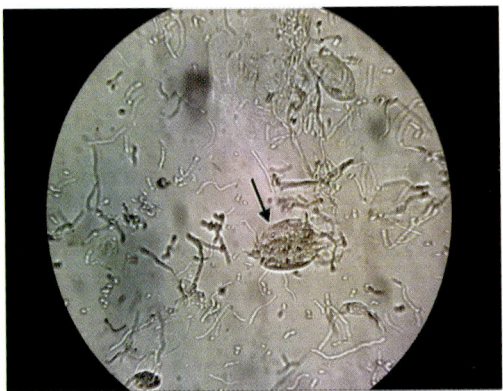

Fig. 2: *Trichomonas* wet smear (arrow).

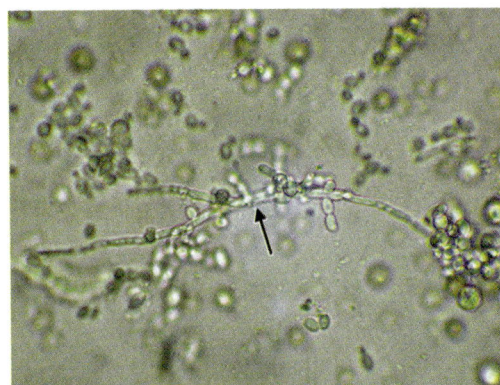

Fig. 3: *Candida* wet smear (arrow).

Wet Smear with Potassium Hydroxide

Vaginal discharge is collected by a similar method as saline smear and a drop of discharge is placed on a slide. A drop of 10% KOH solution is placed on the discharge, covered with a cover slip, and examined for budding yeast cells and hyphae (Fig. 3).

Whiff Test

The whiff test is done for the diagnosis of bacterial vaginosis. A drop of vaginal discharge is mixed with KOH solution on a slide and a characteristic fishy odor is emitted indicating a positive test. This is due to amines produced by anaerobic organisms.

Testing of Vaginal pH

The pH of the vaginal secretions can be obtained by placing a pH paper against the discharge on the lateral vaginal wall. The paper should include a range of pH from 4.0 to >5.0. Cervical mucus, semen, and blood are alkaline, and can interfere with pH testing. The normal vaginal pH in a reproductive age group woman is of 3.8–4.2 and is consistent with normal vaginal flora. In bacterial vaginosis, vaginal pH is characteristically >4.5 due to decrease in lactobacilli.

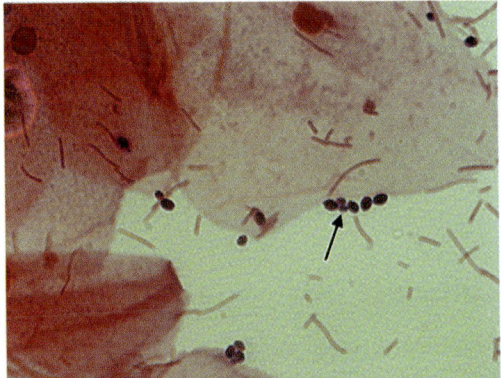

Fig. 4: Gram-stained smear showing budding yeast cell (arrow).

Gram Staining of Discharge

Gram staining of vaginal discharge can be done using standard methods. Yeast is detected (Fig. 4) and the predominant bacterial flora such as normal gram-positive lactobacilli or abnormal gram-negative coccobacilli, and rods can be assessed. Although, *T. vaginalis* is best identified by its characteristic motility, it can be sometimes identified on Gram stain as well (Fig. 5). Clue cells can be identified accurately. They are vaginal epithelial cells with indistinct margins and studded with bacteria (Fig. 6). For the evaluation of

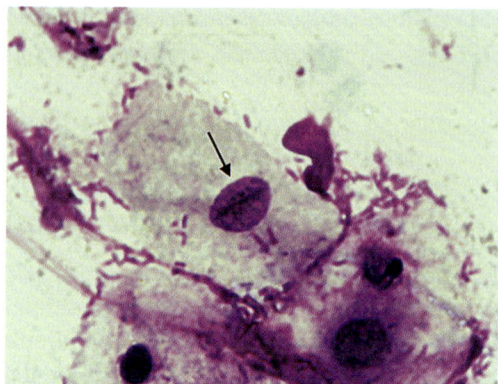

Fig. 5: Gram-stained smear showing *Trichomonas vaginalis* (arrow).

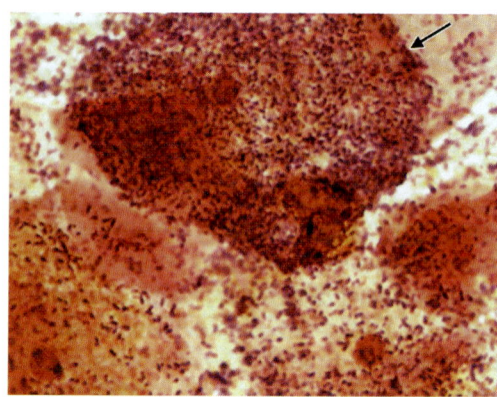

Fig. 6: Gram-stained smear with clue cells in bacterial vaginosis (arrow).

cervicitis, Gram staining of the endocervical mucus may be helpful. Presence of gram-negative diplococci inside the cells is diagnostic for *N. gonorrhoeae*.[6] An excess of leukocytes of >10/HPF in the endocervical mucus suggests chlamydial cervicitis.[7]

Culture of Discharge

Cultures do not substitute a careful history, physical examination, and microscopic examination of the wet smear. Dependence on the results of vaginal culture in the absence of microscopic examination of the vaginal discharge often results in suboptimal treatment. However, cervical cultures are helpful in some cases.

For the diagnosis of vaginal candidiasis and vaginal trichomoniasis, wet smear is usually adequate, except in women with recurrent infection, where culture sensitivity will be desirable. Yeast usually grows on routine culture as well as on specific Sabouraud media. *T. vaginalis* may be cultured, but culture facilities are not available in most laboratories and may take up to 7 days for the report. Endocervical swabs are plated on Thayer-Martin medium soon after collection for growing *N. gonorrhoeae*. It is highly sensitive (>90%) and cost-effective. *Chlamydia* cultures are expensive and require a high level of expertise hence not used in routine practice. Routinely enzyme immunoassays are used for the diagnosis of chlamydial infection. These are less expensive and results are available faster.

Various criteria have been described for the diagnosis of bacterial vaginosis.[5] These include Amsel criteria, Hay/Ison criteria, and Nugent's criteria. For details of Amsel and Nugent criteria, refer to Table 4. The Bacterial Special Interest group of the British Association for Sexual Health and HIV (BASHH) recommend using the Hay/Ison criteria in clinics dealing with genitourinary infections.

Nucleic Acid Amplification Tests

Nucleic acid amplification test (NAAT) is available for the diagnosis of chlamydia and gonorrhoea.[6,7] This is highly sensitive but an expensive test. It has the advantage of testing for both these organisms on the same sample. NAAT offers the highest sensitivity for the detection of Trichomonas

Table 4: The Hay/Ison criteria.

Grades	Characteristics of Gram-stained smear of vaginal discharge
Grade 0	No bacteria present
Grade 1 (normal)	Lactobacillus morphotypes predominate
Grade 2 (intermediate)	Mixed flora with some lactobacilli present, but *Gardnerella* or *Mobiluncus* morphotypes also present
Grade 3 (bacterial vaginosis)	Predominantly *Gardnerella* and/or *Mobiluncus* morphotypes. Few or absent Lactobacilli
Grade 4	Gram-positive cocci predominate

vaginitis. It should be the test of choice where resources are adequate and is becoming the current "gold standard" with sensitivities of 88–97% and specificities of 98%–99%,[3] depending on the specimen and reference standard.

Pap Smear

Papanicolaou (Pap) smear may be helpful in detecting some vaginal and cervical pathogens such as *Trichomonas*, yeast cells, and clue cells.

Additional Investigations

All women presenting with vaginal discharge and their partners should be offered screening for sexually transmitted infections. The investigations advised include:
- Venereal Disease Research Laboratory (VDRL)/*Treponema pallidum* hemagglutination assay (TPHA) for syphilis
- Serology of HIV
- Hepatitis B surface antigen
- Hepatitis C antibodies.

Women with recurrent vaginal candidiasis are advised screening for diabetes mellitus.

Routine urine examination and urine culture sensitivity is advised to women with associated urinary symptoms.

Urethral culture for *N. gonorrhoeae* is indicated in the presence of urethral discharge or if gonorrhoeae is suspected.

In women where a cervical lesion is suspected of malignancy or cervical tuberculosis, relevant investigations such as PAP smear, cervical biopsy for histopathology, and for presence of *Mycobacterium tuberculosis* on smear or culture are advised.

Transvaginal sonography (TVS) is indicated in postmenopausal women with discharge coming out through cervix for any collection or growth in the uterine cavity. Pap smear, endocervical smear, and endometrial sampling may be considered in these women subsequently.

MANAGEMENT (BOX 1 AND FLOWCHARTS 1 AND 2)

The treatment of a woman presenting with vaginal discharge can be either a syndromic approach in low-resource settings or targeted based on the infective organism. For syndromic approach, various kits are provided by the National AIDS Control organization (NACO), Government of India, which can be prescribed to both partners depending upon whether the discharge is due to vaginitis or cervicitis or PID (Flowchart 2).

KEY POINTS

- Vaginal discharge is a common symptom among women in reproductive age group.

Flowchart 1: Algorithm for clinical approach to a woman presenting with discharge per vagina.

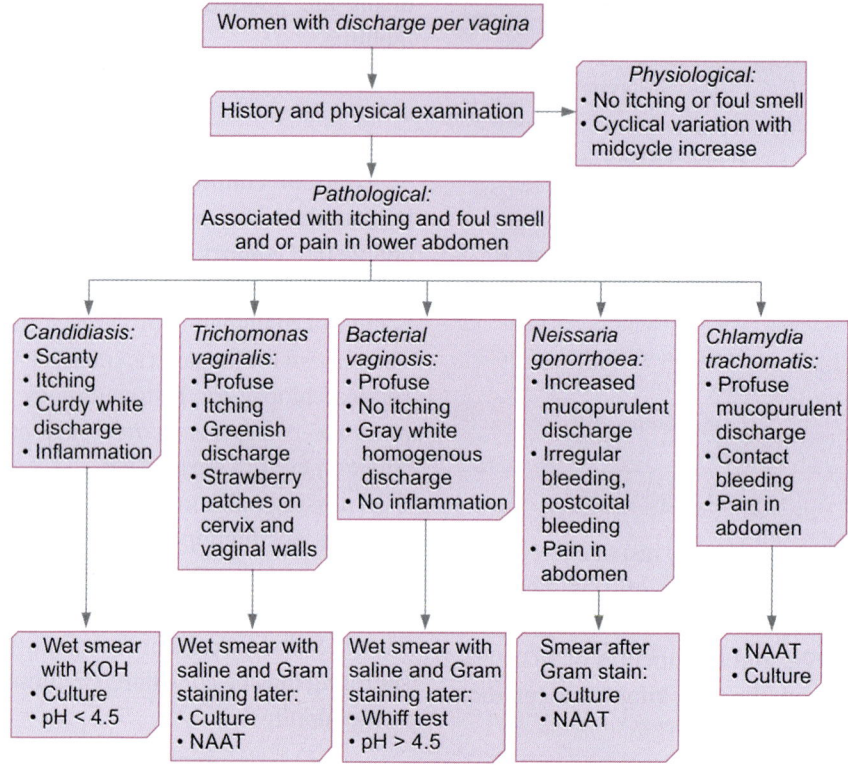

(NAAT: nucleic acid amplification test)

Box 1: General management principles for women with discharge per vagina.

- Safe sexual practices
- Avoid sex until symptoms have improved, particularly if there is fissuring of the skin
- Use of barrier contraceptives (except candidiasis)
- Treat both partners simultaneously
- Contact tracing

- A good history and examination are important to differentiate between physiological and pathological discharge.
- Only reassurance is enough in women with physiological discharge.
- A simple wet smear is a very useful tool in diagnosing common conditions such as candidiasis, trichomoniasis, and bacterial vaginosis.
- Cultures are not required routinely but should be offered to women with recurrent infection or resistant to treatment.
- Appropriate laboratory testing should be performed based on history and examination.
- Management should be specific to patient signs and symptoms and directed to specific infection.

REFERENCES

1. Thulkar J, Kriplani A, Agarwal N, Vishnubhatla S. Aetiology & risk factors of vaginitis &

Flowchart 2: Recommended management of specific infections.

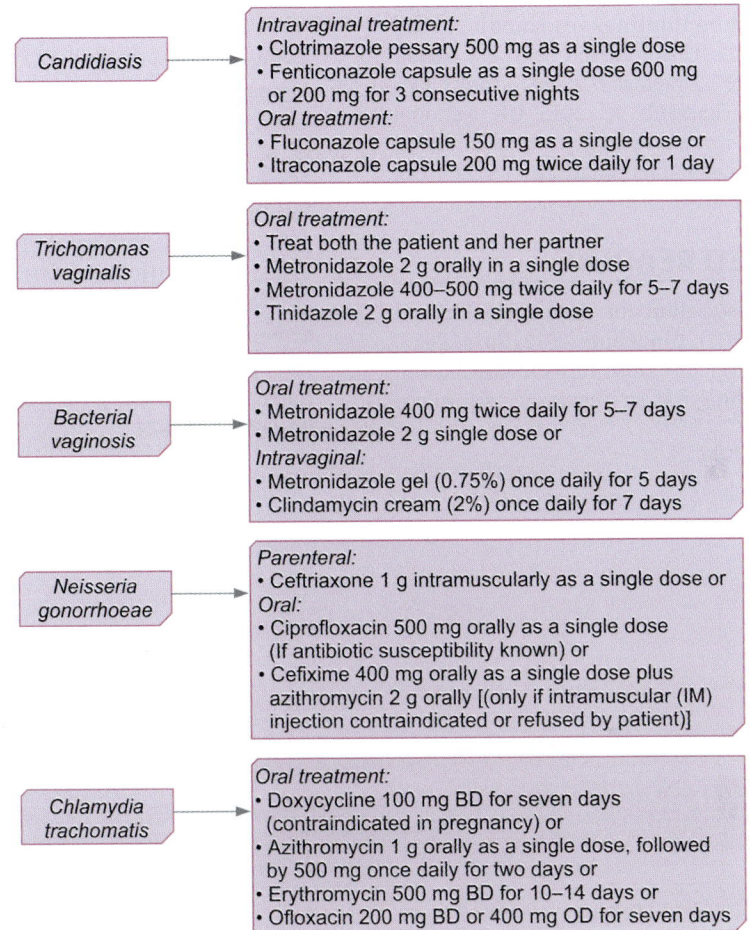

its association with various contraceptive methods. Indian J Med Res. 2010;131:83-7.
2. French L, Horton J, Matousek M. Abnormal vaginal discharge: using office diagnostic testing more effectively. J Fam Pract. 2004; 53(10):805-14.
3. Sherrard J, Ison C, Moody J, Wainwright E, Wilson J, Sullivan A. United Kingdom National Guideline on the Management of Trichomonas vaginalis 2014. Int J STD AIDS. 2014;25(8):541-9.
4. Saxon C, Edwards A, Richardson RR, Owen C, Nathan B, Palmer B, et al. Clinical Effectiveness group, British Association for Sexual Health and HIV national guideline for the management of vulvovaginal candidiasis 2019.
5. Hay P, Patel S, Daniels D. (2012). UK National Guideline for the management of Bacterial Vaginosis 2012. [online] Available from https://www.guidelinecentral.com/summaries/uk-national-guideline-for-the-management-of-bacterial-vaginosis-2012/#section-society. [Last accessed February, 2020].
6. Fifer H, Saunders J, Soni S, Sadiq ST, FitzGerald M (2019). British Association for Sexual Health and HIV national guideline for

the management of infection with Neisseria gonorrhoeae (2019). Available from https://www.bashhguidelines.org/media/1208/gc-2019.pdf. {Last accessed February, 2020].
7. Nwokolo NC, Dragovic B, Patel S, Tong CYW, Barker G, Radcliffe K. 2015 UK National Guideline for the management of infection with Chlamydia trachomatis. Int J STD AIDS. 2016;27(4):251-67.

SUGGESTED READING

1. British Association for Sexual Health and HIV (BASHH): Guidelines 2012, 2014, 2019. [online] Available from https://www.bashh.org/guidelines. [Last accessed February, 2020].
2. Committee on Practice Bulletins—Gynecology. Vaginitis in Nonpregnant Patients: ACOG Practice Bulletin, Number 215. Obstet Gynecol. 2020;135(1):e1-17.
3. Pappas PG, Kauffman CA, Andes DR, Clancy CJ, Marr KA, Ostrosky-Zeichner L, et al. Clinical Practice Guideline for the Management of Candidiasis: 2016 Update by the Infectious Diseases Society of America. Clin Infect Dis. 2016;62(4):e1-50.
4. van Schalkwyk J1, Yudin MH2; INFECTIOUS DISEASE COMMITTEE. Vulvovaginitis: screening for and management of trichomoniasis, vulvovaginal candidiasis, and bacterial vaginosis. J Obstet Gynaecol Can. 2015;37(3):266-74.

31. Approach to a Woman Presenting with Abnormal Uterine Bleeding

Asmita Kaundal, Neha Gami

INTRODUCTION

Menstruation is a regular physiological event occurring in the lives of women in the reproductive age group. Normal menstruation refers to cyclical flow of blood lasting for 2–7 days at an interval of 28 ± 7 days. The average blood loss is <60 mL/cycle.[1] Any deviation in cycle length, duration, or amount of bleeding, bleeding in between normal cycles (intermenstrual bleeding) or bleeding after menopause (postmenopausal bleeding) is grouped under the broad term abnormal uterine bleeding (AUB).

Abnormal uterine bleeding has a significant impact on the quality of life of the women. Prevalence of the disorder varies between different age groups and from region to region ranging from 3 to 35%.[2] AUB can have many causes, some of which may coexist. For this reason, the International Federation of Obstetrics and Gynecology (FIGO) has devised a classification system for AUB, the PALM–COEIN classification system.[3] According to this classification, causes of AUB are either structurally visible such as polyps, adenomyosis, leiomyoma, malignancy, or hyperplasia; or causes which are not structurally visible such as coagulopathy, ovulation dysfunction, endometrial causes, iatrogenic, and not otherwise classified. Use of terms such as menorrhagia, metrorrhagia, oligomenorrhea, and dysfunctional uterine bleeding (DUB) are abandoned as the terms are poorly defined with no consistent meaning.[4] Heavy menstrual bleeding (HMB) for menorrhagia and intermenstrual bleeding (IMB) for metrorrhagia are preferred over the older terminology.

A classification of AUB into chronic, acute, and intermenstrual AUB was also made by the FIGO at the Conference in Cape Town in 2009.[2] Chronic AUB is defined as uterine bleeding that is abnormal for 6 or more months in either volume of blood loss and or regularity. It usually does not require immediate intervention. Acute AUB is defined as an episode of heavy bleeding requiring immediate intervention.[5]

The revised FIGO AUB System 1 terminology used for menstrual patterns is shown in Table 1.[4]

DIFFERENTIAL DIAGNOSIS OF ABNORMAL UTERINE BLEEDING

Box 1 gives the differential diagnosis of AUB in all age groups. However, in adolescents' immature hypothalamic–pituitary axis, endocrinopathies and disorders of hemostasis such as immune thrombocytopenia (ITP) and coagulation disorders are more common. In women of reproductive age group, pregnancy complications, fibroids, pelvic inflammatory

Section 2: Gynecology

Table 1: Terminology used for menstrual patterns as per the revised FIGO AUB system.[1]

Parameter	
Frequency	• Absent (no bleeding) = amenorrhea • Infrequent (>38 days) • Normal (≥24 days to ≤38 days) • Frequent (≤24 days)
Duration	• Normal (≤8 days) • Prolonged (≥8 days)
Regularity	• Regular (shortest-to-longest cycle variation of ≤7–9 days) • Irregular (shortest-to-longest cycle variation of ≥8–10 days)
Flow volume (determined by the patient)	• Light • Normal • Heavy
Intermenstrual bleeding (IMB) Bleeding between cyclically regular menses	• None • Random • Cyclic (predictable: early cycle, mid cycle, late cycle)
Unscheduled bleeding on progestin ± estrogen gonadal steroids (birth control pills, rings, patches, or injections)	• Not applicable (not on gonadal steroid medication) • None (on gonadal steroid medication) • Present

(AUB: abnormal uterine bleeding; FIGO: International Federation of Obstetrics and Gynecology)

Box 1: Differential diagnosis of abnormal uterine bleeding (AUB).

- *Structural abnormalities*:
  – Tumors—benign or malignant
    » *Benign*: Fibroids, fibroid polyp, endometrial polyp, and cervical polyp
    » *Malignant*: Endometrial cancer, cancer cervix or vagina, GTN, estrogen-producing ovarian tumors
  – Cervical erosion
  – Adenomyosis
  – Prolapse with decubitus ulcer
- *Endometrial hyperplasia*:
  – Simple or complex, with or without atypia
- *Endocrinopathies*:
  – Immature HPO axis (adolescents)
  – *HPO dysfunction*: Stress, weight loss/gain
  – Hypothyroidism
  – Hyperprolactinemia
  – PCOS
- *Coagulopathies or bleeding disorders*:
  – von Willebrand disease
  – Idiopathic thrombocytopenic purpera
  – Aplastic anemia
- *Infections*:
  – *PID*: Chlamydia and tuberculosis
  – Iatrogenic following abortion and delivery
- *Iatrogenic*:
  – *Medications*: Hormones, anticoagulants, and antipsychotics
  – Hormonal contraceptives
  – Intrauterine contraceptive device
  – Foreign body
- *Others*:
  – Atrophic endometritis
  – Urinary tract
  – Gastrointestinal tract

(GTN: gestational trophoblastic neoplasia; HPO: hypothalamic-pituitary-ovarian; PCOS: polycystic ovary syndrome; PID: pelvic inflammatory disease)

disease (PID), and endometrial hyperplasia are common causes of AUB whereas in postmenopausal women malignancies are more common.

HISTORY

A detailed menstrual history is important to narrow the differential diagnosis. Age at menarche and menopause is important for early age at menarche (<10 years) or late menopause (>55 years) is associated with increased risk of endometrial malignancy.

It is easy to elicit menstrual history in menstrual abnormalities wherein the cycles are regular but is challenging in patients, where cycles are irregular. In these cases, the menstrual pattern can be described by asking the minimum and maximum number of days the woman bleeds, and the minimum and maximum interval between the 1st day of two consecutive cycles, and describe the menstrual cycles as the range of the number of days she bleeds and range of the interval between the cycles. Sometimes the woman can be asked to keep a menstrual calendar for understanding the menstrual abnormality.

History of prolonged cycles with heavy menstrual flow is suggestive of anovulatory cycles and unopposed estrogen exposure which may be associated with increased risk of endometrial hyperplasia and malignancy.

It is important to differentiate irregular or intermenstrual bleeding from postcoital bleeding. Ask for any association between the sexual act and bleeding episode. Postcoital bleeding may be due to cervical erosion, cervical polyp, or cervical carcinoma.

In women with postmenopausal bleeding, duration of menopause is important. A history of menopause of long duration and vaginal dryness is suggestive of low estrogen levels in the body and may cause bleeding due to atrophic endometritis.

Duration of Illness

To begin with, find out the duration of illness by asking how long back the woman had normal menstrual cycles. What was the pattern of bleeding at that time, i.e., number of days she bled and the interval between two consecutive cycles? It is important to emphasize that the interval in question is between the onset of two consecutive cycles and not between the end of first cycle and the beginning of next cycle.

Severity of Bleeding

Severity of bleeding is assessed in terms of number of pads used each day, whether partially or fully soaked. Flooding and/or passage of clots indicate excessive blood loss. One can assess the blood loss in terms of the percentage of the loss compared to previous normal cycles, e.g., 25%, i.e., one fourth, 50% half, 150%, one and half times the blood lost in previous cycles. This is helpful in assessing the impact of treatment in follow up visits.

Onset of Illness

The onset of illness is important. It is insidious with fibroids and sudden with any pregnancy-related problem, PID or following intrauterine contraceptive device (IUCD) insertion. History of preceding amenorrhea indicates that the episode could either be a pregnancy-related problem or anovulation related.

While eliciting history of amenorrhea, the date of last menstrual period (LMP) is often asked. It is important to find out if the LMP was normal or scanty. Pregnant woman can have implantation bleeding in first 3 months and women with anovulatory cycles may have breakthrough spotting or light bleeding and consider it wrongly as her LMP. So, LMP is essentially the date of last normal menstrual period.

Course of Illness

Progressively increasing menorrhagia with or without dysmenorrhea is usually suggestive of fibroid uterus and/or adenomyosis.

Associated Dysmenorrhea

History of associated secondary dysmenorrhea is an important symptom. Severe dysmenorrhea, which worsens with the onset of periods and persists even after periods, is suggestive of adenomyosis. Congestive dysmenorrhea, which gets relieved with the onset of period, is present in women with PID and fibroids. Spasmodic dysmenorrhea, which is associated with bouts of bleeding and is described by patients as being something similar to labor pains, is present in women with submucosal fibroid in the process of expulsion.

Associated Symptoms

In women with menorrhagia, it is important to enquire about any history of recent medical termination of pregnancy (MTP) or spontaneous abortion suggestive of postabortion complications such as postabortion menorrhagia, incomplete abortion, infection, or gestational trophoblastic neoplasia.

History of pain in the lower abdomen and discharge per vaginum is indicative of PID. Any history of abdominal lump is suggestive of fibroid.

One needs to rule out thyroid dysfunction by asking any history of heat or cold intolerance, any constipation or diarrhea, and any loss or gain of weight. History of galactorrhea should be elicited in women with prolonged cycles, which is suggestive of hyperprolactinemia. Any history of hot flashes suggests premature ovarian failure as a cause of menstrual irregularity.

History of foul-smelling discharge mixed with blood and postcoital bleeding may suggest cervical carcinoma. History of something coming out of vagina (uterovaginal prolapse) may suggest decubitus ulcer. Weight loss, anorexia, and cachexia suggests malignancy (endometrial, cervical, or ovarian). It is important to ask for any history of trauma or injury.

Contraceptive History

Detailed history of contraceptive use, especially history of IUCD insertion or hormonal contraception such as oral contraceptive pills, depot medroxy progesterone acetate, levonorgestrel intrauterine system (IUS), and emergency contraception can cause menstrual abnormality.

Medical History

History of diabetes mellitus and hypertension is a risk factor for endometrial cancer in women of perimenopausal age group. Any history of tuberculosis should be elicited as it may be associated with heavy menstrual bleeding initially and decreased flow subsequently. History of easy bruising is indicative of some coagulation disorder.

Family History

Certain diseases have a familial predisposition. Any history of fibroids, genital or breast cancer in mother or sister should be elicited as these conditions have a familial clustering. History of coagulation disorders in any family member could point to an underlying bleeding disorder in women with heavy periods. Family history of heavy periods or postpartum hemorrhage (PPH) in mother or sister could point toward a coagulation disorder. Family history of diabetes mellitus, hypertension, tuberculosis, and uterine, ovarian, breast or colon cancer in the family is important.

Obstetric History

In the obstetric history, one needs to ask the duration of married life; if the patient has had any difficulty in conceiving or did she ever require ovulation induction to help her conceive. This history, when present, may suggest polycystic ovary syndrome (PCOS). History of nulliparity is associated with endometrial cancer whereas history of early onset of sexual activity, early age at first child birth, multiparity, and reduced spacing between pregnancies is associated with cervical carcinoma.

Each conception with its outcome should be described in detail with special mention of any antepartum, intrapartum, or postpartum complications. Finally, past and present use of any contraceptive should be asked for.

History of Past Illness

History of any myomectomy in past is important as there can be a recurrence of fibroid. History of breast cancer with the use of tamoxifen can be associated with endometrial hyperplasia and endometrial cancer. History of hypertension and diabetes associated with menstrual irregularity could be a part of the corpus cancer syndrome. History of any bleeding disorder should be asked for.

Drug History

History of use of anticoagulants could explain the heavy menstrual bleeding while history of recent use of hormonal pills in the form of oral contraceptive pills, emergency pills, or hormone replacement therapy (HRT) could explain any deviation from the normal menstrual cycle. Unopposed estrogen therapy as HRT or tamoxifen for breast cancer are associated with endometrial carcinoma.

EXAMINATION

General Physical Examination

Height and weight are measured and body mass index (BMI) is calculated. Obese women are at higher risk of endometrial carcinoma. The vitals are assessed as patients presenting with severe bleeding may have tachycardia and hypotension. Women with chronic blood loss may be pale but well compensated. Moreover, recording blood pressure is important because women presenting with postmenopausal bleeding are old and are more likely to be hypertensive. The severity of pallor is assessed and corroborated with the history. Temperature of the patient is recorded as women with AUB due to acute PID may be febrile. Bruising, petechiae, or hemarthrosis may indicate some underlying coagulation disorder or suggest that the woman may be on anticoagulant therapy.

Breast Examination

Careful bilateral breast examination should be carried out to detect any retraction or puckering of skin or nipples, any discharge from nipples, or palpable lump suggestive of breast carcinoma. Any milky discharge from the breast (galactorrhea) could be associated with hyperprolactinemia leading to abnormal menstrual cycles.

Systemic Examination

Systemic examination includes a detailed examination of the respiratory system, cardiovascular system, and abdominal examination.

Per Abdomen Examination

On inspection, there might be distension in lower abdomen due to a large fibroid or ovarian mass. On palpation, deep tenderness in the iliac fossa or hypogastrium may suggest PID. A palpable intra-abdominal lump in lower abdomen with lower margin not reached is likely to be a fibroid; this is as compared to ovarian masses where the lower limit is usually reached and the mass may be lifted out of the pelvis. However, with large ovarian mass, the lower limit may not be reached. Spleen, if palpable, could signify a platelet disorder or chronic anemia. Look for any evidence of ascites, which could be associated with underlying malignancy.

Per Speculum Examination

On per speculum examination, look for rugosities and color of vaginal mucosa; pale vagina with absent rugosities is suggestive of atrophic vagina. Thickened vaginal mucosa with decubitus ulcer indicates a long-standing uterovaginal prolapse (Fig. 1). Unhealthy discharge per vaginum may be due to PID. Sometimes a fibroid polyp or an endocervical or endometrial polyp may be seen coming out of the cervical os (Figs. 2 and 3). The threads of a forgotten IUCD may be visualized and cervical lesions such as cervical erosion (Fig. 4), carcinoma cervix (Fig. 5) may be detected.

If the patient is not bleeding, a Papanicolaou (Pap) smear and endocervical brushing should be taken prior to per vaginal examination. (Fig. 6).

Per Vaginum Examination

On per vaginum examination, assess the size, position, and shape of the uterus, its mobility, and presence of any tenderness or any adnexal mass such as tubo-ovarian

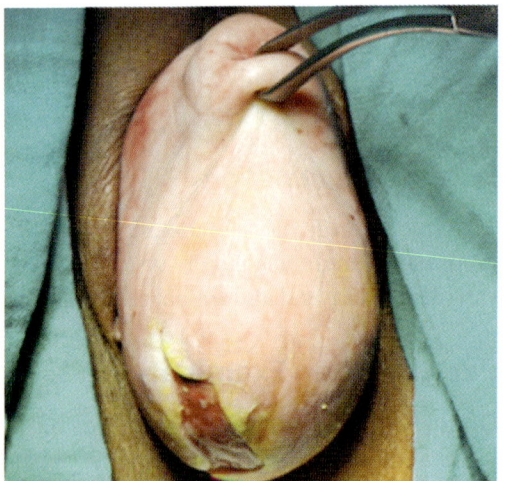

Fig. 1: Prolapse with decubitus ulcer.

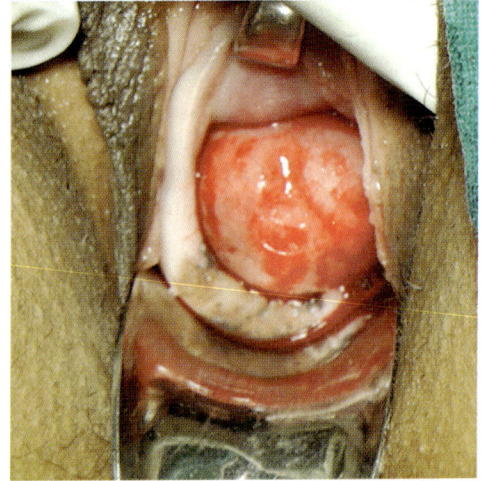

Fig. 2: Per speculum examination—fibroid polyp.

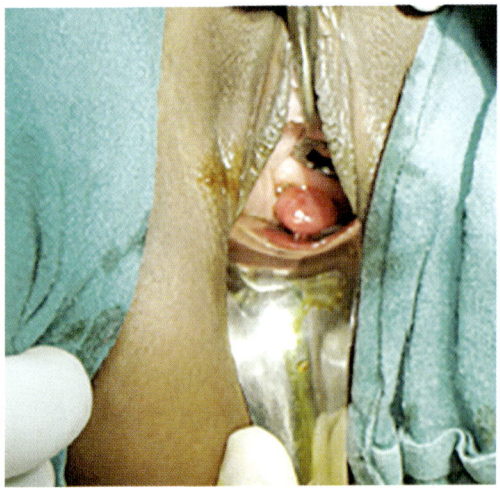

Fig. 3: Per speculum examination—endocervical polyp.

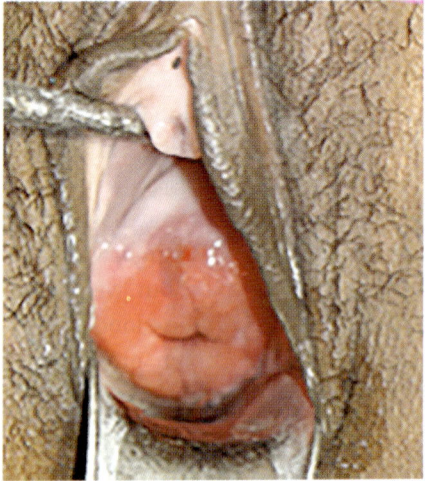

Fig. 4: Per speculum examination—cervical erosion.

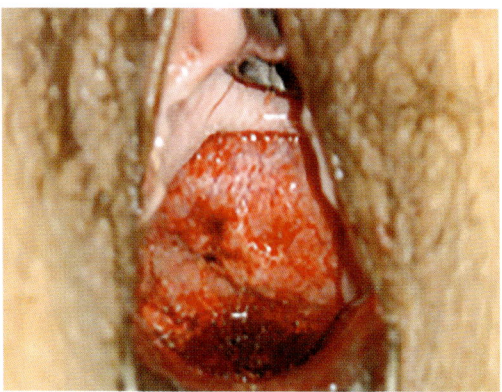

Fig. 5: Per speculum examination—cervical cancer.

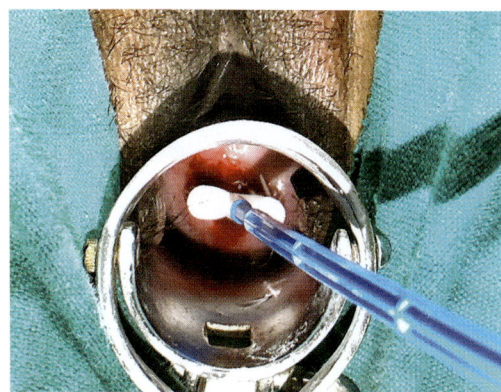

Fig. 6: Endocervical brushing for Pap smear. (Pap: Papanicolaou)

mass or ovarian tumor. The size of the uterus is enlarged in case of pregnancy, fibroid, adenomyosis, and endometrial carcinoma. It is irregular in shape in case of fibroids. Uterine tenderness is present in adenomyosis and PID. Fornices are tender in PID.

INVESTIGATIONS

The investigative workup of these women is essentially guided by the age, history, and clinical examination. The investigations include urine pregnancy test, cervical cytology, a complete blood count, peripheral smear, and reticulocyte count for anemia and any evidence of thrombocytopenia.

In the presence of signs and symptoms of endocrine disease, specific tests such as thyroid profile and serum prolactin should be carried out.

Evaluation for any hematological disorder is not routinely done for all women presenting with AUB. It should only be done if the clinical history is suggestive (positive screen) of bleeding disorder (Box 2). Initial investigations for bleeding disorders include platelet count, prothrombin time and partial thromboplastin time. Special tests for von Willebrand disease or other coagulopathies is

> **Box 2:** Indication for screening for bleeding disorders.[7]
> - Heavy menstrual bleeding since menarche
> - *One of the following*:
>   – Postpartum hemorrhage
>   – Surgery-related bleeding
>   – Bleeding associated with dental procedures
> - *Two or more of the following*:
>   – Bleeding during brushing once or twice per month
>   – Epistaxis once or twice per month
>   – Gum bleeding
>   – History of bleeding disorders in the family

guided by the medical history, family history of bleeding disorders, and the initial tests.

A Pap smear and endocervical brushing should be taken prior to per vaginal examination (Fig. 6). It is a good practice to do VIA and VILI in the clinic after taking Pap smear. Any growth, polyp, or abnormal acetowhite area or unstained areas on VIA or VILI, respectively, should be biopsied. Colposcopy is indicated in case of abnormal Pap Smear (ASCUS-H, LSIL or HSIL), any abnormality on VIA or VILI or when cervical cancer is strongly suspected (Figs. 7 to 9). High-risk HPV DNA is indicated for triaging in women >30 years of age with Pap smear report of atypical

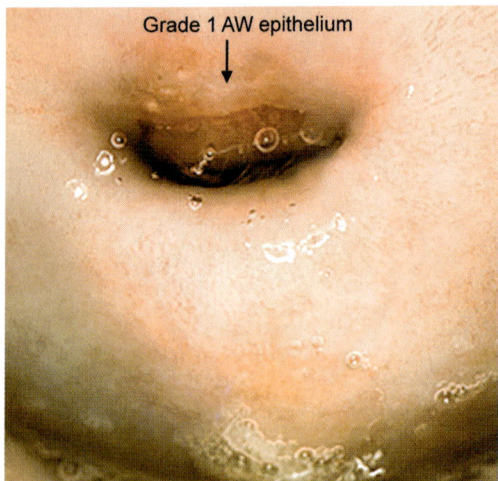

Fig. 7: Negative VIA grade 1 acetowhite area on anterior lip of cervix.
(VIA: visual inspection with acetic acid; AW: acetowhite)

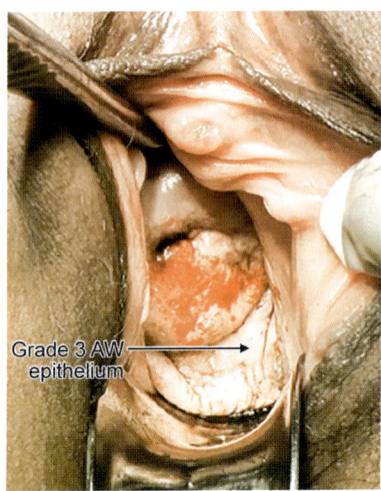

Fig. 8: Positive VIA grade 3 acetowhite area on posterior lip of cervix and posterior vaginal wall.
(VIA: visual inspection with acetic acid; AW: acetowhite)

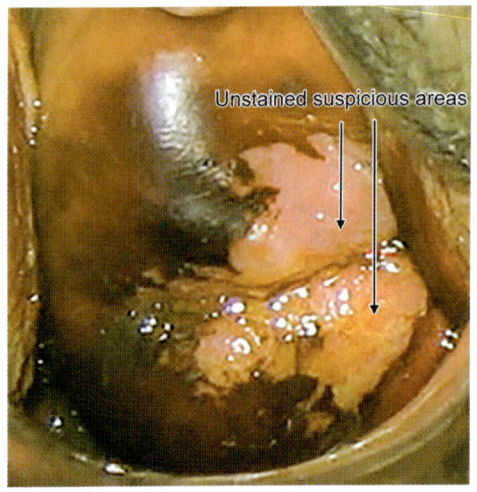

Fig. 9: Visual inspection of the cervix with Lugol's iodine; unstained suspicious area.

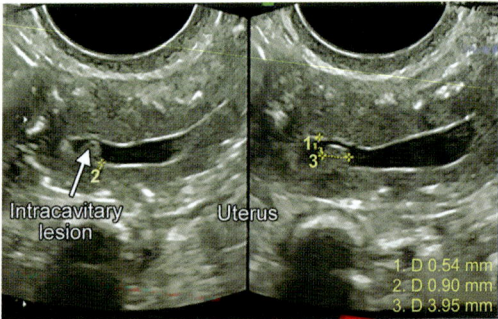

Fig. 10: Saline sonohysterography showing an intrauterine lesion.

squamous cells of undetermined significance (ASCUS). The British Society for Colposcopy and Cervical Pathology (BSCCP) recommends colposcopy in women with postcoital bleeding above the age of 40 with associated intermenstrual bleeding or with persistent vaginal discharge.[6]

Ultrasonography is used to evaluate the uterus and adnexa. The initial scan can rule out pregnancy and other anatomical abnormalities such as polyps and fibroids. Transvaginal ultrasonography TVS can be used as an initial investigation for evaluation of endometrium and to select cases requiring further evaluation by saline infusion sonohysterography (SIS) or hysteroscopy (Fig. 10). In TVS done on day 4–6 of the menstrual cycle, an endometrial thickness of less than

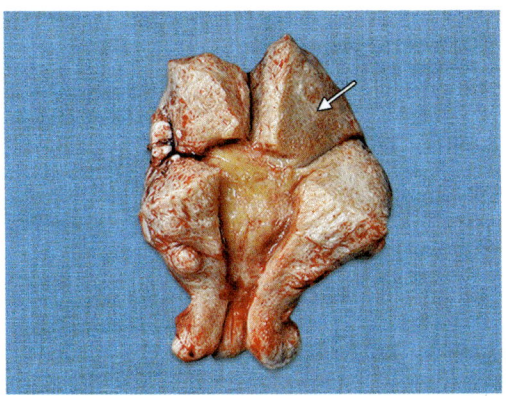

Fig. 11: Adenomyosis on cut section.

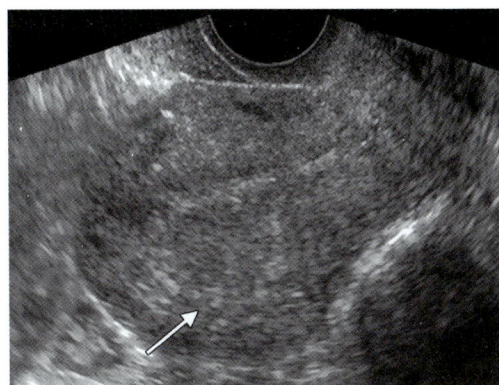

Fig. 12: Ultrasound appearance of adenomyosis.

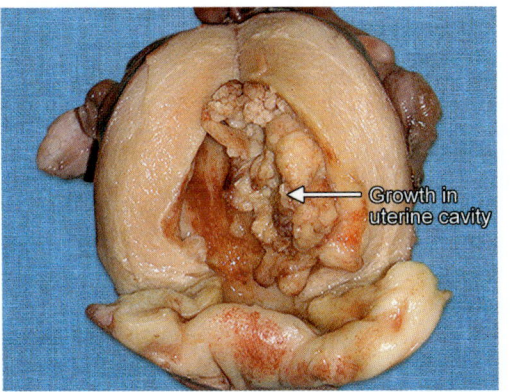

Fig. 13: Carcinoma body uterus—cut section of uterus.

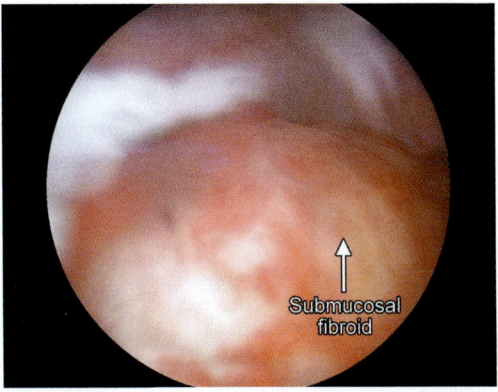

Fig. 14: Hysteroscopic view of submucosal fibroid.

5 mm rules out any significant endometrial pathology (Fig. 11).[9] Any focal thickening is an indication for sonohysterography or hysteroscopy. Adenomyosis can be diagnosed on ultrasonography (Fig. 12) and further confirmed on magnetic resonance imaging (MRI).

Endometrial sampling should be done in all women over 40 years of age and in younger women with high risk factors for endometrial cancer and in those, who show no improvement after 3 months of medical management. It is rarely indicated in adolescents. The sample should be sent for histopathological examination, acid-fast bacilli (AFB) smear and culture. It can be done as an office endometrial biopsy, dilatation and curettage, or hysteroscopy-directed biopsy. Office endometrial biopsy has a sensitivity of 67–96%. It is a relatively safe technique and does not require cervical dilatation or anesthesia. Dilatation and curettage is indicated in cases likely to be technically difficult as in postmenopausal women. Hysteroscopy-directed biopsy has the advantage of diagnosing focal lesions such as carcinoma body uterus (Fig. 13), polyps, and submucosal fibroids (Fig. 14). Diagnosis with supportive history, examination, and investigations is briefly described in Table 2.

Section 2: Gynecology

Table 2: Summary of diagnosis with supportive history, examination, and investigations.

Diagnosis	History	Examination	Investigations
Immature HPO axis	Irregular cycles within 2 years of menarche	Pallor may be present Gynecological examination—normal	Normal
Pregnancy complications	Preceding amenorrhea	PV: Uterus enlarged and soft; internal os may be open	• UPT positive • Ultrasound will show gestational sac or products of conception in uterus
Pelvic inflammatory disease (PID)	Vaginal discharge, pain in lower abdomen, and fever	PS: Mucopurulent discharge PV: Tenderness in fornices and or palpable adnexal masses	Ultrasound may show adnexal mass and free fluid in pouch of Douglas
Fibroid	Regular cyclical heavy periods, secondary dysmenorrhea Heaviness in lower abdomen, abdominal lump, and frequency of urination	PS: Fibroid polyp may be seen coming through the os PV: Uterus enlarged, firm, irregular, mobile and movements transmitted to cervix	Ultrasound, MRI
Adenomyosis	Heavy periods with severe dysmenorrhea	PV: Slightly enlarged and tender uterus	Ultrasound, MRI
Endometrial carcinoma	Irregular heavy bleeding	PS: May be normal PV: Slightly enlarged uterus	• *Ultrasound*: Endometrial thickness increased, endometrial–myometrial junction not clear, irregular growth within the endometrium • Endometrial biopsy with or without hysteroscopy • MRI for staging
Ovulatory dysfunction (O)	Irregular bleeding with variable volume	PS: Normal PV: No abnormality detected PS: Normal	• Ultrasound will rule out organic cause • Endometrial biopsy if age > 40 years, failure of medical management for 3 months or presence of risk factors for endometrial carcinoma
Estrogen-producing ovarian tumors	Heavy cycles	PV: Adnexal mass	Ultrasound, MRI
Trophoblastic disease	History of having been pregnant or molar pregnancy in past, history of irregular bleeding	PS: Bluish nodules in vagina, especially suburethral region PV: Uterus may be normal in size or slightly enlarged, soft, Ovaries may be enlarged	Ultrasound, UPT, serum β-human chorionic gonadotropin (β-hCG) titers, MRI
Intrauterine contraceptive device (IUCD)	History of IUCD insertion Heavy cycles at short intervals	PS: Threads seen PV: Normal	Ultrasound
Drugs (anticoagulants)	History of heart disease with valve replacement, or thrombosis in past with heavy cycles	PS: May be normal PV: Normal	Prothrombin time (PT), partial prothrombin time with kaolin (PTTK), and platelet count

(HPO: hypothalamic–pituitary–ovarian; MRI: magnetic resonance imaging; UPT: urine pregnancy test; PS: per speculum; PV: per vaginum; NAD: no abnormality detected)

Management

Management of the women with abnormal uterine bleeding depands upon age, presentation (acute or chronic), desire for fertility, comorbid conditions, contraindication for a specific treatment modality and preferences of women. Any woman presenting with acute AUB requires stabilization and urgent management with antifibrinolytic agents and hormonal therapy. She should receive appropriate resuscitative and supportive measure to stop the bleeding along with replacement of fluid and blood products, if required. For women who are hemodynamically stable or are presenting with chronic AUB both medical and surgical options are available.

Tranexamic acid and NSAIDs should be considered as a first line of management except in cases of bleeding disorders if it is certain that the women is not pregnant.

LNG-IUS is an excellent option for all age groups . There is significant reduction in the blood loss. In addition it offers contraceptive benefits to women. Unscheduled spotting in the initial months of insertion is a problem and women need to be counseled about that prior to insertion.

Combined hormonal contraceptives are effective in the treatment of AUB for women eligible for contraceptive methods but unsuitable or unwilling for LNG-IUS.

Cyclical progestins are also a good option for those with contraindications for combined hormonal methods.

Centchroman (ormeloxifene) is a non hormonal contraceptive used in women who are unsuitable for hormonal methods.

If the above mentioned methods fail and the women is either unwilling or unfit for surgery, GnRH agonists with add back therapy can be considered.

In the surgical management cause specific management of the structural causes is offered.

Hysterectomy should be considered if all other methods fail or if patient does not want conservative management.

Women with evidence of carcinoma should be referred to a gynecological oncologist as early as possible for further evaluation and management.

KEY POINTS

- Abnormal uterine bleeding significantly affects a woman's quality of life.
- Use of PALM–COEIN system of classification provides a uniform system of classification.
- All the women with AUB should be subjected to meticulous history, examination, and clinical investigations based on initial workup.
- All adolescents' or adult women with positive screen should be investigated for bleeding disorders.
- All postmenopausal women should be evaluated for endometrial carcinoma.
- Medical management should be considered as an initial treatment, and surgical management should be offered if medical management fails, or it is contraindicated or denied by the patient.
- All acute cases of AUB should receive immediate intervention.

REFERENCES

1. Fraser IS, Warner P, Marantos PA. Estimating menstrual blood loss in women with normal and excessive menstrual fluid volume. Obstet Gynecol. 2001;98(5PT 1):806-14.
2. Harlow SD, Campbell OM. Epidemiology of menstrual disorders in developing countries: A systematic review. BJOG. 2004;111(1):6-16.
3. Munro MG, Critchley HO, Broder MS, Fraser IS, FIGO menstural disorder committee.

FIGO classification system (PALM-COEIN) for causes of abnormal uterine bleeding in nongravid women of reproductive age. Int J Gynaecol Obstet. 2011;113(1):3-13.
4. Munro MG, Critchley HO, Fraser IS, FIGO menstural disorder Committee. The two FIGO systems for normal and abnormal uterine bleeding symptoms and classification of causes of abnormal uterine bleeding in the reproductive years: 2018 revisions. Int J Gynaecol Obstet. 2018;143(3):393-408.
5. Munro MG, Mainor N, Basu R, Brisinger M, Barreda L. Oral medroxyprogesterone acetate and combination oral contraceptives for acute uterine bleeding: a randomized controlled trial. Obstet Gynecol. 2006;108(4):924-9.
6. British Society for Colposcopy and Cervical Pathology. Guidelines for colposcopy. [online] Available from www.bsccp.org.uk. [Last accessed March, 2020].
7. Kouides PA, Conard J, Peyvandi F, Lukes A, Kadir R. Hemostasis and menstruation: appropriate investigation for underlying disorders of hemostasis in women with excessive menstrual bleeding. Fertil Steril. 2005;84(5):1345-51.

SUGGESTED READING

1. American College of Obstetricians and Gynecologists. ACOG committee opinion no. 557: Management of acute abnormal uterine bleeding in nonpregnant reproductive-aged women. Obstet Gynecol. 2013;121(4):891-6.
2. Committee on Practice Bulletins—Gynecology. Practice bulletin no. 128: Diagnosis of abnormal uterine bleeding in reproductive-aged women. Obstet Gynecol. 2012;120(1):197-206.
3. Committee on Practice Bulletins—Gynecology. Practice bulletin no. 136: Practice bulletin on management of abnormal uterine bleeding associated with ovulatory dysfunction. Obstet Gynecol. 2013;122(1):176-85.
4. Demers C, Derzko C, David M, Douglas J; Society of Obstetricians and Gynecologists of Canada. Gynaecological and obstetric management of women with inherited bleeding disorders. J Obstet Gynaecol Can. 2005;27(7):707-32.
5. National Institute for Health and Care Excellence (NICE). (2018). Nice Guidelines: Heavy menstrual bleeding: Assessment and management. [online] Available from https://www.nice.org.uk/guidance/ng88/resources/heavy-menstrual-bleeding-assessment-and-management-pdf-1837701412549. [Last accessed March, 2020].
6. Singh S, Best C, Dunn S, Leyland N, Wolfman WL. No. 292-Abnormal uterine bleeding in pre-menopausal women. J Obstet Gynaecol Can. 2018;40(5):e391-415.

32. Approach to a Woman Presenting with Infertility

Seema Singhal, Namita Jain

INTRODUCTION

Infertility is defined as 1 year of unprotected intercourse without conception. Some prefer the term *subfertility* to describe women or couples who are not sterile but exhibit decreased reproductive efficiency.

Table 1 gives the cumulative pregnancy rates in relation to age.

The National Institute for Health and Care Excellence (NICE) and the American Society for Reproductive Medicine (ASRM) recommend initiating infertility investigations after 12 months of unprotected intercourse. Counseling regarding options should be offered to couples who are not physically able to conceive (i.e., same-sex couples or persons lacking reproductive organs).

Early evaluation is indicated in the following:
- Women older than 35 years (due to age-related decline in fertility and poor outcome with assisted reproductive techniques (ART)
- When infertility factor is known or highly suspected in the female (oligo/amenorrhea, uterine or tubal disease, endometriosis, family history of early menopause, and previous ovarian surgery) or in the male (undescended testis, history of orchitis, varicocele, hydrocele) or prior treatment for cancer in either partner.

DIFFERENTIAL DIAGNOSIS

For a woman to conceive spontaneously, there are three essential components—sperm, ovum, and patent fallopian tube. It is essential that woman should ovulate, the ovum should be picked up by fimbrial end of fallopian tube transported to the ampullary part of the tube where sperms reach from the vagina through the cervix and uterine cavity, and fertilization takes place. The fertilized ovum is then transported into the uterine cavity for implantation.

Depending on this basic physiology, the causes of infertility can be divided as given in Table 2.

Table 1: Probability of conceiving a clinical pregnancy by number of menstrual cycles.[1]

Age category (years)	Pregnant after 1 year/12 cycles (%)	Pregnant after 2 years/24 cycles (%)
19–26	92	98
27–29	87	95
30–34	86	94
35–39	82	90

Table 2: Causes of infertility.[2]

Female factor infertility:	
• Ovarian	21–25%
• Tubal	14–20%
• Others (uterine, cervical, vaginal, peritoneal)	10–13%
Male factor	26–30%
Unexplained	25%
Combined	40%

Ideally, initial consultation should be scheduled to allow sufficient time to obtain comprehensive medical, reproductive, and family history and to perform thorough physical examination. Both female and male partners should be evaluated together so that the couple has full understanding of the diagnosis and management.

Initial evaluation also focusses on preconception care (folic acid supplementation, rubella, and chickenpox vaccination) and lifestyle changes (cessation of smoking and toxic exposure). Sexual intercourse every 2–3 days, limiting alcohol to 1–2 units/week, and BMI <30 kg/m² (for both partners) optimize the chances of conception.[1]

HISTORY

Female Partner

Age

Maternal age is inversely related to fecundity. Female fertility declines with age. However, because there is little or no overall measurable decline in male fertility before the age of 45–50 years, male partner generally contributes relatively little to the overall age-related decline in fertility.[2]

Duration and Type of Infertility

Duration of infertility should be elicited. It is inversely proportional to successful treatment in unexplained infertility.

Whether the infertility is primary or secondary is important. Primary infertility is the inability to conceive in a couple who has had no prior pregnancy and secondary infertility is the inability to conceive in a couple who has had at least one prior conception irrespective of the outcome.

Contraceptive History

Previous history of contraceptive use as regards the method, any associated problems and duration of use should be enquired. Sometimes, the return of fertility can take up to 1 year after injection depomedroxyprogesterone acetate (DMPA). Tubal obstruction can be suspected in women using intrauterine contraceptive devices as they are at an increased risk of pelvic inflammatory disease (PID) and resultant tubal damage.

Sexual History

Sexual history should be elaborated in detail. The knowledge of the fertile period, frequency of intercourse, any sexual dysfunction like vaginismus, impotence or premature ejaculation in male partner, any coital difficulties, dyspareunia and use of lubricants need to be elicited, as all these factors can contribute to infertility. History suggestive of sexually transmitted infections (STIs) such as ulcers on genitalia, multiple sexual partners, and recurrent PID is important as it increases the risk of tubal factor infertility.

Menstrual History

Age at menarche, cycle length, duration and amount of flow, associated dysmenorrhea, and date of last menstrual period should be enquired. Ovulatory dysfunction is suggested by late menarche, prolonged periods (oligomenorrhea) and decrease in menstrual blood flow (hypomenorrhea and premenstrual spotting). Periods of amenorrhea followed by a heavy cycle is suggestive of ovulatory dysfunction. Dysmenorrhea and/or deep dyspareunia may be present in endometriosis or PID. Menorrhagia with dysmenorrhea may suggest presence of adenomyosis or a submucosal or intramural uterine fibromyoma.

Obstetric History

A detailed obstetric history, especially in patients with secondary infertility can give important clues to the likely cause of infertility. History of prior pregnancies and complications; fertility in other relationships, abortions, miscarriages, ectopic and molar pregnancies must be recorded. A note should be made of occurrence of any puerperal or postabortal infections, if any, in previous pregnancies.

Gynecological History

Any history suggestive of PID or vaginal infections such as lower abdominal pain, foul-smelling vaginal discharge, menstrual irregularity, itching in vulvar region needs to be elicited. Inquiries should include symptoms of endometriosis such as dysmenorrhea, dyspareunia, or chronic pelvic pain. Recent cervical cytology (Pap test) must be reviewed.

History suggestive of any endocrinopathy is important. This includes history of intolerance to heat or cold, alteration in bowel habits, increase or decrease in sleep or weight, easy fatigability suggestive of thyroid disorder; galactorrhea, oligomenorrhea or amenorrhea, headache and/or any visual disturbances suggestive of hyperprolactinemia; hirsutism, acne, weight gain, and menstrual irregularity suggestive of polycystic ovarian syndrome.

History of Past Illness

History of tuberculosis, thyroid disorder, diabetes mellitus, prolonged treatment or hospitalization, and any surgery should be elicited. Laparotomy increases the risk of infertility due to pelvic adhesions. Previous surgeries such as "complicated" appendectomy, caesarean sections, salpingectomy for ectopic pregnancy, ovarian cystectomy, wedge resection, ovarian drilling, and myomectomy, predispose to adhesion formation and increase the likelihood of tubal dysfunction. Surgeries on the ovaries such as cystectomy, drilling, enucleation, and/or fulguration of endometriosis can decrease the ovarian reserve. Any vaginal or cervical surgeries should be recorded. History of rubella infection or vaccination, use of any medications, and any drug allergies should be elicited.

Personal History

The occupation of the women, any addictions, smoking, or alcohol use should be enquired.

Previous Treatment History

History of previous evaluation for infertility and results thereof should be reviewed and documented in detail. Previous history of treatment for reproductive tract infection (RTI) and STI or tuberculosis should be enquired. Medical treatment with sex steroids may cause temporary cessation and that with cytotoxic agents and abdominal irradiation may cause permanent damage to the ovulatory function of the woman. Neuroleptic, antidepressant, and antihypertensive drugs can cause hyperprolactinemia and related problems.

Family History

Family history of infertility, birth defects, genetic disease, early menopause, reproductive problems, consanguinity, diabetes mellitus, hypertension, tuberculosis, and ovarian, uterine, or breast malignancy should be elicited.

Male Partner

Age, occupation, personal history of smoking, use of alcohol or substance abuse, habit of wearing tight underwear, anosmia or hyposmia suggestive of Kallmann syndrome, any congenital malformation, delayed onset of puberty and cryptorchidism should be elicited. Exposure to heavy metals such as lead and heat have a detrimental effect on semen quality. Intake of corticosteroids or psychotropic drugs causing hyperprolactinemia can affect semen quality.

History of Past Illness

History of infections such as mumps, RTI, and STI should be ascertained. History of sinopulmonary infections (paranasal sinuses and pulmonary airways) may suggest genetic diseases such as Young syndrome, Kartagener syndrome or cystic fibrosis. History of pelvic and inguinal surgeries, major pelvic or head trauma should be elicited. History of metabolic or neurological condition may be related to erectile and ejaculatory dysfunction. History of chemotherapy or irradiation or exposure to toxic substances such as pesticides is important.

Sexual History

The frequency of sexual intercourse, number of sexual partners, premature ejaculation, impotence, or any coital problems should be noted. Use of lubricants can contribute to infertility.

EXAMINATION

Examination of Female Partner

For the female partner, a complete physical and gynecological examination is mandatory at the first visit.

General Physical Examination

Body mass index (BMI) should be calculated at the first visit. Women with a BMI of >30 kg/m² are likely to take longer to conceive and should be advised to reduce weight. Women who have a BMI of <19 kg/m² and irregular menstruation should be advised to increase the body weight so as to improve their chances of conception.[1]

The vital parameters such as pulse and blood pressure should be recorded. Pallor if present should be investigated and treated. Correction of anemia is important prior to initiation of treatment of infertility. Any enlargement of thyroid, any nodules, or presence of exophthalmos may be suggestive of thyroid disorder. Any signs of hyperandrogenism such as hirsutism, distribution and texture of hair, acne and acanthosis nigricans are looked for. Breast examination should be done for presence of any lump or galactorrhea.

Systemic Examination

Cardiovascular and respiratory systems must be carefully examined. Respiratory system is examined for any findings suggestive of tuberculosis.

Per Abdomen Examination

Abdomen is examined for any scars or masses. Any mass or tenderness in lower abdomen, if present should be noted.

Examination of Genitalia

Pelvic examination: A per speculum examination is done to observe any abnormal vaginal discharge or cervical infection or lesion. Pap smear should be taken, as per schedule. Per vaginal examination is done to find out uterine size, shape, position, mobility, any adnexal mass or tenderness, nodules or scarring in pouch of Douglas (POD), and induration or thickening of uterosacral ligaments. Per rectal examination is done for any nodularity or scarring in POD indicating endometriosis. The uterus is usually fixed and retroverted in endometriosis. An enlarged irregular uterus is suggestive of fibroids.

Examination of Male Partner

It is not clear whether physical examination of the male partner is always necessary, if the semen analysis is normal many centers do not routinely examine the male partner.

General Physical Examination

The examination includes BMI, pulse, and blood pressure. Men with a BMI of >30 kg/m² are likely to have reduced fertility. The hair growth and distribution and presence of gynecomastia should be looked for. Testicular dysfunction due to acquired gonadotropin deficiency is associated with symptoms such as asthenia, reduction in growth of beard, libido, and volume of the ejaculate. Whereas men with congenital gonadotropin deficiency have scanty or no body hair, infantile genitalia with small testis, and gynecomastia. Anosmia may be associated in men with Kallmann syndrome.

Examination of Genitalia

A thorough physical examination should focus on general signs such as secondary sex characteristics (hair distribution, absence of gynecomastia, and skeletal muscle development), and on the genitalia. Genital examination includes testicular size, volume, consistency, location of urethral meatus, size, texture, position, and orientation of epididymis and bilateral palpation of vas deferens. Testicular size can be assessed by using Prader orchidometer. The normal range is 12–30 mL. Small testes are related to testicular dysfunction or hypogonadism. Congenital bilateral absence of vas deferens (CBAVD) suggests the presence of mutation of the cystic fibrosis (CF) transmembrane conductance regular gene (*CFTR*). Cysts or nodularity of the epididymis suggests congenital or inflammatory changes that can lead to obstruction.

Examination of the spermatic cord in the upright position is important to evaluate for the presence of varicocele.

Varicocele is classified into three grades: Grade 1 palpable only with Valsalva maneuver, grade 2 palpable without Valsalva maneuver, and grade 3 detectable by visual inspection. Digital rectal examination can detect cysts in the seminal vesicles and prostatic adenoma and neoplasia.

After a detailed history and clinical examination of both partners, presence or absence of an underlying physical problem can be made out and a provisional diagnosis is made. Investigations are planned to confirm the clinical diagnosis.

INVESTIGATIONS

Male Partner

The laboratory evaluation begins with a semen analysis. The sample should be collected in a private room near the laboratory in order to limit the exposure of the semen to fluctuations in temperature and to control the time between collection and analysis. The sample should be collected after a minimum of 2 days and a maximum of 7 days of ejaculatory abstinence and the semen parameters are compared with the World Health Organization (WHO) reference

Table 3: Lower reference limits (5th centiles and their 95% confidence intervals) for semen characteristics [World Health Organization (WHO) Manual of Semen Analysis, 2010].[3]

Semen characteristics	Lower reference limits
pH	>7.2
Semen volume (mL)	1.5 (95% CI 1.4–1.7)
Total sperm count ($\times 10^6$/ejaculate)	39 (95% CI 33–46)
Sperm concentration ($\times 10^6$/mL)	15 (95% CI 12–16)
Total motility (%)	40 (95% CI 38–42)
Progressive motility (%)	32 (95% CI 31–34)
Vitality (live spermatozoa, %)	58 (95% CI 55–63)
Sperm morphology (normal forms, %) using strict Tygerberg criteria	4 (95% CI 3–4)
Peroxidase-positive leukocytes (10^6/mL)	<1
Seminal fructose (μmol/ejaculate)	≥13
Seminal zinc (μmol/ejaculate)	≥2.4
Seminal neutral glucosidase (mU/ejaculate)	≥20

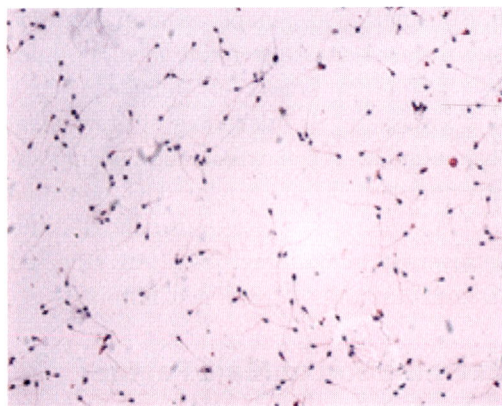

Fig. 1: Slide showing sperms.

values (Table 3). Figure 1 shows a picture of the sperms under microscope. If the values are abnormal according to the WHO criteria, repeat semen analysis is offered. It is ideally undertaken after 3 months of initial analysis. This allows time for one complete cycle of formation of spermatozoa. However, if there is gross abnormality such as azoospermia or severe oligozoospermia, repeat test should be advised at the earliest.

If the semen analysis result is abnormal, further evaluation is indicated. In males with oligospermia or azoospermia, hormonal evaluation [serum testosterone, follicle-stimulating hormone (FSH) and luteinizing hormone (LH)] is indicated. Obtaining morning levels of total testosterone (normal range 240–950 ng/dL) and FSH; (normal range 1.5–12.4 mIU/mL) can help differentiate between primary and secondary hypogonadism. A decreased testosterone level with an increased FSH level points to primary hypogonadism. A low testosterone level with a low FSH level signals a secondary cause.

Other investigations including testicular biopsy, genetic testing, and imaging may be needed based on hormonal profile and physical characteristics of the male partner. Men with low testosterone but high FSH and LH should be offered karyotyping. Those with low testosterone and low or normal FSH and LH hyperprolactinemia should be ruled out which is reversible with proper treatment. Men with azoospermia and normal hormonal profile should be investigated for ejaculatory duct obstruction.

Sperm DNA Fragmentation Index

Sperm DNA integrity is an important component for embryo development. A number of tests have been described to measure sperm DNA fragmentation such as sperm chromatin structure assay (SCSA) and terminal deoxynucleotide transferase-mediated dUTP nick end labeling assays (TUNEL). Threshold values used to define an abnormal test is ≥25–27% for SCSA and ≥36% for TUNEL assays.[4] However, existing data are too limited for an association between abnormal DNA integrity and reproductive outcomes to routinely recommend this test for evaluation of male infertility.

Female Partner

Baseline investigations should be performed to assess ovulatory function, ovarian reserve, uterine cavity, and tubal patency.

Ovulatory Function

Regular menstrual cycle occurring at intervals of 24–38 days exhibiting consistent flow characteristics and accompanied by consistent pattern of molimina symptoms is usually indicative of normal ovulation:
- Historically basal body temperature was used to give presumptive evidence of ovulation. But sometimes it is uninterpretable and cannot accurately predict timing of ovulation.
- Commercially available urinary LH kits identify the mid-cycle LH surge suggesting the presence of ovulation. Its repetitive use may become expensive and frustrating. Also, false-positive LH tests have been estimated to occur in 7% of cases.
- Endometrial biopsy and histological dating have been used to evaluate ovulation (Figs. 2A and B). Their use is limited and they have been abandoned as routine tests.
- Mid-luteal serum progesterone testing is an easy method and is the most commonly used test to confirm ovulation. It is usually done on day 21 of a 28-day cycle or 7 days before the commencement of menses. As the progesterone concentration fluctuates widely among normal women and affects interpretation. Some authors reported that serum progesterone levels >10 ng/mL correlate with a normal "in-phase" endometrial histology. Whether this value is correlated with luteal function is unclear.
- Transvaginal ultrasonography (US) is a noninvasive method for confirming ovulation; however, it is time consuming and costly. Baseline sonography on day

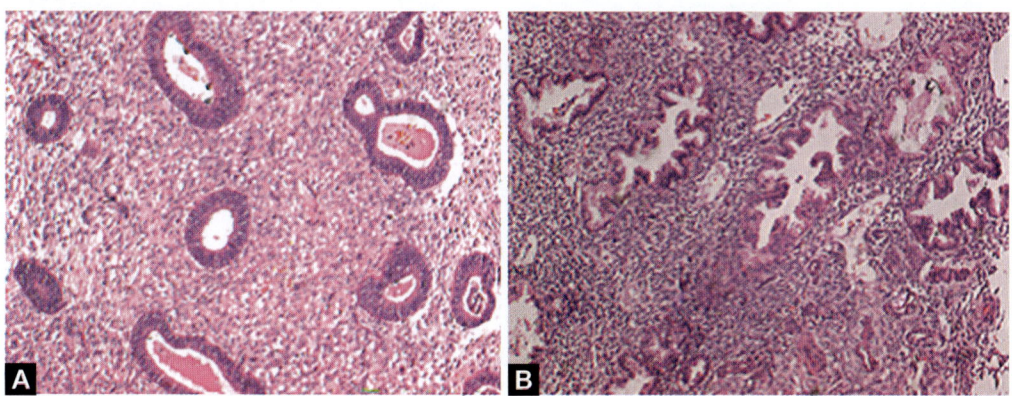

Figs. 2A and B: Histopathology of endometrium—proliferative phase (A) and secretory phase (B).

3 of menstruation should be done to evaluate baseline uterine endometrium, ovarian size and volume, antral follicle count, and residual follicular cyst, if any. Serial US examinations starting on day 10 of the cycle on alternate day can evaluate follicular growth, endometrial thickness, and change in endometrial pattern, disappearance of follicle and appearance of the corpus luteum, indirectly indicating ovulation (Figs. 3 to 5).

Practically, menstrual history is all that is required in women with regular cycles in order to confirm ovulation. Still, the NICE guidelines do recommend measuring mid-luteal progesterone in women undergoing infertility investigation even in the presence of regular cycles.

Patient with abnormal uterine bleeding, oligomenorrhea or amenorrhea generally do not require any specific test to establish anovulation. However underlying cause should

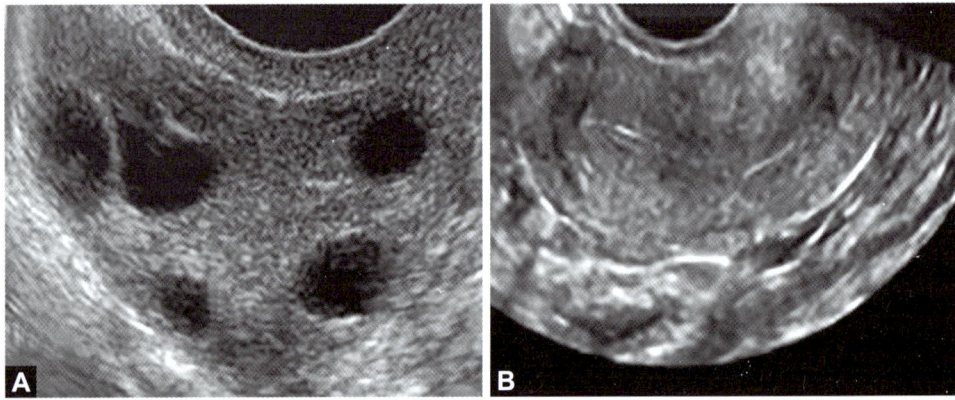

Figs. 3A and B: Baseline D2 or D3 scan of ovary and uterus. (A) Scan showing antral follicles; (B) Scan showing thin endometrium.

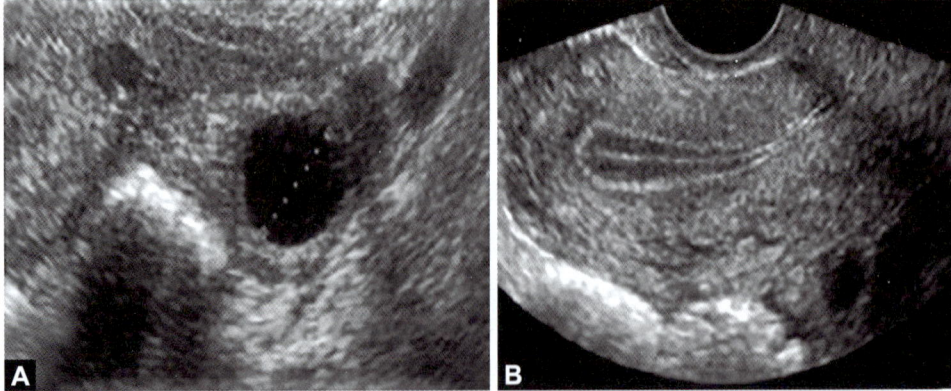

Figs. 4A and B: D12 scan of ovary and uterus. (A) Scan showing dominant follicle; (B) Scan showing proliferative endometrium (triple layer).

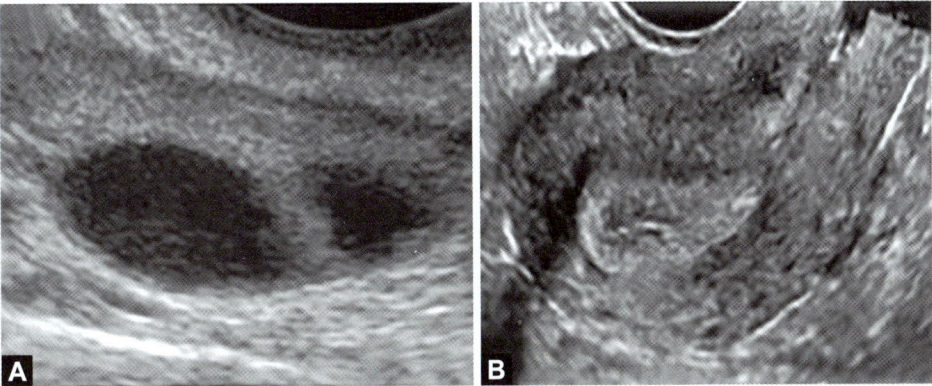

Figs. 5A and B: D15 scan of ovary and uterus. (A) Scan showing corpus luteum; (B) Scan showing secretory endometrium (echogenic).

be sought for targeted treatment. Serum TSH and prolactin levels are assessed in women with anovulation to identify thyroid and prolactin disorders, which may be corrected with the specific treatment.

The WHO categorizes ovulatory disorders into three groups: Group I hypogonadotropic hypogonadism hypothalamic pituitary failure (10%), Group II normogonadotropic normogonadism hypothalamic–pituitary dysfunction (85%), and Group III hypergonadotropic hypogonadism ovarian failure (5%)

Women in group I typically present with amenorrhea and low gonadotropin levels, most commonly due to low body weight or excessive exercise. Women in group II include those with polycystic ovary syndrome. Women in group III include women with premature ovarian failure and can conceive only with oocyte donation and in vitro fertilization.

In women presenting with amenorrhea, a high serum FSH level (>25 mIU/mL with a low estradiol level can distinguish ovarian failure from hypothalamic pituitary failure, which typically reveals a low or normal FSH level (<10 mIU/mL) and a low estradiol level.[5]

Women with signs and symptoms of hyperandrogenism require further investigations (serum testosterone, δ4-androstenedione, dehydroepiandrosterone-sulfate (DHEA-S) and 17-hydroxy-progesterone) to rule out the presence of late-onset congenital adrenal hyperplasia, Cushing syndrome, or androgen-producing tumors.

Ovarian Reserve

Ovarian reserve testing is an important part of infertility evaluation. It describes the reproductive potential as a function of number and quality of oocytes.

These tests helps in prognostication in women with diminished ovarian reserve such as:

- Over 35 years of age
- Family history of early menopause
- Single ovary or history of ovarian surgery or chemotherapy or irradiation
- Poor response to gonadotropin therapy
- Unexplained infertility
- Those planning treatment with assisted reproductive technology.

Tests which are used to predict ovarian reserve are day 3 serum FSH and estradiol E_2 levels, early follicular phase antral follicle count (AFC), and anti-Müllerian hormone

(AMH). It also helps in choosing the optimal stimulation regime to avoid iatrogenic complications. However, poor results do not suggest inability to conceive. Other ovarian tests such as serum inhibin B or estradiol E_2 levels, ovarian volume, ovarian flow measurement, and clomiphene citrate challenge test are not recommended.

- *Day 3 FSH and estradiol*: A serum FSH measured on cycle day 2-4 is used to predict the ovarian reserve. High values (>10-20 IU/L) are associated with poor response to stimulation.[6] However, FSH values shows cycle-to-cycle variation. FSH is downregulated by E2, and these hormonal markers should be interpreted together. Indeed, elevated E2 could otherwise falsely normalize FSH. Basal serum estradiol should not be used alone to predict ovarian reserve but it aids in interpreting a normal serum FSH levels. Limited evidence suggests that women with normal early follicular phase FSH levels with elevated serum estradiol levels (60-80 pg/mL) are associated with poor response to gonadotropin stimulation, higher IVF cancellation rates, and lower pregnancy rates.[5] FSH >8.9 IU/L is an indicator for a low response and <4 IU/L is for a high response.[1]
- *AFC*: It is measured by counting 2-10 mm follicles in both the ovaries by transvaginal US in early follicular phase. It carries little intra- or intercycle variability in experienced hands. A low AFC helps in predicting poor response to stimulation but does not reliably predict failure to conception. According to the NICE guideline, AFC >16 predicts a high response while AFC <4 predicts poor response to stimulation.[1]
- *AMH*: It is a dimeric glycoprotein member of the TGF-β superfamily. AMH expression is observed in pre-antral and small antral follicles. It is found in growing follicles and is gonadotropin independent. Hence, cyclic variation of AMH is minimal, blood sample for AMH can be obtained at any time during the cycle. Yet there has been no international standard for the AMH assay. According to the NICE, AMH levels >3.5 ng/mL are predictive of a high ovarian response, while a level under 0.75 ng/mL is predictive of low response.[1]

Day-3 FSH and E2 are the most used screening tests, but AFC and AMH appear to be more sensitive and specific in the prediction of poor ovarian response. The Bologna criteria for poor ovarian reserve include at least one abnormal ovarian test: AFC <5-7 follicles or AMH <0.5-1.1 ng/mL.[5]

Tubal Patency Test

Evaluation of tubal patency can be carried out by hysterosalpingography (HSG), diagnostic laparoscopy with chromopertubation and/or sonosalpingography.

Hysterosalpingography: Hysterosalpingography is a radiographic evaluation of the fallopian tubes that is performed by injecting radiocontrast of either oil-based or water-soluble media into the uterine cavity via the cervix (Fig. 6). It is usually used as a first-line modality due to its therapeutic and diagnostic benefits, except in cases with comorbidities such as previous history of PID, endometriosis or previous pelvic, or lower abdominal surgery, where laparoscopy with chromopertubation is preferred (Fig. 7). It should be performed in the early follicular phase to ensure the absence of pregnancy and to facilitate maximum uterine visibility. The HSG is done to evaluate the shape, any filling defect of uterine cavity and patency of fallopian tubes (Figs. 8A and B). The site

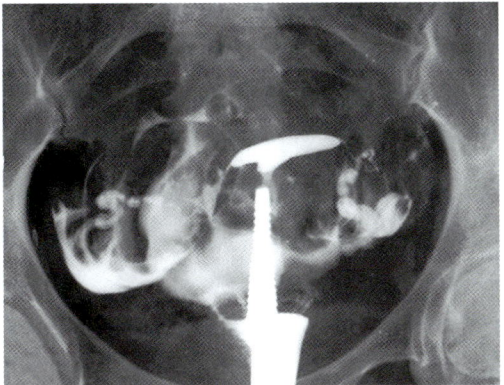

Fig. 6: Normal hysterosalpingography.

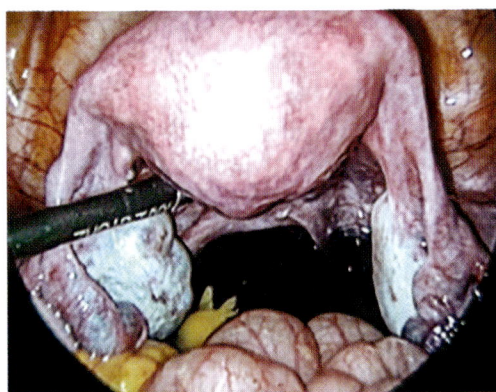

Fig. 7: Diagnostic laparoscopy and chromopertubation.

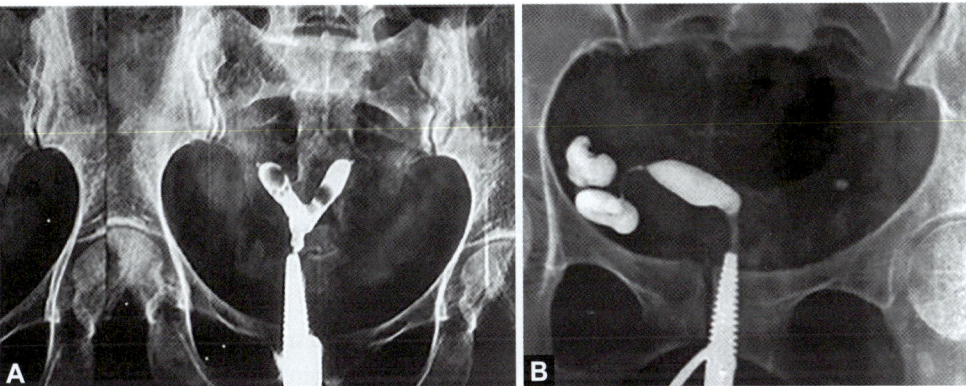

Figs. 8A and B: Abnormal HSG—bicornuate/septate uterus with bilateral cornual block and artifacts (A) and unicornuate uterus with hydrosalpinx (B).

of block can be identified by HSG (Fig. 9). HSG findings of "proximal tubal occlusion" usually require further testing to rule out tubal spasm, collection of debris, or a mucus plug. HSG is more specific for detecting distal as opposed to proximal occlusion and has a high correlation with laparoscopic findings.[6] (Refer to Chapter 49 for details of HSG).

Hysterosalpingo-contrast sonography: Hysterosalpingo-contrast sonography (HyCoSy) shows intratubal flow of contrast media. The presence of fluid in the cul-de-sac after uterine instillation implies patency of at least one

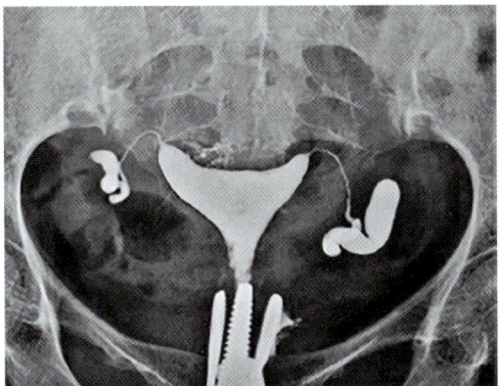

Fig. 9: Abnormal hysterosalpingogram showing bilateral hydrosalpinges.

tube. Pain induced by HyCoSy and its complications are comparable to HSG. Although HyCoSy might have been considered inferior to HSG for evaluating tubal patency, it has been shown to be as reliable as HSG if an appropriate expertise is available.[6]

Laparoscopy with chromopertubation: Laparoscopy with chromopertubation has long been considered as the "gold standard" for evaluating tubal patency. It helps to diagnose and treat conditions that decrease fertility, including endometriosis or periadnexal adhesions. However, it is an invasive procedure that requires general anesthesia. Laparoscopy is indicated when there is evidence or strong suspicion of endometriosis, pelvic/adnexal adhesions, or significant tubal disease requiring treatment.

HSG and HyCoSy are the first-line tests to evaluate the fallopian tubes in infertile women. These procedures are generally well tolerated, inexpensive, and capable of demonstrating tubal patency at rates as high as 80%.[5] The choice between these two techniques depends on availability, operator experience, and whether the patient is allergic to contrast media or iodine. Laparoscopy for diagnostic purposes is rarely needed.

Assessment of Uterine Cavity

Intrauterine abnormalities are relatively uncommon cause of infertility but should be excluded. It includes endometrial polyps, submucosal myoma, adhesions, or a uterine septum.

Transvaginal US and other imaging methods such as 3D-US and magnetic resonance imaging (MRI) help in making a diagnosis.

Hysterosalpingography defines the shape and size of the uterine cavity. It helps in identifying congenital and acquired uterine cavity abnormalities. However, HSG cannot help in differentiating between septate and bicornuate uterus. HSG has a lower sensitivity and specificity and high rates of false-positive and false-negative results for diagnosing intrauterine abnormalities compared to hysteroscopy.

Hysterosonography is a combination of US with saline or contrast media infusion (HyCoSy) into the uterine cavity. It assesses the patency of the fallopian tubes following examination of the uterine cavity. As with US, it is more precise for diagnosing polyps or submucosal fibroids than endometrial hyperplasia or structural abnormalities. 3D-hysterosonography could also be performed and seems to be comparable with hysteroscopy for diagnosing intrauterine lesions.

Hysteroscopy remains the definitive method for evaluation and treatment of intrauterine pathology.[6] Since hysteroscopy is an invasive method for evaluation of the uterine cavity, it is usually reserved for further evaluation and treatment of already suspected anomalies using imaging techniques. It allows direct visualization of endocervical canal, uterine cavity, endometrium, and cornual openings of the uterine cavity but not the uterine contour (Fig. 10). It should be done for intrauterine space-occupying lesions detected on HSG such as intrauterine adhesions or submucous fibroids (Figs. 11A and B). It is not offered as a routine to infertile women during their initial workup.

Congenital uterine anomalies should be investigated by MRI, 3D-US, or a combination of laparoscopy and hysteroscopy.

Peritoneal Factors

Peritoneal factors such as endometriosis or pelvic adhesions may cause infertility.

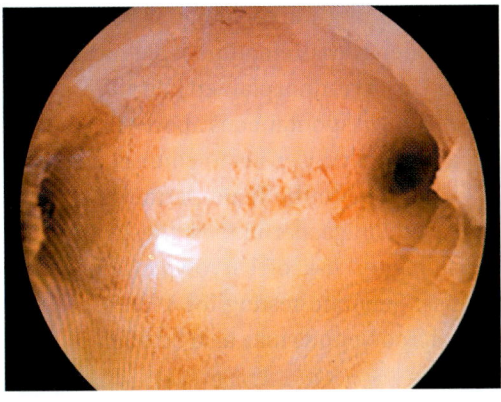

Fig. 10: Normal hysteroscopic findings.

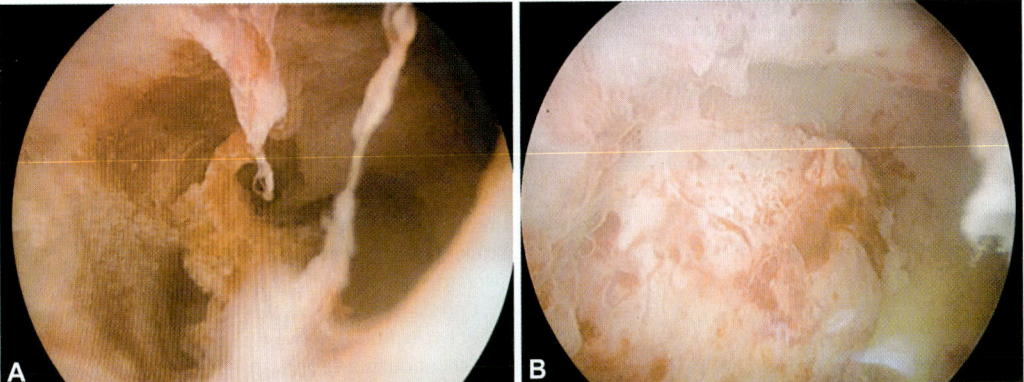

Figs. 11A and B: Abnormal hysteroscopic findings—broken intrauterine adhesions and ragged endometrium (A) and submucous myoma (B).

Suspicion can arise on the basis of history/ or physical examination but needs to be confirmed. It should be considered as one of the factors in unexplained infertility. Laparoscopy with direct visualization of the pelvic organs helps in reaching a diagnosis.

Tests of Limited Clinical Utility

- *Postcoital test*: Postcoital testing of cervical mucus is no longer recommended because it does not affect clinical management or predict the inability to conceive.

- *Endometrial biopsy*: The American Society of Reproductive Medicine highlights the lack of benefit of the endometrial biopsy in the evaluation of the infertile women and does not recommend use of this test unless endometrial pathology is strongly suspected. In women with high index of suspicion of tuberculosis like past history of tuberculosis in self or family, positive findings on examination and or imaging (HSG, X-ray chest, and ultrasound of pelvis) endometrial biopsy is indicated to rule out endometrial tuberculosis. For details of endometrial biopsy, refer to Chapter 49.

- *Antibody testing*: Routine testing for antiphospholipid, antisperm, antinuclear, and antithyroid antibodies is not supported by existing data.
- *Chlamydia antibody test*: Chlamydia trachomatis serology screening has been advocated for patients at high risk of tubal damage and to increase the accurate prediction of tubal disease in conjunction with HSG. However, this test has been shown to have limited clinical value.
- *Mycoplasma cultures*: Obtaining routine Ureaplasma urealyticum and Mycoplasma hominis cultures is of limited value, as there is minimal evidence for a role of these organisms in female infertility.
- *Karyotype*: Karyotyping is offered to women with premature depletion of ovarian reserve, unexplained infertility, and in recurrent spontaneous abortions. There is a general consensus to counsel and offer karyotype to the male partner if there is severe oligospermia as these men are at higher risk of karyotypic abnormalities. Separate testing for Y chromosome microdeletions may also be offered.

MANAGEMENT

The management is based on the cause identified. Table 4 summarizes the options for the management of an infertile couple.

Table 4: Management of an infertile couple.

Male factors	Female factors

• Lifestyle modifications: Cessation of smoking, normalize BMI, healthy life style, and optimization of any metabolic disorders
• Mild male factor: IUI
• Secondary hypogonadism:
  – Hypogonadotropic hypogonadism–Induction of spermatogenesis by Gonadotropin replacement therapy
  – Prolactin adenomas Dopamine agonist therapy, cabergoline
• Varicocele: Surgical repair indicated in grade III varicocele with abnormal semen parameters
• Obstructive azoospermia: Surgical correction microsurgical end-to-end anastomosis or ICSI after sperm retrieval from testis or epididymis PESA, TESA, or TESE
• Genetic counseling and testing prior to ICSI and ART, AID or adoption
	• Lifestyle modifications: Normalize BMI, cessation of smoking, timed contact
	• Ovulatory dysfunction:
	  – Correct reversible causes like hypothyroidism and or hyperprolactinemia
	  – Ovulation induction with letrozole, clomiphene citrate or gonadotropins according to the WHO type
	Tubal factor:
	• Surgical reconstruction for younger women with isolated proximal tubal disease (cornual block) or isolated mild-to-moderate distal tubal disease
	• IVF ET for those with severe tubal disease or older women
	• Hydrosalpinges to be clipped or removed before IVF ET
	• Endometriosis:
	  – Surgical resection, fulguration of endometriotic patches and adhesiolysis followed by COS + IUI
	  – ART
	• Uterine causes: Surgical correction of intrauterine polyps, adhesions, submucous fibroids
	• Cervical factor: OI + IUI

Unexplained infertility:
- COS + IUI
- ART: IVF/ICSI ET

(AID: artificial insemination by donor; ART: assisted reproductive technology; BMI: body mass index; COS: controlled ovarian stimulation; ET: embryo transfer; ICSI: intracytoplasmic sperm injection; IUI: intrauterine insemination; IVF: in vitro fertilization; OI: ovulation induction; PESA: percutaneous epididymal sperm aspiration; TESA: testicular sperm aspiration; TESE: testicular sperm extraction; WHO: World Health Organization)

KEY POINTS

- Infertility is a stressful situation for most couples.
- Infertility can be due to male factor or female factor or both or unexplained.
- A comprehensive history and physical examination of both the partners is a key to reach a correct diagnosis.
- Both the partners should undergo basic infertility investigations including semen analysis, documentation of ovulation, and tubal patency test.
- Further evaluation is based on the results of basic investigations and include hormonal assessment, imaging, karyotyping, and genetic studies.
- Couples should be fully informed, educated, and counseled during evaluation and treatment.
- Treatment is tailored depending upon the cause identified.
- Lifestyle modifications and a healthy lifestyle is an important initial intervention.

REFERENCES

1. National Collaborating Centre for Women's and Children's Health (UK). Fertility: assessment and treatment for people with fertility problems. London (UK): RCOG Press; 2004.
2. Fritz MA, Speroff L. Clinical Gynecologic Endocrinology and Infertility. 8th Edition, Philadelphia: Lippincott Williams & Wilkins; 2011.
3. World Health Organization. (2010). WHO laboratory manual for the examination and processing of semen. [onlie] Available from https://apps.who.int/iris/bitstream/handle/10665/44261/9789241547789_eng.pdf;jsessionid=DB052FAA6465346FF-B0033727A6C7062?sequence=1. [Last accessed March, 2020].
4. Practice Committee of American Society for Reproductive Medicine. Diagnostic evaluation of the infertile male: a committee opinion. Fertil Steril. 2012;98:294-301.
5. Gardner DK, Weissman A, Howles CM, Shoham Z. Textbook of assisted reproductive techniques: Clinical Perspectives (Volume 2), 5th edition. New York: CRC Press; 2018.
6. Practice Committee of American Society for Reproductive Medicine. Diagnostic evaluation of the infertile female: a committee opinion. Fertil Steril. 2015;103(6):e44-50.

SUGGESTED READING

1. Bhasin S, Brito JP, Cunningham GR, Hayes FJ, Hodis HN, Matsumoto AM, et al. (2018). Endocrine Society (ES): Clinical practice guideline on testosterone therapy in men with hypogonadism. J Clin Endocrinol Metab. 2018;103(5):1715-44.
2. Conway G, Dewailly D, Diamanti-Kandarakis E, Escobar-Morreale HF, Franks S, Gambineri A, et al. The polycystic ovary syndrome: A position statement on the polycystic ovarian syndrome. Eur J Endocrinol. 2014;171(4): P1-29.
3. Jungwirth A, Diemer T, Kopa Z, Krausz C, Minhas S, Tournaye H. (2016). European Association of Urology (EAU): Guidelines on male infertility. [online] Available from https://uroweb.org/guideline/male-infertility/. [Last accessed March, 2020].
4. National Institute for Health and Care Excellence (NICE). (2013). Clinical guideline on fertility problems – Assessment and treatment. [online] Available from https://www.nice.org.uk/guidance/cg156. [Last accessed March, 2020].
5. Royal Australian and New Zealand College of Obstetricians and Gynaecologists (RANZCOG). (2018). Fibroids in infertility. [online] Available from https://ranzcog.edu.au/RANZCOG_SITE/media/RANZCOG-MEDIA/Women%27s%20Health/Statement%20and%20guidelines/Clinical%20-%20Gynaecology/Fibroids-in-Infertility-(C-Gyn-27)-March-2018.pdf?ext=.pdf. [Last accessed March, 2020].
6. SOGC clinical practice guideline: The management of uterine fibroids in women with otherwise unexplained infertility. J Obstet Gynaecol Can. 2015;37(3):277-85.

33. Approach to a Woman Presenting with Dysmenorrhea

Manisha Bajaj

INTRODUCTION

Dysmenorrhea is defined as cyclical lower abdominal or pelvic pain that occurs during menstruation. It is commonly classified into two types—*primary* and *secondary*. It is primary when there is no coexistent pelvic pathology and secondary when there is an identifiable pelvic pathology. Occasionally, a third type, *membranous* dysmenorrhea is described, which is intense cramping pain due to passage of endometrial cast. It is the most severe form of primary dysmenorrhea with positive family history and recurrence after pregnancy.

Depending on the nature of pain, dysmenorrhea is also classified as *spasmodic* or *congestive*. Spasmodic dysmenorrhea is characterized by intermittent colicky pain starting with the onset of menstruation, whereas congestive dysmenorrhea is a continuous dull aching pain or heaviness in lower abdomen, starting 2–3 days before the onset of menstruation and gets relieved with the onset of menstruation. Primary dysmenorrhea is usually spasmodic, whereas secondary dysmenorrhea can be either spasmodic or congestive, or a combination of the two.

Dysmenorrhea is one of the most common gynecological complaints with almost 50–90% postmenarcheal females having varying degrees of distress related to it.[1-3] It is assessed that it is a source of recurrent disability in approximately 10% of women due to severe and incapacitating pain that interferes with their daily activities and normal occupation. Although it is not a significant disease in majority but is important in terms of its effect on woman's overall health, both physical and mental, as well as an indicator of underlying gynecological condition in case of secondary dysmenorrhea.

Majority of women have no risk factors but dysmenorrhea is more common in women of age <30 years, BMI <20 kg/m², age of menarche <12 years, smokers, those with longer duration of bleeding during periods, irregular or heavy flow, and history of sexual assault.[4] Primary dysmenorrhea is more common in younger girls and prevalence decreases with age. In view of underreporting all adolescent girls should be screened for dysmenorrhea.

DIFFERENTIAL DIAGNOSIS

The differential diagnosis of dysmenorrhea is as given in Box 1. The common causes are as depicted in Figure 1.

HISTORY

History is vital in establishing the diagnosis of dysmenorrhea and to differentiate between

Box 1: Causes of dysmenorrhea.
- Primary dysmenorrhea
- Secondary dysmenorrhea:
  - *Vaginal*:
    » Imperforate hymen
    » Transverse vaginal septum
  - *Cervical*:
    » Cervical atresia
    » *Cervical stenosis*: After medical termination of pregnancy by surgical method (MTP), conization, cervical amputation, and reconstruction
  - *Uterine*:
    » Obstructing functional Müllerian anomaly: Noncommunicating rudimentary horn (hematometra)
    » Adenomyosis
    » Fibroid (submucous) or fibroid polyp
    » Intrauterine contraceptive device (IUCD)
    » Endometritis
    » Intrauterine adhesions
    » Cervical descent (early stages)
  - *Adnexa*:
    » Ovarian cyst
    » Salpingo-oophoritis (PID)
    » Endometriosis
  - *Others*:
    » Pelvic adhesions
    » Pelvic congestion syndrome
    » Inflammatory bowel disease
    » Irritable bowel syndrome
    » Psychogenic

primary and secondary dysmenorrhea. Further it also helps in identifying the likely etiology of secondary dysmenorrhea. A detailed menstrual history is a must.

Menstrual History

Patient should be asked about the age of menarche and the relation of the onset of dysmenorrhea with menarche. Primary dysmenorrhea usually starts within a few years of onset of periods, when ovulatory cycles begin; whereas secondary dysmenorrhea starts late in third or fourth decades of life, except if it is associated with an obstructed Müllerian anomaly, when it starts with the onset of menarche or in the first few cycles.

The relationship of the pain to onset and cessation of periods is very important. Primary dysmenorrhea begins with the onset of menstruation and lasts for the first 1–2 days, whereas in secondary dysmenorrhea, pelvic heaviness and backache begins before the periods and may get relieved within hours of onset of periods as in pelvic inflammatory disease (PID), or increase in severity with onset of periods and continue throughout

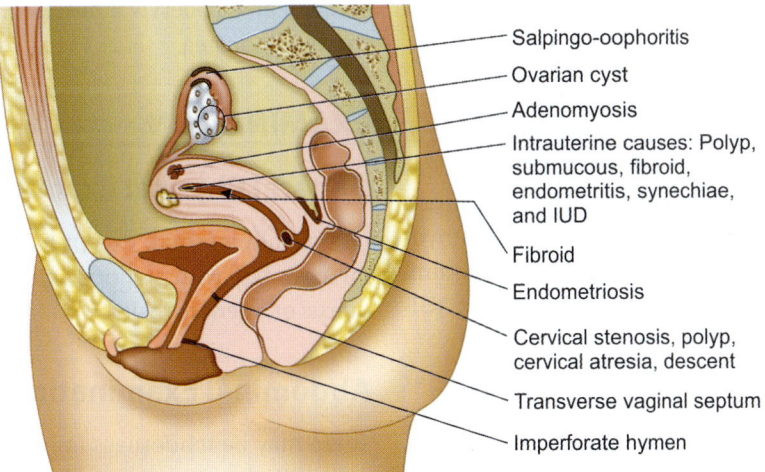

Fig. 1: Common causes of dysmenorrhea.
(IUD: intrauterine device)

periods or sometimes even after the bleeding stops as in endometriosis. Women with dysmenorrhea due to early stages of cervical descent complain of backache and labor-like pains during periods.

The nature of pain, whether intermittent or continuous, helps to differentiate between primary and secondary dysmenorrhea. Pain in primary dysmenorrhea is spasmodic, whereas it can be intermittent, continuous, or mixed in secondary dysmenorrhea depending upon the cause. The radiation of pain toward back and thighs is common with primary dysmenorrhea. However, in secondary dysmenorrhea, there is pelvic heaviness and lumbosacral backache.

History of any aggravating or relieving factors is important. Association of symptoms such as nausea, vomiting, diarrhea, headache, bloating, breast tenderness, mood alterations, and weight gain point toward primary dysmenorrhea. Sometimes, there may be history of syncope or collapse. Dyspareunia, pain during intercourse, indicates some organic pathology in pelvis such as endometriosis or PID. Secondary dysmenorrhea is usually refractory to simple treatments such as non-steroidal anti-inflammatory drugs (NSAIDs).

Presence of symptoms such as infertility, painful defecation, and constant dull aching pain in lower abdomen are suggestive of endometriosis, whereas symptoms such as abnormal uterine bleeding (AUB) or menorrhagia are suggestive of fibroid or adenomyosis. Any history of discharge per vaginum, pain in lower abdomen with or without AUB is suggestive of PID.

The pain is usually midline and suprapubic in location. Rarely dysmenorrhea may be unilateral and should raise the suspicion of a uterine malformation such as a noncommunicating rudimentary horn with hematometra or pain arising from better developed horn of a bicornuate uterus. Other causes of unilateral dysmenorrhea are septate uterus, one-sided endometrial distribution, juvenile cystic adenomyoma, or a small leiomyoma at the uterotubal junction.

The impact of pain on the quality of life, like whether the pain interferes with the daily activities, is important. Any progressive increase in intensity and whether pain is present at other times should be noted.

Obstetric History

It is important to know if previous delivery has resulted in any relief of pain as in patients with primary dysmenorrhea and endometriosis. Adenomyosis is more common in middle-aged multiparous women. The history of contraception is significant, as use of intrauterine contraceptive device (IUCD) can sometimes cause dysmenorrhea whereas use of oral contraceptive pills (OCPs), Depot medroxyprogesterone acetate (DMPA), progestin intrauterine system relieves dysmenorrhea due to endometriosis and adenomyosis. Any history of difficult childbirth may suggest some degree of cervical descent contributing to dysmenorrhea.

EXAMINATION

General Physical Examination

It is usually normal, except presence of pallor in women with menorrhagia due to fibroid uterus or adenomyosis.

Abdominal Examination

There may be tenderness in lower abdomen, as in PID or a mass may be felt in case of fibroid or adenomyosis.

Pelvic Examination

In young unmarried girls, who are not sexually active and where the history is suggestive of primary dysmenorrhea, it is not essential to carry out a pelvic examination. However, if these girls do not respond to simple treatment with NSAIDs and OCPs, and there are features suggestive of some coexistent pathology, a per rectal examination is carried out for evaluation of the pelvic organs.

In sexually active women, per speculum and per vaginum examination should be offered. Per speculum examination can help in diagnosing first-degree cervical descent, hypertrophied cervix and nabothian follicles suggestive of chronic cervicitis, discharge, and any vaginal or cervical abnormality suggestive of obstructed Müllerian anomaly.

Bimanual examination is done to assess the size, shape, position, mobility, and tenderness of the uterus. Fornices are palpated for any adnexal mass, tenderness, induration, thickness, and scarring. The uterosacral ligaments and pouch of Douglas are assessed for any nodularity, tenderness, or scarring, suggestive of endometriosis. Further adnexal enlargement and lateral displacement of cervix may suggest endometriosis. Uterus is enlarged in case of fibroids and adenomyosis. Enlargement is usually symmetrical in adenomyosis but irregular with fibroids. The cervical motion tenderness, uterine tenderness with restricted mobility, thick tender fornices, and uterosacrals suggest PID.

INVESTIGATIONS

Careful analysis of history and clinical examination usually helps in making a provisional diagnosis as regards the type and cause of dysmenorrhea, the investigations are offered accordingly. No specific investigations are needed to confirm the diagnosis of primary dysmenorrhea. Investigations are useful in women of primary dysmenorrhea not responding to simple measures, women with secondary dysmenorrhea, and those with progressively increasing dysmenorrhea.

Complete blood count with peripheral smear is indicated in women with menorrhagia and suspected PID to diagnose anemia and raised counts, respectively. Ultrasonography is a useful tool for diagnosing conditions like fibroids, adenomyosis, tubo-ovarian (TO) masses, and endometriomas. Transabdominal ultrasound can be performed for adolescents if they do not respond to initial treatment. Transvaginal ultrasound is more sensitive for detecting adnexal masses, fibroids, and uterine anomalies, especially if coupled with sonohysterography for the diagnosis of intracavitary lesions such as polyps. Magnetic resonance imaging (MRI) is very sensitive and specific in diagnosing adenomyosis, endometriosis, and obstructed Müllerian anomalies. Hysterosalpingography (HSG) or hysteroscopy is sometimes indicated for confirming the diagnosis of intrauterine adhesions and uterine malformations. Microbiological cultures for chlamydia and gonorrhea from endocervix or peritoneal fluid in suspected cases of PID is indicated.

Laparoscopy is rarely required. It is indicated for those with a provisional diagnosis of endometriosis, chronic pelvic pain, and PID and in cases where etiology is unknown and routine treatment with NSAIDs and OCPs fails, it often detects unsuspected mild endometriosis, even in teenage girls.

Flowchart 1 summarizes the workup of a woman with dysmenorrhea.

MANAGEMENT

The principle of management in primary dysmenorrhea is pain management whereas in secondary dysmenorrhea, the principle is to treat the cause.

Flowchart 1: Algorithm for clinical approach to a woman presenting with dysmenorrhea.

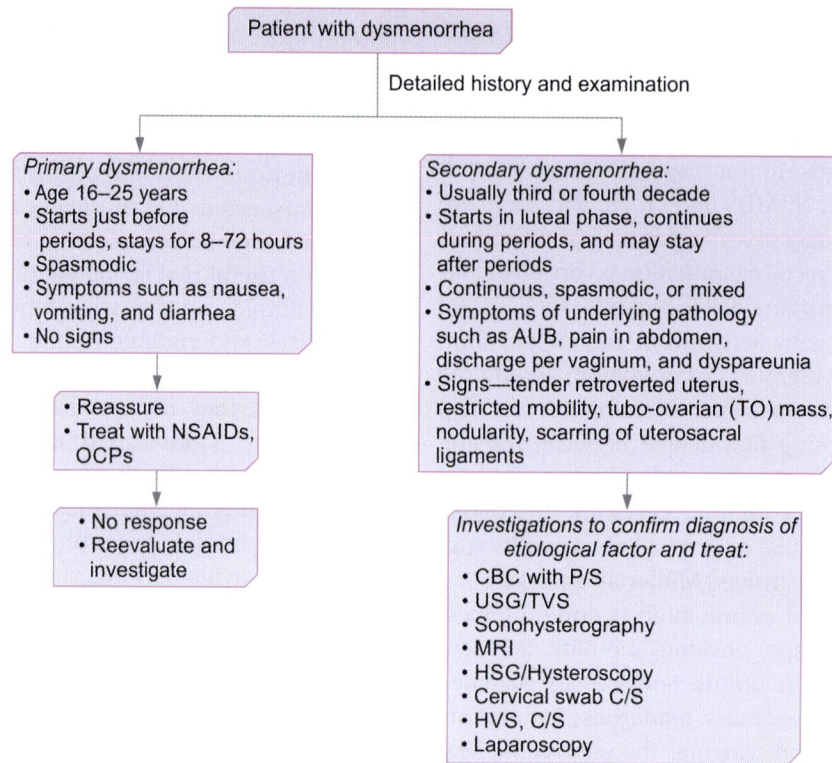

(AUB: abnormal uterine bleeding; CBC: complete blood count; C/S: culture sensitivity; HSG: hysterosalpingography; HVS: high vaginal swab; MRI: magnetic resonance imaging; NSAIDs: nonsteroidal anti-inflammatory drugs; OCPs: oral contraceptive pills; P/S: peripheral smear; TVS: transvaginal scan; USG: ultrasonography)

First-line intervention: Advice general measures such as exercise and topical heat for 1–2 cycles. Continue if the response is good.

Second-line intervention: Start on NSAIDs, mefenamic acid or cyclooxygenase-2 inhibitor, selective NSAIDs, or acetaminophen if NSAIDs are not tolerated with or without hormonal therapy for 3–4 cycles. NSAIDs are started just prior to or with the onset of periods for 2–3 days or till the periods last. It is continued if the woman responds to it. Hormonal treatment can be offered in the form of OCPs, DMPA, progestin intrauterine system depending upon the patient's choice, profile, and need.

If there is no response, investigate for other cause such as endometriosis, fibroid, hematometra, and adenomyosis, and treat the cause.

Third-line intervention: Transcutaneous electrical nerve stimulation (TENS) is an option for those not willing to take or not responding to hormonal therapy. For those not responding to hormonal therapy, empiric treatment with gonadotropin agonists or antagonists can also be tried. Dysmenorrhea due to endometriosis responds to these. Woman may be considered for laparoscopy and treatment of endometriosis as gonadotropin agonists cannot be given for >6 months due to its side effects.

Refractory dysmenorrhea: In these cases, hysterectomy may be considered after the family is completed. Nerve transection procedures are not advocated.

Supportive therapies such as behavioral counseling, dietary modifications, and alternative therapies may have a limited role.

KEY POINTS

- A detailed and a comprehensive history is a must to diagnose the type and cause of dysmenorrhea.
- Primary dysmenorrhea is a diagnosis of exclusion. All the causes of secondary dysmenorrhea should be ruled out.
- Investigations are guided by the history and examination.
- Endometriosis, pelvic infection, and malformations have significant impact on woman's health and future reproductive functions; hence diagnosing them at the earliest is best for preventing further complications.
- The impact of dysmenorrhea on woman's quality of life is important and guides her management.
- A sympathetic approach with consideration of psychological and behavioral aspects will help in better patient management.

REFERENCES

1. Jamieson DJ, Steege JF. The prevalence of dysmenorrhea, dyspareunia, pelvic pain and irritable bowel syndrome in primary care practice. Obstet Gynecol. 1996;87(1):55-8.
2. Andresch B, Milson I. An epidemiologic study of young women with dysmenorrhea. Am J Obstet Gynecol. 1982;144(6):655-60.
3. Marc Fritz A, Leon Speroff. Clinical gynecologic endocrinology and infertility. Philadelphia: Lippincott Williams & Wilkins; 2010. p. 579.
4. Sundell G, Milsom I, Andersch B. Factors influencing the prevalence and severity of dysmenorrhoea in young women. Br J Obstet Gynaecol. 1990;97(7):588-94.

SUGGESTED READING

1. ACOG Practice Bulletin No. 110: noncontraceptive uses of hormonal contraceptives. Obstet Gynecol. 2010;115(1):206-18.
2. Burnett M, Lemyre M. No. 345-Primary dysmenorrhea consensus guideline. J Obstet Gynaecol Can. 2017;39(7):585-95.

34

Approach to a Woman Presenting with Dyspareunia

Manisha Bajaj

INTRODUCTION

Dyspareunia or female sexual dysfunction refers to recurrent or persistent genital pain that is experienced just before, during, or after penile-vaginal intercourse and interferes with sexual pleasure. It also includes difficult and incomplete penetration. It may be present in both partners but is more common in females. As many women do not seek treatment for this problem, it is difficult to assess the true prevalence. However, it is the most common form of sexual dysfunction with a significant negative impact on quality of life and has a wide prevalence ranging from 8 to 21%.[1]

It is estimated that at least two thirds of women experience dyspareunia at some point of time in their life.[2] It is not a disease, but rather a symptom of underlying disease having multifactorial etiology and pathogenesis spanning a continuum from physical to psychogenic factors. The current concept regarding the initiation of pain suggests an initial inciting event that is then perpetuated by confounding factors. Dyspareunia initially may be due to lesions of external genitalia and introital area causing severe pain or difficulty when penetration is attempted, which may then lead to spasm of pelvic floor muscles. Subsequently, the anticipation or memory of pain may lead to spasm even when the organic lesion has healed. Thus, it creates a self-perpetuating cycle.

In 2015, the Fourth Consultation on Sexual Medicine (ICSM) reviewed the existing systems and included dyspareunia as a part of female genital–pelvic pain dysfunction, others being genital sexual pain, vulvodynia, and vaginismus.[3] The risk factors for the sexual dysfunction include biological, psychological, and sociocultural factors. Women with pelvic inflammatory disease (PID), peri- and post-menopause, anxiety, depression, and history of sexual abuse are at high risk for dyspareunia.[4]

Dyspareunia can be classified depending upon the onset and location. Based on the onset, it is classified into *primary* or *secondary* dyspareunia, primary when it occurs with the onset of first sexual contact and secondary when it follows previously normal sexual relations. Primary is often psychosocial and secondary is usually due to organic cause.

Depending on the site, it can be classified into *superficial* or *deep* dyspareunia. Superficial or insertional dyspareunia is pain on initial attempt at penetration and due to local cause at or around the introitus or may be a conditioned response to a previous unpleasant experience. Deep dyspareunia is pain during penile thrusting deep within the vagina and is usually due to gynecological problems such as endometriosis, infection, and previous surgery. If the pain persists or occurs several hours later, then it is mostly

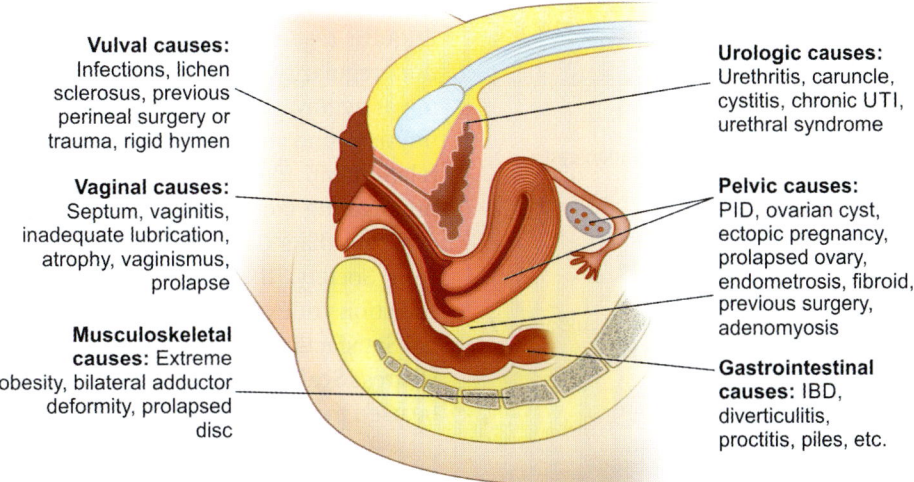

Fig. 1: Organic causes of dyspareunia.
(IBD: inflammatory bowel disease; PID: pelvic inflammatory disease; UTI: urinary tract infection)

psychological in origin. The differentiation is useful to arrive at an appropriate diagnosis, referral, treatment, and ultimately prognosis.

Dyspareunia can also be broadly divided in to *organic* or *nonorganic*. Organic dyspareunia is usually due to an underlying pathology whereas nonorganic dyspareunia is psychogenic in origin. Nonorganic or psychogenic dyspareunia has been classified as *type I intrapersonal*, which involves guilt, misinformation, previous traumatic experience, and prior organic lesions, and *type II interpersonal*, which is due to relationship issues, wherein dyspareunia is an excuse to avoid sex.

DIFFERENTIAL DIAGNOSIS

Differential diagnosis of dyspareunia is as given in Box 1. The common causes are depicted in Figure 1.

HISTORY

A careful history directed toward chronology of discomfort, its magnitude, and its effect is

Box 1: Differential diagnosis of dyspareunia.

- Organic causes:
  - Vulval:
    » *Vulval infections*: Candidiasis and genital herpes
    » Infection of Bartholin's gland
    » *Dermatological conditions*: Lichen sclerosus, lichen planus, and lichen simplex chronicus
    » *Previous perineal surgery*: Episiotomy, perineorrhaphy, and circumcision
    » Previous trauma
    » Burns
    » *Congenital disorders*: Imperforate hymen, rigid hymen, and painful and hymenal tags
    » *Idiopathic*: Vulvodynia and vestibulitis
  - Vaginal:
    » Vaginitis
    » *Congenital disorder*: Transverse vaginal septum
    » *Vaginal adhesion/stricture*: Postsurgery and postradiation
    » Inadequate lubrication (sympathomimetic drugs, OCPs, menopause, radiotherapy, and chemotherapy)
    » Irritants (contraceptives and douches)
    » Prolapse
    » Vaginal atrophy as in menopause

Contd...

Contd...

- » Vaginismus
- » Sjögren's syndrome
- *Pelvic (uterine and ovarian)*:
  - » Retroverted uterus
  - » *Pelvic mass*: Fibroid and ovarian cyst
  - » Adenomyosis
  - » Pelvic endometriosis
  - » Prolapsed ovaries
  - » Pelvic inflammatory disease
  - » Ectopic pregnancy
  - » *Previous pelvic surgery*: McCall culdoplasty
  - » Pelvic congestion syndrome
- *Gastrointestinal*:
  - » Inflammatory bowel disease
  - » Diverticulitis
  - » Proctitis
  - » Fissure in ano
  - » Hemorrhoids
- *Urological*:
  - » Urethritis
  - » Urethral caruncle
  - » Cystitis
  - » Interstitial cystitis
- *Others*:
  - » *Inaccessibility of vulva*: Extreme obesity, bilateral adductor deformity, and myofascial pelvic pain syndrome
  - » Neurological—multiple sclerosis, Parkinsonism, and fibromyalgia
- *Psychological causes*:
  - » Fear of pain (phobic reaction) and guilt
  - » Shame
  - » Traumatic sexual experience/rape
  - » Relationship distress
  - » Fear of penetration
  - » Unresolved anger/conflict
  - » Inadequate precoital stimulation or foreplay
  - » Pregnancy fear
  - » Hysterical hyperesthesia of vulva and thighs
  - » Major anxiety conflicts
  - » Hostility
  - » Sexual aversions

(OCPs: oral contraceptive pills)

essential from both the partners. The communication skills play a vital role; the physician should take care that both the partners are comfortable and assure them of strict confidentiality. It is important to ask direct questions as well as open-ended questions. Enquire regarding the site, intensity, duration, regularity, associated symptoms, relieving or aggravating factors, and impact on the physical and emotional aspects of life and relationship. Identification of the inciting and propagating factors is necessary to reach an accurate diagnosis. The International Pelvic Pain Society, the validated Female Sexual Function Index, the Global Measure of Sexual Satisfaction Scale, and the Female Sexual Distress Scale are the questionnaires that can be used to evaluate the woman.[5]

History of Present Illness

A patient's own narrative of the problem is quite helpful in pointing out the cause and magnitude. Ask her to define specifically what she perceives. It is important to know the onset and duration of dyspareunia and character of the pain whether burning, stinging and sharp, dull aching, throbbing, or stabbing. Whether the pain is with every act of coitus, or it is before, during, or after the intercourse?

Pain before genital touch is suggestive of vulvodynia. Pain occurring at the very beginning of intercourse is suggestive of vestibulodynia or active vaginal infection. Pain on deep penetration may be due to PID, endometriosis, or interstitial cystitis. Pain occurring after sex may be related to generalized vulvodynia or pudendal neuralgia. Pain that get aggravated with exercise or sitting is suggestive of pudendal neuralgia.

It is important to know the exact site of pain. Pain on vulva suggests vulvar dermatosis or vulvodynia, pain in perianal area may be related to fissures or nerve trapment, and pain at entry may be due to infection or vulvar pain syndrome.

It is important to note if the symptom dates to delivery, vaginal surgery, menopause, hip injury, radiotherapy, chemotherapy, or occurrence of any lesions at introitus. Any history of drug intake such as sympathomimetic, gonadotropin-releasing hormone (GnRH) agonists, etc., should be elicited as these can reduce lubrication.

Sexual History

Most patients and doctors are not very comfortable, while eliciting sexual history. So, it is important that a proper professional atmosphere is created during consultation. Sexual history may carry the clues to the cause of dyspareunia. It is important to know if the libido of the woman is good and does she has lubrication during foreplay. She should be asked if she has had pain-free period of sexual contact or not. As decreased libido and inadequate lubrication are common causes of dyspareunia. It is important to know the number of partners she has and whether she has pain with a specific or all partners. Explore the relationship issues and find whether dyspareunia is affecting her relationship with her partner or not. Enquire regarding emotional factors and whether she and her partner have done anything regarding the problem? History of any traumatic sexual experience should be elicited. Any problem with the male partner such as impotence, penile deformity, and premature ejaculation should be excluded.

History of Past Illness

Ask for any history of vaginal discharge, pain in lower abdomen, or dysmenorrhea suggestive of PID or endometriosis. History of any perineal, vaginal or abdominal surgery, sexually transmitted diseases (STDs), pelvic radiation should be elicited. Any history of gastrointestinal or urological disorder, any autoimmune or neurological disorder should be noted.

Obstetrical History

Childbirth can have significant impact on the sexual health of a woman. Perineal trauma and instrumental delivery can result in postpartum dyspareunia. So, enquire regarding mode of delivery and any complications therein. Any history of operative vaginal delivery, episiotomy repair, perineal tears, or infection should be asked for. Enquire about current contraceptive usage as lactation and progesterone are methods that can result in dyspareunia due to dryness. History of use of other methods such as intrauterine device (IUD), spermicides, jellies, foams, and douches should also be elicited as they can act as irritants. Latex in condoms and diaphragm can also cause allergic reaction. No differences were found in the use of combined oral contraceptive pills between the women who had dyspareunia and those who did not.[6]

Menstrual History

Note the details of menstrual cycles and ask for presence of dysmenorrhea, and if present, then whether it is primary or secondary. The dysmenorrhea coexisting with dyspareunia is mostly secondary.

Personal History

History of alcohol and recreational drug abuse should be asked for.

Family History

Enquire if there was negative family attitude toward sex.

EXAMINATION

It is very important to be gentle and understanding while examining a woman presenting with dyspareunia. A thorough examination should be performed in the presence of a female attendant or the partner. Examination should not aim toward reproducing the symptoms. Examination, which is painful for the patient, will not provide much information to the doctor. The patient should be taken into confidence and assured that the examination will be interrupted as soon as the patient feels any discomfort. An eye-to-eye contact and good communication should be maintained all through the examination and the examination should be stopped immediately as soon as the patient feels any discomfort. Patient should be encouraged to point to the area where it pains the most. She can be provided with picture or diagram of the perineal area to point at the exact site of pain. Before proceeding to the local examination, a general physical and systemic examination is done.

Per Abdomen Examination

Abdomen is inspected for any scars or lumps. Presence of scars may indicate previous surgery. This is followed by palpation for any tenderness or mass. In case a mass is palpable, it should be assessed for its size, location, margins, mobility, and tenderness.

Examination of Genitalia

Inspection of Vulva

The vulva is examined for pubic hair, for labial fullness, and for any evidence of vulvar atrophy. The labia are gently separated, and vulva is looked for the presence of any lesions such as ulcers, pustules, vesicles, growth, warts, cysts, hypo- or hyperpigmentation, scarring, keratinization, and erythema. Any discharge, if present at the introitus, is noted. Intense redness at the ostia of Bartholin's and Skene's gland suggests vestibulodynia. The perineum and perianal area are inspected for any of the above-mentioned lesions. Ask the patient to strain and observe for any uterovaginal prolapse.

Palpation

The pressure point testing is first done on external genitalia with a moistened cotton swab moving from medial thighs, buttocks, mons pubis, labia majora, clitoris, labia minora, and vulvar vestibule. The clinician also assesses the clitoris and bulbocavernosus reflexes, and appearance of the tissues along with pain mapping.

This is followed by a systematic palpation of the labia majora, clitoral prepuce, perineum, interlabial sulci, and labia minora for any tenderness or induration. As per speculum examination is not well tolerated by most of the women with dyspareunia, one should first introduce a single finger without touching the vestibule and carry out a monomanual examination.

If the patient tolerates it well, a gentle palpation of the vaginal walls and cervix is carried out followed by palpation of levator ani muscles for its tone, tenderness and trigger points. Vaginismus can occur during examination and approximately 25% women tolerate the examination well but have spasm during intercourse. The pudendal nerve is palpated medial to the ischial spine at its entry into pudendal canal for pudendal neuralgia. It is important to palpate the posterior fourchette for any suture knots or granulomata in women with postnatal dyspareunia and postperineorrhaphy dyspareunia. This is followed by a per speculum examination if the patient allows.

Per Speculum Examination

Per speculum examination is done with a narrow well-lubricated speculum. It is inserted taking care that it does not touch the vestibular area. The vagina is examined for any evidence of atrophy, ulcers, growth, infection, discharge, trauma, prolapse, and any anatomical abnormality such as septae and synechiae. Pale mucosa, decreased rugosity, elasticity, and vaginal depth indicate vaginal atrophy.

Cervical inspection may reveal cervicitis, erosion or growth, which requires further evaluation. A Pap smear and cervical or vaginal swab should be collected for culture sensitivity. The discharge is subjected to pH testing, wet mount, potassium hydroxide (KOH) preparation, and culture. Thick white curdy discharge is suggestive of candidiasis, copious malodorous yellow–green discharge of trichomoniasis, and gray or yellow discharge with positive whiff test of bacterial vaginosis.

Bimanual Examination

Bimanual examination is done at the last and provides the most useful information, especially in women with deep dyspareunia. Here, specifically look for any rectovaginal nodules, pelvic masses, tenderness, and cervical motion tenderness. The size, shape, and mobility of the uterus is assessed. Vaginal fornices are palpated for adnexal pathology. Rectovaginal examination is done to assess the rectovaginal septum and uterosacral ligaments for any evidence of endometriosis in the form of nodularity and tenderness.

INVESTIGATIONS

History and examination usually lead to diagnosis in most cases and any further investigations depend upon the findings on examination. Investigations are usually indicated when nongynecologic causes are suspected. Vaginal and cervical swabs for culture sensitivity, wet smear with saline and KOH, abdominal and pelvic ultrasound, and diagnostic laparoscopy are carried out whenever indicated. The genital ulcers are examined for syphilis, chancroid, lymphogranuloma venereum (LGV), granuloma inguinale, and herpes simplex virus (HSV). Wet mount prepared with vaginal discharge using saline or KOH is examined for the presence of increased leukocytes, *Trichomonas*, clue cells, and *Candida*. Whiff test is done by mixing the discharge with KOH, which in the presence of bacterial vaginosis produces fishy smell. Cervical or vaginal biopsy is indicated in case of suspicion of dermatoses, intraepithelial lesion, or neoplasia. Urine analysis, urine culture, and cystoscopy are indicated in cases of suspected bladder pathology or diverticulum. Transabdominal and transvaginal ultrasound is carried out in cases of suspected pelvic and abdominal pathology. Diagnostic laparoscopy may be required, if suspicion of endometriosis is there. Keeping in view the morbidity and complications, invasive investigations such as laparoscopy should be ordered judiciously.

Flowchart 1 summarizes the workup of a woman presenting with dyspareunia.

MANAGEMENT

The management depends upon the initial assessment and the likely cause. Most of the cases are treated at the level of gynecologists but some may require a multidisciplinary approach and referral to various specialists including dermatologists, urologist, gastrointestinal specialist, neurologist, psychiatrist, and psychologist. Those with vulvar pain syndrome need to be managed by an integrated approach.

The common causes of dyspareunia include endometriosis, adenomyosis, and

Flowchart 1: Algorithm for clinical approach to a woman presenting with dyspareunia.

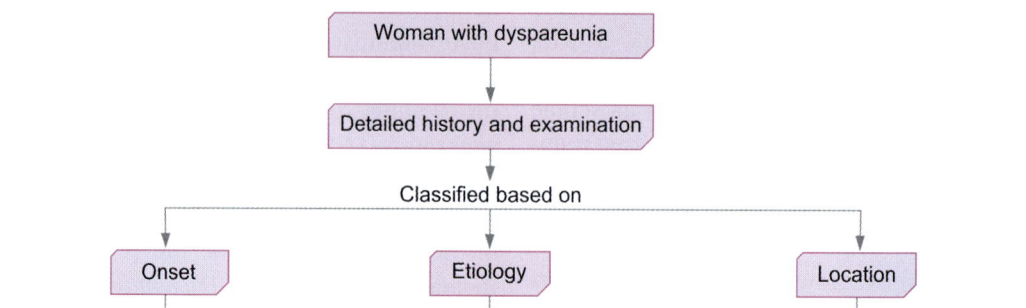

PID in younger women and vaginal atrophy in perimenopausal and postmenopausal women. Treatment is targeted to specific disorder. Application of intravaginal estrogen creams is very useful in women with atrophic vagina. Sexual counseling is an important intervention which is a simple but effective intervention.

KEY POINTS

- Dyspareunia is a common, but underreported problem significantly influencing a woman's health, relationships, and quality of life.
- It is not a disease, but a symptom of an underlying disease with both organic and psychological factors contributing to it.
- Although the current treatment approach favors it as a pain disorder, the knowledge of the causative organic factor must be integrated with an understanding of the ongoing psychological factors and attitudes that perpetuate the pain cycle.
- The identification of the initiating and propagating factors is necessary to reach a correct diagnosis and successful treatment.
- A thorough examination in conjunction with a detailed history almost always reveals the diagnosis and rarely any further investigations are required to confirm it.
- Management of dyspareunia is best done by a multidisciplinary team, especially of women where no specific disease can be identified.

REFERENCES

1. Latthe P, Latthe M, Say L, Gülmezoglu M, Khan KS. WHO systematic review of prevalence of chronic pelvic pain: a neglected reproductive health morbidity. BMC Public Health. 2006;6:177.
2. Jonathan S Berek. Berek & Novak's Gynecology, 14th edition. Philadelphia: Lippincott Williams & Wilkins; 2007. p. 314.

3. McCabe MP, Sharlip ID, Atalla E, Balon R, Fisher AD, Laumann E, et al. Definitions of sexual dysfunctions in women and men: A consensus statement from the fourth international consultation on sexual medicine 2015. J Sex Med. 2016;13(2):135-43.
4. Latthe P, Mignini L, Gray R, Hills R, Khan K. Factors predisposing women to chronic pelvic pain: systematic review. BMJ. 2006; 332(7544):749.
5. Verit FF, Verit A. Validation of the female sexual function index in women with chronic pelvic pain. J Sex Med. 2007;4(6):1635-41.
6. Danielsson I, Sjöberg I, Stenlund H, Wikman M.. Prevalence and incidence of prolonged and severe dyspareunia in women: results from a population study. Scand J Public Health. 2003;31(2):113-8.

SUGGESTED READING

1. American College of Obstetricians and Gynecologists' Committee on Gynecologic Practice; American Society for Colposcopy and Cervical Pathology (ASCCP). Committee Opinion No 673: Persistent Vulvar Pain. Obstet Gynecol. 2016 Sep;128(3):e78-84.
2. Female Sexual Dysfunction: ACOG Practice Bulletin Summary, NUMBER 213. Obstet Gynecol. 2019;134(1):203-5.
3. Royal College of Obstetricians and Gynaecologists (RCOG) (2012). Green-top guideline on the initial management of chronic pelvic pain. [online] Available from https://www.rcog.org.uk/globalassets/documents/guidelines/gtg_41.pdf. [Last accessed March, 2020].

35
Approach to a Woman Presenting with Lower Abdominal Pain

Manisha Bajaj

INTRODUCTION

Lower abdominal pain or pelvic pain is a common complaint in women. There are numerous causes of pain in lower abdomen mostly related to the genital tract, occasionally to intestinal and urinary tract. Rarely neurological, vascular, musculoskeletal, and psychological factors may be responsible for pain in lower abdomen. The provisional diagnosis is often based on the clinical history and examination but confirmed with the aid of investigations.

The intensity of pain can range from mild discomfort to severe debilitating pain. Pelvic pain can be acute or chronic in onset and may be recurrent in nature. Acute pelvic pain is usually severe, often associated with nausea, vomiting, diaphoresis, apprehension, etc. Timely meticulous examination and accurate diagnosis is vital to prevent significant morbidity and occasional mortality associated with it.

Chronic pelvic pain (CPP) is insidious in onset or may follow acute pelvic pain. It can affect both physical and psychological aspects of the woman. The American College of Obstetricians and Gynecologists (ACOG) define CPP as a noncyclical pain in lower abdomen or pelvis of longer than 6 months' duration not occurring solely with menstrual periods or sexual intercourse, and not related to pregnancy and is of sufficient severity to interfere with daily routine activities or result in seeking medical advice.[1] It may be intermittent or continuous. The prevalence of CPP varies from 4 to 25%, but only a few seek medical advice. It is an indication for approximately 20% hysterectomies for benign causes.[2] Tender love and care along with a multidisciplinary approach is essential for definitive diagnosis and management of this condition.

DIFFERENTIAL DIAGNOSIS

The diagnosis of pelvic pain in women can be challenging. The genital tract, lower ileum, sigmoid colon, and rectum share common nerve supply. So, distinction between gynecologic and gastrointestinal pain is often difficult. The various differential diagnoses of lower abdominal pain are as listed in Table 1.

HISTORY

A detailed history should be elicited as it clinches the probable diagnosis in most cases. It is supplemented with a thorough general physical and systemic examination. Completing a daily pain diary for two to three menstrual cycles may help the woman and the doctor identify provoking factors or temporal associations.

Table 1: Differential diagnosis of lower abdominal pain.		
Acute	Chronic	Recurrent
Gynecological causes		
Ectopic pregnancy	Chronic pelvic inflammatory disease (PID)	Premenstrual tension
Abortion (threatened/inevitable)	Pelvic congestion syndrome	Dysmenorrhea (primary/secondary)
Acute PID	Pelvic adhesions	Obstructed Müllerian anomaly
Tubo-ovarian abscess	Endometriosis or adenomyosis	Mittelschmerz pain
Ruptured ovarian cyst	Ovarian remnant syndrome	Adenomyosis
Twisted ovarian cyst	Early stages of uterine prolapse	Endometriosis
Twisted/pedunculated subserous		
Submucous/degenerating fibroids		
Corpus luteum hematoma		
Gastrointestinal causes		
Terminal ileitis	Irritable bowel syndrome	Constipation
Appendicitis	*Inflammatory bowel disease*: Ulcerative colitis	Appendicitis
Gastroenteritis	Crohn's disease	Diverticulitis
Bowel obstruction	Gastrointestinal infection	
	Gastrointestinal malignancy	
Urological causes		
Ureteral/Vesical calculus	Urethral syndrome	Ureteral/Vesical calculus
Urinary tract infection	Interstitial cystitis	
Acute retention of urine	Cystourethritis	
	Pyelonephritis	
	Carcinoma	
Others		
	Fibromyalgia	Myofascial pain
	Spondylolysis	Abdominal angina
	Coccydynia	Hernia
	Degenerative changes	Aortic aneurysm
	Osteitis pubis	
	Abdominal wall hematoma	
	Somatic manifestation of depression	
	Physical or sexual abuse	
	Idiopathic pain	

History of presenting illness is taken as follows:
- What is the site of pain? The patient can be given the pictures of the body and asked to point at the exact site of pain. Whether it is present all over the lower abdomen or localized in left or right iliac fossa or suprapubic region or occurs at different places at different times? Gynecological pain due to pelvic inflammatory disease (PID), fibroid, or endometriosis may be present in whole lower abdomen whereas pain in right iliac fossa may be due to appendicitis and in left iliac fossa due to diverticulitis or colitis. Suprapubic pain is suggestive of cystitis, PID, endometriosis, degenerating fibroid, gastroenteritis, or irritable bowel syndrome. Pain moving from one quadrant to another is typical of gastrointestinal causes and unlikely to be gynecological in origin.
- Was the onset of pain sudden or gradual? Sudden onset of pain is typically associated with ruptured ectopic pregnancy, rupture or torsion of ovarian cysts, mittelschmerz, renal colic, intestinal colic, gastroenteritis, and irritable bowel syndrome. While gradually developing pain is suggestive of conditions such as PID and endometriosis.
- What is the duration of pain? If the pain has been there for months, it is likely to be due to conditions such as chronic PID and endometriosis and unlikely to be due to conditions such as appendicitis, ectopic pregnancy, gastroenteritis, or renal colic.
- How severe is the pain? It can be scored on a visual analog scale which allows the patient to scale the pain on a scale of 0–10 with 10 being the worst possible pain. Mild pain is suggestive of pathologies such as mittelschmerz, endometriosis, degeneration of uterine fibroid, chronic PID, cystitis, gastroenteritis, amebiasis, and irritable bowel syndrome. Moderate pain, one that interferes only with some activities, is associated with all nongynecological conditions such as appendicitis, gastroenteritis, and pyelonephritis. Severe pain can be due to acute PID, ruptured ectopic pregnancy, torsion of ovarian cysts or adnexa, degenerated fibroids, pyelonephritis, renal stones, gastroenteritis, bowel obstruction, and diverticulitis.
- What is the nature of the pain? The pain can be colicky or cramping, dull aching, burning, intense needle-like or feeling of tearing. Colicky pain is rhythmic due to smooth muscle contractions and occurs when bowel, uterus, or ureter is involved. Pain due to appendicitis and diverticulitis may be both cramping and continuous. PID may cause dull aching steady pain ensuing from inflammation and stretching of the peritoneum, and colicky pain due to local irritation of the bowel. Dragging pain in the lower back and abdomen, which increases with activity, may be due to stretching of nerve fibers in uterosacral ligaments in early stages of uterine descent. Typically, the woman is pain free in the morning, but has pain after doing her daily activities and progressively increases as the day passes by. Burning, aching or shooting pain of long-standing duration with previous history of surgery, trauma, and inflammation can be neuropathic pain. Highly localized, sharp, stabbing or aching pain, exacerbated by movements in nerve distribution area and persisting beyond 5 weeks may be due to nerve entrapment in scar tissue, fascia, or a narrow foramen.
- Is the pain increasing? Constantly increasing pain indicates serious conditions requiring immediate attention such as

ectopic pregnancy, appendicitis, ovarian torsion, acute PID, abscess, etc. Pain that improves gradually requires observation or conservative management.
- What are the associated symptoms? Nausea and vomiting are associated with causes such as appendicitis, gastroenteritis, intestinal obstruction, ectopic pregnancy, and torsion of ovarian cyst. CPP with menstrual exacerbation can also be due to pelvic venous congestion.
- Are there any associated urinary or bowel symptoms? Gynecological conditions do not usually affect the bladder and bowel functions. Presence of symptoms related to bowel or bladder indicates involvement of gastrointestinal or urinary systems. Both constipation and diarrhea characterize irritable bowel syndrome. Women with bowel obstruction present with constipation whereas diarrhea is associated with gastroenteritis, diverticulitis, etc. The urinary symptoms indicate presence of cystitis, pyelonephritis, or ureteric stones. Renal colic due to ureteric stones presents with severe colicky pain and hematuria whereas conditions such as cystitis and pyelonephritis present with dysuria, rarely hematuria.

In conditions such as ruptured ectopic pregnancy and ruptured corpus luteal hematoma, there is hemoperitoneum, which causes referred pain in the right shoulder due to irritation of subdiaphragmatic area and stimulation of phrenic nerve.

Aggravating and relieving factors provide a clue to the possible etiology of pain. The pain, which gets aggravated with the movement, suggests peritoneal irritation as in patients with ruptured ectopic pregnancy, torsion ovarian cyst, acute PID, appendicitis, diverticulitis, and bowel perforation. The patient tries to lie still in this situation. The pain that is aggravated by food intake suggests presence of gastrointestinal problems such as gastric ulcer, gastroenteritis, diverticulitis, and irritable bowel syndrome or bowel obstruction.

The impact of pain on the quality of life is important and can be done by using various questionnaires.

Treatment History

History of any previous diagnostic test done or treatment received should be elicited.

History of Past Illness

A detailed history of a similar complaint in the past provides an insight into the present condition. Cyclical recurrence of symptoms suggests conditions such as endometriosis and mittelschmerz. Recurrent episodes are also common with diverticular disease and irritable bowel syndrome. The risk of repeat ectopic is more in women with previous history of ectopic pregnancy.

Previous history of ovarian cyst, endometriosis, or PID increases the likelihood of recurrence of these diseases. A history of cystitis or pyelonephritis increases the risk of cystitis and pyelonephritis in future. Women, who have undergone hysterectomy in the past, are unlikely to suffer from pain due to pregnancy-related problems. Any previous history of surgery may suggest adhesions as a possible cause of pain. History of diagnostic laparoscopy with normal pelvic findings within last 1 year decreases the likelihood of conditions such as uterine fibroids and endometriosis as a cause of lower abdominal pain.

History suggestive of depression should be elicited as CPP can be a manifestation of depression. In some individuals, child sexual abuse may initiate a cascade of events or reactions which makes an individual more vulnerable to the development of CPP as an adult. Women who continue to be abused are particularly at risk.

Menstrual History

The relation of pain with menstrual cycle should be carefully elicited as in many conditions such as endometriosis, adenomyosis, PID, and early stages of uterine descent there is associated dysmenorrhea. Mid-cycle pain is characteristic of mittelschmerz.

Contraceptive History

The risk of PID is increased with use of intrauterine device (IUD). Current use of the IUD increases the risk of ectopic pregnancy by decreasing the chances of intrauterine pregnancy. Oral contraceptive pills (OCPs) prevent functional ovarian cysts, PID, mittelschmerz, dysmenorrhea, and endometriosis. Tubal ligation reduces the risk of pregnancy-related problems and lower the risk of PID. However, ligated women can have ectopic pregnancy.

Sexual History

A detailed psychosocial history is important, especially in reference to dyspareunia. Deep dyspareunia points toward endometriosis. Sexual or physical abuse has been associated with CPP.

EXAMINATION

General Physical Examination

A careful general physical examination is done with special reference to patient's vitals, temperature, and any pallor. Presence of pallor may point toward blood loss due to ectopic pregnancy or incomplete abortion. A woman presenting with acute abdominal pain due to ruptured ectopic pregnancy may present in hemorrhagic shock. Similarly, woman with acute abdomen consequent to surgical conditions such a perforated appendix or bowel may present in endotoxic shock. Patients with an infective cause of abdominal pain, such as PID, cystitis, gastroenteritis, and appendicitis, may have fever or be in septic shock.

Systemic Examination

General physical examination is followed by a meticulous systemic examination including respiratory and cardiovascular systems and a detailed abdominal examination.

Per Abdomen Examination

Inspection of abdomen is followed by palpation. Abdomen may be distended on inspection. Superficial palpation for any tenderness is followed by deep palpation. Diffused tenderness is elicited with ruptured ectopic pregnancy, gastroenteritis, and bowel obstruction. Appendicitis is suspected, if there is tenderness in right lower quadrant and diverticulitis, if there is tenderness in left lower quadrant. Ectopic pregnancy, ovarian cyst, and mittelschmerz may present with tenderness in any quadrant in lower abdomen. Suprapubic pain suggests cystitis, PID, endometriosis, dysmenorrhea, complicated ovarian cyst, or abortion.

The presence of voluntary guarding suggests ectopic pregnancy, tubo-ovarian abscess, appendicitis, or PID. Involuntary guarding and marked rebound tenderness are characteristics of peritonitis as seen with appendicitis, diverticulitis, acute PID with pelvic peritonitis, ruptured ectopic pregnancy, and torsion of ovarian cyst.

Enlarged uterus of >12 weeks pregnancy size may present as a midline lower abdominal mass. Uterus may be enlarged because of pregnancy, fibroid or collection in uterine cavity, hematometra, or pyometra. Both appendicitis and diverticulitis can present as a mass, but they are usually in the right and left lower quadrants, respectively, and may be either ill-defined or may not be felt abdominally.

The costovertebral angle (CVA) tenderness is characteristically appreciated with pyelonephritis and sometimes renal colic and is usually unilateral.

Pelvic Examination

An intact hymen usually indicates absence of pregnancy-related complications and PID. On per speculum examination, bleeding through the cervical os may be present in cases with ectopic pregnancy, or threatened or inevitable abortion. Other causes of bleeding through the cervical os include endometrial and fibroid polyps. Dirty purulent discharge may be seen in PID, septic abortion, and infected fibroid polyp. Sometimes, products of conception or a fibroid polyp may be seen protruding through a dilated cervical os.

Bladder is normally nontender. Suprapubic tenderness may be present in cystitis or endometritis. In pregnancy, cervix is soft on palpation. Mild cervical motion tenderness or cervical excitation pain is nonspecific, however, moderate-to-severe cervical excitation pain is present in ectopic pregnancy and torsion of ovarian cyst.

Uterine enlargement is present in pregnancy and pregnancy-related complications such as ectopic pregnancy and fibroids. An irregular contour almost always indicates the presence of fibroids. Pregnancy complications, PID, and endometriosis can cause uterine tenderness.

It might be difficult to palpate adnexal masses, particularly when the patient cannot relax due to tenderness or if she is obese. In women with PID, the fornices may be thick and tender. It is very unlikely for the patient to have PID in the absence of significant tenderness in the fornices. A tender adnexal mass is suggestive of ectopic pregnancy, torsion of ovarian cyst, adnexa, or tubo-ovarian abscess, and a nontender mass is suggestive of an ovarian cyst, tubo-ovarian cyst, hydrosalpinx, or an endometrioma. A tender mass in the pouch of Douglas (POD) suggests appendicitis, diverticulitis, acute PID with tubo-ovarian abscess, complicated ovarian cyst, or ectopic pregnancy. Nontender masses are usually ovarian cysts or fecaliths in the colon. Tender nodules in the POD on the uterosacral ligaments are distinctive of endometriosis; however, they are best felt through combined vaginal and rectal examination.

INVESTIGATIONS

Complete Blood Count

High total leukocyte count ($>15,000/mm^3$) and neutrophilia usually indicate the presence of an infectious process in the body. Hemoglobin may be low in women with ectopic pregnancy, abortion, and fibroid uterus with menorrhagia.

Pregnancy Test

As ectopic pregnancy is an important differential diagnosis in any woman presenting with acute abdominal pain in reproductive age group, urine pregnancy test is mandatory to rule it out. If the pregnancy test is positive and ectopic pregnancy is suspected, then quantitative estimation of serum β-human chorionic gonadotropin (β-hCG) hormone is done. If the serum β-hCG level is >1,500 IU, an intrauterine gestational sac should be visible on transvaginal ultrasound.

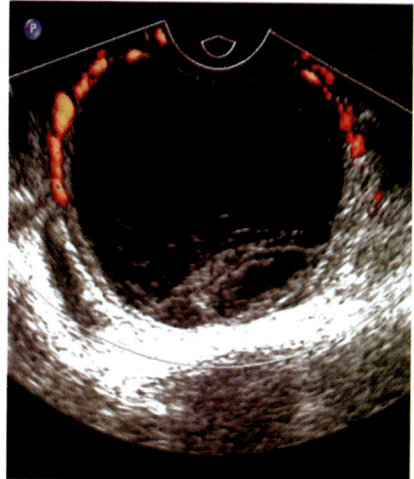

Fig. 1: Transvaginal ultrasound showing hemorrhagic cyst.

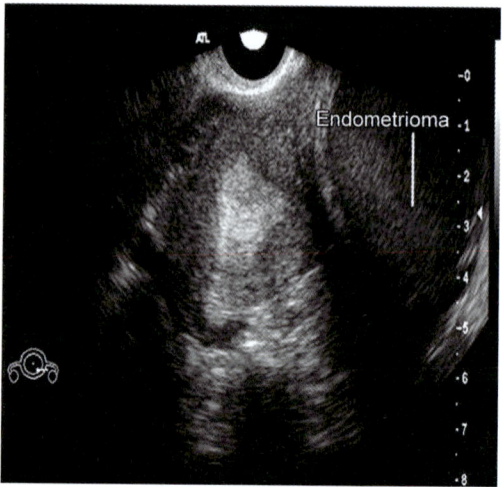

Fig. 2: Transvaginal ultrasound showing uterus with endometrioma.

Ultrasound of Abdomen and Pelvis

Ultrasound is helpful in diagnosing ovarian cysts (Fig. 1), endometriomas (Fig. 2), fibroids (Fig. 3), intrauterine pregnancy, and free fluid in the pelvis. It can identify an inflamed appendix but is not a very sensitive tool for diagnosing appendicitis.

Computed Tomography of Abdomen

Computed tomography (CT) of abdomen is very useful in the diagnosis of gastrointestinal problems such as appendicitis, diverticulitis, bowel obstruction, renal stones, adnexal masses, and intra-abdominal abscesses.

Magnetic Resonance Imaging

Magnetic resonance imaging (MRI) is a useful investigation for diagnosing endometriosis (Fig. 4) and helps in differentiating a dermoid cyst from endometrioma.

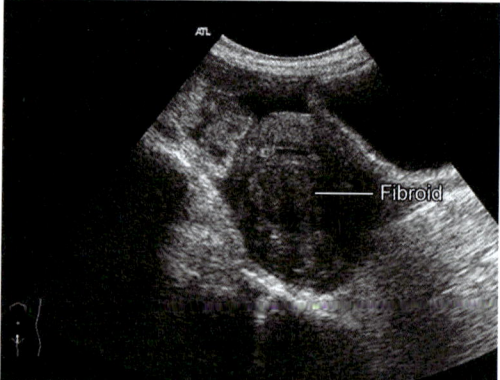

Fig. 3: Transvaginal ultrasound showing posterior wall fibroid of uterus.

Gonorrhea/*Chlamydia* Cultures

Chlamydia culture is helpful in supporting the diagnosis of PID. A positive culture, however, does not necessarily mean that the pelvic or abdominal pain is solely because of gonorrhea or *Chlamydia*.

Culdocentesis or paracentesis is a useful diagnostic aid for identifying hemoperitoneum or pyoperitoneum whenever there is free fluid in pelvis or abdomen, respectively

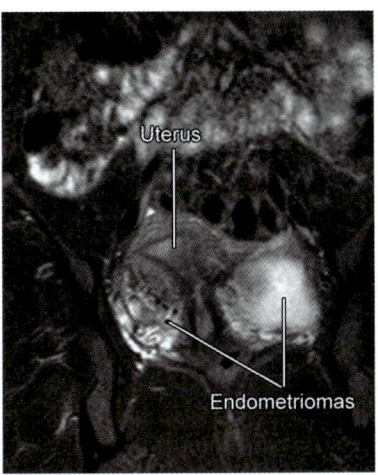

Fig. 4: Magnetic resonance imaging showing bilateral endometriomas.

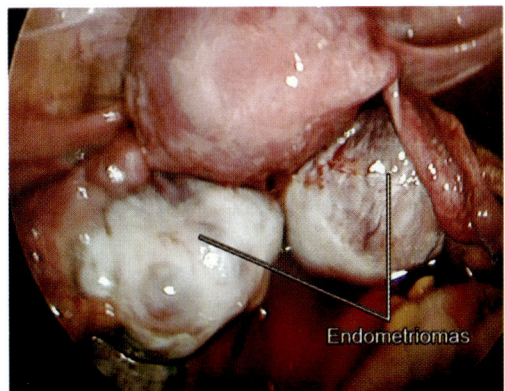

Fig. 5: Diagnostic laparoscopy—bilateral endometriomas adherent to posterior wall of uterus.

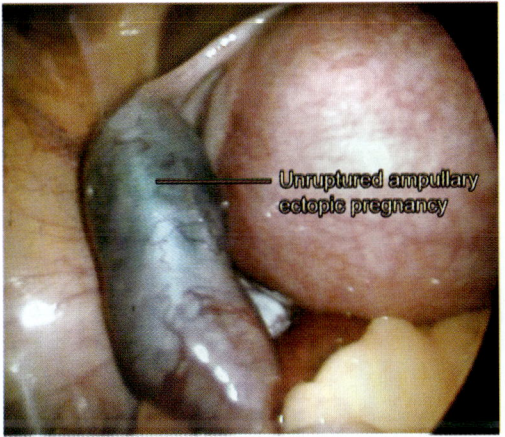

Fig. 6: Diagnostic laparoscopy—unruptured ectopic pregnancy.

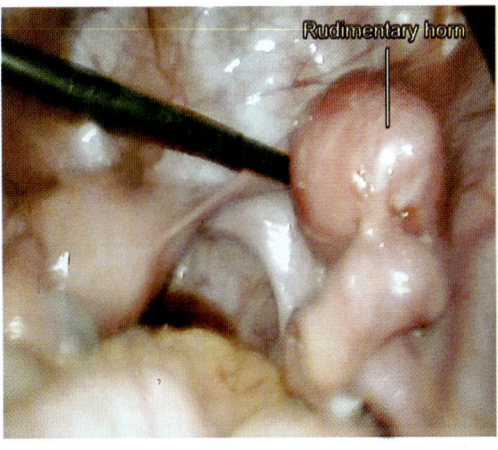

Fig. 7: Diagnostic laparoscopy—rudimentary horn.

on clinical examination or ultrasound. In the presence of a positive pregnancy test, aspiration of unclotted blood from abdomen or pelvis indicates hemoperitoneum due to ectopic pregnancy. In the absence of a positive pregnancy test, fresh blood suggests a corpus luteum hemorrhage and old blood suggests a ruptured endometrioma. Aspiration of purulent fluid is suggestive of peritonitis or sometimes sebaceous fluid of dermoid cyst. However, nowadays, culdocentesis has a limited role due to easy availability of imaging modalities such as ultrasonography, CT scan, and MRI.

Diagnostic Laparoscopy

Diagnostic laparoscopy is useful to diagnose and manage conditions such as endometriosis (Fig. 5), ectopic pregnancy (Fig. 6), rudimentary horn (Fig. 7), torsion of ovarian

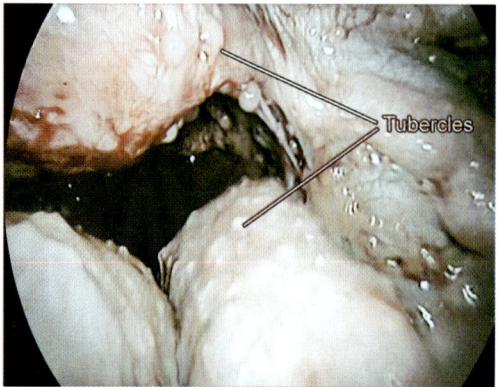

Fig. 8: Diagnostic laparoscopy—pelvic inflammatory disease (tubercular).

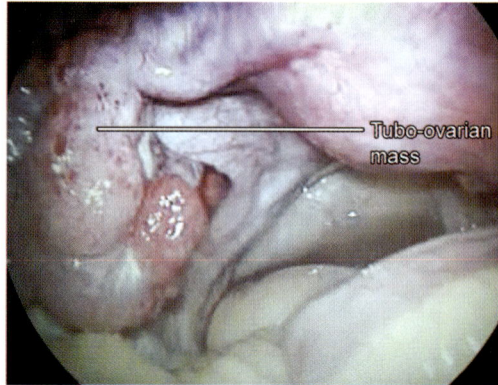

Fig. 9: Diagnostic laparoscopy—tubo-ovarian mass.

Flowchart 1: Algorithm for initial approach to a woman presenting with lower abdominal pain.

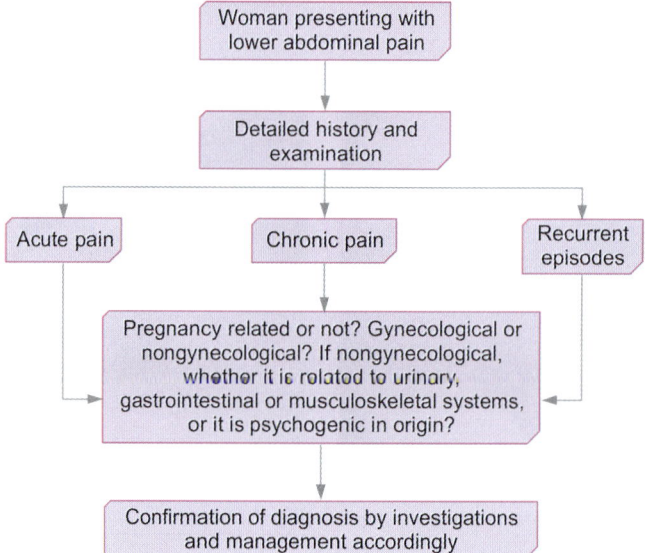

cyst, PID (Fig. 8), tubo-ovarian mass (Fig. 9), and adhesions. Diagnostic laparoscopy has been the "gold standard" in the diagnosis of CPP but it may be better seen as a second-line of investigation if other therapeutic interventions fail. Women with cyclical pain should be offered a therapeutic trial using the combined oral contraceptive pill or a gonadotropin-releasing hormone (GnRH) agonist for a period of 3–6 months before having a diagnostic laparoscopy. The levonorgestrel-releasing intrauterine system could also be considered.

Micro-laparoscopy or "conscious pain mapping" has been proposed as an alternative to diagnostic laparoscopy under general anesthesia. Although, the technique seems to provide an opportunity to confirm particular lesions as the source of the woman's pain, it has not been widely adopted.

Flowchart 1 describes the initial approach to a woman presenting with pain lower

Flowchart 2: Management of a woman presenting with pain lower abdomen.

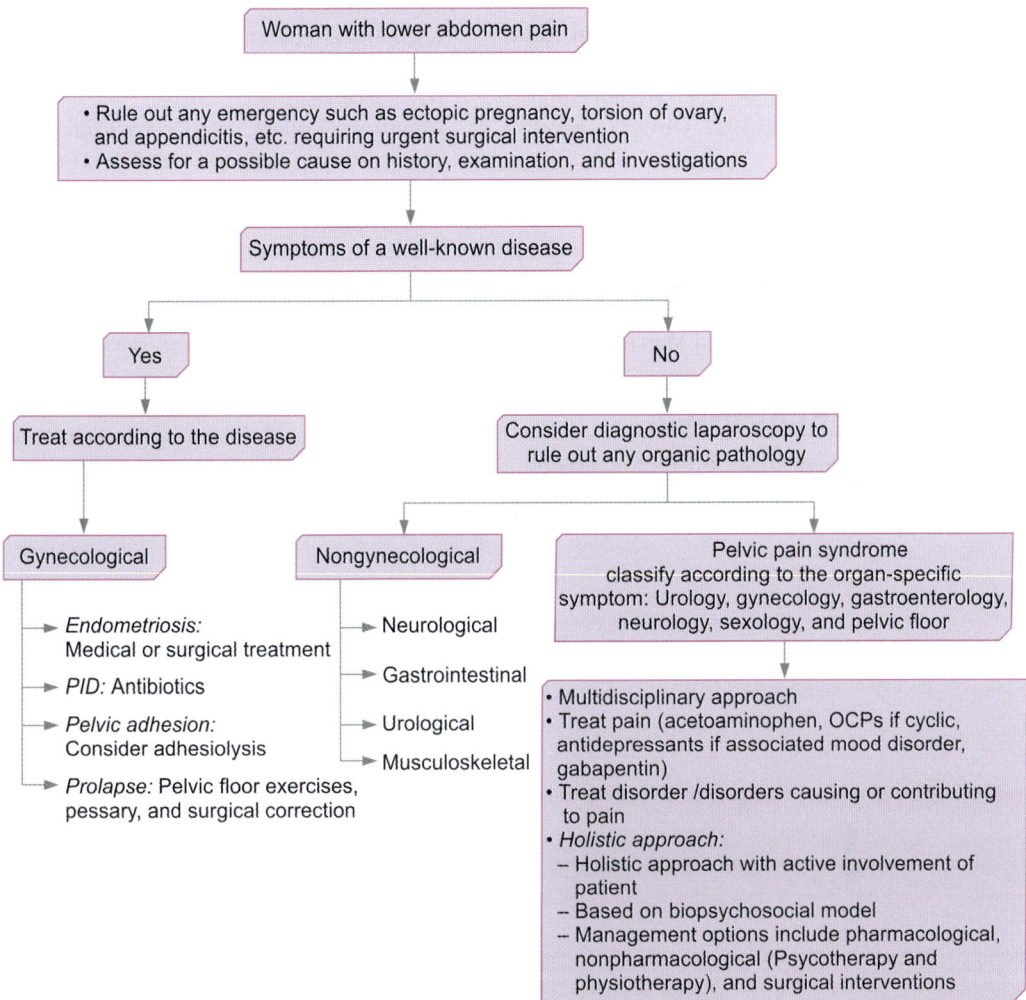

abdomen. Flowchart 2 describes the detailed management of a woman presenting with pain lower abdomen.[3]

KEY POINTS

- Lower abdominal pain is a common problem in women.
- It can be acute or chronic pain.
- The differential diagnosis, workup, and management of the patient essentially depend upon the nature of the pain.
- The approach should consider all the major sources of pain such as gynecological, gastrointestinal, urological, psychological, musculoskeletal, and neurological.
- Careful history and examination of all these systems can help in the identification of the exact source of pain.
- CPP is poorly understood and difficult to manage. It requires a sympathetic and supportive approach.

REFERENCES

1. Ortiz DD. Chronic pelvic pain in women. Am Fam Physician. 2008;77(11):1535-42.
2. Farquhar CM, Steiner CA. Hysterectomy rates in the US 1990-1997. Obstet Gynecol. 2002;99(2):229-34.
3. Engeler D, Baranowski AP, Borovicka A, Cottrell A, Dinis-Oliveria P, Elneil S, et al. (2014). Guidelines on Chronic Pelvic Pain. [online] Available from https://uroweb.org/wp-content/uploads/26-Chronic-Pelvic-Pain_LR.pdf. [Last accessed March, 2020].

SUGGESTED READING

1. ACOG and American Society for Colposcopy and Cervical Pathology (ASCCP) (2016). Committee opinion number 673: Persistent vulvar pain. [online] Available from acog.org/clinical-guidance/committee-opinion/articles//2016/09/persistent-vulvar-pain. [Last accessed March, 2020].
2. American College of Obstetricians and Gynecologists (ACOG). ACOG Practice Bulletin, Number 218: Chronic pelvic pain. 2020;135(3):e98-109.
3. European Association of Urology (EAU) (2019). Chronic pelvic pain. [online] Available from uroweb.org/guideline/chronic-pelvic-pain/?=summary-of-change. [Last accessed March, 2020].
4. Jarrell JF, Vilos GA, Allaire C, Burgess S, Fortin C, Gerwin R, et al. Consensus guidelines for the management of chronic pelvic pain. J Obstet Gynaecol Can. 2005;27(8):781-826.

36. Approach to a Woman Presenting with Abdominal Lump

Shilpa Dhingra

INTRODUCTION

Abdominal lump is defined as a palpable mass arising from the pelvis or abdomen, diagnosed clinically on abdominal or pelvic examination. It may be asymptomatic and diagnosed incidentally on routine checkup or ultrasound; or it may be symptomatic with the patient presenting with abdominal lump, abdominal pain, abnormal uterine bleeding or any bowel or urinary problem. Lump abdomen can be genital or extragenital in origin. Lump that is genital in origin may arise from uterus, fallopian tube or ovary and extragenital may arise from conditions related to bowel, bladder or other abdominal organs or structures.

DIFFERENTIAL DIAGNOSIS

The differential diagnosis of lump abdomen is tabulated in Table 1.

Table 1: Differential diagnosis of lump abdomen.

Genital causes	
Uterine	Ovarian

Neoplastic:
• *Benign:*
  – Myoma
  – Adenomyoma
• *Malignant:*
  – Endometrial cancer
  – Sarcoma
  – Advanced cervical cancer due to associated pyometra
	Neoplastic:
	• *Benign:*
	  – Epithelial tumor
	  – Germ cell tumor
	  – Stromal cell tumor
	  – Sex cord tumor
	• *Malignant:*
	  – Epithelial carcinoma
	  – Germ cell carcinoma
	  – Sex cord tumor
	  – Metastatic tumor

Nonneoplastic:
• Pyometra
• *Hematometra*:
  – Obstructed Müllerian anomaly
  – Post-surgery cervical stenosis
• *Pregnancy*:
  – Intrauterine
  – Molar
  – *Ectopic*: Rudimentary horn
	Nonneoplastic:
	• Follicular cyst
	• Theca lutein cyst
	• Corpus luteum cyst
	• Endometriotic cyst

Contd...

Contd...

Fallopian tube	Para-ovarian cyst

• Neoplastic:
  – Fallopian tube carcinoma
• Nonneoplastic:
  – Chronic ectopic pregnancy
  – Tubo-ovarian mass or abscess
  – Hydrosalpinx/Pyosalpinx
	• Broad ligament:
	  – Tumor
	  – Cyst

Extragenital causes	

• Urinary system related:
  – Distended bladder
  – Pelvic kidney
  – Bladder carcinoma
  – Urachal cyst
• Retroperitoneal masses:
  – Hematoma
  – Abscess
  – Sarcoma
  – Lymphoma
  – Leiomyoma
	• Bowel related:
	  – Appendicular lump
	  – Encysted ascites
	  – Ileocecal tuberculosis
	  – Crohn's disease
	  – Diverticular abscess
	  – Carcinoma colon
	  – Volvulus

HISTORY

The history of present illness will depend upon the presenting complaints. If the woman presents with the complaint of lump abdomen, then the history starts with the details of the lump, duration since when noticed, site, size, any increase or decrease in size, rate of progress, and any associated symptoms like fever, pain, trauma, any menstrual, urinary or bowel problem. Then the details of each associated symptoms such as pain, menstrual irregularity, fever, urinary or bowel problem need to be elicited in detail keeping in mind the differential diagnosis.

If the lump is diagnosed incidentally, leading history of symptoms pertaining to various causes of lump abdomen is elicited. Any urinary problems like frequency, dysuria, dribbling, hematuria, etc. need to be inquired. Any alteration in bowel habits such as constipation, diarrhea, tenesmus, feeling of incomplete evacuation, and melena need to be inquired. Any loss of weight or appetite is important, as it is present in patients with malignancy or tuberculosis (TB).

Menstrual History

A detailed menstrual history is important, as any abnormal uterine bleeding or postcoital bleeding is suggestive of a genital tract abnormality such as fibroid uterus, adenomyosis, endometrial carcinoma, and carcinoma cervix. Any history of amenorrhea may suggest a pregnancy-related problem such as intrauterine pregnancy, molar pregnancy or ectopic pregnancy, or a hormone-producing ovarian tumor. History of dysmenorrhea is an important symptom in women with adenomyosis or hematometra.

Obstetrical History

Obstetrical history is important as certain diseases such as fibroids and endometrial carcinoma are more common in nulliparous women; whereas cervical and ovarian carcinoma are more common in multiparous women.

Past History

Any past history of prolonged illness or treatment such as TB and inflammatory bowel disease is important. Any past history of surgery such as conization, transcervical resection of endometrium, Manchester repair, and even sometimes suction and evacuation for medical termination of pregnancy (MTP) can result in cervical stenosis with resultant hematometra.

Family History

Any family history of TB, malignancy of ovary, breast, uterus, colon, etc. needs to be elicited.

This should be followed by personal history of any allergies and treatment history.

EXAMINATION

Examination includes general physical examination, breast examination, systemic examination, per abdomen examination, and pelvic examination including per speculum, per vaginal, and per-rectal examination.

General Physical Examination

The general physical examination should include any significant cervical or supraclavicular lymphadenopathy, which is present in TB or malignancy of breast and gastrointestinal tract, respectively. Pedal edema, especially unilateral pedal edema, is an important finding in cases with ovarian malignancy.

Breast Examination

Breast examination for any lump or discharge should be carried out as a routine in all women attending the outpatient department (OPD), whether pregnant or not. Care should be taken not to miss the palpation of the axillary tail of breast for any lump and axillary lymph nodes.

Per Abdomen Examination

On per abdomen examination, as regards the lump, following points are to be noted:

- *Size*: Both in terms of actual measurement in centimeters or inches and in terms of uterine height corresponding to weeks of pregnancy
- *Margins*: Well-defined or ill-defined
- *Surface*: Smooth or irregular
- *Consistency*: Soft, cystic, firm, hard or variegated
- *Mobility*: Both side-to-side and above downward
- *Tenderness*: Whether tender or not
- *Lower limit*: Whether lower limit can be reached or not

In addition, it is important to look for any hepatosplenomegaly or free fluid in abdomen.

Uterine Lumps

Lumps of uterine origin are midline, well defined with a smooth or irregular surface, usually mobile from side-to-side and not above downward and cannot be lifted out of pelvis.

Ovarian Lumps

Ovarian lumps may or may not be midline, are well defined or ill defined, surface is usually smooth if benign and may be irregular, hard or variegated if malignant; mobile in all directions if benign, but mobility is restricted if complicated or malignant.

It is difficult to differentiate between ascites and a big ovarian cyst occupying whole of the abdomen, as fluid thrill can be elicited in both. In a big ovarian cyst, the flanks are resonant on percussion due to presence of displaced bowel loops, whereas flanks are dull in case of ascites.

Pelvic Examination

Pelvic examination includes both per speculum, per vaginal, and per rectal examination if indicated.

Per Speculum Examination

The per speculum examination describes the condition of cervix and vagina, and presence or absence of any vaginal discharge. It also provides an opportunity to take a Pap smear.

Per Vaginal Examination

The per vaginal findings should be described systematically starting from the direction and consistency of the cervix to the size, position, consistency, and mobility of the uterus whether it is tender or nontender. The fornices are examined for any mass, induration, thickening, scarring or tenderness.

On per vaginal examination, fibroids are usually felt in continuity with the uterus, whereas the ovarian tumors are felt separate from the uterus and a groove can be appreciated between the two. The movement of the cervix is not transmitted to the lump in ovarian masses, whereas it is transmitted in cases of uterine masses and vice versa. A few exceptions are there such as movements of a pedunculated, subserous fibroid may not be transmitted to the cervix and likewise the movements of a complicated ovarian mass like endometrioma, inflammatory tubo-ovarian mass or malignant ovarian adherent to the uterus, may be transmitted to the cervix.

All ovarian masses are tipped through one or more fornices. If not, then it is likely that the origin of the mass is extragenital. A retroverted uterus with restricted mobility, scarring, tenderness, and nodularity in pouch of Douglas (POD) is pathognomonic of endometriosis, whereas nontender nodules in POD without any scarring may be present in case of ovarian malignancy due to peritoneal deposits. In case of large masses filling up the pelvis, it is important to assess the free space available between the lateral border of the mass and the lateral pelvic wall, so as to assess the likely difficulty during surgery and need for intravenous pyelography or CT pyelography to delineate the course of ureter. In patients with chronic ectopic pregnancy, the uterus is mostly normal in size and pushed anteriorly due to collection of blood in POD, i.e., pelvic hematocele.

It is important to clinically differentiate a uterine mass from a broad ligament mass. In patients with broad ligament mass, the uterus is usually pushed on to the opposite side, the lower limit of the mass reaches below the level of internal os and the mobility of the mass is restricted.

Per Rectal Examination

Per rectal examination is carried out to confirm the per vaginal findings. Any collection or nodules in POD and/or the induration of Mackenrodt's ligaments are better felt on per rectal examination. Sometimes, when the uterus is acutely retroverted or pushed backward by a mass occupying the anterior fornix, the appreciation of the size of the uterus is enhanced on per rectal examination, compared to per vaginal examination. Condition of rectal mucosa, any rectal mass, and whether the rectum is empty or loaded, can be assessed by per rectal examination. In young girls who are not sexually active and in those with vaginal atresia, assessment of uterus and adnexa is possible only through per rectal route.

INVESTIGATIONS

In women of reproductive age group presenting with a lump abdomen, pregnancy and related complications should be ruled out by doing a urine pregnancy test or serum-human chorionic gonadotropin (hCG).

Ultrasound

Ultrasound is a powerful tool to differentiate a uterine from an extrauterine mass, a genital from an extragenital mass, and possibly a benign from a malignant mass. This provides a further direction for investigations. A transabdominal ultrasound with a full bladder is always done before proceeding with a transvaginal (TVS) ultrasound, because with TVS, the depth of visualization is limited and one may not be able to visualize the whole mass if it is big and may miss out on some findings. Use of color Doppler increases the sensitivity and specificity of differentiating benign from malignant ovarian masses.

The various details observed on ultrasound are whether the lesion is unilateral or bilateral, unilocular or multilocular, if any solid areas are present, any evidence of ascites or metastasis, thickness of septae, and their vascularity. Malignant lesions are usually bilateral, multilocular with solid areas, thick septae, increased vascularity, and presence of ascites and metastasis.

Specific Tumor Markers

Specific tumor markers are useful in differentiating malignant from benign ovarian tumors. If the ovarian tumor is present in a child or young girl, germ cell tumors should be suspected and tumor markers such as hCG, alpha-fetoprotein (AFP), lactic dehydrogenase (LDH), and placental alkaline phosphatase (PALP) should be done. Of these, LDH and PALP are specific for dysgerminoma. Cancer antigen 125 (CA 125) is used when serous epithelial cell tumor is suspected; CA 19-9 and carcinoembryonic antigen (CEA) are specific for mucinous epithelial tumors; and inhibin and estradiol for granulosa cell tumors. The serum levels of these markers are significantly raised in the presence of malignancy.

Computed Tomography

Computed tomography is useful in assessing the lymph nodes and omentum and is useful in evaluation of adnexal masses.

Magnetic Resonance Imaging

Magnetic resonance imaging is useful in differentiating a uterine from an ovarian mass and diagnosing dermoid, endometrioma, and adenomyosis. It is also useful in defining the number and sites of fibroids, and their relation to the endometrial cavity. It helps in identifying the level and nature of obstruction in women with Müllerian duct anomalies.

Positron Emission Tomography

Positron emission tomography is useful in the diagnosis of nodal disease or recurrences.

Fine Needle Aspiration Biopsy

In some selected cases, if the diagnosis is not clear, fine needle aspiration biopsy may be offered for making the diagnosis.

The approach to a woman presenting with a lump in the abdomen is summarized in Flowchart 1.

MANAGEMENT

The management of a mass felt per abdomen as a lump is mostly surgical. The common causes of lump lower abdomen in women are fibroid or ovarian tumor.

For ovarian tumors, the surgical procedure depends upon the age of the woman, whether benign or malignant, and any associated complication like infection, torsion or hemorrhage in the cyst. The aim is to conserve as much of ovarian tissue as

Flowchart 1: Algorithm for clinical approach to a woman with a lump in lower abdomen.

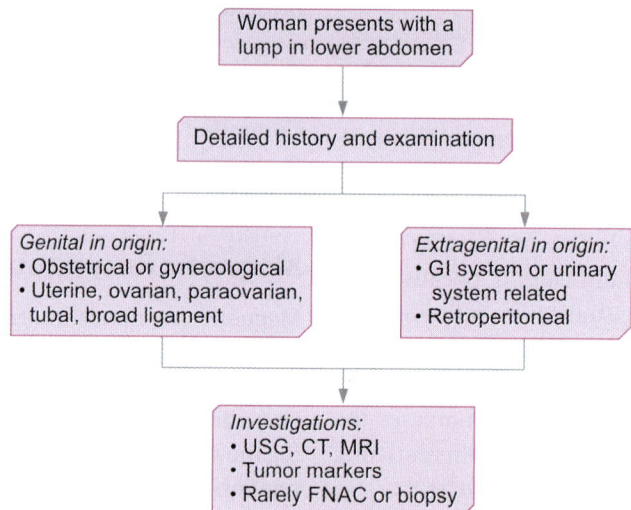

(CT: computed tomography; FNAC: fine needle aspiration cytology; GI: gastrointestinal; MRI: magnetic resonance imaging; USG: ultrasonography)

Table 2: Treatment options according to the condition.

Condition	Management
Ovarian tumor	• *Benign*: Ovarian cystectomy, oophorectomy or salpingo-oophorectomy • *Malignant*: Staging laparotomy with total abdominal hysterectomy with bilateral salpingo-oophorectomy and omentectomy followed by chemotherapy or neoadjuvant therapy followed by surgery in advanced cases • In younger women, conservative surgery may be offered in selected cases and early stage tumors
Fibroids	• *Younger women*: Myomectomy • *Older women*: Hysterectomy ± Salpingo-oophorectomy or myomectomy, if uterus preservation is desired • *Other options*: Uterine artery embolization and magnetic resonance guided focused ultrasound in selected cases
Adenomyosis	• Hysterectomy • Adenomyomectomy
Chronic ectopic pregnancy	• Exploratory laparotomy with salpingectomy and evacuation of pelvic hematocele • Laparoscopic salpingectomy and evacuation of pelvic hematocele
Endometriosis	• Enucleation of endometrioma, adhesiolysis, fulguration of endometriotic patches • TAH ± Salpingo-oophorectomy in older women

(TAH: total abdominal hysterectomy)

possible if the ovarian tumor is benign and the woman is young.

For fibroids present as lump abdomen, the management depends on the age of the woman, whether woman wishes to preserve her fertility and or her uterus. Table 2 describes the various treatment options according to the condition.

KEY POINTS

- Lump abdomen is a common symptom with which a woman presents to the gynecology OPD.
- Pregnancy should be ruled out if the woman is in the reproductive age group.
- Careful history quite often provides clues to the origin of lump whether it is genital or extragenital in origin.
- The exact site of origin and nature of lump can be ascertained by the help of imaging, USG, MRI, and CT scan.
- Rarely, fine needle aspiration biopsy may be required to clinch the diagnosis.

SUGGESTED READING

1. American College of Obstetricians and Gynecologists. ACOG Practice Bulletin. Management of adnexal masses. Obstet Gynecol. 2007;110(1):201-14.
2. Brun JL, Fritel X, Aubard Y, Borghese B, Bourdel N, Chabbert-Buffet N, et al. Management of presumed benign ovarian tumors: updated French guidelines. Eur J Obstet Gynecol Reprod Biol. 2014;183:52-8.
3. Chen HT, Athreya S. Systematic review of uterine artery embolization practice guidelines: are all the guidelines on the same page? Clin Radiol. 2018;73(5):507.e9-507.e15.
4. National Institute for Health and Clinical Excellence. Ovarian Cancer. The recognition and initial management of ovarian cancer. NICE Clinical Guidelines 122. London: NICE; 2011.
5. Royal College of Obstetricians and Gynaecologists (2013). Clinical recommendations on the use of uterine artery embolization (UAE) in the management of fibroids. [online] Available from https://www.rcog.org.uk/globalassets/documents/guidelines/23-12-2013_rcog_rcr_uae.pdf [Last accessed March, 2020].
6. Younas K, Hadoura E, Majoko F, Bunkheila A. A review of evidence-based management of uterine fibroids. TOG. 2016;18:33-42.

37
Approach to a Woman Presenting with Pelvic Organ Prolapse

Nidhi Malhotra, Karishma Thariani

INTRODUCTION

Pelvic organ prolapse (POP) is the downward displacement of the pelvic organs from their normal anatomical position due to a congenital or acquired defect in the pelvic supports. This can involve the uterus, vaginal walls, or posthysterectomy vaginal cuff. The cervix may descent alone or along with bladder, rectum or bowel herniating through the anterior or posterior vaginal walls resulting in vaginal wall protrusion or bulge. The incidence of prolapse increases with age, parity and chronically increased intra-abdominal pressure.[1]

Historically, the vaginal prolapse is named according to the structure herniating through the vaginal wall. Cystocele is the descent of bladder base through the upper two-thirds of the anterior vaginal wall and urethrocele is herniation of the urethra through the lower one-third of anterior vaginal wall. Herniation of the pouch of Douglas through the upper one-third of posterior vaginal wall is known as enterocele and of the rectum through the lower two-thirds of posterior vaginal wall is known as rectocele.

These terms imply an unrealistic certainty as to the structures on the other side of the vaginal bulge, particularly in women who have had previous prolapse surgery. These have hence been replaced by the compartments along with stage of prolapse as per the POP quantification system (POP-Q).

The present concept of female pelvic support divides the pelvis into three compartments anterior, posterior, and middle compartment. The urethra and bladder lie in anterior compartment, anal canal, and rectum in the posterior compartment, uterus or vault in the middle compartment. The suspension system has been described by De Lancey.[2] It has been divided into three levels:
1. Level I consists of uterosacral and cardinal ligaments supporting the cervix and upper part of vagina or vault.
2. Level II comprises of connective tissue attachments to the middle part of vagina.
3. Level III comprises of perineal body (PB) and supports to the urethra.

Defects of support at each of these levels result in a specific type of prolapse such as apical, anterior, or posterior vaginal wall.

DIFFERENTIAL DIAGNOSIS

Usually, there is no difficulty in the diagnosis of uterovaginal prolapse, but sometimes the mass protruding outside vagina may be confused with conditions such as uterine inversion, a fibroid or a vaginal cyst (Table 1).

HISTORY

Pelvic organ prolapse involves various anatomic and functional alterations related to the three vaginal compartments (anterior, apical, and posterior). Detailed history involving

Table 1: Differential diagnosis of pelvic organ prolapse.

Conditions	Differentiating features
Uterine inversion	Cervical os is not visible, a cervical rim is felt all around the mass and fundus of the uterus is not felt on bimanual per vaginum examination. Uterine sound cannot be negotiated due to inversion of the uterine fundus. Ultrasonography (USG) can confirm the findings.
Pedunculated myoma	The pedicle of the myoma may be felt through the cervix. The uterine fundus can be appreciated on bimanual per vaginum examination. Uterine sound can be negotiated by the side of the myoma into the uterine cavity.
Gartner's cyst	Unlike cystocele, this has well-defined margins and is irreducible. The overlying vaginal mucosa is stretched out with loss of rugosities. The cough impulse is absent.

complaints related to each of the three compartments is of vital importance because treatment is decided based on the symptoms. Incidental detection of asymptomatic prolapse does not warrant any treatment in most situations.

History of Presenting Complaints

It is important to understand that the symptomatology of prolapse may not be proportional to the severity of prolapse. The duration of symptoms and disease progression should be asked for.

The patients may present with symptoms directly related to prolapse, such as vaginal bulge, feeling of something coming out of vagina, heaviness, or dragging sensation in pelvis or pelvic discomfort. These symptoms may be associated with prolapse of any compartment. The symptom of vaginal bulge is the most specific symptom for predicting the presence of prolapse beyond the hymen on examination.

Women with anterior compartment prolapse may complain of urinary symptoms such as urgency, frequency, or urge incontinence. However, obstructive urinary symptoms such as voiding difficulties may be present in women with severe anterior compartment or apical prolapse. These women may require vaginal pressure, splinting, or manual replacement of the prolapse to accomplish voiding. They may complain of hesitancy, intermittency and dysuria. They are at a risk of increased postvoid residual urine volume consequent to incomplete voiding with resultant recurrent urinary tract infection (UTI).

History of stress urinary incontinence (SUI) should be asked. Often women with progressive prolapse complain of SUI initially, which gets better with increasing severity of prolapse due to obstruction of bladder neck due to prolapsed organ. Such women should always be examined for occult SUI as they are at risk of manifesting SUI after repair of prolapse.

Women with posterior compartment prolapse may suffer from defecatory dysfunction, such as pain during defecation, need for manual reposition of prolapse for defecation, and anal incontinence of flatus, liquid, or solid stool. These patients often have outlet-type constipation secondary to the trapping of stool within the rectal hernia necessitating the need for splinting or applying manual pressure in the vagina to reduce the prolapse aiding in defecation. Some of these patients may keep their pelvic muscles contracted and push from above to pass stools leading to worsening of posterior compartment prolapse. It is of vital importance to teach these patients pelvic floor relaxation exercises to prevent constipation and recurrence following surgery.

Although the relationship between sexual function and POP is not clearly defined, questions regarding sexual dysfunction must be included in the evaluation of all patients with prolapse. Patients may report symptoms of dyspareunia, decreased libido and orgasm, and increased embarrassment with altered anatomy that affects her body image. Moreover in older frail women if a patient is not sexually active or does not desire to be sexually active in future, she may be offered vaginal obliterative procedures.

History of any discharge or irregular bleeding or spotting per vaginum should be elicited. It may be due to presence of decubitus ulcer in longstanding prolapse.

Symptoms of urinary and or anal incontinence and prolapse and their impact on the woman's health and quality-of-life (QOL) can be measured objectively or quantified using several easy-to-use and validated questionnaires measuring symptom severity, QOL, and sexual function.

OBSTETRICAL HISTORY

A detailed obstetrical history is important as multiparity and vaginal delivery both predispose to prolapse. Details of all pregnancies and deliveries especially with respect to the duration of labor whether prolonged or precipitate labor, duration of second stage, interval between active bearing down efforts and birth of the baby, birthing position, whether it was an instrumental delivery, weight of the baby, and interval between delivery and resumption of heavy work should be elicited. Multiparity, prolonged second stage or prolonged bearing down efforts, precipitate labor, difficult instrumental delivery, birth of a big heavy baby, delivery in a squatting position, and early resumption of work in postnatal period all predispose to POP.

MENSTRUAL HISTORY

In postmenopausal women, the duration since menopause is important as the estrogen deficiency results in aggravation of prolapse consequent to weakening of connective tissue and uterine and vaginal supports. Postcoital or postmenopausal spotting may be present in women, with prolapse and decubitus ulcer. Spasmodic dysmenorrhea may be present in early stage of prolapse in younger premenopausal women, described as pain similar in character to labor pains by parous women.

Past History

Any history of diabetes mellitus, hypertension, neurological disease, chronic constipation, and chronic cough due to bronchitis or asthma should be elicited. Any treatment of prolapse in the form of vaginal pessary, pelvic floor exercises, or surgery should be recorded.

Personal History

Personal history should include the profession of the woman and whether it involves heavy manual work or not. It is important to know if she is a smoker and if she has any drug allergies.

EXAMINATION

The examination includes general physical, breast and systemic examination with special attention to abdominal and local examination of genitalia.

General Physical Examination

The general condition of the patient and her nutritional status is observed. Her pulse, blood pressure, pallor, and presence of any significant lymphadenopathy are noted. The height and weight are recorded and body mass index (BMI) is calculated. Overweight and obese women are at a higher risk of prolapse. Any evidence of presence of a tuft of hair in the sacral region is noted as this suggests spina bifida, a condition, which predisposes to prolapse.

Per Abdomen Examination

Per abdomen examination includes inspecting all the hernial sites. The presence of hernia suggests weakness of fascia at other sites. Look for any scar marks of previous surgery. Palpate for the tone of abdominal muscles, divarication of recti, any abdominal lump, or free fluid in the abdomen with resultant increase in intra-abdominal pressure.

Local Examination

The patient should be examined in dorsal position with buttocks at the edge of the table and legs drawn. The patient may also be examined in standing position, if the physical findings do not correspond to symptoms or if maximum extent of prolapse is not confirmed by the patient.

Local examination includes a systematic examination of external genitalia, perineum, neurological examination for sacral reflexes, details of the prolapsed mass, any evidence of SUI, a per speculum examination, bimanual per vaginum examination, assessment of levator tone, and examination of the anal sphincter using the pill-rolling maneuver on per rectal examination.

Examination of External Genitalia

External genitalia should be inspected for vulvar atrophy or presence of any lesions, rashes, ulcers, atrophy, or any scar marks (Figs. 1 and 2). Any suspicious lesions should be biopsied and treated. The size of the introitus is noted whether lax or not (Fig. 3).

Examination of Perineum

Perineum is examined for the length of the perineal body (PB), any old healed perineal

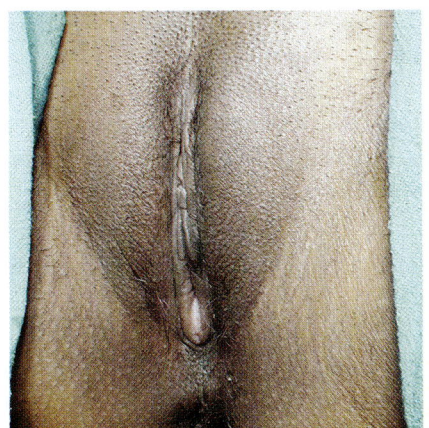

Fig. 1: Normal external genitalia.

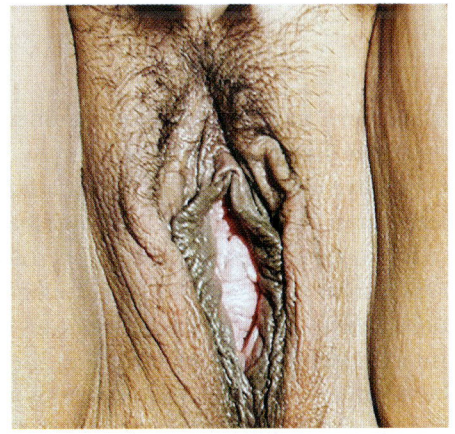

Fig. 2: Atrophic external genitalia.

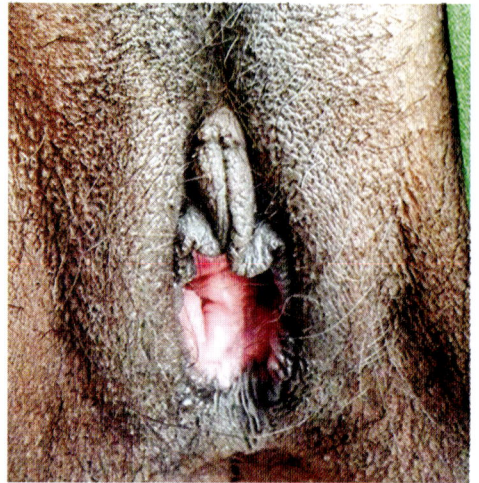

Fig. 3: Lax introitus.

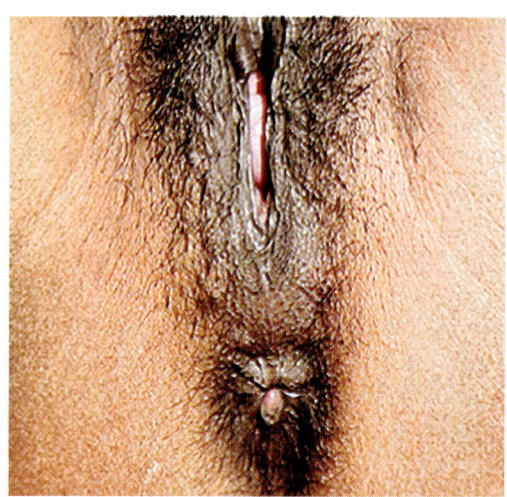

Fig. 4: Intact perineum.

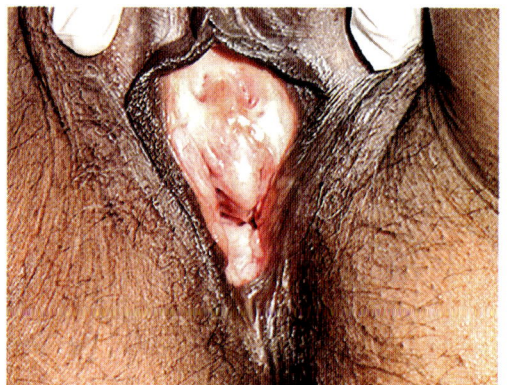

Fig. 5: Deficient perineum.

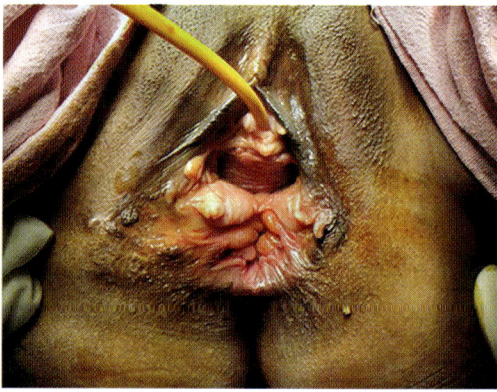

Fig. 6: Torn perineum—complete perineal tear.

tear, and anal morphology. When perineum is intact the posterior vaginal wall is not visible without separating the labia minora whereas with old healed perineal tears lower part of posterior vaginal wall may be visible on inspection (Figs. 4 to 6). The patient is asked to cough or do Valsalva maneuver, the perineum normally gets elevated and shows an inward or cephalad movement of the vulva, perineum, and the anus because of the guarding action of the pelvic floor muscles. However, in patients with perineal descent, there is an outward or caudal movement of the vulva, perineum, and anus.

Demonstration of Stress Urinary Incontinence

Patient should be examined full bladder and asked to cough, any leakage of urine during coughing should be noted (Fig. 7A). If SUI is present, Bonney's test may be performed. In

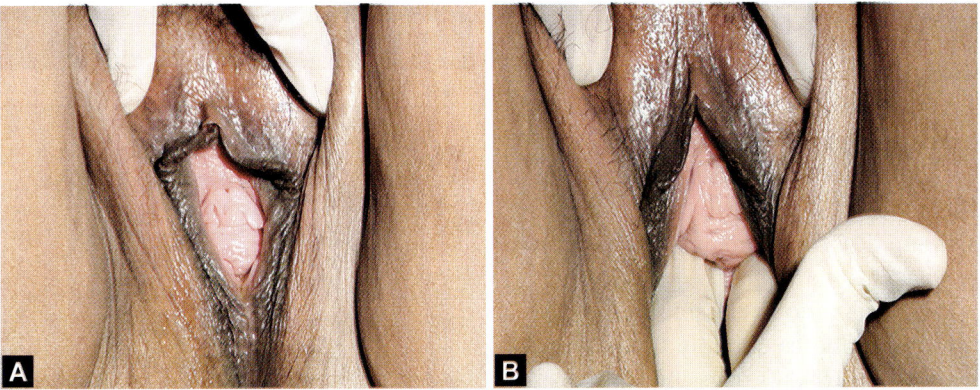

Figs. 7A and B: Stress urinary incontinence: Examination—(A) demonstration of stress urinary incontinence; (B) Bonney's test.

this test, the bladder neck is elevated with index and middle finger on either side of urethra without compressing it. It is positive, if leakage of urine stops on raising bladder neck (Fig. 7B). In women with stage II or more prolapse, if SUI is not demonstrable, it is prudent to look for occult SUI by asking the patient to cough after reposting the prolapse and straightening the urethrovesical angle.

Test for Urethral Hypermobility (Q-tip Test)

It is important to look for urethral hypermobility as it aids in the diagnosis of urodynamic SUI and in planning appropriate treatment for this condition. It is difficult with physical examination to differentiate between cystocele and rotational descent of the urethra and the two often coexist. Historically, Q-Tip test has been done to test the urethral hypermobility, which is often present in cases of poorly supported urethra. For this, a cotton swab lubricated with 1% lignocaine jelly is placed in urethra right up to urethrovesical junction. The woman is asked to strain or do Valsalva maneuver and swab angle

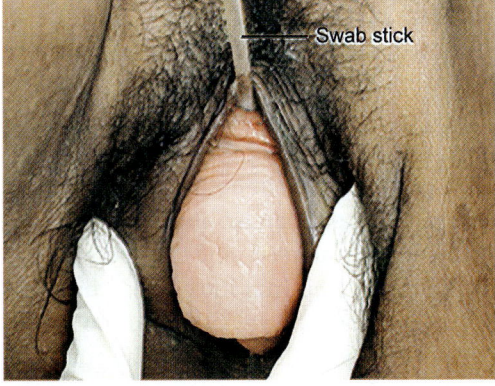

Fig. 8: Q-tip test.

excursion from its position at rest and with Valsalva maneuver is measured with the help of goniometer. An angle excursion of greater than 30° above the horizontal indicates urethral hypermobility (Fig. 8). It has been shown that in most women with stage II and more prolapse have a Q-tip angle greater than 30°. Therefore, measure of urethral mobility may be of importance in women with stage 0 or 1 prolapse or in women with history of prior surgery for incontinence. Ultrasonography may be used as a reliable method for assessing urethral hypermobility where skill and expertise are available.

Examination of Prolapse

A woman with prolapse should be examined, with maximum descent of prolapse. In case, the prolapse is not visible the woman should be asked to perform Valsalva maneuver or asked to cough or do whatever will cause maximum descent of prolapse. The next step is to stage the prolapse.

There are various classification systems used to describe or quantify the severity of prolapse. The Shaw's classification system uses introitus as the reference point; Baden-Walker Halfway system takes hymen as the reference point.[3] Recently, the International Continence Society defined a pelvic organ prolapse quantification system (POP-Q) in 1996.[4] It has a low intraobserver and interobserver variation and is a standardized and reproducible method for quantification of prolapse. In POP-Q, the measurements can be obtained quickly in both experienced and nonexperienced hands. Prolapse in each segment is evaluated and measured relative to the hymen (not introitus), which is a fixed anatomic landmark that can be identified consistently and precisely. The anatomic position of the six defined points for measurement is measured in centimeters above or proximal to the hymen (negative number) or centimeters below or distal to the hymen (positive number), with the plane of the hymen being defined as zero (Table 2). In addition to the measurement of the distances of these points from the hymen, three more measurements are recorded; the genital hiatus (GH), PB and total vaginal length (TVL). GH is measured anteroposteriorly from the middle of external urethral meatus to posterior midline of hymen. PB is measured from posterior point of GH to mid anal opening. All the points except for TVL are measured during maximum straining in centimeters and charted in a 3 × 3 Table.

Table 2: Pelvic organ prolapse quantification system.[4]

Point	Description
Anterior wall (Aa)	Position of a point on the anterior vaginal wall in midline is 3 cm above external urethral meatus corresponding to the suburethral sulcus. Normal position at −3 cm and ranges are −3 cm to +3 cm
Anterior wall (Ba)	Position of most distal point on upper anterior vaginal wall in midline. Normal position at −3 cm, range is −3 cm to a positive value depending on the degree of prolapse of anterior vaginal wall
Posterior wall (Ap)	Position of a point on the posterior vaginal wall in midline 3 cm above hymen, normal position at −3 cm and ranges are −3 cm to +3 cm
Posterior wall (Bp)	Position of a most distal point on upper posterior vaginal wall in midline. Normal position at −3 cm, range is −3 cm to a positive value depending on the degree of prolapse of posterior vaginal wall
Cervix or cuff (C)	It is the apical point or the distal most point on the cervix or vaginal vault after hysterectomy
Posterior fornix (D)	It is a point corresponding to the posterior vaginal fornix in women with a cervix; however, this point is nonexistent in hysterectomized women

TVL is measured by reducing point C or D to most superior position by a sponge holder or a swab.

Accordingly, the prolapse is staged. The description of the stages is as given below.[4]

- *Stage 0*: There is no prolapse; all anterior and posterior wall points are at −3 cm and apical vaginal point C (cervix) equals or nearly equals TVL [−TVL cm to − (TVL − 2) cm].
- *Stage I*: It is when criteria for stage 0 are not fulfilled, and the most distal point of prolapse is >1 cm above the level of the hymenal ring.

- *Stage II*: It is when the most distal point of prolapse is between 1 cm above and 1 cm below the hymenal ring.
- *Stage III*: It is when the most distal point on prolapse is between >1 cm below the hymen, but less than TVL −2 cm.
- *Stage IV*: It is when there is complete vault eversion; the most distal prolapse protrudes to more than or equal to TVL − 2 cm.

Per Speculum Examination

After inserting the speculum observe both anterior and posterior vaginal walls for the status of vaginal mucosa. It is usually atrophic pale, thin, dry, parched, and without rugosities in postmenopausal women consequent to lack of estrogens. The vaginal mucosa may be thick, dry, and hypertrophied in long standing prolapse. Healthy, estrogenized tissue without significant evidence of prolapse, will be well perfused and have rugosities and physiologic moisture. Women with atrophic or hypertrophied dry vaginal mucosa should first be treated with local estrogen creams before repair.

After the resting vaginal examination, observe how far the cervix and the anterior and posterior vaginal walls descend when the patient strains. The leading part of the prolapse should be observed and noted. Prolapse of each compartment should be examined after reposting the other compartments. Depress the posterior vaginal wall with Sims speculum to visualize the anterior vaginal wall completely and ask the patient to strain maximally and look for the descent of anterior vaginal wall (Fig. 9). Prolapse of upper two-thirds of anterior vaginal wall is called cystocele and prolapse of lower one-third of anterior vaginal wall is called urethrocele. It is also important to identify the site of anterior vaginal wall defect whether it is paravaginal, central, or transverse. In case of paravaginal defect lateral vaginal sulci sag when the central portion of anterior vaginal wall is lifted with anterior vaginal wall retractor and the vaginal rugosities are intact (Fig. 10). In midline or central defect there is a central bulge with loss of vaginal rugae and in transverse defect loss of support arise from detachment of anterior vaginal wall from the apex.

Rotate the speculum to elevate the anterior vaginal wall and the cervix, sometimes an anterior vaginal wall retractor may be used along with the Sims speculum to lift the

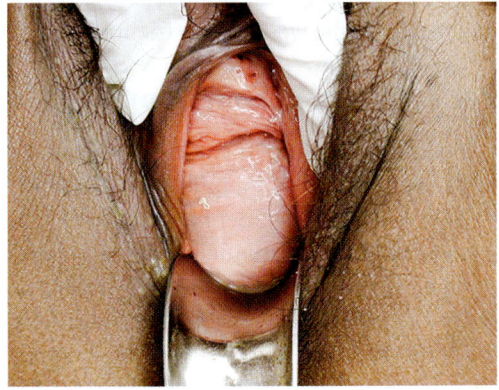

Fig. 9: Visualization of anterior vaginal wall.

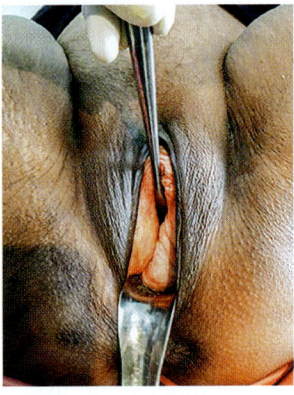

Fig. 10: Demonstration of lateral vaginal wall defect.

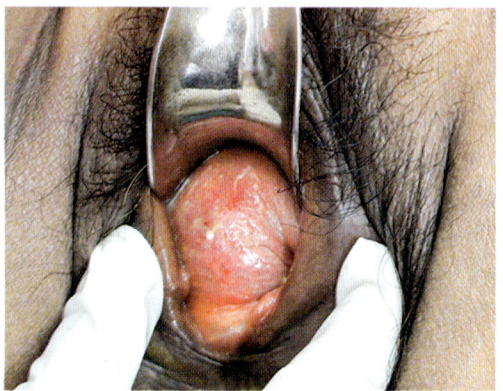

Fig. 11: Visualization of posterior vaginal wall.

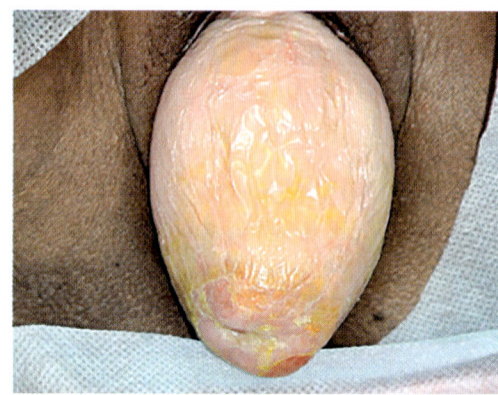

Fig. 12: Dry, atrophic vaginal mucosa.

Table 3: Differentiating features between enterocele and rectocele.

Type of examination	Enterocele	Rectocele
Per speculum examination	Bulge is present at upper one-third of posterior vaginal wall	Bulge is present at lower two-thirds of posterior vaginal wall
Cough impulse on per rectal examination	The impulse is felt at the tip of the finger in case of enterocele	The impulse is felt at the pulp of the finger in case of rectocele
Per rectal examination	In enterocele, bulge is close to cervix and cannot be reached by finger inside the rectum	In case of rectocele, bulge can be reached and insinuated in the vagina by the finger inside the rectum
Rectovaginal examination	Small bowel can be palpated between the rectum and vagina	Small bowel cannot be palpated between the rectum and vagina

cervix to visualize the posterior vaginal wall (Fig. 11).

Prolapse of upper one-third of posterior vaginal wall is called enterocele and prolapse of lower two-thirds of posterior vaginal wall is called rectocele. There are various methods to differentiate between enterocele and rectocele (Table 3).

Condition of cervix is observed whether there is hypertrophy, elongation, congestion, presence of decubitus ulcer, keratinization, or pigmentation.

The condition of vaginal mucosa is noted whether it is atrophied or hypertrophied, dry (Fig. 12), congested, pigmented, or have any decubitus ulcers (Figs. 13A and B) on most dependent part of prolapse due to poor drainage of blood and nondecubitus ulcers on lateral vaginal walls due to friction.

Per Vaginum Examination

Vaginal examination includes examination of vaginal length, its mobility, and presence of any scarring. Procidentia should be differentiated from third degree uterovaginal prolapse. In procidentia, whole of the uterus lies outside the introitus, one can approximate the thumb and fingers and get above the uterus through prolapsed vaginal walls (Fig. 14).

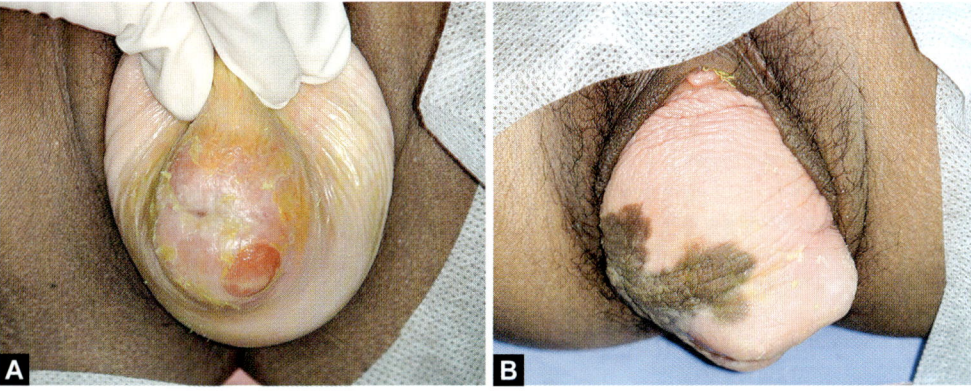

Figs. 13A and B: Vaginal mucosa. (A) Decubitus ulcer; (B) Pigmentation.

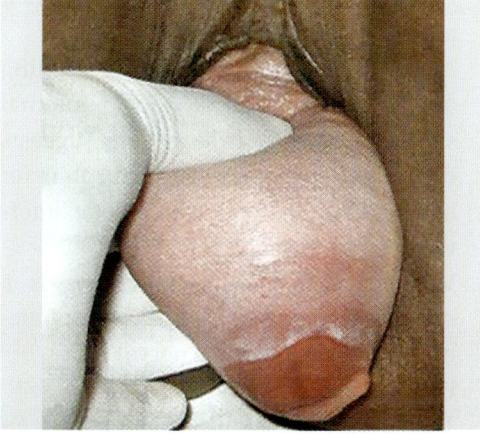

Fig. 14: Procidentia.

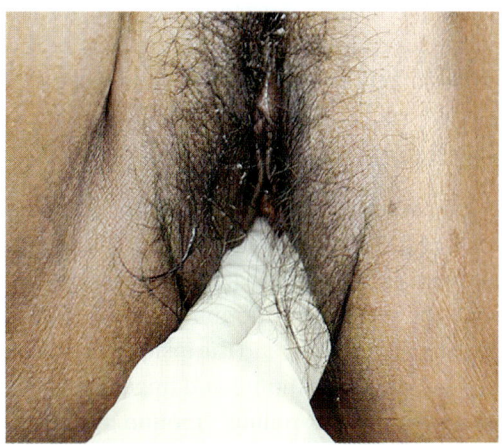

Fig. 15: Assessment of tone of levator ani.

Bimanual Pelvic Examination

Bimanual pelvic (per vaginal) examination should be done to look for the position, size, mobility, and any tenderness of the uterus. Any adnexal mass and/or forniceal tenderness, thickness, scarring, and depth are looked for. Fornices are deep in women with congenital elongation of the cervix whereas they are shallow in postmenopausal women as the cervix is flushed with vaginal vault. In postmenopausal women, there is difficulty in assessing the exact size of uterus on per vaginal examination due to small size of uterus, flushed cervix, shallow fornices, and thick and hypertrophied vaginal mucosa, per rectal examination is helpful in such cases for assessment of the size of the uterus.

Assessment of Levator Tone

In order to assess the levator tone, one should palpate the posterior vaginal wall 2–4 cm above the hymen at 5 and 7o' clock position (Fig. 15). Patient is asked to squeeze her vaginal muscles as though she is holding urine or

Table 4: Modified Oxford scale for grading strength of levator ani muscle.[5]

Grade	Response
0	No discernible muscle contraction
1	A flicker under the finger
2	A weak contraction or increase in the tension without any discernible lift or squeeze
3	A moderate contraction with partial lifting of postvaginal wall and squeezing of finger
4	Good pelvic contraction causing elevation of posterior vaginal wall against resistance and indrawing of perineum
5	Strong contraction of pelvic floor against resistance

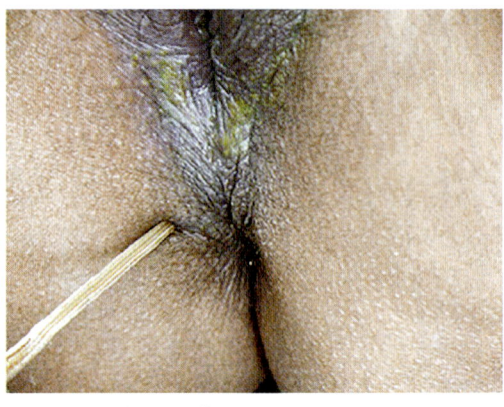

Fig. 16: Anal wink reflex.

stool. The levator muscle strength is graded from 0 to 5 using a modified Oxford scale. The grades of power are as described in Table 4.

Per Rectal Examination

Per rectal examination is done to assess the tone of the anal sphincter. Any anal sphincter tear can be identified, if palpation is done with the examiner's dominant index finger inserted in the anus, and the ipsilateral thumb in the vagina. The thumb and finger then palpate with a "pill-rolling" motion to assess thickness and integrity of the anal sphincter. The presence and absence of rectocele and its differentiation from enterocele is also possible on per rectal examination.

Neurological Examination

Urinary incontinence, fecal incontinence, and rarely uterovaginal prolapse may be the first sign of neurological abnormality. The screening neurologic examination should evaluate mental status, sensory, and motor function of both lower extremities, and include a screening lumbosacral neurologic examination.

The screening lumbosacral examination should include assessments of:

- Pelvic floor muscle strength (as described above)
- Anal sphincter resting tone (85% of resting anal sphincter tone is due to internal sphincter, loss of resting tone suggests disruption of the internal anal sphincter and/or an injury to its sympathetic innervation)
- Voluntary anal contraction (this is a marker of integrity of external anal sphincter and hence pudendal nerve)
- Perineal sensation.

This simple screening examination can be performed quickly and easily as part of gynecologic examination.

Additionally, two reflexes may help in the examination of sacral reflex activity. These are the bulbocavernosus reflex, demonstrated by tapping or stroking an area lateral to clitoris with a cotton swab and observing for the bilateral contraction of bulbocavernosus. This reflex is coordinated at S2–S4 level. The afferent of this reflex is clitoral branch of pudendal nerve and efferent is inferior hemorrhoidal branch of pudendal nerve.

Anal wink reflex is elicited by stroking the perianal skin with cotton swab and observing reflex contraction of anal sphincter (Fig. 16).

INVESTIGATIONS

Diagnosis of uterovaginal prolapse is essentially a clinical diagnosis, no specific investigations are required to confirm the diagnosis. As majority of the women are postmenopausal, they should be offered screening for cervical cancer by Pap smear and endocervical brushing. The smear is usually unsatisfactory as the cervix is constantly lying outside the vagina but moistening the Ayre's spatula and the endocervical brush with saline before taking the smear may improve the yield. Women with urinary complaints are advised to get their urine tested for routine, microscopic examination, and culture sensitivity.

In patients planned for surgery certain investigations are required for preanesthetic fitness. These include a complete blood count, blood sugar test fasting and postprandial, liver and kidney function tests, urine routine examination and culture sensitivity, electrocardiogram (ECG), and chest X-ray. Some gynecologists prefer to get an ultrasound for endometrial thickness and ovaries preoperatively. Endometrial sampling is not indicated as a routine; it is indicated in patients with abnormal uterine bleeding, increased endometrial thickness of >5 mm in postmenopausal women and in patients with postmenopausal bleeding (Flowchart 1).

Management of Pelvic Organ Prolapse

The management of prolapse is decided based on the symptoms, type of prolapse, severity of prolapse, age of the woman seeking treatment young or old, whether sexually active or not, whether she desires fertility preservation or not.

Outline of management of POP is shown in Flowchart 2.

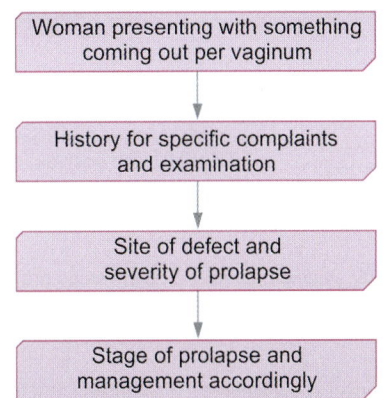

Flowchart 1: Algorithm for clinical approach to a woman presenting with pelvic organ prolapse.

KEY POINTS

- Pelvic organ prolapse is essentially a clinical diagnosis.
- Treatment is indicated only if the patient is symptomatic.
- A detailed evaluation should identify treatable predisposing and aggravating factors like chronic cough, constipation, etc. which should be treated before the prolapse is treated.
- Examination should aim at diagnosing specific defects, so that the treatment can be tailored accordingly.
- Treatment depends upon the symptoms, type of prolapse, stage of prolapse, age of patient, family completed or not, whether desirous of uterine and fertility preservation and sexually active or not.

Flowchart 2: Management of pelvic organ prolapse (POP).

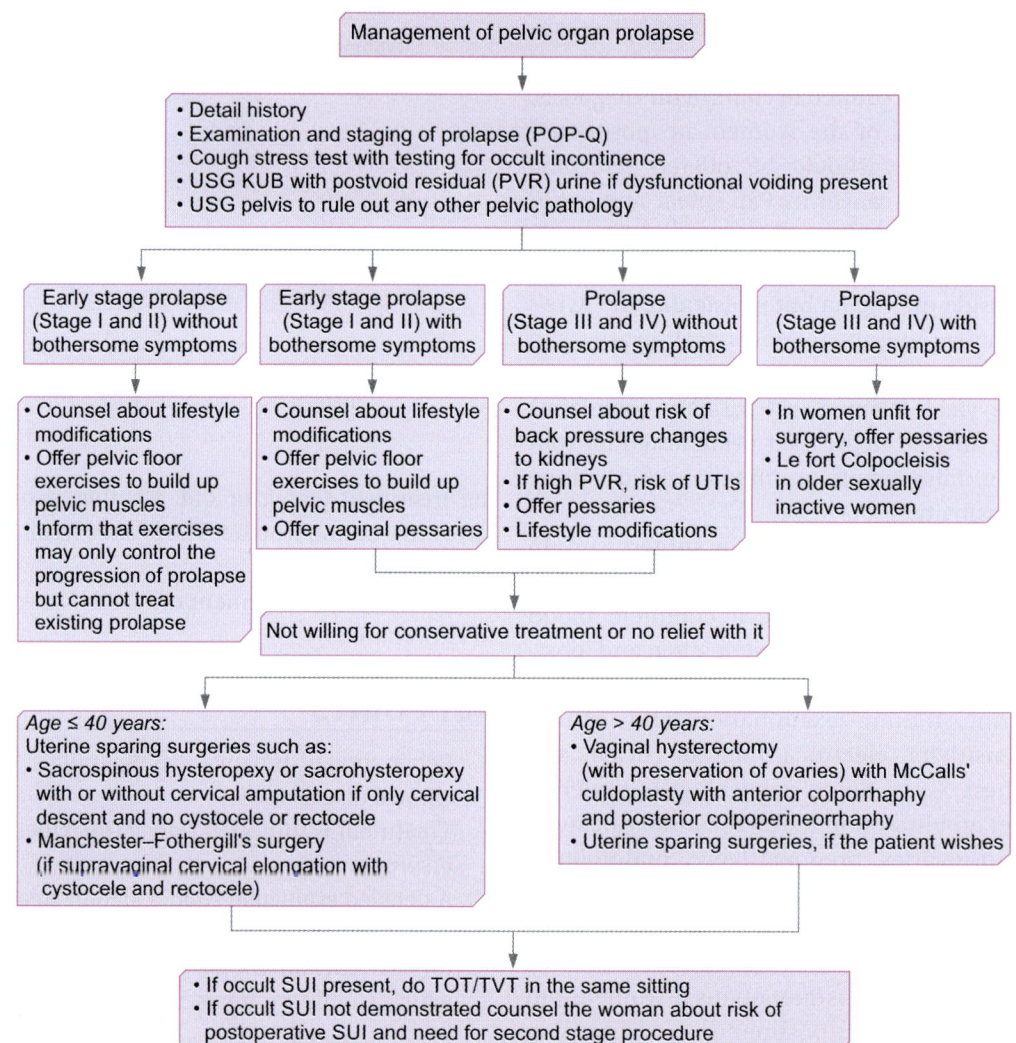

REFERENCES

1. Swift S, Woodman P, O'Boyle A, Kahn M, Valley M, Bland D, et al. Pelvic Organ Support Study (POSST): the distribution, clinical definition, and epidemiologic condition of pelvic organ support defects. Am J Obstet Gynecol. 2005;192(3);795-806.
2. DeLancey JO. Anatomic aspects of vaginal eversion after hysterectomy. Am J Obstet Gynecol. 1992;166:1717-24.
3. Baden WF, Walker T. Surgical Repair of Vaginal Defects. Philadelphia: Lippincott Williams & Wilkins; 1992.
4. Bump RC, Mattiasson A, Bø K, Brubaker LP, DeLancey JO, Klarskov P, et al. The standardization of terminology of female pelvic organ protapse and pelvic floor dysfunction. Am J Obstet Gynecol. 1996;175(1):10-7.
5. Laycock J. Clinical evaluation of the pelvic floor. In: Schussler B, Laycock J, Norton P (Eds). Pelvic Floor Re-education. London: Springer; 1994. pp. 42-8.

SUGGESTED READING

1. AAGL. Practice guidelines on the prevention of apical prolapse at the time of benign hysterectomy. J Minim Invasive Gynecol. 2014;21(5):715-22.
2. ACOG. (2017. Committee opinion on choosing the route of hysterectomy for benign disease. [online] Available from https://www.acog.org/-/media/Committee-Opinions/Committee-on-Gynecologic-Practice/co701.pdf [Last accessed January, 2020].
3. ACOG and American Urogynecologic Society (AUGS). (2017). Committee opinion on management of mesh and graft complications in gynecologic surgery. [online] Available from https://www.acog.org/-/media/Committee-Opinions/Committee-on-Gynecologic-Practice/co694.pdf?dmc=1&ts=20191024T1859470567 [Last accessed January, 2020].
4. Meriwether KV, Antosh DD, Olivera CK, Kim-Fine S, Balk EM, Murphy M, et al. Uterine preservation versus hysterectomy in pelvic organ prolapse surgery – A systematic review with meta-analysis and clinical practice guidelines. Am J Obstet Gynecol. 2018;219(2):129-46.
5. RCOG. (2015). Green top Guideline No. 46 Post-hysterectomy vaginal vault prolapse. [online] Available from https://www.rcog.org.uk/en/guidelines-research-services/guidelines/gtg46/ [Last accessed January, 2020].

38 Approach to a Woman Presenting with Urinary Incontinence

Nidhi Malhotra, Karishma Thariani

INTRODUCTION

Urinary incontinence (UI) is defined by the International Continence Society as "the complaint of involuntary leakage of urine."[1] Epidemiological studies have demonstrated that UI is a very common, but underreported condition, with a reported prevalence of 34% in women aged 40 years and over.

It can be a symptom that the patient complains of, a sign demonstrated on examination, or a condition/diagnosis that can be confirmed by definitive studies. A patient with urinary incontinence needs a thorough examination which should include a detailed history and physical examination.

DIFFERENTIAL DIAGNOSIS

At the initial clinical assessment, UI should be categorized as stress, urge, mixed, overflow, or true incontinence. This is followed by looking for a possible etiology for the same. Close consideration to explicit aspects of the patient's history including type of leakage, its frequency, severity, precipitating factors, and associated symptoms can significantly contribute to clinch the correct diagnosis.

The various types of UI and their details are as listed in Table 1.

Among the various types of UI, prevalence of stress urinary incontinence (SUI) is highest 33% in women of any age, mixed

Table 1: Types of urinary incontinence.

Types of urinary incontinence	Description
Stress incontinence	Involuntary leakage of urine on effort, or exertion, or any increase in intra-abdominal pressure such as sneezing, coughing, and lifting weight. This happens because the intravesical pressure increases more than the urethral pressure with any increase in intra-abdominal pressure. It is the most common type of incontinence.
Urge urinary incontinence	Involuntary leakage of urine accompanied by or preceded by urgency, i.e., a sudden compelling desire to urinate. It may present as escape of a small amount of urine or complete emptying of bladder. It is more common in older women.
Mixed incontinence	Involuntary leakage of urine associated with both urgency and physical activity resulting in an increase in intra-abdominal pressure such as exertion, sneezing, or coughing.
Overflow incontinence	It occurs as a result of obstruction to the bladder neck caused by large fibroids, especially cervical, imperforate hymen with hematocolpos or a hypotonic bladder (neurogenic bladder) as a result of diabetes mellitus.

Contd...

Contd...

Types of urinary incontinence	Description
Extra urethral incontinence	It is related to some anatomical abnormality such as ectopic ureter, vesicovaginal fistula, or ureterovaginal fistula.
Transient and functional incontinence	Functional incontinence is more common in elderly women and refers to incontinence that occurs because of factors unrelated to the physiologic voiding mechanism. A woman who cannot get to the bathroom quickly enough may often become incontinent. Transient incontinence happens in response to reversible conditions such as medications. These conditions can be memorized using the mnemonic "DIAPPERS". D—Delirium I—Infection A—Atrophic urethritis and vaginitis P—Pharmacologic causes P—Psychological causes E—Excessive urine production R—Restricted mobility S—Stool impaction

incontinence is about 50%, pure urge incontinence is only about 13% among adult women, and other types of incontinence is 4%.[2] It is important to differentiate UI from sweating and vaginal discharge.

The differential diagnosis of UI in women based on etiology is as listed in Table 2.

HISTORY

History of Presenting Complaint

A thorough history is essential for the evaluation of UI to assess the type and severity of UI and its impact on the quality of life. As with any other symptoms, the onset and duration of complaint are important.

For knowing the type of urinary incontinence, it is important to ask the following questions:
1. Do you leak when you cough, sneeze, or laugh?
2. Do you ever have an uncomfortably strong urge to urinate such that if you do not reach the toilet you will leak?
3. If yes to 2, then have you ever leaked before you have reached the toilet?
4. How many times during the day do you urinate?
5. How many times during the night do you wake up to urinate?
6. Have you ever wet the bed in the past 1 year?
7. Do you develop an urgent need to urinate when you are stressed, nervous, or in a hurry?
8. Do you ever leak during sexual intercourse?

Table 2: Differential diagnosis of urinary incontinence based on etiology.

Genitourinary etiology	Nongenitourinary etiology

• Filling and storage disorders:
   – Urodynamic stress incontinence
   – Detrusor overactivity (idiopathic and neurogenic)
   – Mixed types
 • Fistula:
   – Vesicovaginal
   – Ureterovaginal
   – Urethrovaginal
   – Uterovesical
 • Congenital:
   – Ectopic ureter
	• Functional:
	   – Neurologic
	   – Cognitive
	   – Psychologic
	   – Physical impairment
	 • Environmental
	 • Pharmacologic
	 • Metabolic

9. How often do you leak?
10. Do you have to wear a pad/diaper to stay dry?
11. Do you have recurrent urinary infections?
12. Do you have blood in urine?
13. Do you have pain on passing urine?
14. Do you find it hard to initiate urination?
15. Do you suffer from thin urinary stream, intermittent stream, and feeling of incomplete bladder emptying?
16. Do you dribble urine, as you stand or walk after passing urine?

Question 1 helps in evaluating for SUI, questions 2 to 8 help in eliciting the symptoms of detrusor overactivity, questions 9 and 10 help in determining the severity of problem, questions 11 to 13 help in screening for bladder neoplasia or UTI, and questions 14 to 16 help in eliciting the symptoms of voiding dysfunction.

In patients with continuous dribbling, it is important to rule out conditions such as vesicovaginal fistula (VVF) or ectopic ureter. A large volume of vaginal leak with no normal voiding indicates presence of a large VVF whereas a small amount of leak with normal voiding indicates the presence of a small fistula; one who leaks intermittently indicates a vesicouterine or vesicocervical fistula. Vaginal leaking at the time of voiding is suggestive of an urethrovaginal fistula.

In patients with true incontinence due to urogenital fistula, a detailed history of any inciting event, obstetric or gynecological such as obstructed labor, difficult operative vaginal delivery, any destructive operation, cesarean section, rupture of uterus, scar dehiscence or symphysiotomy, traumatic fracture of pelvis, prolonged use of or impacted vaginal pessary, gynecological surgery, malignancy, and irradiation, should be elicited.

Prolonged second stage and obstructed labor can lead to compression of bladder and urethra between fetal head and pubic symphysis with resultant ischemic necrosis and formation of fistula after 7–10 days of delivery.

In a cesarean section, trauma to bladder or ureter can occur during pushing the bladder down by blunt dissection when it is densely adherent, inadvertent opening of the bladder in advanced labor, lateral extension of uterine incision, and accidental injury to ureter. Rupture of the uterus or scar dehiscence may involve the bladder or ureter. Broad ligament hematoma associated with these conditions may pose a risk for accidental ureteric injury. In symphysiotomy, the bladder neck is particularly predisposed to injury if pubic bones are separated too widely by forcible abduction of thighs, as the bladder neck loses its support.

Gynecological surgeries such as hysterectomy, pelvic floor reconstructive procedures, vaginoplasty, paravaginal cyst excision, and surgery for tubo-ovarian masses, especially in patients with ovarian tumors, pelvic inflammatory disease, and endometriosis predispose to bladder and ureteric injuries. Any prior history of urologic procedures, spinal or central nervous system (CNS) surgery may predispose to incontinence.

In malignancies, fistulas may form due to direct malignant infiltration, surgery, and or irradiation. Spinal injury and metabolic disorders such as diabetes can result in neurogenic incontinence. History of drug intake like antihypertensives, e.g., diuretics, calcium channel blockers, and angiotensin-converting enzyme inhibitors, is important as a cause of incontinence, especially in older women.

Any restriction of mobility due to arthritis or otherwise can also cause incontinence due to the inability of the old woman to be able to reach the toilet and remove her clothes to relieve herself.

Any history of uterovaginal prolapse, insertion of vaginal pessary for prolapse, constipation, fecal impaction, and fecal incontinence should also be elicited.

Menstrual History

In the postmenopausal women, estrogen deficiency leads to weakening of connective tissue and prolapse and predisposes to UI and recurrent urinary tract infections. Atrophic vaginitis can cause burning on passing urine.

Women with urogenital fistula may have secondary amenorrhea, which is hypothalamic in origin. The periods resume, once incontinence due to fistula is cured.

Some women with uterovaginal fistula consequent to obstetrical trauma may have menouria or cyclical hematuria as a result of an abnormal communication between the uterus and the urinary bladder. A triad of menouria, amenorrhea, and urinary continence is known as Youssef's syndrome.

Obstetric History

The obstetric history should include gravidity, parity, number of vaginal deliveries, any instrumental delivery, and/or cesarean section. Any history of difficult delivery, vaginal lacerations or cervical tears, birth of a large baby, and the time interval between deliveries should be recorded. Pregnancies and deliveries per se predispose to SUI. In case patient complains of continuous incontinence after childbirth, then the interval between the delivery and onset of symptoms should be noted. In case of direct injury to the urinary tract, the patient starts dribbling soon after delivery or cesarean section. However, in case of ischemic injury due to obstructed labor, the woman becomes incontinent after 7–10 days.

Medical History

The clinical assessment should seek to identify relevant coexistent predisposing and precipitating factors. The medical history should identify contributing factors such as diabetes mellitus, chronic lung disease, stroke, lumbar disc disease, fecal impaction, cognitive impairment, congestive heart failure, obesity, connective tissue disorders, chronic urinary tract infection, urinary tract stones, and cancer of pelvic organs. History of all the drugs that the patient is taking should be obtained as certain medications cause incontinence. UI can be cured or considerably improved by discontinuation or substitution of appropriate alternative medications.

Medications that may be associated with UI are listed in Table 3.

Table 3: Drugs that influence bladder function.

Drugs	Side effects
Antidepressants, antipsychotics, and sedatives/hypnotics	Sedation and retention (overflow)
Diuretics	Frequency, urgency [overactive bladder (OAB)]
Caffeine	Frequency, urgency (OAB)
Anticholinergics	Retention (overflow)
Alcohol	Sedation and frequency (OAB)
Narcotics	Retention, constipation, and sedation (OAB and overflow)
α-adrenergic blockers	Decreased urethral tone (stress incontinence)
α-adrenergic agonists	Increased urethral tone and retention (overflow)
β-adrenergic agonists	Inhibited detrusor function and retention (overflow)
Calcium channel blockers	Retention (overflow)
Angiotensin-converting enzyme (ACE) inhibitors	Cough (stress incontinence)

Personal History

The effect of UI on the quality of life of the woman should be assessed. Lifestyle issues such as smoking, alcohol or caffeine abuse, and occupational and recreational factors causing repeated increase in intra-abdominal pressure should be inquired.

Bladder Diary

Every patient with UI should be instructed to maintain a bladder diary. A bladder diary is a daily record of the patient's fluid intake and urinary frequency. It is a useful supplement to the medical history of the patient as the frequency and severity of symptoms are often misleading and inaccurate.

Bladder diaries should record the volume and type of fluid intake and the frequency and volume of each void. Incontinence or nocturia should be noted both as regards the number of episodes and volume voided in each episode. Any associated activities resulting in raised intra-abdominal pressure such as coughing, straining, and lifting weight and associated symptoms such as incontinence and urgency should be recorded.

Bladder diaries are not only helpful for pretreatment assessment but they help in objective assessment of posttherapy outcomes. Bladder diaries are reproducible and correlate well with urodynamic diagnosis. Most authors recommend documentation of symptoms for a period of 3–7 days. However, as the results of the first 3-day period and the last 4-day period are comparable , it is suggested that a 3-day chart may be adequate to document symptoms, thus improving compliance.

EXAMINATION

General Physical Examination

The general condition of the patient and her nutritional status is observed. Her pulse, blood pressure, pallor, and presence of any significant lymphadenopathy are noted. The height and weight are recorded and body mass index (BMI) is calculated. Overweight and obese women are at a higher risk of UI. Any evidence of presence of a tuft of hair in the sacral region is noted as this suggests spina bifida, a condition, which predisposes to prolapse and incontinence. Foot drop can be rarely seen in case of urogenital fistula developing after obstructed labor. Foot drop may be present secondary to prolonged sacral nerve root compression by fetal head in cases of obstructed labor.

Breast Examination

Breast examination is done as a routine for screening of breast cancer in all women attending the outpatient department. Any changes in the overlying skin or retraction of nipple, presence of any lump in the breast, or discharge from the nipple are looked for to detect any suspicious lesion.

Cardiovascular System and Respiratory System

Pulmonary and cardiovascular assessment is indicated in patients with chronic cough or other symptoms such as dyspnea. It is indicated in patients planned for surgery as a part of preanesthetic checkup.

Per Abdomen

Per abdomen examination includes inspection of all hernial sites, divarication of recti, and any surgical scars. The presence of hernia suggests weakness of fascia at other sites as well. Look for any palpable abdominal lump, organomegaly, or free fluid in the abdomen causing increase in intra-abdominal pressure.

Local Examination

There may be ammonical or uriniferous smell from the clothing or body of patient.

Demonstration of Stress Urinary Incontinence

Stress urinary incontinence is demonstrated by Cough Stress Test that involves examining the patient with a full bladder and asking the patient to cough or perform Valsalva maneuver while the examiner watches for leakage of urine per urethra. Patient is asked to lie in a dorsal position with buttocks at the edge of the table, the examiner separates the labia of the patient with thumb and index finger (Fig. 1) or retracts the posterior vaginal wall with a Sims' speculum (Fig. 2) and the patient is asked to cough. Urethral meatus is observed for any escape of urine. Women in whom leakage of urine is observed with an empty bladder the stress incontinence is severe and likely to be due to intrinsic sphincter deficiency, this test is called empty supine stress test.

Bonney's test, which is elevation of bladder neck with index and middle finger on either side of urethra at the level of bladder neck to observe whether leakage of urine stops or not is no longer advocated (Fig. 3).

Assessment of Postvoid Residual Urine

The patient is asked to void and the voided volume is recorded. Postvoid residual volume is then assessed within a few minutes by catheterization or ultrasound examination. A residual volume of less than one third of the

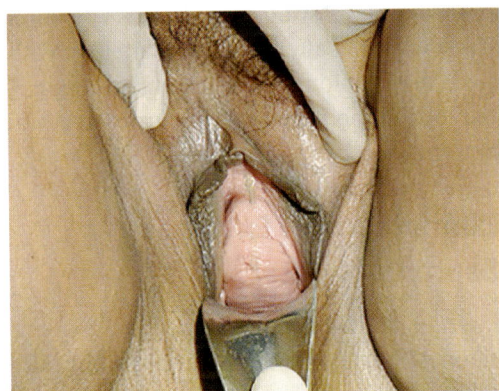

Fig. 2: Demonstration of stress urinary incontinence using Sims' speculum.

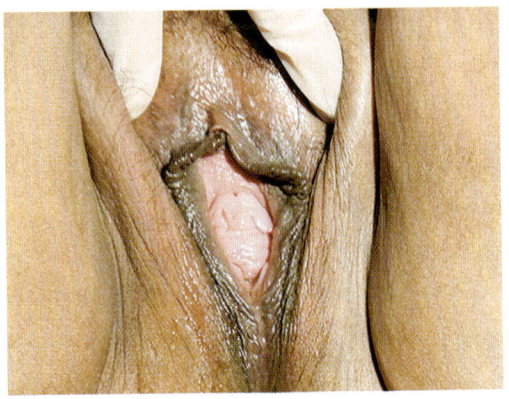

Fig. 1: Demonstrating stress urinary incontinence.

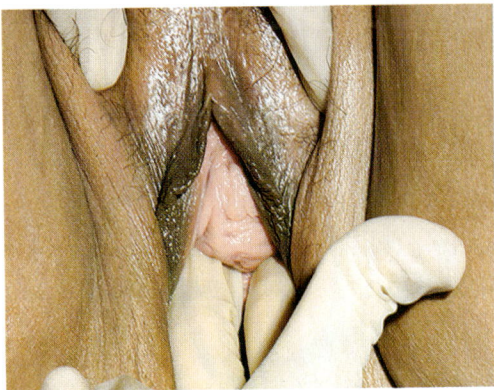

Fig. 3: Bonney's test.

prevoid volume is considered normal. Use of a catheter to assess the residual urine also provides a clean urine sample for culture and urinalysis.

Test for Urethral Hypermobility (Q-Tip Test)

Q-Tip test is done to test for urethral hypermobility, which is present in cases of poorly supported urethra. To elicit this test, a cotton swab lubricated with 1% lignocaine jelly is placed in urethra up to the urethro-vesical junction. This is followed by Valsalva maneuver by the patient and measurement of the excursion of the swab angle from its position at rest with that after Valsalva maneuver with the help of goniometer. An excursion angle of >30° above the horizontal indicates urethral hypermobility (Fig. 4).

Examination of External Genitalia

External genitalia are examined for the condition of vulvar skin and vulvar atrophy. The vulvar skin may be moist, red, inflamed, sodden, and have vulvar lesions such as excoriations, rashes, ulcerations, and white deposits in patients with continuous incontinence due to VVF. Vaginal flora splits urea, leading to alkaline pH and precipitation of phosphate with resultant skin irritation.

The urine may be seen flowing out through the vagina. The patient is asked to strain and observe for any prolapse and any descent or straightening of urethro-vesical angle.

Per Speculum Examination

In women with UI, per speculum examination should be done with a Sims' speculum to visualize the cervix and vagina. Cusco's speculum limits the visualization of vaginal walls. The anterior vaginal wall is better visualized in Sims' lateral position (Fig. 5).

The vaginal walls are inspected for any signs of estrogen deficiency in the form of pale vaginal mucosa with loss of rugosities, and presence of any inflammation or discharge (Fig. 6). The anterior vaginal wall is specially looked for the presence of any urethral diverticulum, any descent, any defect, growth, puckering, and any leakage of urine. The cervix is examined for any defect of the anterior lip, any hypertrophy, erosion, inflammation, or growth.

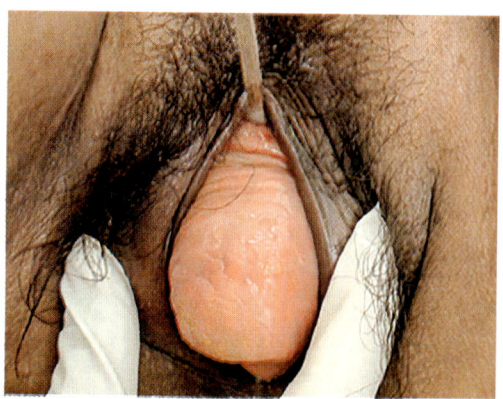

Fig. 4: Q-Tip test.

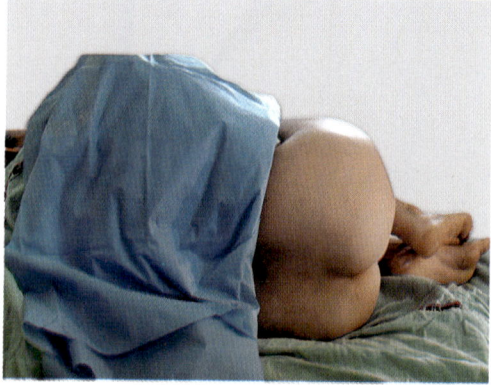

Fig. 5: Sims' position for visualizing vesicovaginal fistula.

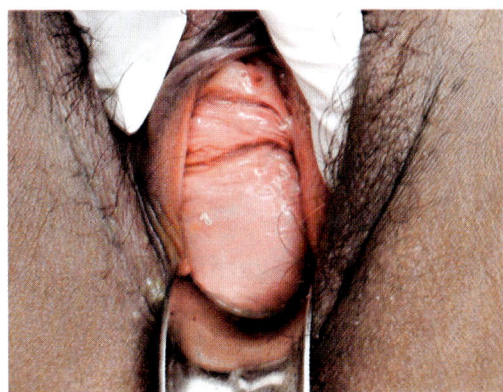

Fig. 6: Normal well-estrogenized vaginal mucosa with normal urethrovesical angle.

In cases with prolapse, a detailed examination is carried out as described in Chapter 37 "Approach to a Woman Presenting with Pelvic Organ Prolapse."

In the presence of a urogenital fistula, the vagina is specifically examined for any scarring or stenosis. The urine collected over the sterile speculum is transferred in a sterile container and sent for urine routine examination and culture and sensitivity. The detailed description of the fistula is recorded. This includes looking for the number, size, and location of fistula, any mucosa protruding through the fistula, any growth from the margin of the fistula, any associated vaginal stenosis, scarring or rectovaginal fistula, whether ureteric openings can be visualized at the edges of the fistula.

Per Vaginal Examination

In Cases Where There is No Fistula

Position of cervix and uterus, size of uterus, its mobility, any adnexal mass and tenderness in bilateral fornices should be looked for. Assessment for the presence of any pelvic mass such as uterine fibroid or ovarian tumor is done. Anterior vaginal wall is palpated for any scarring or fibrosis and its mobility.

In Case of Urogenital Fistula

Findings of per speculum examination are confirmed and number of fistulae, their size, margins, fibrosis, and fixity to underlying bone are assessed. Any vaginal stenosis or scarring is looked for. Examiner must assess mobility of cervix and size, consistency, mobility, and tenderness of uterus. Presence of any tenderness or palpable mass in the bilateral fornices is assessed. In cases where fistula has developed after surgery or delivery and patient presents soon after surgery, a detailed per vaginum examination to localize the fistula should be avoided as it can increase the damage.

Per Rectal Examination

Per rectal examination is useful to check for the tone of anal sphincter, presence of any fecaliths, any rectal growth or rectovaginal fistula.

Assessment of Pelvic Floor Muscles

Assessment of tone of the pelvic floor muscle should be undertaken as a routine. It is done by asking the woman to contract her "vaginal muscles" and hold; normally muscle contraction can be sustained for 5–10 seconds. Very weak or absent voluntary levator ani muscle contractions indicate the need for pelvic floor strengthening exercises.

Neurological Examination of Sacral Reflexes

Neurologic control of voiding should be assessed to determine the presence of any deficits related to the autonomic reflex arc. The lumbosacral nerve roots should be assessed by checking deep tendon reflexes, strength of lower limbs, and the bulbocavernosus and clitoral sacral reflexes. Presence of any abnormal findings such as deep tendon hyperreflexia or absence of the bulbocavernosus reflex suggests a possible underlying neurologic lesion.

Bulbocavernosus Reflex

Bulbocavernosus reflex is coordinated at S2–S4 level through pudendal nerve. The afferent of this reflex is clitoral branch of pudendal nerve and efferent is inferior hemorrhoidal branch of pudendal nerve. It is elicited by stroking labia majora with a cotton swab lateral to the clitoris and looking for reflex bilateral equal contraction of labia majora. Its presence indicates integrity of the reflex arc whereas its absence suggests interruption.

Anal Wink Reflex

Anal wink reflex (S2–S4) is elicited by stroking perianal skin with cotton swab and observing reflex contraction of anal sphincter.

The arc can also be indirectly tested by noting the tone of anal sphincter on per rectal examination, as control of the anal sphincter and bladder are related. Loss of sphincter tone in a patient, who retains sensation, suggests a motor neuron lesion within the arc.

Examination for Perineal Sensation

Perineal sensation is tested; absence of perineal sensation in the presence of sacral reflexes suggests a lesion above the arc like in conditions such as diabetes mellitus, multiple sclerosis, or spinal cord injury. Patients with loss of both perineal sensation and sacral reflexes are likely to have overflow incontinence consequent to neurologic injury to the reflex arc. In patients, where both the reflexes and sensation are present, detrusor instability, stress or overflow incontinence, or a functional problem should be suspected.

Mental Status Examination

A detailed mental status examination is generally not required to detect underlying dementia as it is quite evident by the time the patient presents with UI.

INVESTIGATIONS

Urine Analysis

Urine routine, microscopy, and culture sensitivity are common methods of urine analysis. Urine routine and microscopy should be undertaken in all women presenting with UI. Presence of nitrites and/or leukocyte esterase indicates urinary tract infection. All women presenting with incontinence with or without symptoms of urinary tract infection should have a midstream urine sample sent for culture and sensitivity. Bacteriuria is considered significant if there are >10^5 organisms/mL urine. In symptomatic women with urine routine examination showing leukocytes and nitrites, empirical antibiotic treatment can be started after sending urine for culture sensitivity and reviewed after the report.

Pyridium Test

Phenazopyridine or pyridium turns the urine orange but does not stain the vaginal discharge. Sometimes in obese women, it may be difficult to differentiate UI from vaginal discharge. The woman is given a tablet of pyridium orally and asked to wear a sanitary pad. The pad will stain orange in case of incontinence whereas there is no color in case of vaginal discharge.

Ultrasonography

Pelvic ultrasonography (USG) offers a noninvasive method of assessing postvoid residual urine as in cases, where either poor detrusor activity or outflow obstruction is suspected. Any abdominal or adnexal mass can also be detected on ultrasound.

Transperineal USG and endovaginal USG may be used to document urethral hypermobility and other pelvic floor defects.

Urodynamic Studies

Urodynamic studies are done after ruling out or treating urinary tract infection, if present. Urodynamics is the study of relationship between pressure and flow in the urinary tract. Urodynamic studies include uroflowmetry, urethral pressure profilometry, cystometry, and pressure flow studies. The aim of urodynamics is to replicate symptoms and record the pressure and flow changes in the bladder and recognize the basic cause for the symptoms. It is an invasive investigation, involving catheterization of the bladder and pressure transducer in the rectum to measure pressures in the urethra, bladder, and rectum.

Uroflowmetry

Uroflowmetry is a noninvasive, inexpensive, and is best used as a screening test in patients who may have a voiding dysfunction. It should ideally be done before the other urodynamic studies. It measures the urine flow rate and its pattern. Normally, the maximum flow rate of urine is 15 mL/s and the pattern is bell shaped with an early peak flow rate. In women with obstruction, the flow rate is slow. Uroflowmetry combined with postvoid residual urine can be used for diagnosing voiding dysfunction. Since small voided volumes may affect the shape of the curve, only voided volumes of >150 mL are interpretable. A normal uroflowmetry and a residual volume of <100 mL rule out voiding dysfunction.

Cystometry

Cystometry is the urodynamic study used to describe the pressure/volume relationship of the bladder. It is used to evaluate bladder sensation in relation to volume and its capacity. It also determines the presence or absence of involuntary detrusor contractions. Cystometry can be simply done on outpatient basis. It is not indicated in all women with UI. Women with uncomplicated SUI need not be subjected to cystometry. However, it is indicated if there it is mixed UI to rule out detrusor overactivity prior to surgical management of SUI, previous failed surgery for SUI in patients of pelvic organ prolapse with SUI or any other symptom suggestive of bladder dysfunction.

Normal findings on cystometry include first sensation between 100 and 200 mL, first desire to void at 250–350 mL and strong desire at 400–550 mL. With an atonic bladder, the capacity of bladder is increased due to poor sensation and contractility whereas in a spastic bladder, the capacity is reduced and there are intermittent unrestrained detrusor contractions.

Cystourethroscopy

Cystourethroscopy may help in identifying bladder and urethral lesions such as urethral diverticulum, stricture, fistulas, bladder wall inflammation, and foreign bodies. Bladder mucosal biopsy may be coupled with this investigation to diagnose interstitial cystitis. It is used for the evaluation of incontinence suspected to be due to surgical trauma.

Special Tests for Patients with Urogenital Fistula

Dye Test

About 100 mL of diluted methylene blue or indigo carmine solution is instilled in bladder with Foley catheter and the dye can be seen coming through the opening of VVF in the vagina. The same test can be done after giving oral phenazopyridine.

Three Swab Test or Tampon Test of Moir

Three swab test is indicated in patients, who present with continuous leakage of urine, but the abnormal communication between the bladder and anterior vaginal wall cannot be visualized on per speculum examination. In this test, three cotton swabs are placed in the vagina; one at the vault, one in the middle, and one just above the introitus. Dilute methylene blue solution (100–250 mL) is instilled in bladder by retrograde filling with Foley catheter and patient is asked to walk about for 5 minutes. She is then made to lie down and swabs are removed for inspection. The interpretation is as described below:
- *Urethrovaginal fistula*: The upper two swabs remain dry, but lower swab is stained with dye.
- *VVF*: The lower swab remains dry, but middle and uppermost swabs may be stained with dye.
- *Ureterovaginal fistula*: Only the upper most swab is soaked with urine, but unstained with dye.

Double Dye Test

Oral tablet of phenazopyridine is given to the patient, a tampon is inserted in the vagina and bladder is filled with 200 mL of diluted methylene blue dye. Presence of blue staining is suggestive of VVF or urethrovaginal fistula and presence of red staining is suggestive of ureterovaginal fistula. Dyes are an excellent way of documenting a fistula in the office setting, but further testing is essential to define the fistula completely.[3]

Cystoscopy

Cystoscopy may be performed to visualize the number, size, and site of fistulae; assess the relation of fistula to ureteric openings, bladder neck, and trigone; assess the condition of bladder mucosa for the presence of tissue edema, infection and/or slough; ensure bilateral ureteral patency; identify and remove any foreign body or suture from the bladder. The bladder neck should be examined carefully, and any associated loss of urethral tissue should be made a note of. It also rules out urethral stenosis.

This procedure is best combined with vaginal examination under anesthesia (EUA). In case of large fistula distension of bladder with saline for viewing is possible only when fistula is occluded with vaginal tampon or an inflated bulb of Foley catheter introduced in the bladder through the vaginal opening.

Combined Vaginoscopy-cystoscopy

Combined vaginoscopy-cystoscopy has been described by Andreoni et al.[4] In this technique, the cystoscope is introduced in the bladder and a speculum and laparoscope in vagina simultaneously to enhance the visualization of VVF. Transillumination of the bladder or vagina by turning off the vaginal or bladder light source allows for easier recognition of the fistula in difficult cases.

Color Doppler Ultrasound

Color Doppler ultrasound with contrast media has been described as a diagnostic tool for VVF.[5] Color Doppler ultrasound with contrast media in the urinary bladder may be considered in cases, where cystoscopic evaluation is suboptimal such as in those patients with a small contracted bladder and mucosal changes such as bullous edema or diverticula. The VVF is demonstrated by observing a jet phenomenon through the bladder wall toward the vagina on color Doppler. It has a short learning curve, it is noninvasive, there is no radiation exposure and correlates well with intravenous urography (IVU), cystogram, cystoscopy, and surgical findings.[6]

Radiological Studies

Intravenous Pyelogram

Radiological studies are done prior to planning a surgical repair of VVF. An IVU is necessary to confirm the functioning of kidneys, exclude any ureteral injury or fistula, because 10% of VVFs have associated ureteral fistulas. It has now been replaced by CT urography (Fig. 7).

Computed Tomography

The use of computed tomography (CT) with intravaginal contrast media to detect a VVF has been reported with limited success. CT scanning may be most beneficial in discerning the etiology and the extent of existing disease prior to surgical correction.

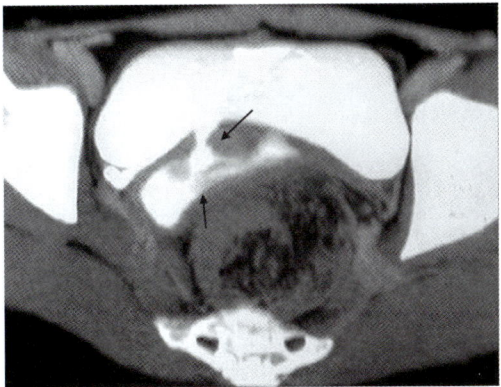

Fig. 7: Vesicovaginal fistula as shown by CT urography. (CT: computed tomography)

Biopsy

In patients with a history of local malignancy, or history of two or more failed repairs, a biopsy of the fistulous tract and microscopic evaluation of the urine for any malignant cells is warranted.

Flowchart 1 outlines the approach to a woman presenting with urinary incontinence.

MANAGEMENT

The outline of the management of urinary incontinence is shown in Flowchart 2.

KEY POINTS

- Urinary incontinence is a common but distressing problem for women.
- A detailed history is a very useful tool to diagnose the type of incontinence whether it is true, stress, urge, or mixed UI.
- A systematic clinical examination can help in making the correct diagnosis.
- Depending upon the type of incontinence, the investigations can be carried out in order to plan the management.

Flowchart 1: Algorithm for clinical approach to a woman presenting with urinary incontinence.

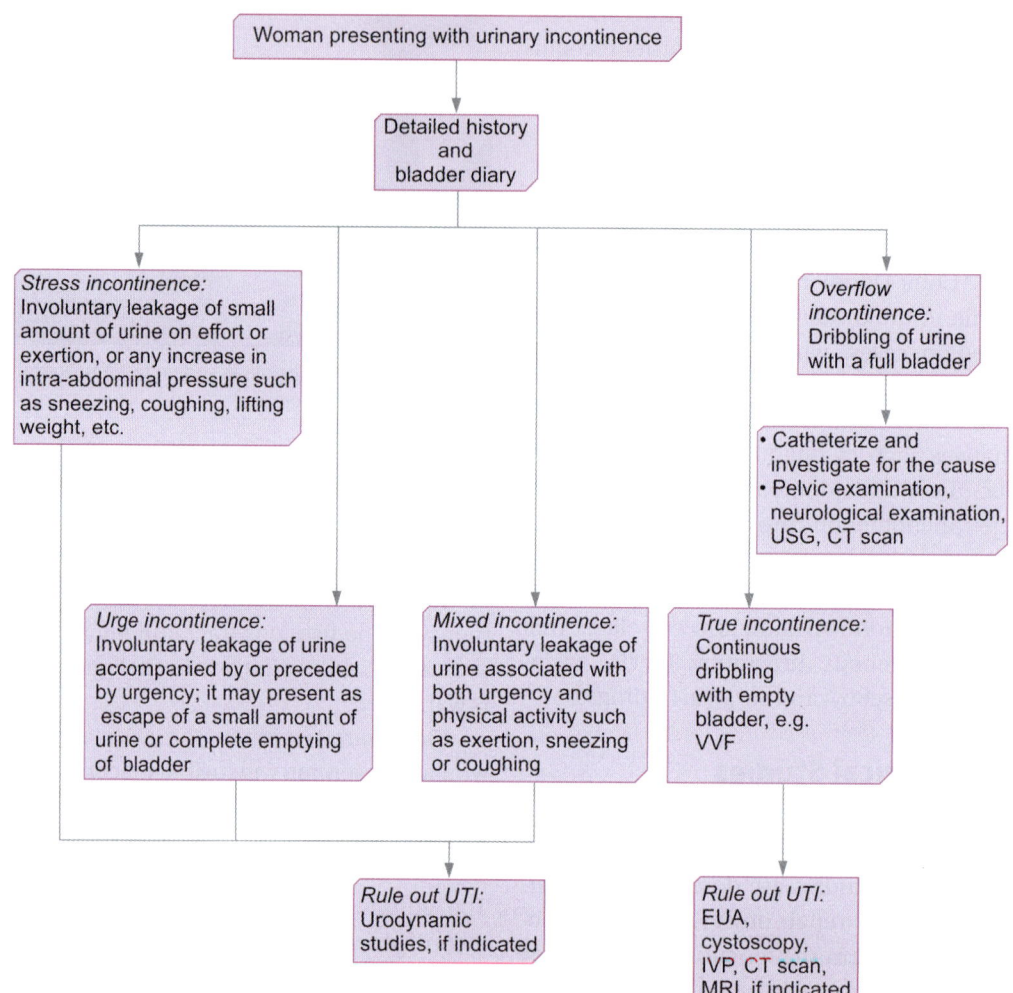

(CT: computed tomography; EUA: examination under anesthesia; IVP: intravenous pyelogram; MRI:, magnetic resonance imaging; USG: ultrasonography; UTI: urinary tract infection; VVF: vesicovaginal fistula)

REFERENCES

1. National Institute for Health and Care Excellence (2006). Urinary incontinence: the management of urinary incontinence in women. NICE clinical guideline 40. [online] Available from https://www.nice.org.uk/guidance/cg40/documents/urinary-incontinence-nice-guideline2.[Last accessed February, 2020].
2. MacLennan AH, Taylor AW, Wilson DH, Wilson D. The prevalence of pelvic floor disorders and their relationship to gender, age, parity and mode of delivery. BJOG. 2000;107(12):1460-70.
3. Hanash KA, Al Zahrani H, Mokhtar AA, Aslam M. Retrograde vaginal methylene blue injection for localization of complex urinary fistulas. J Endourol. 2003;17(10):941-3.

Chapter 38: Approach to a Woman Presenting with Urinary Incontinence

Flowchart 2: Management of urinary incontinence.

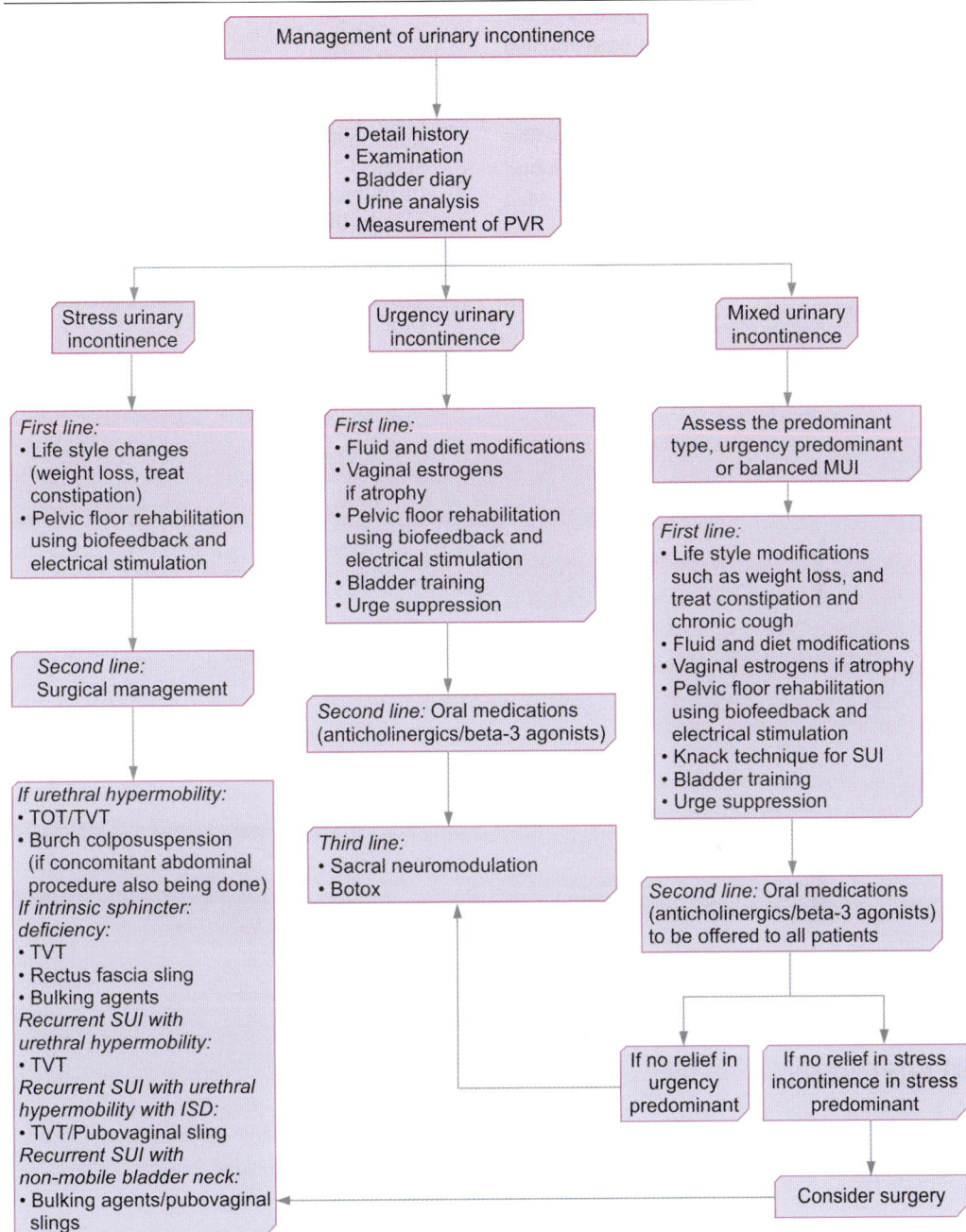

(ISD: intrinsic sphincter deficiency; MUI: mixed urinary incontinence; PVR: post residual void; SUI: stress urinary incontinence; TOT: tension-free obturator tape; TVT: tension-free vaginal tape)

4. Andreoni C, Bruschini H, Truzzi JC, et al. Combined vaginoscopy-cystoscopy: a novel simultaneous approach improving vesicovaginal fistula evaluation. J Urol. 2003;170 (6 Pt 1): 2330-2.
5. Volkmer BG, Kuefer R, Nesslauer T, Loeffler M, Gottfried HW. Colour Doppler ultrasound in vesicovaginal fistulas. Ultrasound Med Biol. 2000;26(5):771-5.
6. Sohail S, Siddiqui KJ. Trans-vaginal sonographic evaluation of vesicovaginal fistula. J Pak Med Assoc. 2005;55(7):292-4.

SUGGESTED READING

1. Capobianco G, Madonia M, Morelli, Desole F. Management of female stress urinary incontinence: A care and update pathway. Maturitas. 2018;109:32-8.
2. Kobashi KC, Albo ME, Dmochowski RR, et al. Surgical Treatment of Female Stress Urinary Incontinence (SUI): AUA/SUFU Guideline. J Urol. 2017;198(4):875-83.
3. Nambiar AK, Bosch R, Cruz F, et al. EAU guidelines on assessment and nonsurgical management of urinary incontinence. Eur Urol. 2018;73(4):596-609.

39. Approach to a Woman Presenting with Anal Incontinence

Harvinder Kaur, Karishma Thariani

INTRODUCTION

Anal incontinence is one of the most devastating symptoms. It is defined as involuntary passage of solid stool, liquid stool, or flatus. Patients feel embarrassed about their symptoms and are often reluctant to discuss their problem. They become confined to their homes, reluctant to interact with their friends, attend any social events, and lose their self-esteem.

The prevalence of incontinence is difficult to estimate because of underreporting and lack of proper definition. The prevalence of anal incontinence varies from 2 to 24%.[1] It affects women of all ages, but the incidence increases with the advancing age.

The maintenance of continence is a complex mechanism and is a function of the anal sphincter complex. It consists of the internal anal sphincter (IAS) muscle, the external anal sphincter (EAS) muscle and the puborectalis (PR) sling. The smooth muscle of the IAS is innervated by the autonomic nervous plexus and is responsible for more than half of the resting anal tone. The striated muscle of EAS is innervated by the inferior branch of pudendal nerve and is responsible for one third of resting tone. Defecation is the result of voluntary relaxation of the EAS and PR that is innervated by the S3, S4 nerves in response to rectal distension that is dictated by the receptors in the pelvic floor and anal transition zone. The most common cause of anal incontinence is obstetric trauma (Fig. 1). The other causes are neurological, posttraumatic, and postsurgical.

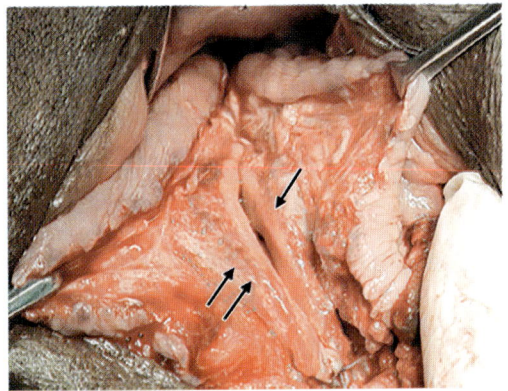

Fig. 1: Fresh perineal tear involving rectum.
(↑: rectal mucosa; ↑↑: internal longitudinal sphincter)

DIFFERENTIAL DIAGNOSIS

Anal incontinence can be due to congenital causes such as Hirschsprung's disease, anorectal agenesis, meningocele, or acquired causes where there is some problem with the anatomic, neurological, or functional factors. The anal incontinence due to congenital causes is treated by pediatric surgeons, hence we will focus on the workup of a woman presenting with acquired incontinence. The acquired causes are as listed in Table 1.

Table 1: Differential diagnosis of acquired anal incontinence.

Anatomic	Neurogenic	Functional
Traumatic: • Obstetric injury • Perineal trauma • Operative trauma or complication • Anal intercourse *Rectovaginal fistula:* • Neoplasm of rectum, anal canal, vulva, vagina or cervix	*Central nervous system:* • Dementia • Mental retardation • Stroke • Oversedation • Injury to brain and spinal cord • Multiple sclerosis • Tabes dorsalis *Peripheral nervous system:* • Polyneuropathy • Diabetes mellitus • Toxic neuropathy • Injury to cauda equina *Traumatic:* • Obstetric trauma • Perineal descent • Chronic straining at stool • Rectal prolapse *Impaired sensation:* • Aging • Muscular dystrophy • Myasthenia gravis	*Abnormal rectal compliance:* • Radiation proctitis • Inflammatory bowel disease *Diarrhea:* • Inflammatory bowel disease • Radiation enteritis • Laxatives *Overflow:* • Fecal impaction • Rectal neoplasm

HISTORY

History of Present Illness

A thorough history is essential for assessing a patient with anal incontinence. The woman should be asked about the duration of problem, frequency of incontinence, time of the day when incontinence occurs, quality of stools lost, control of flatus, need to use pads, frequency of daily bowel movements, constipation, and diarrhea. Fecal urgency may occur because of inability of rectal reservoir to store stool as in proctitis. Sometimes, soiling of clothes may occur without true incontinence such as purulent discharge from fistula in ano or sexually transmitted diseases, blood-stained offensive discharge per rectum in carcinoma of rectum, mucus as in colitis and Crohn's disease, and blood in hemorrhoids.

Duration

It is important to know the duration of complaint as it is helpful in deciding the severity of disease as it affects the patient. If the duration of complaint is short, it means that the problem is severe in nature and the patient is very distressed.

In patients reporting incontinence after obstetric injury, it is prudent to give some time, at least 2 months, to allow for the inflammation to subside, and return of adequate blood supply, and viability of the perineal tissues, before proceeding with any surgical intervention. It also allows for some reinnervation to occur in the cases following childbirth with associated neurological injury.

Awareness Regarding Incontinence

Incontinence may be passive resulting in passage of feces without the patient being aware of it. It suggests loss of central awareness as in dementia, cerebrovascular accident, and mental retardation or sensory loss as in patients with spinal cord injury, cauda equina syndrome, pudendal nerve injury, and diabetes mellitus.

Active incontinence means incontinence despite a patient's awareness and active efforts to retain stools. It suggests sphincter damage with normal neuromuscular innervation. These patients frequently have EAS defect and reduced anal tone as a result of it.

Frequency

Frequency reflects the severity of disease. The patient may become incontinent once or twice in a month due to some altered bowel habit, but if the frequency is more it indicates a problem with the continence mechanism.

Progression of Symptoms

Severity of incontinence may increase or decrease. A patient, who is incontinent initially to flatus, progresses on to incontinence of liquid stools or vice versa. Incontinence following childbirth due to stretching of nerves may improve with time due to some amount of reinnervation. However, in senile incontinence, the problem may worsen with passage of time.

Consistency

It is important to know whether the consistency of the material to which the woman is incontinent is "formed," "semisolid," or "liquid." Incontinence may be present only to liquid if fluid feces are entering the rectum under high pressure, which even a competent continent mechanism cannot handle.

Association with Urgency

In urgency, the patient is unable to hold the passage of feces. It is seen in patients with internal anal sphincter (IAS) and/or EAS defect. It is also seen in patients with a narrow or inflamed rectum with reduced compliance, as in inflammatory bowel disease or radiation proctitis. It is a feature of irritable bowel disease, where stools enter under pressure causing urgent defecation that even a normal sphincter cannot hold.

Preceding Event

Incontinence may follow childbirth, trauma, or surgery. It is helpful to know the exact etiology of the problem for planning management.

Soiling

Soiling may be due to a defect in IAS with intact external sphincter in the absence of neuropathy. It may be evident in patients with hemorrhoidectomy, where the anal cushions are removed, but the external sphincter is normal. Soiling observed after bowel movements may be due to poor hygiene. Soiling with urgency and increased frequency are observed in patients with irritable bowel disease and inflammatory bowel disease.

History of excoriation or perianal discomfort is reported by patients with soiling, who are usually continent but have small leaks.

Any history of genital prolapse (descending perineal syndrome), i.e., descent of anocutaneous junction by >3 cm in relation to ischial tuberosity during straining, less with not. In this, a weakened pelvic floor is not able to withstand the intra-abdominal pressure leading to further descent and stretch injury. Any history of rectal prolapse is also asked for.

The patient needs to be asked, if she is using anything for prevention of incontinence. Some patients modify their diet to maintain continence. So, the exact severity of the problem may be masked in these patients.

Anal incontinence may be associated with incontinence of urine. Urinary and fecal incontinence coexist in certain conditions such as dementia and old age.

Past History

This should include any history of diabetes mellitus, scleroderma, multiple sclerosis, and dermatomyositis indicating a possibility of neuropathy as a cause of incontinence. Any history of bowel problem in the form of alternating diarrhea and constipation is suggestive of inflammatory bowel disease. History of chronic constipation with straining at stool leads to descent of pelvic floor and straightening of anorectal angle. This further stretches the pudendal nerve. Any history of trauma to the spinal cord or pelvis and any history of surgery such as fistulectomy, hemorrhoidectomy, and vulvectomy should be noted. History suggestive of sexually transmitted disease such as discharge per vaginum or urethra, and lesions on genitalia, both in patient and her partner, should be recorded.

Obstetric History

Obstetric history is very important as denervation is more frequent in multiparous women and increases with each subsequent pregnancy. The mode of delivery, whether normal, instrumental, or by cesarean section, is noted as anal sphincter injuries are more common with instrumental vaginal deliveries. The factors associated with increased risk of third-degree tears are birth weight >4 kg, nulliparity, induction of labor, forceps delivery, midline episiotomy, shoulder dystocia, persistent occipitoposterior position, second stage of >1 hour, and epidural analgesia.

Drug History

The patient should be asked about the drugs she is taking. Certain drugs such as use of laxatives may lead to fecal incontinence.

Sexual History

History of anal intercourse may traumatize the anal sphincter with resultant fecal incontinence.

EXAMINATION

General Physical Examination

An overall assessment of the patient is important. This includes her general state of health, mobility, and cognitive status. A brief focused neurological examination is recommended to screen for neurological diseases, but this has a lower detection rate in patients with no history of neurological disease. If history or general physical examination suggests a neurological disease, then a thorough neurological examination is required by a physician.

Breast Examination

Breast examination is done for all women, irrespective of the complaint, to screen for breast cancer.

Systemic Examination

Systemic examination includes examination of respiratory, cardiovascular, and neurological systems and per abdominal examination.

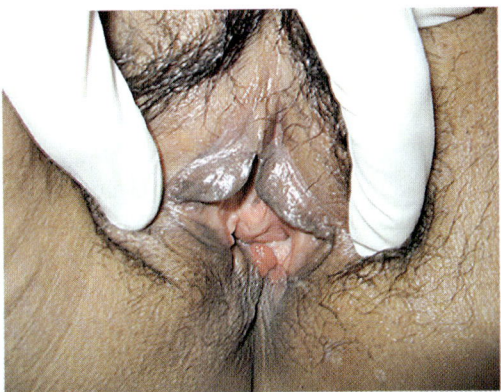

Fig. 2: Old healed complete perineal tear.

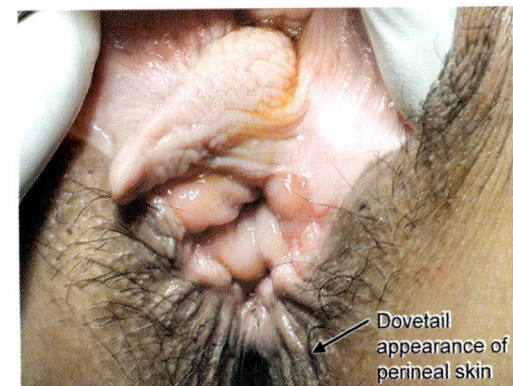

Fig. 3: Dovetail appearance.

Flowchart 1: Interpretation of anal wink reflex.

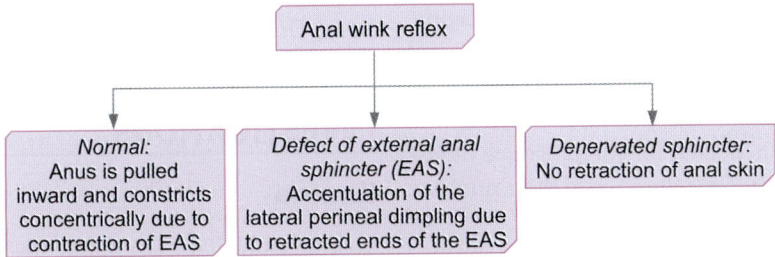

Local Examination

The external genitalia are examined for presence of any atrophic changes, any genital or rectal prolapse, length of perineum whether it is short or absent due to previous obstetric trauma, whether there is evidence of any old healed perineal tear (Fig. 2). We look for the presence of any fistula, hemorrhoids, skin tags, or any excoriation marks.

The anus is carefully inspected for anal rugosities. Normally, rugosities are present all around the anus, but in women with injury to the EAS, there is a dovetail appearance, i.e., the radial distribution of anal creases present laterally and inferiorly but is absent anteriorly due to deficient EAS (Fig. 3). Most obstetric injuries are associated with anterior segmental defect. If the anus is gaping, it indicates loss of sphincteric action. This is followed by anal wink reflex to assess the integrity of S2–S4 dermatome. This is done by stroking the perianal skin with a cotton swab or touching the skin with a pin or asking the patient to cough. The interpretation of the test is as shown in Flowchart 1.

Bulbocavernosus reflex is elicited by light stroking of inferolateral margin of labia majora with a cotton swab and in normal circumstances it causes contraction of bulbocavernosus muscle.

Both these reflexes assess the integrity of pudendal nerve. The afferent limb of bulbocavernosus is through the clitoral branch of the pudendal nerve and efferent limb is through the inferior hemorrhoidal branch of the pudendal nerve. The absence of this reflex reflects central or peripheral neurological deficit. To ensure the integrity of the anal sphincter, insert the index finger into the anal canal and the thumb into the vagina and perform a pill-rolling movement to palpate the anal sphincter. If this technique is inconclusive, ask the woman to contract her anal sphincter with your fingers still in place. When the sphincter is disrupted, you feel a distinct gap anteriorly. If the perineal skin is intact, there may be an absence of puckering on the perianal skin over any underlying defect.

Per Speculum Examination

Per speculum examination is done to inspect the cervix and vagina and look for the presence of any fecal matter or discharge in the vagina, any descent of cervix and or vagina, and any evidence of atrophy or inflammation of vaginal mucosa. The posterior vaginal wall is carefully inspected for the presence of any fistula with special reference to their number, size, site, and margins.

Per Vaginal Examination

Per vaginal examination helps in assessing the uterus and adnexa. In case a rectovaginal fistula is present, its size and margins can be palpated for any fibrosis and its mobility. The levator bulk and tone is assessed (refer to Chapter 37 "Approach to a Woman Presenting with Pelvic Organ Prolapse").

Per Rectal Examination

After lubricating the index finger, the per rectal examination is gently performed to feel for any thickening or irregularity of the anal canal mucosa, detection of any growth, mass, ulcer, or polyp in rectum and assess the consistency of stools and rule out fecal impaction.

The tone of anal musculature is assessed. Examination during relaxation tells about the resting tone, which is mainly due to IAS. Then the patient is asked to squeeze the finger in the anus or cough to assess the maximum squeeze pressure, which is mainly the action of EAS.

The anorectal axis can be evaluated on per rectal examination. Puborectalis muscle is palpable posteriorly at the junction between the rectum and anal canal. By directing the finger posteriorly, the angle between the rectum and anus can be evaluated. The puborectalis muscle pulls the anorectal junction anteriorly to create an angle of 90° approximately between rectum and anal canal. When the patient is asked to squeeze, the puborectalis pulls the finger anteriorly toward the pubic bone. On withdrawing the finger, look for any evidence of mucus, pus, or blood on the finger.

INVESTIGATIONS

Enema

To determine if the woman really has incontinence, an enema may help clarify the problem. About 100 mL of tap water is given and it is observed if the patient can hold this for more than a few minutes. Patients who can hold the enema generally do not have significant incontinence as liquid is more difficult to be held than solid. Such patients may be questioned further to understand their symptoms correctly.

Proctosigmoidoscopy

Proctosigmoidoscopy is useful in diagnosing hemorrhoids, fissure, or fistula and rule out rectal carcinoma or proctitis.

Anal Imaging

Anal imaging is a radiological technique for evaluation of the anatomy of the anal sphincter. It can be endoanal, transvaginal, or transperineal ultrasound depending upon the expertise of the operator. It is easy to carry out, inexpensive, requires no preparation, and causes minimal discomfort. Endoanal ultrasound is performed using 360° rotating 7 MHz endoprobe. The probe is inserted into the anal canal and it provides serial images while withdrawing it slowly (Fig. 4). Anatomic defect can be identified as loss of continuity of muscle rings. The IAS is well visualized because the hypoechogenic smooth muscle is clearly differentiated from the echogenic subepithelial tissue. In contrast, the EAS is of mixed and variable echogenicity, so its boundaries are more difficult to define. The images obtained on endoanal USG act as a roadmap for the repair of sphincter. It gives visualization of the ends of the anal sphincter muscle and the gap between those ends.

Anal Manometry

Anal manometry has two parts—the first part of this test is a pressure profile of the anal canal, which tells about the functional status of external and internal sphincters, and the second part evaluates the rectal sensation. It is performed with the patient in left lateral decubitus position without any bowel preparation. The pressure-sensitive catheter measures the anal canal pressure during rest and voluntary contraction of anal sphincter. The pressure is recorded while slowly withdrawing the catheter or at static points while withdrawing. The parameters measured are as follows:

- *Maximum resting pressure*: It is the highest pressure recorded with the patient at rest. It ranges between 60 and 120 cm H_2O; 85% of this pressure is due to IAS and rest is due to EAS.
- *Maximum squeeze pressure*: It is the maximum increase in pressure over the basal canal pressure initiated by voluntary contraction of the anal sphincter; it ranges between 100 and 200 cm H_2O. It is due to EAS.
- *Anal canal length*: It is measured from a point at which anal sphincter pressure continuously exceeds the average intrarectal pressure by 4 mm Hg.

Rectal sensation is checked by placing a balloon and incrementally distending it. The minimum perceived volume, volume causing urge, maximum tolerable volume, and rectoanal inhibitory reflex (reflex anal contraction and return to normal baseline pressure) are measured. A higher threshold for rectal sensitivity perception is associated with autonomic neuropathy.

Anal manometry cannot distinguish whether the underlying pathology is mechanical disruption of anal sphincter muscle or neurological trauma to pudendal nerve.

Pudendal Nerve Terminal Motor Latency

Pudendal nerve terminal motor latency assesses the pudendal nerve function and measures

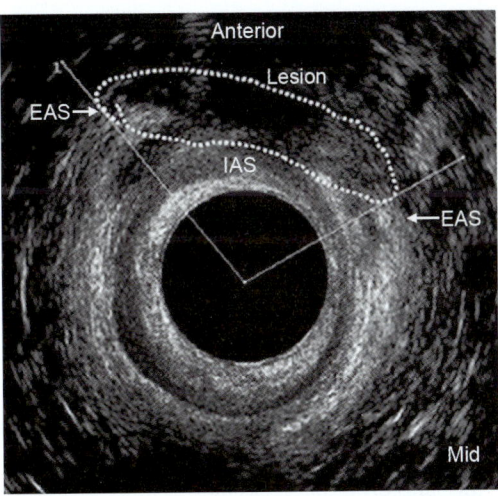

Fig. 4: Endoanal imaging showing a defect in the EAS. (EAS: external anal sphincter; IAS: internal anal sphincter)

conduction velocity of nerve action potential through the terminal part of pudendal nerve between Alcock's canal and EAS. Prolonged conduction time indicates nerve damage, demyelination of nerve sheath due to direct trauma of fetal head, or stretching of the nerve during labor. However, normal latency does not exclude nerve damage because only the fastest conducting fibers are recorded. This test is useful from a research point of view, but not of clinical usefulness. Therefore, this test is not recommended as a routine during evaluation of patients with incontinence.

Defecography

Defecography is the radiological evaluation of the lower gastrointestinal tract. It will tell us about the anorectal angle, pelvic floor descent, length of anal canal, and rectal prolapse. There is significant intraobserver variation and wide overlap between an incontinent and a normal patient. Defecography has a limited role in evaluating the patients with anal incontinence.

Flowchart 2 describes the approach to a woman presenting with anal incontinence.

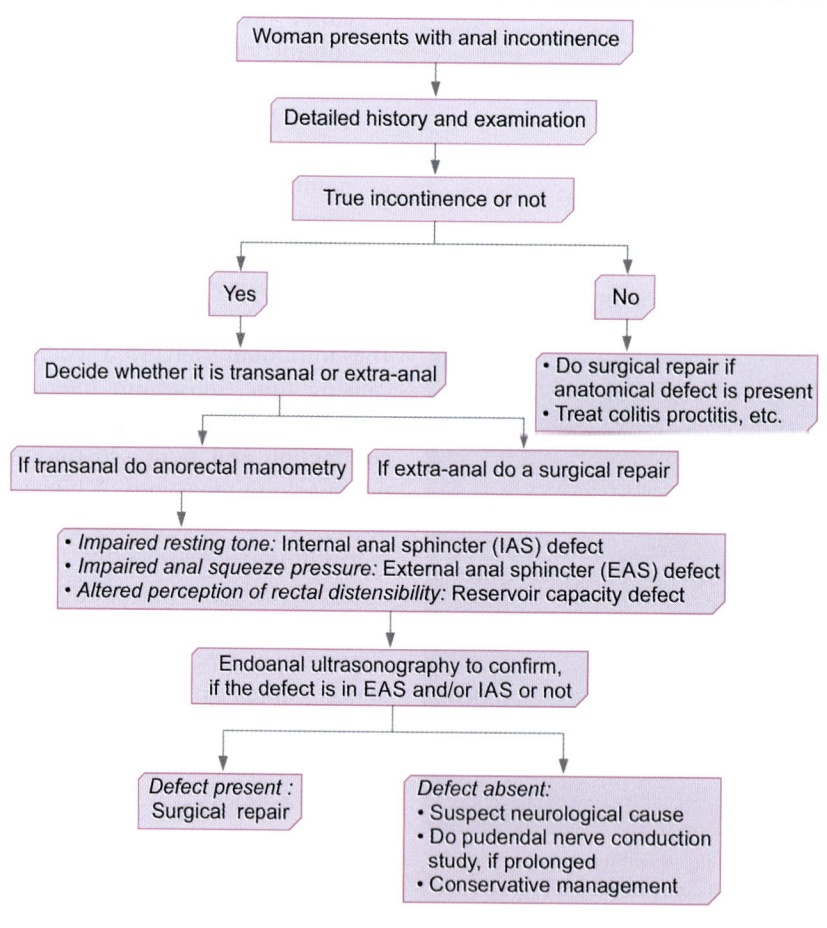

Flowchart 2: Algorithm for a clinical approach to a woman presenting with anal incontinence.

Flowchart 3: Management of fecal incontinence.

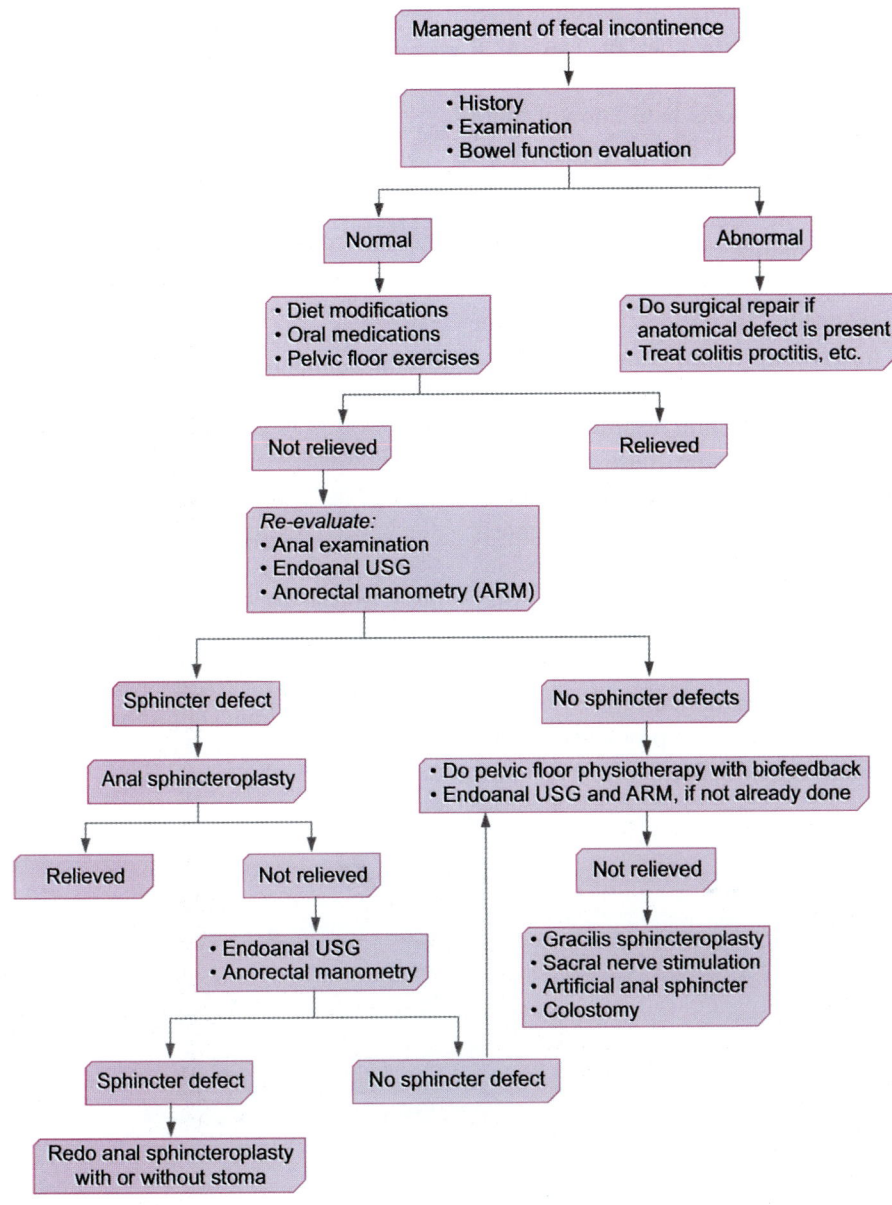

MANAGEMENT

The management depends upon the cause of anal incontinence. Flowchart 3 outlines the principles of management of women with anal incontinence.

KEY POINTS

- The management of a patient with anal incontinence is complicated as fecal continence depends on many factors.

- It is important to first identify whether it is true incontinence or not and then whether it is trans-anal or extra-anal through a fistula.
- The aim of diagnosis is to know if there is any anatomical defect; if yes, then whether it is involving EAS or IAS.
- If there is no anatomical defect, then find out whether the reservoir function of rectum, i.e., sensation, compliance, and capacity, is normal and whether the innervation maintaining continence mechanism is intact or not?
- A careful history and examination are enough in addressing these issues and guiding the treatment (*see* Flowchart 2).
- In certain patients in whom the diagnosis is doubtful or in those with previous treatment failures, further testing may be advised according to the history and examination. No single test is ideal in evaluating such patients.
- There are no standard protocols; testing should be individualized.

REFERENCE

1. Macmillan AK, Merrie AE, Marshall RJ, Parry BR. The prevalence of fecal incontinence in community-dwelling adults: a systematic review of the literature. Dis Colon Rectum. 2004;47(8):1341-9.

SUGGESTED READING

1. Abrams P, Andersson KE, Birder L, Brubaker L, Cardozo L, Chapple C, et al. Fourth International Consultation on Incontinence: Recommendations of the International Scientific Committee: Evaluation and treatment of urinary incontinence, pelvic organ prolapse, and fecal incontinence. Neurourol Urodyn. 2010;29(1):213-40.
2. ACOG Practice Bulletin No. 210 Summary: Fecal incontinence. Obstet Gynecol. 2019;133(4):837-9.
3. National Institute for Health and Care Excellence (NICE). (2014). Interventional procedures guidance: Insertion of a magnetic bead band for faecal incontinence. [online] Available from https://www.nice.org.uk/guidance/IPG483. [Last accessed February, 2020].

40: Approach to a Woman Presenting with Pruritus Vulvae

Shalini Singh, Vibhu Mendiratta

INTRODUCTION

Pruritus vulvae present as persistent vulvar itching. It usually affects up to 1 in 10 women in their life. It is an acute or chronic disorder of the skin around the vulva and the anal region. It is very distressing when persistent. The vulva comprises a mixture of hair-bearing and non-hair-bearing keratinized skin covering mons pubis, labia majora and labia minora, and it meets vaginal mucosa at the introitus.

Pruritus vulvae can either be a manifestation of a generalized skin disorder or due to a local cause. It is most often a symptom of an underlying condition rather than a primary condition. It can affect a woman at any age, although it is more common in females at extremes of age. It should be distinguished from vulvodynia, which refers to chronic vulvar discomfort or pain characterized by burning or stinging sensation, irritation, or redness of the female genitalia in the absence of any infection or skin disease of the vulva or vagina. Vulvar irritation can be caused by any moisture left on the skin in the form of perspiration, urine, vaginal discharge, or even small amounts of feces by virtue of its close proximity with the urethral meatus and anal opening and closed, humid microenvironment.

Causes of pruritus vulvae are summarized in Box 1.[1] Regardless of the cause, pruritus vulvae often leads to scratching which perpetuates the itch. This so-called itch-scratch cycle can itself change the appearance of vulvar skin. Usually, there is a delay in seeking medical advice, and women

Box 1: Causes of pruritus vulvae.

- *Infections*:
  - *Fungi*: Candidiasis (Fig. 1)
  - *Protozoal*: Trichomoniasis
  - *Parasitic*: Pediculosis pubis, scabies, and threadworm
  - *Viral*: Genital herpes
- *Dermatological conditions*:
  - Vulval dermatitis and lichen simplex chronicus
  - Lichen sclerosus (Fig. 2)
  - Squamous hyperplasia of skin
  - Lichen planus
  - Psoriasis
  - Hidradenitis suppurativa
  - Syringomas
  - Fox Fordyce disease
  - Irritant and allergic dermatitis
- *Neoplastic causes*:
  - Vulval intraepithelial neoplasia (VIN)
  - Vulval cancer
  - Paget's disease
- *Pregnant women*:
  - Vulvar varicosities and engorgement
- *Menopausal women*:
  - Dryness
  - Soiling of vulva with urine or feces
  - Atrophic vaginitis
- *Systemic causes of generalized pruritus*:
  - Iron-deficiency
  - Renal or hepatic impairment
  - Diabetes
  - Thyroid dysfunction
  - Stress or psychosis
  - Foreign body in children

often self-medicate with over-the-counter preparations before seeing their physician.

HISTORY

Whenever a patient presents with vulvar itch, a thorough history is helpful in establishing the likely cause of symptoms. The duration of illness; the pattern, whether it is local or generalized, continuous or episodic, or recurrent; any aggravating or relieving factors; and any diurnal variation are to be recorded. Any history of vaginal discharge, vulvar soreness, dysuria, dyspareunia, and itching at other sites is noted. Recent use of new fabric, condoms, and jellies and history of hygiene practices, such as vaginal washes, soaps, shower gels, sanitary products, and hygiene wipes, should be ascertained. Exposure or use of any drug must be recorded. Use of oral contraceptive pills and steroids predisposes to candidiasis.

The patient should be asked as regards history of use of any medications, previous or current, for treatment of this problem and her response to the same. Ask directly about urinary or fecal incontinence as women may be reluctant to disclose it. Enquire about any history of skin disease or similar symptoms at other sites. It is important to take a sexual, gynecological, and medical history. Enquire about the presence of pruritus in other family members for excluding scabies.

Medical History

A history suggestive of diabetes mellitus (DM), thyroid disorder, anemia, and atopy should be asked. Pruritus can be secondary to iron deficiency, renal and liver failure or an underlying psychiatric problem such as depression. A detailed note of drugs being used needs to be made as drugs such as antibiotics, corticosteroids, and oral contraceptives can cause vulvovaginal candidiasis. Drugs such as thiazides, nonsteroidal anti-inflammatory drugs (NSAIDs), antimalarials, and beta blockers are known to aggravate lichen planus. Medications such as lithium, beta blockers, and antimalarials trigger psoriasis.

Menstrual History

Menstrual history is important to know if the woman is pregnant. Pregnancy predisposes to vulvovaginal candidiasis. If the woman is postmenopausal, she is more likely to have thinning and dryness of vaginal mucosa coupled with urinary or fecal incontinence that can cause pruritus vulvae. Postmenopausal women are more likely to have lichen sclerosis.

Family History

Certain vulval diseases such as lichen sclerosus, lichen planus, psoriasis, autoimmune diseases, and atopy have a genetic predisposition, so it is important to elicit a family history of these disorders.

EXAMINATION

We should offer a chaperone and ensure the patient's privacy and dignity. The woman should ideally be examined with a good light source on an examination couch. The vulva should be examined systematically, followed by inspection of the perianal region and natal cleft. A detailed examination of external genitalia including mons pubis, labia majora, labia minora, urethral meatus, vaginal opening, anus and perineum should be carried out in all patients. One should look for any erythema, rash, scaling, white patch, scarring, fissures, thickening, hyperpigmentation, excoriation, any warts, ulcers, swelling, discharge, lice in pubic hair, and threadworms around anus.

Oral mucosa is examined for presence of lichen planus, scalp, elbows, knees, and nails for psoriasis and lichen planus. Whole-body examination is done for any eczema or dermatitis. Per speculum, per vaginal, and/or per rectal examination should be done wherever indicated. Per rectal examination is useful to detect foreign body in vagina in small children. It is important to look for any enlargement of inguinal lymph nodes.

INVESTIGATIONS

Investigations are planned based on the provisional diagnosis on history and examination. Microscopic examination of saline smears from the discharge and scrapings from the lesions, swabs, and culture of vaginal discharge for fungal, bacterial, and viral infections should be done in cases of suspected vulvovaginitis.

Papanicolaou (Pap) smear is taken and colposcopic examination of cervix, vagina, and vulva should be done in cases of suspected premalignant and malignant lesions. Vulvar biopsies are indicated, where the diagnosis is in doubt or the patient does not respond to treatment or there is suspicion of vulvar intraepithelial neoplasia (VIN) or vulvar cancer as in women presenting with induration, condyloma, plaques, or persistent erosions on the vulvar skin. Toluidine blue test is helpful in identifying the site for biopsy. Toluidine blue (1%) is applied to the vulva from mons pubis to perianal area and allowed to dry, and then sponged with 3% acetic acid for colposcopic examination to detect darkly stained areas for biopsy.[2]

Patch test for allergic contact dermatitis can be done. Most common allergens are cosmetics, preservatives in topical medications, washing detergents, soaps, conditioners, textile dyes, rubber, sanitary pads, panty liners, etc.

Complete blood count (CBC) and serum ferritin levels are done to detect iron-deficiency anemia. Fasting and postprandial blood sugar levels and thyroid function tests are done if indicated on history. Blood tests such as enzyme-linked immunosorbent assay (ELISA) for human immunodeficiency virus (HIV) and Venereal Disease Research Laboratory (VDRL) test are indicated if sexually transmitted infection is suspected. Urine is subjected to routine and microscopic examination and urine culture is sent in case of suspected urinary tract infections. Stool examination is done for ova or cyst. Flowchart 1 depicts the algorithm of the workup of a woman presenting with pruritus vulvae.

MANAGEMENT

Management of pruritus vulvae depends on treating the underlying cause. Most patients

Flowchart 1: Algorithm for clinical approach to a woman presenting with pruritus vulvae.

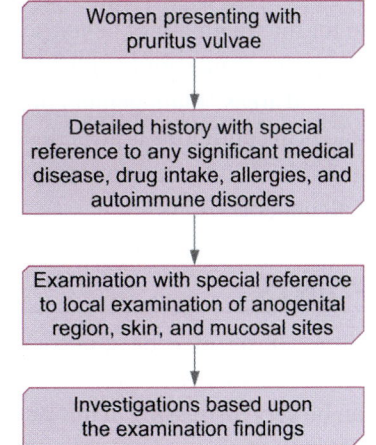

benefit from general advice regarding care of the vulvar skin. Patient education and general advice should be given which can help reduce itching. When washing, avoid using water alone or water and soap as this cause dryness of skin which makes it itchier. Use an emollient as a soap substitute with water to wash the vulvar area once daily. This should be applied by hand. The same emollient can also be used as a moisturizer several times a day. Avoid using bubble baths, shower gels, deodorants, perfumes, talcum powder, over-the-counter creams, antiseptics, and cleansing wipes on the vulvar skin. After washing, dry the vulvar area by dabbing gently (not rubbing) with a soft towel or using a hairdryer on a cool setting held away from the skin. Avoid colored toilet paper. Avoid using condoms that are lubricated with spermicide. Avoid wearing tight-fitting underwear or other close-fitting clothes, e.g., tights. Wear cotton/silk underwear and avoid wearing underwear made from synthetic fibers. At night, consider sleeping without underwear. Topical steroids are used to treat several vulvar conditions, and patients should be given clear instructions on their use, together with written information. Very potent topical steroids (e.g., clobetasol propionate 0.05%) are used for the treatment of lichen sclerosus and lichen planus and should only be applied to the affected areas.[3] Management of specific dermatological conditions is given in Table 1. Antihistaminic is indicated for symptomatic relief in all patients.

Table 1: Management of specific dermatological conditions.

Disease	Treatment
Lichen planus	Very potent topical steroids (e.g., clobetasol propionate)
Lichen sclerosus (Fig. 1)	Very potent topical steroids (e.g., clobetasol propionate) for 3–4 weeks followed by topical tacrolimus (0.1%)
Lichen simplex chronicus	Potent topical steroids along with keratolytic agent, e.g., salicylic acid
Vulvar dermatitis	• Avoidance of potential allergens and irritants • General care of the vulva • Topical steroids
Psoriasis	• Topical steroids emollients • Vitamin D analogs (e.g., calcitriol) • Topical steroids
Hidradenitis suppuravita	• Skin hygiene measures • Long-term antibiotics such as doxycycline 100 mg daily for 6 months
Vulvovaginal Candidiasis (Fig. 2)	• Topical antifungal application (e.g. clotrimazole) along with vaginal pessary 100 mg OD for 7 days or • Oral antifungal fluconazole 150 mg stat • Sexual partner not treated • No abstinence *Recurrent cases*: • Fluconazole 150 mg every 2–3 days for three doses then every week for 6 months
Trichomonas vaginitis	• Tab metronidazole 2 gm oral single dose or Tab metronidazole 400–500 mg twice a day for 5–7 days • Tab tinidazole or Tab secnidazole 2 gm stat treat both patient and her partners

KEY POINTS

- Pruritus vulvae may be due to local or systemic causes.
- It can be very distressing, if it is persistent and recurrent.
- The history should essentially include similar symptoms at other sites, any

Chapter 40: Approach to a Woman Presenting with Pruritus Vulvae

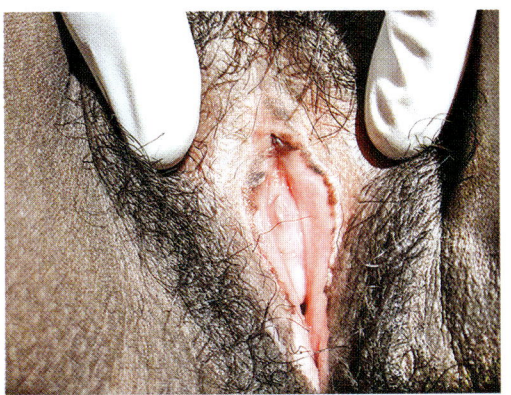

Fig. 1: Lichen sclerosus.

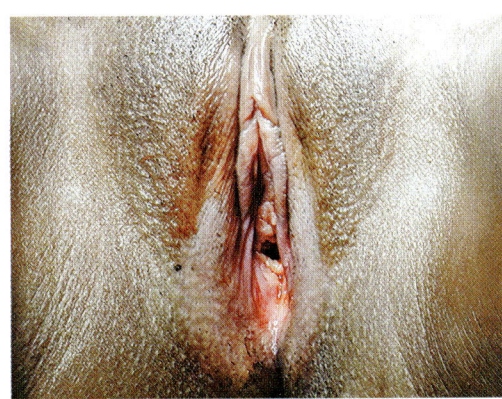

Fig. 2: Candida vulvovaginitis.

significant medical, drug, family and personal history of autoimmune or allergic disorders.
- The treatment includes maintenance of local hygiene, keep the area dry, symptomatic relief with antihistaminic and specific treatment depending on the disorder.

REFERENCES

1. Solone M, Hillard PJA. Adult Gynecology: Reproductive Years. Berek and Novak's Gynecology, 16th edition, Chapter 10, pp. 193-219.
2. Hoffman BL, Schorge JO. Preinvasive lesions of lower genital tract. Williams Gynaecology, 3rd edition, Chapter 29, pp. 624-52.
3. Horowitz IR, Buscema J, Majmudar B. Surgical conditions of Vulva. Te Linde's Operative Gynecology, 11th edition, Chapter 23, pp. 802-46.

SUGGESTED READING

1. ACOG Practice bulletin no. 93: diagnosis and management of vulvar skin disorders. Obstet Gynecol. 2008;111(5):1243-53.
2. Committee on Practice Bulletins—Gynecology. Vaginitis in nonpregnant patients: ACOG Practice Bulletin, Number 215. Obstet Gynecol. 2020;135(1):e1-17.
3. Edwards SK, Bates CM, Lewis F, Sethi G, Grover D. British Association for Sexual Health and HIV (BASHH): UK national guideline on the management of vulval conditions. Int J STD AIDS. 2015;26(9):611-24.
4. van der Meijden WI, Boffa MJ, Ter Harmsel WA, Kirtschig G, Lewis FM, Moyal-Barracco M, et al. 2016 European guideline for the management of vulval conditions. J Eur Acad Dermatol Venereol. 2017;31(6):925-41.

41 Approach to a Woman Presenting with Vulvar Lesion

Shilpa Singla, Anuja Rao

INTRODUCTION

The symptoms associated with vulvar skin dermatoses, primarily pruritus, irritation, and pain, are very distressing for the patients. The exact prevalence of vulvar dermatoses is unknown; however, it is well accepted that vulvar symptoms are a common problem for women.[1,2] An extensive range of lesions may involve the vulva. These can be benign, premalignant or malignant, and present as a pigmentary change, ulcer or growth. The pigmentary changes can be inflammatory or noninflammatory.

Genital ulcer is an ulcerative, erosive, pustular or vesicular lesion of the skin or mucous membrane of genitalia that may be caused by sexually transmitted infection (STI) or non-STI-related conditions. Sexually transmitted diseases (STDs) are the most common cause of genital ulcers.

In order to make a correct diagnosis and appropriately manage a case of genital lesion, it is necessary to be aware of all the differential diagnoses and their characteristics.

DIFFERENTIAL DIAGNOSIS

Differential diagnosis of genital ulcers, pigmented lesions, and vulval growth is as given in Tables 1 to 3, respectively.

Table 1: Differential diagnosis of genital ulcers.

Nature of ulcer	Common	Rare
Sexually transmitted infections (STIs)		
	• Genital herpes (Fig. 1) • Syphilis • Mollescum contagiosum • HPV genital wart	• Lymphogranuloma venereum • Chancroid • Granuloma inguinale
Non-STI related		
• Infectious	• Fungal: *Candida* (Fig. 2), *Tinea* (Fig. 3) • Bacterial: Staphylococcus, Streptococcus, Mycobacterium, Salmonella	• Viral: Cytomegalovirus (CMV), Varicella-zoster, Epstein-Barr (EB) virus
• Infestations	• Scabies	• Thread worm, enterobiasis

Noninfectious:
• Bullous:
  – Nonautoimmune
 	
  – Autoimmune
	• Contact dermatitis
	• Erythema multiforme
		• Toxic epidermal necrolysis
		• Pemphigus vulgaris
		• Cicatricial pemphigoid

Contd...

Contd...

Nature of ulcer	Common	Rare
Nonbullous	• Lichen sclerosus (Fig. 4) • Inflammatory bowel disease (ulcerative colitis, Crohn's disease) • Nonspecific vulvitis • Aphthous ulcers • Seborrheic keratosis	• Erosive lichen planus (Fig. 5) • Behçet's disease • Fixed drug eruption
Malignancy	• Squamous cell carcinoma • Vulval intraepithelial neoplasia	• Extramammary Paget's disease • Basal cell carcinoma • Langerhans cell histiocytosis • Mammary like gland adenoma (Hidradenoma papilliferum)
Systemic diseases	• Crohn's disease • Systemic lupus erythematous	Acrodermatitis enteropathica

Table 2: Differential diagnosis of pigmented lesions.

Inflammatory	Noninflammatory
• Lichen planus • Lichen sclerosus • Lichen simplex chronicus • Vulval intraepithelial neoplasia • Dermatitis (contact irritant/atopic/primary irritant) (Fig. 6) • Psoriasis (Fig. 7) • Intertrigo • Lupus erythematosus • Other rare conditions (Behçet's disease, Reiter's disease, Crohn's disease)	• Acanthosis nigricans • Vitiligo (Fig. 8) • Lentigo, lentiginosis • Melanocytic nevus • Postinflammatory hyperpigmentation • Leukoplakia • Benign vulvar melanosis

Table 3: Differential diagnosis of vulval growth.

Cysts	Benign growth	Malignant growth
• Mucous cysts • Bartholin and Skene's duct cysts (Fig. 9) • Sebaceous cyst (Fig. 10) • Epidermal inclusion cyst	• Acrochordon (fibroepithelial polyp) • Fibroma, fibromyoma, and dermatofibroma • Lipoma (Fig. 11) • Hidradenoma • *Vascular lesion*: Hemangioma • Lymphangioma • Angiokeratoma • Warts (Fig. 12)	• Squamous cell carcinoma (Fig. 13) • Adenocarcinoma • Sarcoma • Basal cell carcinoma • Melanoma

HISTORY

A good clinical history is very important and helpful in making a correct diagnosis. A detailed history of vulvar lesion is elicited. The personal profile and hygiene of the affected individual, incubation period, duration over which the lesion has evolved, and the course of progress of disease can predict the underlying etiological agent in STIs (Table 4). Any preceding or associated signs and symptoms, such as itching, pain, fever, and glandular enlargement should be noted. Whether there is any past history of similar lesions is important as recurrence is common with herpes simplex infection.

Besides, a good medical history such as history suggestive of any autoimmune

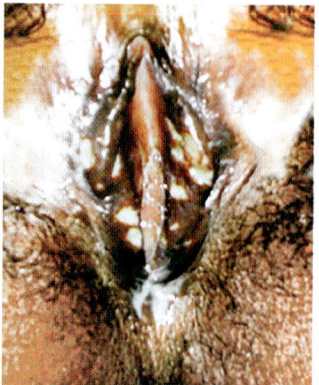

Fig. 1: Genital herpes.

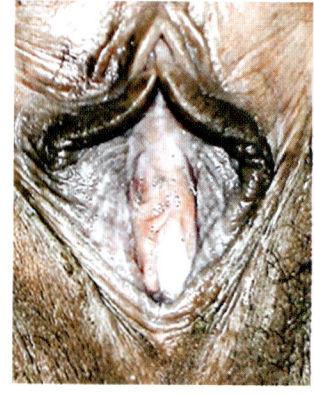

Fig. 2: Candida vulvovaginitis.

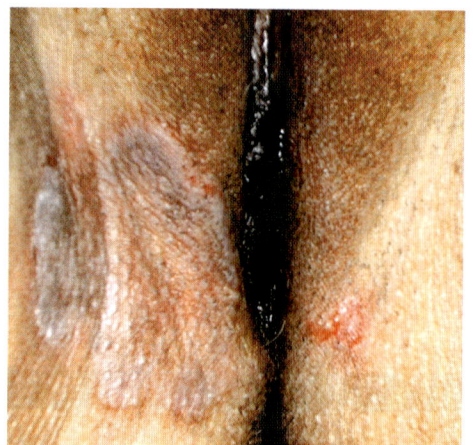

Fig. 3: Tinea.

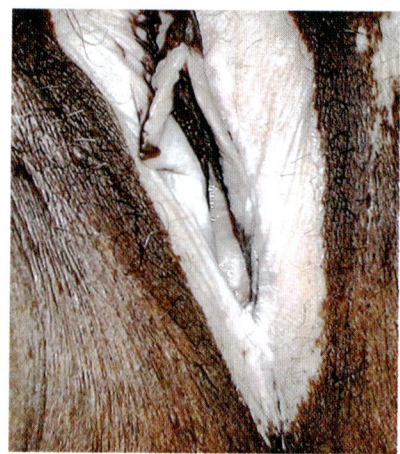

Fig. 4: Lichen sclerosus.

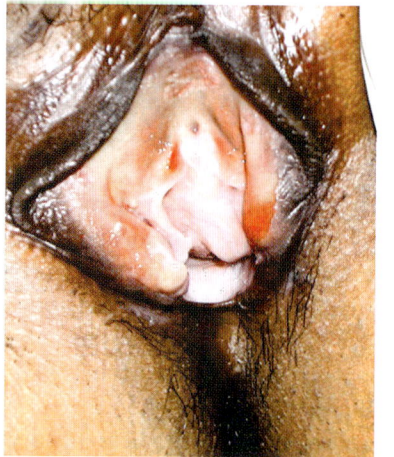

Fig. 5: Erosive lichen planus.

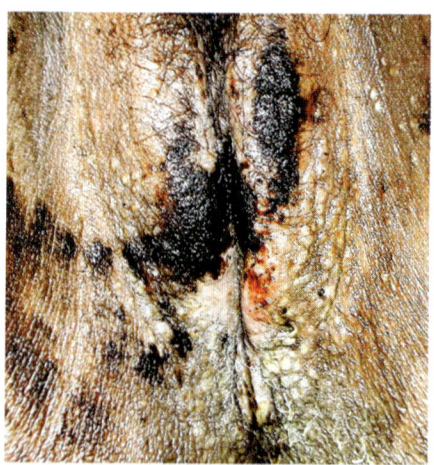

Fig. 6: Contact dermatitis.

Chapter 41: Approach to a Woman Presenting with Vulvar Lesion

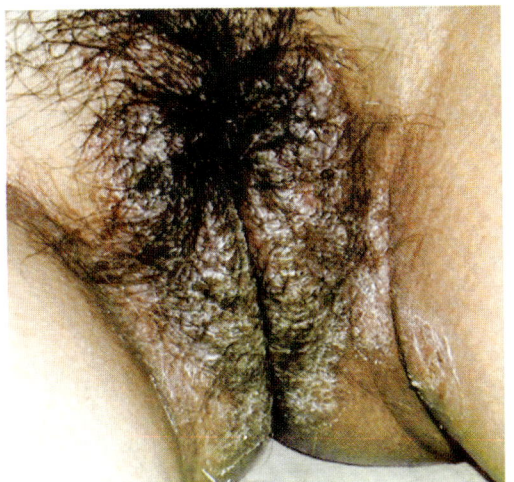

Fig. 7: Psoriasis.

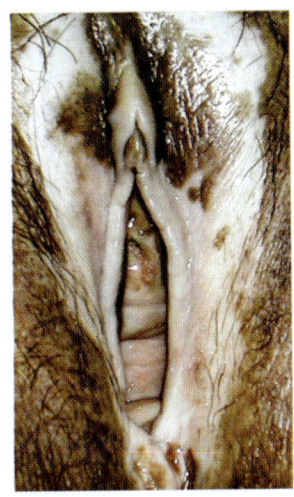

Fig. 8: Vitiligo.

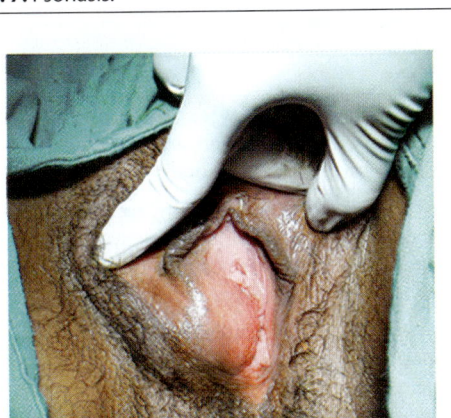

Fig. 9: Bartholin's cyst.

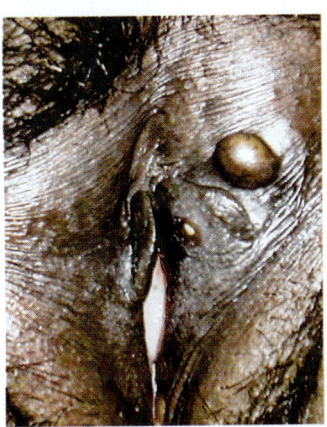

Fig. 10: Sebaceous cyst.

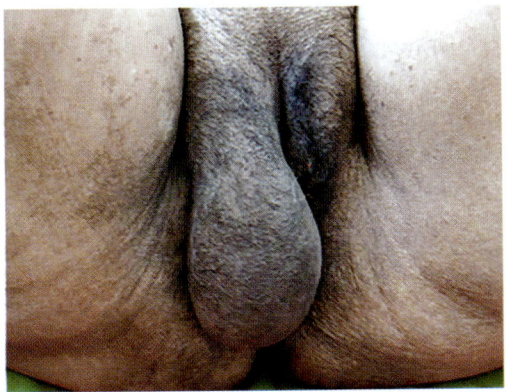

Fig. 11: Vulval lipoma.

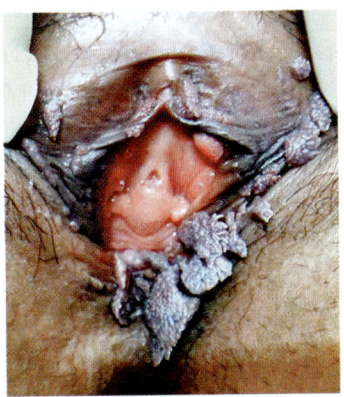

Fig. 12: Vulval warts.

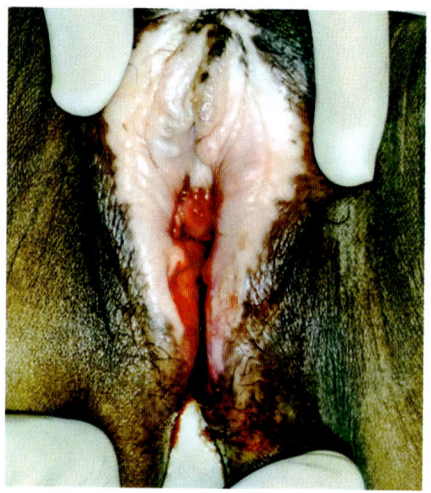

Fig. 13: Vulval dystrophy with squamous cell carcinoma of vulva.

Table 4: Clinical features of sexually transmitted infection on history.

Disease	Incubation period	Course of illness
Syphilis	3–90 days	Most lesions appear within 2–6 weeks of exposure; primary lesion heals often without treatment and is followed by rash of secondary syphilis in 1–4 months
Genital herpes	2–7 days	Primary painful multiple vesicular lesions appear within a week of exposure associated with systemic symptoms like fever, myalgia; after healing, recurrent lesions appear within 1–4 months with 4–7 episodes per year
Lymphogranuloma venereum	3–30 days	Genital ulcer self-limiting, tender inguinal and femoral lymphadenopathy; in those with anal contact proctocolitis with anal pain, rectal discharge, tenesmus, constipation, and fever may be present
Chancroid	5–14 days	Painful genital ulcer with suppurative inguinal lymphadenopathy
Granuloma inguinale	1–180 days	Painless ulcerative lesions, which bleed on touch

disorder such as inflammatory bowel disease, drug intake, any local application of medication or chemical, and presence of lesions at non-genital sites at present or in the past, can provide clues in cases with noninfectious causes of genital ulcer. Any history of local trauma is also important.

Sexual History

The likelihood of genital herpes, syphilis, chancroid, and lymphogranuloma venereum (LGV) increases when the patient has been engaged in sexual diversions with multiple partners. It is important to know the profession of the patient and her spouse or partner, as certain professions like sex workers, drivers, policemen, etc. are at an increased risk of STDs. The history of any genital ulcers and lesions in the partner should also be inquired.

It is important to know whether the ulcers are restricted to the genital area or not. Ulcers involving both genital and non-genital sites suggest nonvenereal origin such as psoriasis, lichen planus (LP), Behçet's disease, dermatitis herpetiformis, erythema multiforme, aphthous ulcerations, and pemphigus or pemphigoid.

The differential diagnosis of ulcers limited to the genital area in sexually active patients includes not only STIs but also other causes such as local trauma, drug reactions, nonulcerative skin lesions with secondary excoriation, and rarely squamous cell carcinoma of vulva. Careful history helps in excluding these diagnoses. Sometimes women presenting with lesions due to trauma may be suffering from herpes genitalis. The differentiation is made by the difference in incubation periods. Traumatic ulcers come up soon after intercourse (0–24 hours), whereas herpetic lesion will have a long incubation period.

Tetracyclines, sulfonamides, methaqualone, and sometimes phenolphthalein laxatives and barbiturates cause fixed drug reactions.

EXAMINATION

General Physical Examination

Stigmata of systemic involvement as in immunocompromised conditions such as human immunodeficiency virus (HIV), uncontrolled diabetes, diseases with multiorgan involvement such as Behçet's disease, lichen planus, and drug eruptions should be looked for. A detailed dermatological examination for similar lesions elsewhere is important.

Local Examination

A thorough systematic examination of lesions is very essential to establish the exact etiology. This should include the distribution, number, margins, depth and base of ulcers, and any associated discharge. The lymph node involvement should be looked for, whether unilateral or bilateral and presence or absence of any signs of inflammation and/or suppuration or discharge. The lower limbs should be examined for any involvement like elephantiasis in case of LGV. Sometimes, multiple pathogens may occur concurrently in the same ulcer.

Other than the examination of the ulcers, a detailed examination of the external genitalia including mons pubis, labia majora, labia minora, urethral meatus, vaginal opening, anus, and perineum should be carried out. One should look for any erythema, rash, scaling, white patch, scarring, fissures, thickening, hyperpigmentation, excoriation, any warts, ulcers, swelling, discharge, lice in pubic hair, and threadworms around anus. Per speculum, per vaginal, and per rectal examination should be done wherever indicated specially in cases with suspected vulvar intraepithelial neoplasia (VIN) or squamous cell carcinoma. Any evidence of regional lymphadenopathy including the inguinal and femoral lymph nodes should be recorded.

The clinical examination characteristics of sexually transmitted genital ulcers are as described in Table 5.

Inguinal lymphadenopathy often accompanies genital ulceration and is of some help in distinguishing the various types of genital ulcers. Patients with primary herpes generally have very painful inguinal lymphadenopathy, patients with chancroid and LGV often have tender, but less painful, lymphadenopathy, and those in chancroid may suppurate with erythema and edema of overlying skin. Patients with syphilis usually have painless, firm lymphadenopathy. These distinctions, however, do not permit a definitive diagnosis.

Table 5: Diagnostic characteristics on examination of genital ulcers with sexually transmitted infections.

Features	Genital herpes	Syphilis	LGV	Chancroid	Granuloma inguinale
Primary lesion nature	Vesicle, papules, ulcers, typically bilateral in primary and unilateral in recurrent	Papule, ulcer	Papule, ulcer	Ulcer	Ulcer
Number	Multiple, may coalesce	Usually single	Single	Single or multiple	Single or multiple
Genital distribution	Vulva, vagina, cervix, perineum, legs, and buttocks	At the site of inoculation	At the site of inoculation	At the site of inoculation	At the site of inoculation
Painful/Painless	Painful	Painless	Painless	Painful	Painless
Margins	Erythematous, punched out	Sharply demarcated	Variable	Violaceous, undermined	Hypertrophic or sclerotic
Depth	Superficial	Superficial	Superficial	Excavated	Superficial
Base	Red and smooth	Red and smooth	Variable	Yellow to gray exudate	Beefy red (bleeds on touch)
Induration	None	Firm	Rare	Rare; usually soft	
Secretion	Serous	Serous	Variable	Purulent to hemorrhagic	Bloody

(LGV: lymphogranuloma venereum)

INVESTIGATIONS

Investigations include blood sugar, total and differential leukocyte count, erythrocyte sedimentation rate, serology, Gram staining, and culture of the smear obtained from the base of ulcers and discharge and immunological tests to detect antigen–antibody complexes. The specific tests indicated for the diagnosis of different infections are given in Table 6.

A scraping from the base of the herpetic lesion stained by Giemsa or Wright's stains (Tzanck smear) may show characteristic multinucleated giant epidermal cells. The various techniques for demonstration of viral antigen include immunofluorescence or immunoperoxidase, demonstration of viral DNA (DNA hybridization technology) or

Table 6: Investigations for diagnosis of specific infections.

Etiological agent	Investigation
Herpes	Culture, cytology (Tzanck smear), viral antigen detection, viral DNA, serology, histopathology
Syphilis	Dark field examination, direct immunofluorescence, serology, histopathology
Chancroid	Culture, Gram stain of tissue scraping
LGV	Culture, micro-indirect fluorescence (MIF), complement fixation test, histopathology
Granuloma inguinale	Giemsa or Wright's stain of tissue smears and sections, histopathology

(DNA: deoxyribonucleic acid; LGV: lymphogranuloma venereum)

demonstration of viral particles by electron microscopy. Viral culture is the most sensitive and specific method of diagnosis.

Serologic tests are used in the diagnosis of primary infection, as well as for sero-epidemiologic studies. Sera are obtained at time of presentation and after 2 weeks; a fourfold rise in serum antibody titer suggests a primary infection.

The tests used for diagnosis of syphilis are demonstration of *Treponema pallidum* (*T. pallidum*) by dark field examination of the exudate of infectious lesions, fluorescent methods, silver staining methods of biopsy specimens, and serological tests. Most widely used methods to diagnose syphilitic infection are demonstration of *T. pallidum*. The important serologic tests are of two types; antitreponemal tests that is detecting specific antibodies to treponemal antigens usually demonstrable 2 weeks after infection and nonspecific antibodies to cardiolipin antigen in the antilipoidal tests positive after approximately 4 weeks. The most widely used tests are treponemal tests such as the microhemagglutination assay for *T. pallidum* (MHA-TP), the fluorescent treponemal antibody-absorption (FTA-ABS) test, and nontreponemal tests such as the rapid plasma reagin (RPR) card test or the Venereal Disease Research Laboratory (VDRL) test.

For diagnosis of chancroid to culture the *Haemophilus ducreyi* (*H. ducreyi*), special sensitive and selective culture media should be obtained. In some cases, Gram staining of a scraping of the exudate from the ulcer base may demonstrate the characteristic "railtrack" or "school of fish" appearance of *H. ducreyi*. Techniques such as enzyme immunoassay (EIA), DNA probes, dot immunobinding, and immunofluorescence assays have a limited role.

For LGV, a swab from infected tissue (bubo, genital or rectal tissue) to culture for *Chlamydia trachomatis* (*C. trachomatis*) is required. Identification of the isolate as a LGV strain must be performed in a reference laboratory. At present, the most used serologic tests are the complement fixation test and the microimmunofluorescence test. Apart from the clinical presentation, laboratory confirmation by demonstration of typical Donovan bodies in direct tissue smears from tissue scrapings using Giemsa or Wright's staining methods/in biopsy material stained by hematoxylin and eosin/silver staining method or slow-Giemsa stain. The microorganisms exhibit bipolar staining and resemble closed safety pins. *Calymmatobacterium granulomatis* is extremely difficult to grow in vitro.

Biopsy from the lesion is indicated in hypertrophic lesions not responding to initial treatment or are suspicious of malignancy.

Clinical approach to a woman presenting with vulval lesion is as shown in Flowchart 1.

MANAGEMENT

The management of vulvar lesions is multimodal. The principles of management are:
- General hygiene and appropriate skin care
- Treatment of coexistent infection
- Control of pruritus by topical or systemic medication
- Condition specific treatment of STIs
- Partner tracing and treatment and sexual counseling.

General Hygiene and Skin Care

The area should be kept clean and dry. Repeated washing with soap can worsen dermatitis. Cotton undergarments and loose-fitting clothes should be used. Scented soaps, shampoos, douches, sprays etc. should be avoided. After washing, the area should be dried with a soft absorbent cloth or paper

Flowchart 1: Algorithm for clinical approach to a woman presenting with vulval lesion.

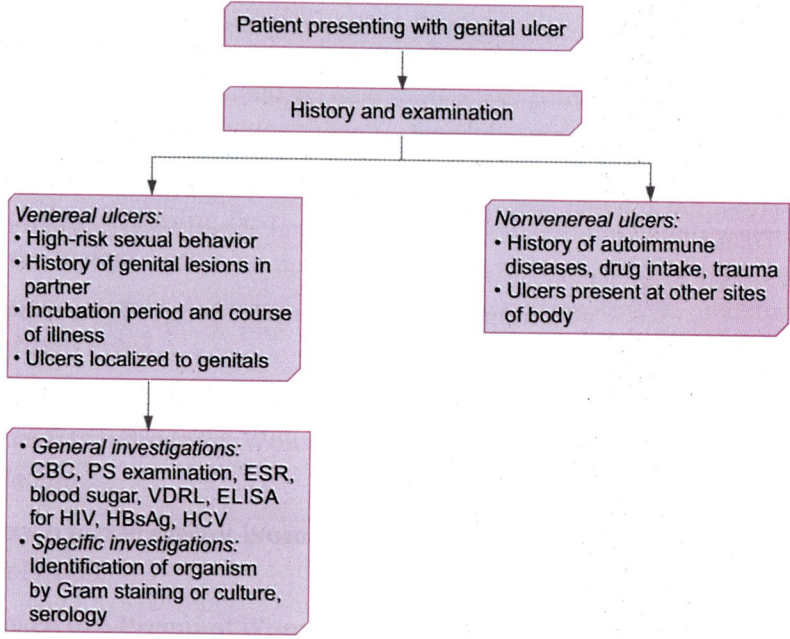

(CBC: complete blood count; ELISA: enzyme-linked immunosorbent assay; ESR: erythrocyte sedimentation rate; HBsAg: hepatitis B surface antigen; HCV: hepatitis C virus; HIV: human immunodeficiency virus; PS: peripheral smear; VDRL: Venereal Disease Research Laboratory)

by gentle patting and not rubbing. The moisture in the area can then be sealed with nonallergic emollient like petroleum jelly or a topical steroid ointment. This maintains a skin barrier.

Treatment of Coexistent Infections

Infections like candidiasis, genital herpes simplex or bacterial infection should be diagnosed with smears and cultures and treated with appropriate agent. Candidiasis with antifungal agents, tablet fluconazole 150 mg single dose; Herpes simplex with antivirals, acyclovir 400 mg 5 times a day for 5–7 days; and bacterial infections with antibiotics, amoxicillin clavulanic acid 625 mg every 8 hours or cephalexin 500 mg every 6 hours for 5–7 days.

Treatment of Pruritus

Nonsedating antipruritic agents are usually not effective in pruritus due to vulvar lesions. Oral sedating antipruritic agents such as doxepin and hydroxyzine are effective for nighttime itching.[3] Doxepin is tricyclic antidepressant with antihistaminic action whereas hydroxyzine is first-generation H1 antihistamine. Patients are usually started on a low dose of 5 to 10 mg amitriptyline taken at night to minimize side effects. Doxepin can be started at a dose of 25 mg nightly and increased to 75 mg as needed.

First-line local treatment with women with mild symptoms is application of low-to-medium potency steroid ointment that is hydrocortisone 1–2% or triamcinolone 0.1% ointment 1–2 times a day for 10–14 days. For those with moderate-to-severe symptoms, high potency corticosteroid ointment clobetasol propionate 0.025 or 0.05% is prescribed every night for 1 month. In those with corticosteroid-dependent dermatitis, use of the topical calcineurin inhibitors (TCIs) tacrolimus 0.03% ointment or pimecrolimus 1% cream is advised.[4] Compared to topical steroids as anti-inflammatory agents, TCIs carry the advantage of lack of risk of atrophy, striae, and steroid dermatitis.

While atopic dermatitis and contact dermatitis are expected to resolve relatively quickly with topical corticosteroids, these conditions can be recurrent if the skin barrier is not continually maintained.

Vulvar lichen sclerosus (LS) is commonly treated with a super potent topical steroid, such as clobetasol. Recalcitrant lesions should be biopsied to rule out squamous cell carcinoma. Long-term maintenance treatment of topical steroid application 1 to 3 times weekly and ongoing follow-up is recommended to minimize recurrence, sexual dysfunction from scarring, and malignancy transformation.

The first-line treatment of vulvar LP is super potent topical steroids with a long-term focus, as described above for vulvar LS. Erosive mucosal LP tends to be more difficult to control. Any hypertrophic lesion that does not respond to treatment should be biopsied to exclude neoplasia.

Sexually transmitted infections need to be treated with specific agents. It is important to trace the partners of the patient and treat them. Sexual counseling is important and use of condoms should be promoted.

KEY POINTS

- Vulvar symptoms and lesions are a common problem for women.
- Most clinicians seek the assistance of dermatologists for the diagnosis and management of vulvar lesions because most of the STDs present as vulval lesions and gynecologists see such patients infrequently.
- Vulvar lesions can be benign, premalignant or malignant, and present as a pigmentary change, ulcer or growth.
- A thorough knowledge of the differential diagnosis is important for early diagnosis and appropriate management.
- The principles of management include general hygiene and appropriate care of skin, treatment of coexistent infection, control of pruritus, and condition specific treatment of STIs.

REFERENCES

1. Pathak D, Agrawal S, Dhali TK. Prevalence of and risk factors for the vulvar diseases in Nepal: a hospital based study. Int J Dermatol. 2011;50(2):161-7.
2. Harlow BL, Wise LA, Stewart EG. Prevalence and predictors of chronic lower genital tract discomfort. Am J Obstet Gynecol. 2001; 185(3):545-50.
3. Aoki T, Kushimoto H, Hishikawa Y, Savin JA. Nocturnal scratching and its relationship to the disturbed sleep of itchy subjects. Clin Exper Dermatol. 1991;16(4):268-72.
4. Weisshaar E. Successful treatment of genital pruritus using topical immunomodulators as a single therapy in multimorbid patients. Acta Derm Venereol. 2008;88(2):195-6.

SUGGESTED READING

1. American College of Obstetricians and Gynecologists (ACOG) (2008). Practice bulletin for diagnosis and management of vulvar skin disorders.
2. British Association for Sexual Health and HIV (BASHH) (2014). 2014 UK National Guideline on the Management of Vulval Conditions. [online] Available from http://content.guidelinecentral.com/guideline/get/pdf/3010 [Last accessed March, 2020].
3. British Association of Dermatologists (BAD) (2002). Guidelines for the management of lichen sclerosus.
4. European Academy of Dermatology and Venereology (EADV) (2017). 2016 European guideline for the management of vulval conditions.

42. Approach to a Woman Presenting with Amenorrhea

Ritu Sharma, Jasmeet K Monga

INTRODUCTION

Amenorrhea is the absence or cessation of menses.[1] The normal menstrual cycle is the result of interaction between hypothalamic–pituitary–ovarian axis, the outflow tract, and various environmental factors. A disruption at any level along this axis can lead to amenorrhea (Flowchart 1). Amenorrhea can be physiological or pathological. Physiological amenorrhea includes pregnancy, lactation, menopause, and prepubertal period. Pathological amenorrhea is further classified into primary and secondary amenorrhea.

Primary amenorrhea is defined as the absence of onset of periods by the age of 13 years in the absence of normal growth or secondary sexual development or as the absence of onset of periods by the age of 15 years in the presence of normal growth and secondary sexual development. Secondary amenorrhea, in a woman who has been previously menstruating, is defined as the cessation of periods for an interval of time equivalent to a total of at least three previous cycles or 6 months.[2-4] In the United States of America, the incidence of primary amenorrhea is < 1% and that of secondary amenorrhea is 5–7%.

Flowchart 1: Hypothalamic–pituitary–ovarian axis.

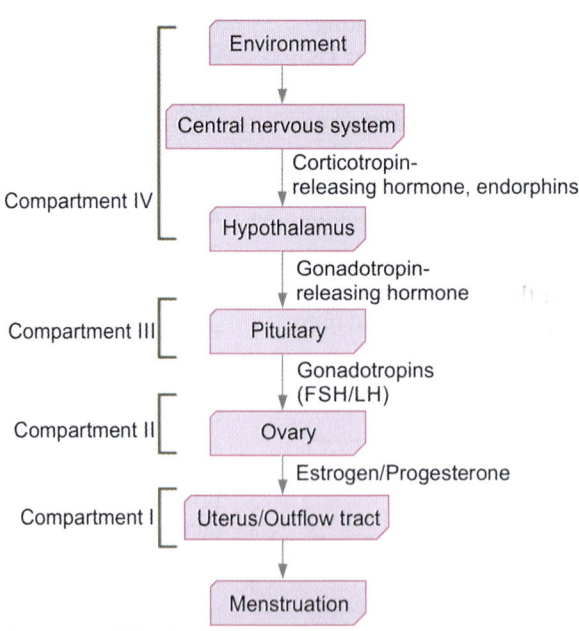

(FSH: follicle-stimulating hormone; LH: luteinizing hormone)

DIFFERENTIAL DIAGNOSIS

The causes of amenorrhea as per involvement of various compartments of the hypothalamic–pituitary–ovarian–uterine axis have been enumerated in Table 1. Though many factors responsible for amenorrhea are common, the most prevalent and unique cause of primary amenorrhea is gonadal dysgenesis followed by Mullerian agenesis whereas pregnancy is the most common cause of secondary amenorrhea. For identifying the underlying cause, systematic evaluation including a detailed history, thorough examination, and relevant investigations plays a pivotal role.

HISTORY

Since good history can reveal diagnosis in 85% of the cases, the following areas in the history need thorough evaluation.

History of Present Illness

History of childhood growth pattern: Evaluate growth, pubic hair, and breast development patterns in a woman with primary amenorrhea. Pubarche, thelarche, and adrenarche are delayed or absent in hypothalamic–pituitary failure. In isolated ovarian failure, adrenarche is normal, while pubarche and thelarche are delayed or absent. Early pubarche is associated with polycystic ovary syndrome (PCOS).

History of excessive weight loss or gain: This suggests that amenorrhea could be related to thyroid disorders, hypothalamic disorder, PCOS, or some chronic disease.

History of excessive exercise: Since excessive exercise can cause hypothalamic amenorrhea, inquire about the type of exercise and duration per week.

History of galactorrhea: This is present in association with hyperprolactinemia.

History of hirsutism, acne, alopecia, and deepening of voice: These features are associated with hyperandrogenic states such as PCOS, congenital adrenal hyperplasia, and adrenal or functioning ovarian tumor.

History of heat or cold intolerance, palpitations, altered bowel habit such as constipation or diarrhea: These are suggestive of thyroid disorders.

History of visual disturbances, vomiting, or headache: These are suggestive of raised intracranial tension which can be due to tumors such as pituitary macroadenomas and craniopharyngiomas.

History of hearing loss: This is one of the symptoms of Perrault syndrome. These patients have normal karyotype, gonadal dysgenesis, and neurosensory deafness. Hearing loss as a result of chronic suppurative otitis media (CSOM) may be associated with Turner's syndrome and Müllerian agenesis.

History of anosmia: This is the manifestation of Kallmann's syndrome or congenital gonadotropin-releasing hormone (GnRH) deficiency.

History of cyclical abdominal pain: This symptom is associated with outflow tract obstruction or cryptomenorrhea.

History of vasomotor symptoms: Symptoms such as hot flashes, dry vagina, dyspareunia, and sleep disturbances are suggestive of premature ovarian failure.

Past Medical and Surgical History

History of chronic illnesses such as chronic liver or kidney disorder, diabetes, epilepsy, tuberculosis, and irritable bowel syndrome is elicited as these can cause hypothalamic amenorrhea. Previous chemotherapy or

Table 1: Differential diagnosis of amenorrhea.[2,3,5]

Disorders of compartment I (uterus and outflow tract) Normal FSH, LH (Normogonadotropic)	Disorders of compartment II (ovary) Raised FSH, LH (Hypergonadotropic)	Disorders of compartment III (pituitary) Low FSH, LH (Hypogonadotropic)	Disorders of compartment IV (hypothalamus, central nervous system) Low FSH, LH (Hypogonadotropic)	Others
Müllerian agenesis Androgen insensitivity syndrome Asherman's syndrome: Cervical stenosis Surgical removal of uterus	Gonadal dysgenesis: • Turner's syndrome: Most common (50%) • Turner's mosaic syndrome • Perrault syndrome • Swyer syndrome Vanishing testes syndrome Premature ovarian failure: • Chromosomal abnormality: Turner's mosaic syndrome • Autoimmune • Post chemotherapy/post radiotherapy/postsurgical • Infections (mumps and tuberculosis) • Galactosemia • Idiopathic Premature menopause	Hypopituitarism: • Infections, radiotherapy, surgery • Sheehan's syndrome • Congenital: Mutation of β-subunit of follicle-stimulating hormone (FSH) • Intracranial tumors (unclassified pituitary adenoma) Hyperprolactinemia: • Prolactin >100 ng/mL • Pituitary adenoma • Prolactin <100 ng/mL • Drugs (oral contraceptives, antidepressants, antiepileptics, antipsychotics, opiates, and cocaine) • Increased ectopic production (prolactin-secreting tumor in hypopharynx, ovarian dermoid, teratoma, gonadoblastoma, renal cell carcinoma, and bronchogenic carcinoma) • Disturbed metabolism (chronic liver and renal disease) • Breastfeeding/breast stimulation	Congenital abnormalities: • Isolated gonadotropin-releasing hormone (GnRH) deficiency Kallmann's syndrome Constitutional delay: Eating disorder (anorexia/bulimia) Excessive exercise/psychological stress: Intracranial tumors (craniopharyngioma) Hypothalamic destruction (due to infections, neurosarcoidosis, tuberculosis, radiotherapy, surgery), Thalassemia major Chronic diseases (liver, kidney, or thyroid disorder, and diabetes) Drugs (oral contraceptives, antidepressants, antiepileptics, antipsychotics, opiates, and cocaine)	Physiological: (Pregnancy, lactation, menopause) Thyroid disorder Hyperandrogenic states: • PCOS • Androgen-secreting tumors • Cushing's syndrome • Congenital adrenal hyperplasia • Adult-onset congenital adrenal hyperplasia • Acromegaly Immunodeficiency states

radiotherapy may result in premature ovarian failure or hypothalamic amenorrhea due to related stress. Any history of psychiatric illness is important as amenorrhea can be due to the disease itself or drugs being used for treatment.

Surgical procedures such as transcervical endometrial resection, thermal balloon ablation, or repeated uterine curettage may lead to destruction of the basal layer of endometrium and surgeries such as Manchester's repair and conization can result in cervical stenosis and ultimately amenorrhea.

Menstrual History

Menstrual history is relevant while evaluating secondary amenorrhea. Ask the age of menarche, date of last menstrual period, duration of cycle, flow, and any associated dysmenorrhea. PCOS is associated with oligomenorrhea or amenorrhea without dysmenorrhea, whereas in Asherman's syndrome, the menstrual cycles are usually regular with scanty flow which may be painful. Secondary amenorrhea due to premature ovarian failure may be preceded by progressive decrease in flow and or infrequent menstrual cycles.

Sexual History

Pregnancy must be excluded in all sexually active women even in girls with primary amenorrhea.

Obstetric History

Obstetric history is relevant while evaluating secondary amenorrhea. Previous history of postpartum hemorrhage and failed lactation suggests Sheehan's syndrome. History of repeated abortions and/or curettage, post-abortion, or puerperal sepsis is suggestive of Asherman's syndrome. History of suction and evacuation followed by amenorrhea and cyclical abdominal pain may be suggestive of cervical stenosis and associated cryptomenorrhea. History of use of hormonal contraceptives such as combined pills, centchroman, depot-medroxyprogesterone acetate (DMPA), norethindrone enanthate (NETEN), or levonorgestrel-intrauterine system (LNG-IUS) is important, as their use may lead to hypomenorrhea or amenorrhea.

Dietary History

A detailed dietary history is important, as eating disorders such as anorexia nervosa and bulimia are associated with hypothalamic amenorrhea.

Family History

The pubertal and menstrual history of the mother and sisters of the patient is important, as it can point toward constitutional delay in puberty. History of infertility and genetic disorders in the family can help in making the diagnosis in women with primary amenorrhea.

Drug History

Antipsychotics, antiepileptics, hormonal contraceptives, antitubercular drugs, opiates, and cocaine all can cause amenorrhea.

History of Head Injury

Head injury can result in involvement of hypothalamus or pituitary leading to amenorrhea.

EXAMINATION

Good history combined with thorough general physical and local examination is required to clinch the important diagnostic clues.

General Physical Examination

Observe the stature of the patient; stature abnormalities are associated with chromosomal abnormalities. Women with Turner's syndrome are short stature whereas those with androgen insensitivity syndrome are usually tall. Body mass index is calculated which is usually high in PCOS and Cushing's syndrome but low in anorexia nervosa.

Look for somatic stigmata such as webbed neck, low-set hair line and ears, short fourth metacarpal and metatarsals, broad shelf-like chest, and widely spaced nipples, which are associated with Turner's syndrome; buffalo hump, central obesity, hypertension and proximal muscle weakness are typical of Cushing's syndrome.

Note the features suggestive of hyperandrogenism such as acne, hirsutism, alopecia, deepening of voice and oily skin.

Thyroid swelling, exophthalmos and palpitations, if present, point toward thyroid disorders.

Hypothermia, bradycardia, hypotension and decreased subcutaneous fat raise suspicion of anorexia nervosa.

Skin examination should be done carefully, as its state can arouse suspicion of certain diseases. Yellow skin is associated with anorexia, oily skin with hyperandrogenic states, thin parchment skin and striae with Cushing's syndrome, vitiligo or increased pigmentation of palmer creases with primary adrenal insufficiency, warm and moist skin with hyperthyroidism, and acanthosis nigricans with PCOS and diabetes mellitus.

Cardiovascular abnormalities such as coarctation of aorta may be present in patients with Turner's syndrome. Chest findings can be there in case of neurosarcoidosis and tuberculosis.

Examination of ears should be done as neurosensory deafness is present in Perrault syndrome and chronic otitis media in Turner's syndrome. Auditory involvement is also observed in patients with Müllerian agenesis.

Examination of eyes is done in women presenting with associated visual disturbance or other features suggestive of pituitary tumor.

Secondary Sex Characters and Breast Examination

Axillary and pubic hair development is dependent on adrenal and ovarian androgens. Tanner staging is done. Axillary and pubic hair may be normally developed in Mullerian agenesis, gonadal dysgenesis and secondary amenorrhea. They may be sparse or absent in panhypopituitarism, androgen insensitivity syndrome, autoimmune premature ovarian failure, and autoimmune primary adrenal insufficiency.

Breast examination is done carefully. Tanner staging will help in assessing the developmental stage of breasts. Breasts are well developed in Mullerian agenesis and androgen insensitivity syndrome, not developed in Turner's syndrome, gonadal dysgenesis and underdeveloped in constitutional delay. Galactorrhea, if present, is suggestive of hyperprolactinemia.

Abdominal Examination

Presence of hepatosplenomegaly may point toward some chronic disease, suprapubic mass due to hematocolpos and hematometra suggests obstructed Mullerian abnormalities and inguinal hernia with palpable undescended testis may be found in androgen insensitivity syndrome.

Examination of External Genitalia

External genitalia are examined and any signs of virilization are noted. External genitalia are normally developed in Mullerian agenesis and gonadal dysgenesis. Labia minora are underdeveloped in androgen insensitivity syndrome. Enlargement of clitoris is suggestive of hyperandrogenism.

Pelvic Examination

Pelvic examination is done to determine the patency of vagina, and presence and size of uterus. The vagina may be absent or there may be an imperforate hymen or transverse vaginal septum indicating outflow tract obstruction (Figs. 1 and 2). In case of hematocolpos due to imperforate hymen, there will be a bluish bulge at the introitus with positive cough impulse sign, which is not seen in case of transverse vaginal septum. Vaginal mucosa is thin and pale with absent rugosities due to estrogen deficiency in premature ovarian failure. Uterus and vagina are normal in Asherman's syndrome and chronic diseases, rudimentary or absent in Mullerian agenesis and androgen insensitivity syndrome, and enlarged in pregnancy and hematometra.

Per Rectal Examination

Per rectal examination is indicated to find out the size of uterus or a pelvic mass in a young unmarried girl who is not sexually active. It also helps in appreciating the level of obstruction in genital tract by the distance of the bulge from the anal or vaginal opening as felt on per rectal examination.

INVESTIGATIONS[2,3,6,7]

Pregnancy test is the initial step in the diagnostic evaluation of secondary as well as primary amenorrhea associated with well-developed secondary sexual characters and intact uterus. Provisional diagnosis made on the basis of history and examination directs further workup. It is essential to determine the compartment which is affected and then to establish the precise cause so as to initiate the specific treatment. Algorithms for clinical approach to patients with primary and secondary amenorrhea are shown in Flowcharts 2 and 3, respectively, and various investigations that are required to confirm the diagnosis are discussed in the following text.

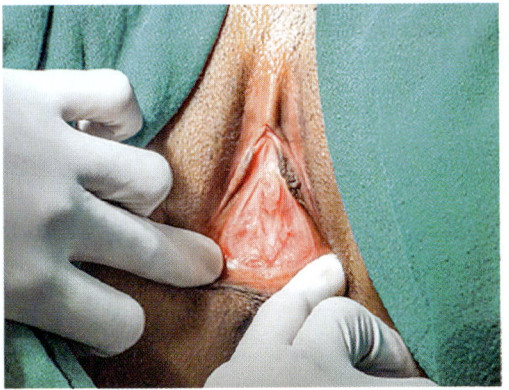

Fig. 1: Absent vaginal opening in vaginal agenesis.

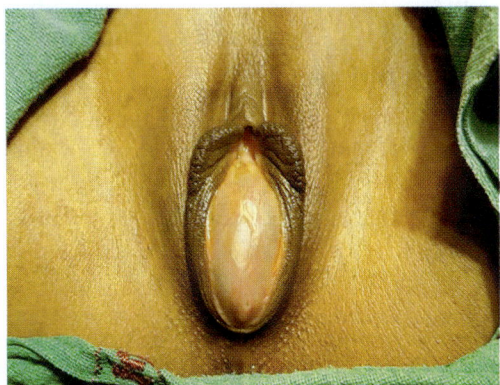

Fig. 2: Imperforate hymen.

Section 2: Gynecology

Flowchart 2: Algorithm for clinical approach to primary amenorrhea.[2,3,5]

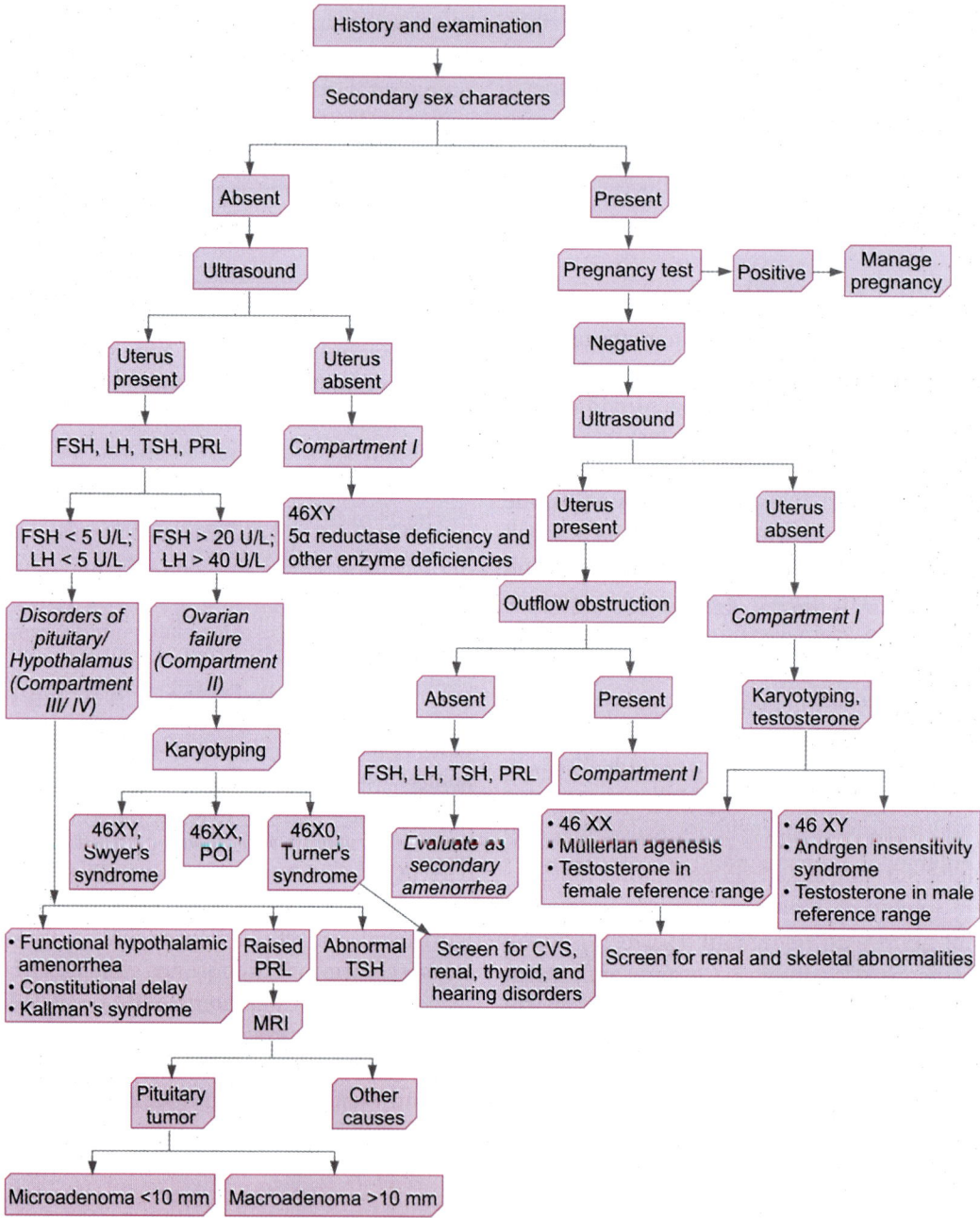

(FSH: follicle-stimulating hormone; LH: luteinizing hormone; MRI: magnetic resonance imaging; POI: primary ovarian insufficiency; PRL: prolactin; TSH: thyroid-stimulating hormone)

Flowchart 3: Algorithm for clinical approach to secondary amenorrhea.[2,3,5]

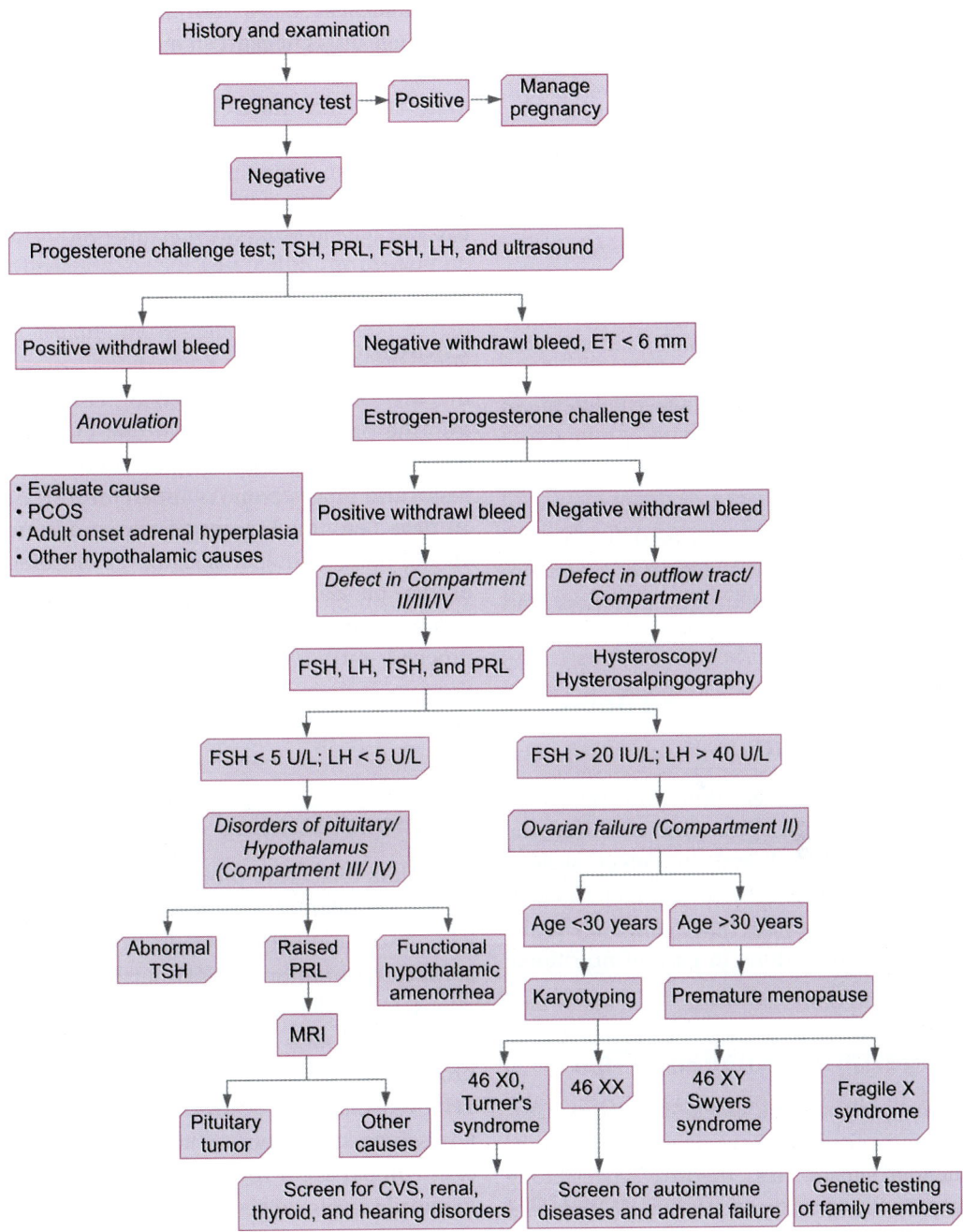

(FSH: follicle-stimulating hormone; LH: luteinizing hormone; MRI: magnetic resonance imaging; PCOS: polycystic ovarian syndrome; PRL: prolactin; TSH: thyroid-stimulating hormone)

Urinary Pregnancy Test

Urinary pregnancy test is done in both primary and secondary amenorrhea.

Basic Blood Investigations

Basic blood investigations are done to diagnose underlying chronic systemic diseases such as diabetes mellitus and liver and renal disorders. These include complete blood count, erythrocyte sedimentation rate (ESR), liver function test (LFT), kidney function test (KFT), urinalysis and blood sugar levels and glucose tolerance test. Other blood investigations such as serum calcium and phosphorous, antinuclear antibodies, thyroid antibodies, rheumatoid factor, and galactose-1-phosphate uridyltransferase deficiency are offered, if indicated (suspicion of premature ovarian failure, autoimmune disorders, and galactosemia).

Skeletal Skiagrams and Bone Mineral Density

Skeletal skiagrams are done to assess bone age (delayed bone age implies constitutional delay in puberty) and to detect skeletal abnormalities (present in 12% of cases of Mullerian agenesis[2]). Bone mineral density measurement is done in case of nutritional disorders.

Progesterone Challenge Test

In the progesterone challenge test, progesterone is given for 7–10 days in the recommended doses (e.g. medroxyprogesterone acetate 10 mg orally once a day). Withdrawal bleeding occurs within 2 weeks of conclusion of drug administration. Positive withdrawal test indicates anovulation and is suggestive of estrogen-primed endometrium (serum estradiol level is ≥ 50 pg/mL and endometrial thickness is ≥ 6 mm). If progesterone challenge test is negative, it means that estrogen priming of endometrium is lacking or there is outflow tract obstruction. To differentiate between the two, we should proceed with estrogen progesterone challenge test. However, withdrawal bleed has poor sensitivity and specificity for ovarian function.

Estrogen–progesterone Challenge Test

In the estrogen–progesterone challenge test, the patient is prescribed oral estrogen daily for 21 days (e.g., 2 mg estradiol orally daily) and progesterone is added for the last 10 days (e.g., medroxyprogesterone acetate 10 mg orally daily). If withdrawal bleeding occurs, the defect lies in either the ovaries or the pituitary–hypothalamic axis and we proceed further to differentiate between the two. If there is no bleeding, it indicates outflow tract abnormality and we proceed accordingly.

Hormonal Studies

The initial endocrine profile includes serum follicle-stimulating hormone (FSH), luteinizing hormone (LH), prolactin, and thyroid-stimulating hormone (TSH); further testing needs to be decided. The hormonal levels should be done 2 weeks after the estrogen-progesterone challenge test, as the FSH and LH levels may be suppressed. Gonadotropin levels help to diagnose whether the defect is in compartment II, III, or IV. Raised gonadotropin levels suggest ovarian failure while low levels indicate pituitary or hypothalamic disorder. Gonadotropin-releasing hormone stimulation test can be done to assess whether the defect lies in compartment IV or III.

Raised serum levels of prolactin are indicative of hyperprolactinemic states responsible for amenorrhea (compartment III). High levels of prolactin inhibit normal GnRH pulse rhythm resulting in low levels of gonadotropin. Amenorrhea in thyroid disorders is associated with raised levels of thyrotropin-releasing hormone (TRH) and thyroxin. Raised levels of TRH stimulate lactotropes which lead to increased secretion of prolactin. High levels of thyroxin inhibit FSH release leading to amenorrhea.

Hyperandrogenic states are diagnosed by elevated serum levels of testosterone, dehydroepiandrosterone sulfate, and 17-hydroxyprogesterone (Table 2). Etiology in PCOS is

Table 2: Hormonal assays.[2,3,8]

Hormone	Serum levels	Evaluate
Prolactin: Normal level—0–20 ng/mL	• *Raised level*: <100 ng/mL • *Raised level*: >100 ng/mL	• Drugs, chronic diseases, and ectopic production • Prolactinoma (compartment III)
Thyroid-stimulating hormone (TSH): Normal level—0.34–4.25 μIU/mL	• Raised TSH level • Low TSH level	• Hypothyroidism • Hyperthyroidism
Follicle-stimulating hormone (FSH) Luteinizing hormone (LH): Normal level—5–20 IU/L	• Low level <5 IU/L or normal level • Raised level FSH >20 IU/L, LH >40 IU/L	• Pituitary and hypothalamus (compartment III/IV) • Ovaries (compartment II)
Serum estradiol: Normal level—20–443 pg/mL (follicular phase—30–120 pg/mL; Preovulatory—130–370 pg/mL, at times >400 pg/mL)	Low estradiol levels	Ovaries (compartment II)
Testosterone: Normal level—20–80 ng/dL	• *Raised level*: ≤150 ng/dL • *Raised level*: ≥150 ng/dL	• Hyperandrogenic chronic anovulation • Androgen-secreting tumor
Dehydroepiandrosterone sulfate: Normal level—80–350 μg/dL	• *Raised level*: ≤ 700 μg/dL • *Raised level*: ≥ 700 μg/dL	• Hyperandrogenic chronic anovulation • Adrenal or ovarian tumor
17-Hydroxyprogesterone Normal morning levels (in follicular phase): <200 ng/mL	• *Raised level*: ≥200–800 ng/dL • *Raised level*: >800 ng/dL	• Do adrenocorticotropic stimulation test to diagnose congenital adrenal hyperplasia • Nonclassical congenital adrenal hyperplasia
*Dexamethasone suppression test	Level >1.8 μg/dL is significant	Cushing's syndrome

Low dose: Early morning cortisol levels at 8.00 am; give 1 mg of dexamethasone orally at 11.00 pm and measure plasma cortisol level at 8.00 am next morning (normal expected value of plasma cortisol is <1.8 μg/dL).
High dose: Plasma cortisol levels at 8.00 am; give 8 mg of dexamethasone at 11.00 pm and measure plasma cortisol levels at 8.00 am next morning (>50% reduction in plasma cortisol is normal).

complex related to insulin resistance, raised LH levels, and failure of normal follicular development and ovulation.

Imaging Studies

Pelvic ultrasonography is done to find out if the outflow tract is normal or there are any congenital abnormalities of the uterus, cervix, vagina, and ovaries. We can also diagnose hematocolpos or hematometra. Magnetic resonance imaging is required to confirm the findings of ultrasonography; for a better understanding of the nature, type, and level of the defect; to rule out urinary tract abnormalities such as ectopic kidney, horseshoe kidney, or renal agenesis, which are seen in one third of patients of Mayer–Rokitansky–Kuster–Hauser syndrome[2] and in Kallmann's syndrome; and to evaluate central nervous system for any tumor if there are signs and symptoms of raised intracranial tension (headache and visual disturbances) or elevated levels of prolactin are present.

Karyotyping

Karyotyping is indicated in women presenting with primary amenorrhea with absent uterus and premature ovarian failure at an age of <30 years to find out any associated chromosomal anomalies and offer screening to family members accordingly. In women with primary amenorrhea and presence of Y chromosome, as in androgen insensitivity syndrome, gonadectomy is indicated after complete physical growth to prevent gonadal malignancy. It also diagnoses Turner's syndrome.

Hysteroscopy or Hysterosalpingography

Hysteroscopy or hysterosalpingography is required to confirm the diagnosis of Asherman's syndrome.

Biopsy of Endometrium and Ovaries

Endometrial biopsy is indicated in secondary amenorrhea to know about the state of endometrium and rule out endometrial tuberculosis. Ovarian biopsy is rarely required to know about the exact state of folliculogenesis in primary and secondary amenorrhea.

Leptin

Leptin is a cytokine secreted by adipocytes, hypothalamus, and pituitary gland, which in turn affect neuroendocrine and reproductive function. Its levels are decreased in malnutrition and eating disorders.

Describes the comparison between three common causes of primary amenorrheas (Table 3).

MANAGEMENT[9-12]

Table 4 lists the various treatment options according to the cause of amenorrhea. Surgery is the treatment of choice for obstructive causes and intracranial tumors such as craniopharyngioma and macroadenoma. In women with premature ovarian failure and planned gonadectomy, the treatment is directed toward hormone replacement therapy till the age of menopause to prevent harmful effects on the heart and bones. Diseases such as hypothyroidism and hyperprolactinemia can be treated medically. PCOS is treated by lifestyle modification and hormonal therapy.

KEY POINTS

- Detailed workup including a comprehensive history and a thorough examination is essential to reach the most probable cause of amenorrhea.

Table 3: Comparison between Turner's syndrome, androgen insensitivity syndrome and mullerian agenesis.

Clinical features	Turner's syndrome	AIS	Mullerian agenesis
Primary amenorrhea	+	+	+
Kary type	45 × O	46 × Y	46 × X
Breast	Absent	Developed	Developed
Pubic and axillary hair	Sparse	Absent	Present
Vagina	Present	Blind	Blind
Uterus	Small streak	Absent	Absent
Gonads	Ovaries	Testis	Ovaries

Table 4: Management of amenorrhea.[9-12]

Level of abnormality	Differential diagnosis	Treatment
Compartment I	• Imperforate hymen • Transverse vaginal septum • Absent uterus	• Hymenoplasty • Vaginoplasty • Creation of neovagina if absent vagina Gonadectomy after 16 years if Y chromosome detected
	• Tubercular endometritis • Asherman's syndrome • Cervical stenosis	• ATT • Hysteroscopic adhesiolysis • Cervical dilatation
Compartment II	• Premature ovarian failure • Gonadal dysgenesis	• HRT • Gonadectomy after 16 years if Y chromosome detected • IVF with donor oocyte for infertility
Compartment III	• Hyperprolactinemia • Tumors (adenoma)	• Bromcriptine or cabergoline • Surgery if macroadenoma • HRT
Compartment IV	Anorexia nervosa	• HRT • Ovulation induction with gonadotropins in infertile women

(ATT: antitubercular treatment; HRT: hormone replacement therapy; IVF: in vitro fertilization)

- Stepwise approach plays a vital role as it systematically excludes causes related to various compartments and helps to initiate the basic treatment accordingly.
- Cause of amenorrhea should be accurately diagnosed and treated as its future implications on fertility, risk of endometrial cancer, and osteoporosis can significantly affect the quality of life.
- In androgen insensitivity syndrome, gonadectomy is warranted after complete physical growth to prevent gonadal malignancy.
- Infertility in premature ovarian failure requires egg donation and surveillance is needed in these patients for other autoimmune diseases and adrenal failure.
- Anovulation due to hyperprolactinemia is managed medically (cabergoline/bromocriptine) or surgically (pituitary tumor).
- PCOS treatment involves lifestyle modifications, weight reduction, and symptomatic treatment.
- Androgenic tumors must be managed surgically.
- Eating disorders, excessive exercise, and constitutional delay are managed by counseling, dietary supplements and psychiatrist consultation. The treatment

may be multidisciplinary involving endocrinologist, neurosurgeon, physician, and psychiatrist, if needed.

REFERENCES

1. Stedman TL. Stedman's Medical Dictionary, 28th edition. Philadelphia: Lippincott Williams and Wilkins; 2013.
2. Taylor HS, Pal L, Seli E. Amenorrhea. In: Speroff L, Fritz Marc A (Eds). Clinical Gynecologic Endocrinology and Infertility, 8th edition. Wolter Kluwer: Lippincott Williams and Wilkins; 2018. pp. 435-94.
3. Berek JS. Amenorrhea. Berek & Novak's Gynecology, 16th edition. Wolters Kluwer Health/Lippincott Williams and Wilkins; 2019. pp. 866-88.
4. Practice Committee of American Society for Reproductive Medicine. Current evaluation of amenorrhea. Fertil Steril. 2008;90(5 suppl):S219-25.
5. Klein DA, Paradise SL, Reeder RM. Amenorrhea: a systematic approach to diagnosis and management. Am Fam Physician. 2019;100(1):39-48.
6. Nelson LM. Clinical practice. Primary ovarian insufficiency. N Engl J Med. 2009;360(6):606-14.
7. Nakamura S, Douchi T, Oki T, Ijuin H, Yamamoto S, Nagata Y. Relationship between sonographic endometrial thickness and progestin-induced withdrawal bleeding. Obstet Gynecol. 1996;87(5 pt 1):722-5.
8. Cunningham FG, Leveno KJ, Bloom SL, Hauth JC, Rouse D, Spong CY. William Obstetrics, 25th edition. New York: McGraw Hill; 2018. pp. 1258-9.
9. Capito C, Leclair MD, Arnaud A, et al. 46, XY pure gonadal dysgenesis: clinical presentations and management of tumor risk. J Pediatr Urol. 2011;7(1):72-5.
10. Committee on Gynecologic practice. American College of Obstetricians and Gynecologists. Committee opinion No 698: Hormone therapy in primary ovarian insufficiency. Obstet Gynecol. 2017;129(5):e134-41.
11. Committee on adolescent health care. American College of Obstetricians and Gynecologists. Committee opinion No 702: Female athelete triad. Obstet Gynecol. 2017; 129(6):e160-7.
12. Kyriakidis M, Caetano L, Anastasiadou N, et al. Functional hypothalamic amenorrhea: leptin treatment, dietary intervention and counseling as alternatives to traditional practice-systematic review. Eur J Obstet Gynecol Reprod Biol. 2016;198:131-7.

SUGGESTED READING

1. Committee on adolescent health care. American College of Obstetricians and Gynecologists. Committee opinion No 728: Mullerian agenesis—Diagnosis, management and treatment. Obstet Gynecol. 2018;131(1):e35-42.
2. Gordon CM, Ackerman KE, Berga SL, Kaplan JR, Mastorakos G, Misra M, et al. (2017). Endocrine Society (ES): Clinical practice guideline on functional hypothalamic amenorrhea. [online] Available from https://www.endocrine.org/clinical-practice-guidelines/hypothalamic-amenorrhea. [Last accessed February, 2020].
3. Webber L, Davis M, Anderson R, et al. ESHRE Guideline: management of women with premature ovarian insufficiency. Human Reproduction. 2016;31(5):926-37.

43. Approach to a Woman Presenting with Hirsutism

Jasmeet K Monga

INTRODUCTION

Hirsutism is defined as the presence of excessive terminal coarse hair in females in a male-like pattern, i.e., in androgen-dependent areas. This includes areas such as upper lip, chin, midsternum, upper and lower abdomen, upper and lower back, and buttocks. It can be a result of either increased production of androgens or increased sensitivity of receptors to circulating androgens. It affects between 5 and 15% of women surveyed.[1,2] Hirsutism needs to be differentiated from hypertrichosis, which is a generalized vellus, fine lightly pigmented nonsexual hair growth that may be hereditary or due to some medications. This extremely disturbing condition can have a huge negative impact on the patient's psychological, social, and emotional well-being. It is important to understand that hirsutism is a symptom and not a diagnosis. It can be a manifestation of a serious underlying disorder that may have implications in terms of treatment, counseling, or prognosis. The fundamental concern, while handling these patients, is to decide whether hirsutism is due to an underlying disorder or it is idiopathic or familial. However, in both cases, this condition needs to be managed sensitively as it is primarily a cosmetic and psychological problem.

DIFFERENTIAL DIAGNOSIS

Differential diagnosis of hirsutism is given in Box 1.

HISTORY

An in-depth history in most instances can point toward the etiology. The onset and progression are important as sudden onset at a later age, rapid progression, and severe hirsutism and presence of symptoms of virilism are suggestive of an androgen-producing tumor of ovarian or adrenal origin.

> **Box 1:** Differential diagnosis of hirsutism.
> - Polycystic ovary syndrome (PCOS)
> - Nonclassic congenital adrenal hyperplasia (NCAH)
> - Hyperandrogenism, insulin resistance, and acanthosis nigricans (HAIR-AN) syndrome
> - Ovarian hyperthecosis
> - *Androgen-secreting tumors*:
>   - Ovarian origin:
>   » Sertoli–Leydig cell tumors (arrhenoblastoma and androblastoma)
>   » Granulosa-theca cell tumor
>   » Hilus cell tumor
>   - Adrenal origin:
>   » Adenoma or carcinoma
> - *Endocrine disorders*:
>   - Cushing's syndrome
>   - Acromegaly
>   - Hypothyroidism
>   - Hyperprolactinemia
> - *Drug induced*: Danazol
> - Idiopathic hirsutism

> **Box 2:** Drugs causing hirsutism.
> - Testosterone
> - Danazol
> - Anabolic steroids
> - Progestins
> - Phenothiazines
> - Sodium valproate
> - Alpha-methyldopa
> - Reserpine
> - Metoclopramide

Changes in weight and facial contour, disproportionate fat distribution, and appearance of purple striae are all features of cortisol excess. Hair loss or male-pattern balding and acne point toward androgen excess. Details of pubertal development and its relation to onset of excessive hair growth need to be elicited, as excessive hair growth around the time of puberty is common in polycystic ovary syndrome (PCOS) and non-classic congenital adrenal hyperplasia (NCAH).

It is important to elicit a thorough history of any medications or local application of hair-stimulating drugs that can lead to hirsutism. In athletes, in patients with endometriosis, or in those with history of sexual dysfunction, inquiry must be made into the use of anabolic or androgenic steroids. Use of testosterone gel by a partner must be inquired into. Drugs that can cause hirsutism are listed in Box 2.

Certain food supplements contain dehydroepiandrosterone or androstenedione, which can cause hirsutism in women. History of any treatment taken or hair removal method used.

Menstrual History

History of menstrual irregularity, such as oligomenorrhea or amenorrhea, is suggestive of ovulatory dysfunction and requires further evaluation. Infertility, family history of type 2 diabetes mellitus (DM), hypertension, and obesity may be associated with ovarian dysfunction even in the absence of obvious menstrual disturbances.

Menopause is associated with increase in facial hair growth in the absence of any other pathology. But hirsutism associated with other features of hyperandrogenism developing for the first time, or rapidly progressing in the postmenopausal period, needs to be evaluated as it may be a manifestation of an underlying androgen-secreting tumor or ovarian hyperthecosis.

Obstetric History

A detailed reproductive history is important. History of infertility may point toward PCOS. The treatment of hirsutism by oral contraceptive pills can prevent pregnancy. Moreover, women who are being treated with antiandrogens need to be counseled regarding avoiding pregnancy during treatment to prevent adverse effects on the growing male fetus.

Family History

A familial predisposition is seen with PCOS, NCAH, type 2 DM, and idiopathic hirsutism.

EXAMINATION

The physical examination of the patient aims at an assessment of the severity of hirsutism, i.e., the extent, type, and pattern of the hair growth, any signs of virilization, any underlying medical disorders, and presence of any ovarian or adrenal tumor.

Hypertrichosis, or generalized excessive hair growth in a nonsexual pattern, may be hereditary or drug induced (e.g., phenytoin and cyclosporine) and should not be confused with hirsutism.

As far as the evaluation of severity of hirsutism is concerned, a visual score, Ferriman-Gallwey (FG) score, is used.[2] This involves

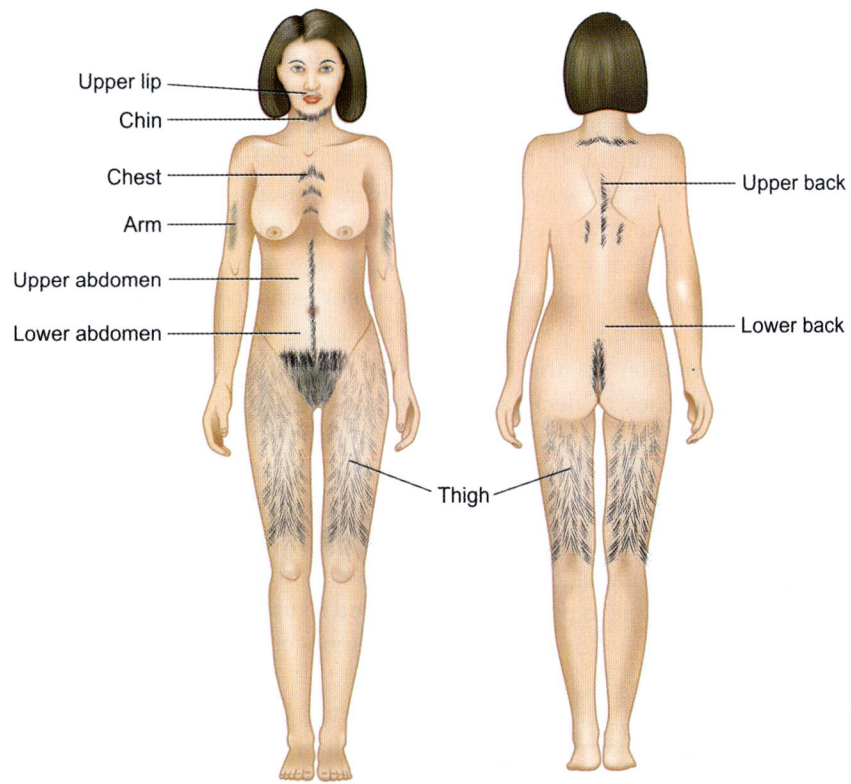

Fig. 1: Sites for assessment of hair growth in Ferriman–Gallwey scoring.

scoring the hair at nine androgen-sensitive body areas (Fig. 1) from 0 to 4 depending on the texture, thickness, and pigmentation of the hair. The total score is calculated by adding the scores from all nine areas. FG total scores that define hirsutism vary according to ethnicity. A score of 8 or more is generally diagnostic of hirsutism. Unwanted, localized, excessive hair growth in the absence of an abnormal visual score is a common normal variant. But in the presence of menstrual disturbances, even a low visual score is important as it might be associated with hyperandrogenism. The shortcomings of this scoring system include noninclusion of certain important areas such as buttocks and sideburns, lack of importance to focal hair growth, and lack of objectivity.

General physical examination should include height, weight, body mass index (BMI), and waist–hip circumference ratio (WHR). To calculate BMI, weight in kilograms is divided by square of height in meters (kg/m^2). BMI and waist–hip ratio are reflective of presence of obesity and the pattern of fat distribution. In android obesity, i.e., central or apple-shaped obesity, waist–hip ratio is >0.85 and it is associated with significant morbidity. A waist circumference of >35 inch is associated with increased risk of DM and cardiovascular disease. Any other signs of androgen excess such as presence of acne, signs of defeminization such as decrease in breast size and loss of female body contour, and signs of virilization such as deepening of voice, balding, clitoromegaly, and increase in size of muscles of shoulder girdle should be looked for. Plethora, centripetal obesity, purple striae, and enlarged dorsocervical and supraclavicular fat pads are all suggestive of cortisol excess in the patient. Clitoromegaly is suspected when the clitoris protrudes beyond the hood. Clitoromegaly is defined as a clitoral index, i.e. the product of sagittal and transverse diameters of glans, of >35 mm^2. In normal women, it is <25 mm^2. Acanthosis nigricans, i.e., pigmentation on the crural folds such as side and back of neck, axilla, underneath breasts, and acrochordons or skin tags are suggestive of insulin resistance.

The patient also needs to be evaluated for thyroid enlargement and galactorrhea. A careful abdominal and bimanual pelvic or per rectal examination is done to pick up any adrenal or ovarian mass.

INVESTIGATIONS

Investigations are based on history and examination. The aim is to find out specific androgen involved, its circulating levels, organ of origin, cause, and its metabolic effects.

Androgen levels should be evaluated in all women with an abnormal visual score. In women with unwanted hair growth restricted to local areas, in the absence of any menstrual disturbances, and absence of an abnormal visual score, testing for elevated androgen levels is not required. In these women, the likelihood of picking up an underlying disorder is low.[3]

In the initial assessment, early morning serum hormone levels are assessed in the first week of onset of periods and include serum testosterone levels both total and free, sex hormone-binding globulin (SHBG), dehydroepiandrosterone sulfate (DHEA-S), 17 hydroxyprogesterone (17-OHP), follicle-stimulating hormone (FSH), and luteinizing hormone (LH). The normal levels of serum testosterone are 20–80 ng/dL and levels of >150 ng/dL suggests androgen-producing tumor. Serum testosterone levels may be normal in majority of women with mild hirsutism. Moreover, serum testosterone levels may not correlate well with the severity of hirsutism due to variations in individual's hair receptor sensitivity to testosterone. Raised plasma-free testosterone levels in patients with normal levels of circulating testosterone may result in subtle hyperandrogenism. Obese woman may have a high free testosterone value because of reduced SHBG attributable to hyperinsulinemia.

A high DHEA-S level is suggestive of excess androgen production of adrenal origin and if substantially elevated, the presence of adrenocortical neoplasm should be ruled out.

Serum DHEA levels are markedly raised (Flowchart 1) in women with hirsutism due to adrenal cause such as congenital adrenal hyperplasia (CAH) or adrenal tumor.

Measurement of 17-OHP levels is useful in diagnosing NCAH due to 21-hydroxylase deficiency. A level of <200 ng/mL excludes the disorder with 90% certainty. A high level of >800 ng/dL suggests presence of this enzyme deficiency. If the result is equivocal (200–800 ng/dL), then the baseline 17-OHP levels are followed by 250 µg of synthetic adrenocorticotropic hormone (ACTH) intravenously and a repeat sample of 17-OHP is collected after 1 hour; a level of >1,500 ng/dL is diagnostic of NCAH.

In women with clinical evidence of cortisol excess, overnight dexamethasone suppression test can help to diagnose Cushing's syndrome. Plasma cortisol level of >1.8 mcg/dL at 8 AM after 1 mg dexamethasone at midnight is significant. Measuring 24 hours urine free cortisol can help in

Flowchart 1: Algorithm for clinical approach to a woman presenting with hirsutism.

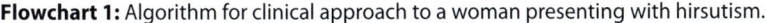

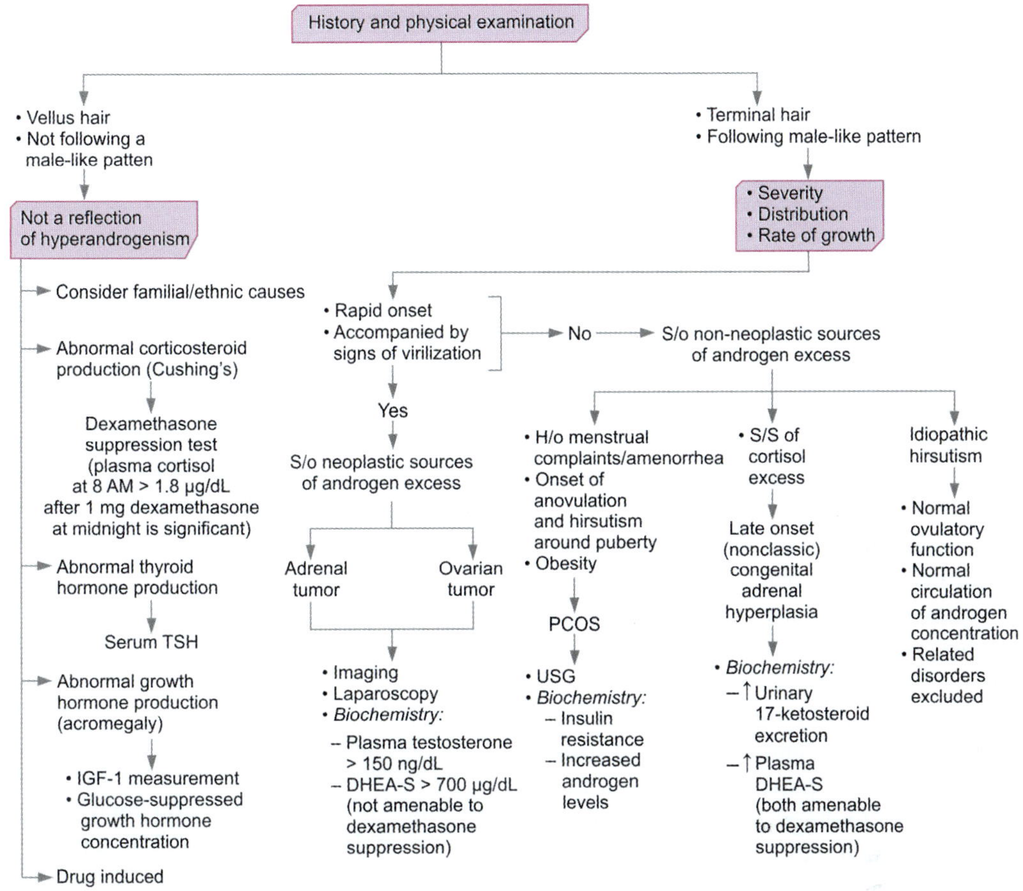

(DHEA-S: dehydroepiandrosterone sulfate; H/o: history of; IGF-1: insulin-like growth factor-1; PCOS: polycystic ovary syndrome; S/o: suggestive of; S/S: signs and symptoms; TSH: thyroid-stimulating hormone; USG: ultrasonography)

confirming the diagnosis of Cushing's syndrome in these women.

In clinical practice, in women presenting as adult hirsutism with virilization and oligomenorrhea, the priority is to separate the ovarian from the adrenal androgen overproduction as the underlying cause. This is possible by dexamethasone suppression test. Oral dexamethasone 0.5 mg is administered orally every 6 hour for 2 days. Blood sample is obtained pre- and postadministration of dexamethasone for measuring the level of DHEA-S, Testosterone and Cortisol. The results are interpreted to differentiate between adrenal and ovarian source of androgens (Table 1).

The usefulness of FSH and LH levels and deranged LH:FSH ratio is limited for the diagnosis of PCOS in women with hyperandrogenism. The LH:FSH ratio is normal, i.e., 1:1 in 50% of women with PCOS. However, a high LH level is associated with a poor response to attempted induction of ovulation and an increased risk of abortion in women with PCOS.

Table 1: Interpretation of dexamethasone suppression test.

Source of androgen	DHEA-S	Testosterone	Cortisol
Adrenal	>60% suppression	>40% suppression	
Ovarian	Suppressed	Not suppressed	Suppressed
Combined	Suppressed	<40% suppression	Suppressed
Cushing's syndrome or adrenal cancer	Not suppressed		

In women with irregular cycles and hirsutism, thyroid function tests and serum prolactin levels should be assessed. In women with regular cycles, serum progesterone levels on day 21 of onset of menstruation may be assessed for excluding any ovulatory dysfunction. A value of >4 ng/mL indicates ovulation.

Postmenstrual ultrasound is done to assess the endometrial thickness, any evidence of polycystic ovaries such as ovarian volume, number of follicles, nature of ovarian stroma, and rule out presence of any ovarian neoplasm.

The presence of 12 or more follicles ranging from 2 to 9 mm and an increased stroma are suggestive of polycystic ovaries. These morphologic findings are nonspecific and may be seen in other conditions such as NCAH, hyperprolactinemia, and thyroid dysfunction or even in normal women. Ultrasound is useful in excluding any adrenal tumor.

Other imaging modalities such as computed tomography (CT) scan or magnetic resonance imaging (MRI) may be used for diagnosing small androgen-secreting tumors. MRI can exclude adrenal masses of <5 mm diameter and detect bilateral adrenal hyperplasia. Rarely, selective venous catheterization or scintigraphy with iodomethylnorcholesterol is used to detect small tumors not picked up on imaging.

Metabolic abnormalities are common among women with PCOS and hyperandrogenism, insulin resistance, and acanthosis nigricans (HAIR-AN) syndrome. They need to be screened for insulin resistance and dyslipidemia. They are subjected to a standard 2-hour oral glucose tolerance test (OGTT) measuring both fasting blood sugar and 2 hours level after 75 gm glucose load. According to the World Health Organization (WHO) criteria, impaired glucose tolerance (IGT) is diagnosed by a normal fasting blood glucose ≤ 110 mg/dL and a 2-hour value between 140 and 199 mg/dL, while frank DM is diagnosed when fasting blood glucose is >126 mg/dL or a 2-hour value is >200 mg/dL.

Serum lipid profile is ordered after 12 hours of fasting state and we look specifically for the levels of triglycerides and high-density lipoprotein (HDL). A level ≥150 mg/dL of triglycerides and/or a value of <50 mg/dL of HDL points toward metabolic syndrome.

MANAGEMENT[3]

Patient-important hirsutism, or unwanted sexual hair-growth of any degree that distresses the woman enough to seek treatment, is the criterion for starting treatment for hirsutism.

The various options include pharmacotherapy, cosmetic measures, and lifestyle modifications (Flowchart 2). Pharmacotherapy is the first-line treatment with or without cosmetic measures. Pharmacologic agents target androgen production and action. Lifestyle modification is initiated in those with higher BMI or metabolic derangement. For all agents, a trial of at least 6 months

Flowchart 2: Management of woman with hirsutism.

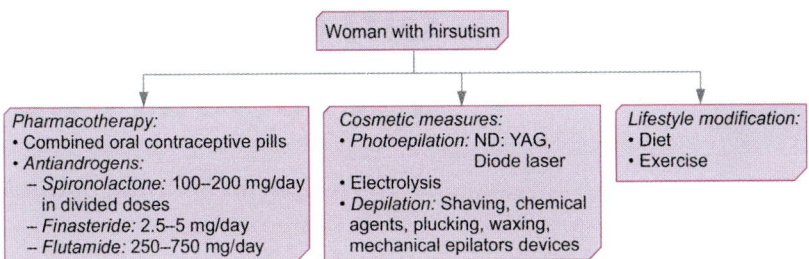

is suggested before making dose changes, adding a new medication, or changing to a new medication.

Combined oral contraceptives: OCs containing ethinyl estradiol are generally recommended as the first-line treatment in patients not desiring fertility. All OCs appear to be equally effective. In women at high risk of venous thromboembolism (VTE), OCs with ethinyl estradiol at the lowest effective dose of 20 µg, and a low-risk progestin are preferred. OCs containing levonorgestrel (LNG) are the safest in terms of VTE risk (as compared to those containing norgestimate, desogestrel, gestodene, or the antiandrogenic progestin, and cyproterone acetate), but the effect of LNG on metabolic biomarkers is a concern in women with possibility of metabolic syndrome. OCs containing antiandrogenic progestins such as cyproterone acetate do not offer any clinically important advantages.

Antiandrogens are recommended as the second-line therapy because of their teratogenic potential, unless the woman is not sexually active or is using effective contraception. These agents can be used as an add-on along with OCs if patient-important hirsutism persists after 6 months of treatment with OCs.

Spironolactone is an aldosterone antagonist. It may cause menstrual irregularity, postural hypotension, and dizziness. It is contraindicated in women with renal impairment.

Finasteride inhibits type 2 5-alpha-reductase activity. Flutamide is an androgen receptor inhibitor; it is not recommended due to hepatotoxic potential.

For obese women with PCOS, lifestyle changes including diet, exercise, and behavioral modification may improve hirsutism by helping in weight loss, decreasing serum testosterone, and fasting insulin levels.

KEY POINTS

- Hirsutism is a distressing condition with significant psychological morbidity.
- In most cases, there is underlying hyperandrogenism.
- The initial assessment should include an attempt to find out the source of excess androgens if any, impact of the problem on fertility, and psychosocial well-being of the patient.
- The treatment is tailored according to the cause and the related problems.

REFERENCES

1. McKnight E. The prevalence of 'hirsutism' in young women. Lancet. 1964;1(7330):410-3.
2. Ferriman D, Gallwey JD. Clinical assessment of body hair growth in women. J Clin Endocrinol Metab. 1961;21:1440-7.
3. Martin KA, Anderson RR, Chang RJ, et al. Evaluation and Treatment of Hirsutism in Premenopausal Women: An Endocrine Society Clinical Practice Guideline. J Clin Endocrinol Metab. 2018;103(4):1233-57.

44

Approach to a Girl Presenting with Precocious Puberty

K Aparna Sharma, Sadia Mansoor

INTRODUCTION

Puberty is a series of predictable events varying in timing, sequence, and tempo resulting in the development of secondary sexual characteristics and attainment of ability of sexual reproduction. It marks the change from childhood to adolescence. Understanding the aberrations of pubertal development warrants basic working knowledge of the timing and sequence of normal pubertal changes. The pubertal development typically takes place over 4.5 years. The age of onset of puberty has been declining gradually over the past century consequent to the increasing prevalence of obesity. Breast budding is usually the first recognized pubertal change, followed by appearance of pubic hair, peak growth velocity, and menarche. The most frequently utilized staging system for puberty is published by Marshall and Tanner, and the sequence of changes is commonly referred to as "Tanner stages" or sexual maturity ratings (SMRs) (Table 1).[1]

Precocious puberty is defined as pubertal development occurring more than 2.5 standard deviations (SD) earlier than the average age and warrants a battery of expensive and time-consuming investigations. Traditionally, precocious puberty has been defined as the development of secondary sexual characteristics before the age of 8 years. However, in view of the declining age at onset of puberty over the past few decades, the exact age at which the diagnosis should be considered and evaluated is still under speculation. The application of traditional definition of puberty could result in a large number of potentially normal girls undergoing costly testing (PROS study).[2] A lower age threshold could result in a failure to identify children with pathological disease.[3] To draw a balance between safety and cost-effectiveness, the

Table 1: Tanner stages of secondary sexual characteristics development (Figs. 1 and 2).

Stage	Stages of breast development	Stages of pubic hair development
1	Prepubertal	Prepubertal
2	Enlargement of areola and elevation of breast and papilla (breast bud)	Growth of few long hair, straight or curly, slightly pigmented hair along labia
3	Further enlargement of breast and areola	Growth of a few darker, coarser, and curly hair on junction of pubes
4	Areola and papilla form a separate mound on the breast	Adult type hair, but covering smaller area and no spread to medial side of thighs
5	Areola recedes resulting in a mature breast with only papilla projecting	Adult type with horizontal distribution on mons pubis

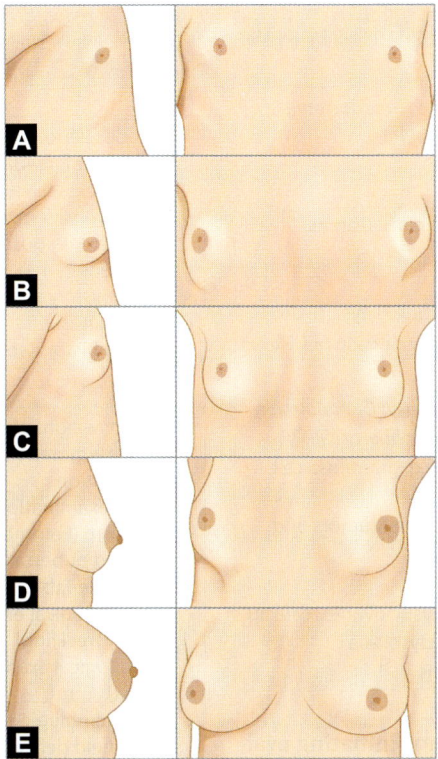

Figs. 1A to E: Tanner stages of breast development. (A) Tanner stage 1 prepubertal breast; (B) Tanner stage 2 breast; (C) Tanner stage 3 breast; (D) Tanner stage 4 breast; (E) Tanner stage 5 mature breast.

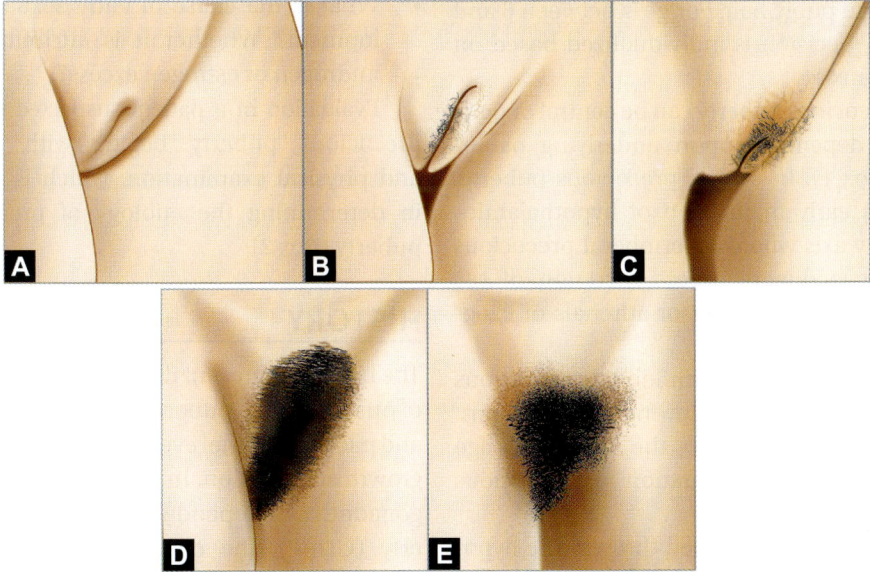

Figs. 2A to E: Tanner stages of pubic hair development. (A) Tanner stage 1 prepubertal pubic hair; (B) Tanner stage 2 pubic hair; (C) Tanner stage 3 pubic hair; (D) Tanner stage 4 pubic hair; (E) Tanner stage 5 adult feminine pubic hair.

> **Box 1:** Differential diagnosis of precocious puberty.
>
> *Causes of precocious puberty*
>
> *Central or true precocious puberty: Gonadotropin-dependent precocious puberty (GDPP):*
> - Idiopathic
> - Genetic/familial
> - Central nervous system (CNS) hamartomas
> - Other CNS tumors
> - CNS irradiation
> - Other lesions such as subarachnoid cyst, hydrocephalus, trauma, inflammatory disease of CNS, and tuberous sclerosis
>
> *Peripheral or pseudo precocious puberty: Gonadotropin-independent peripheral precocious puberty (GIPP):*
> - Functioning ovarian tumors, e.g. granulosa cell tumor and functional cysts
> - Adrenal pathology such as adrenal tumors and congenital adrenal hyperplasia
> - Primary hypothyroidism
> - McCune–Albright syndrome: Cystic ovaries, café au lait spots, polyostotic fibrous dysplasia
> - Intake of exogenous estrogens

> **Box 2:** Salient points in workup of precocious puberty.
>
> *History*
> - Age, sequence and pace of pubertal changes
> - Presence of headaches, seizures, abdominal lump or pain, excessive mental or physical stress
> - *Past history*: Central nervous system (CNS) disease or trauma, exposure to exogenous androgens or estrogens
> - *Family history*: Age of onset of puberty in parents and siblings
> - Dietary history, socioeconomic history
>
> *Examination*
> - Height, weight and height velocity (cm/year), facial asymmetry or dysmorphism, thyroid examination
> - Breast examination (galactorrhea)
> - Hirsutism (Ferriman-Gallwey scoring)
> - Detailed pubertal staging sexual maturity rating (SMR) (*see* Table 1)
> - Dermatological examination (cafe-au-lait spots, axillary freckling)
> - Neurological examination (focal neurological deficit)
> - Ophthalmologic examination (lisch nodules, visual field deficits)
> - Abdominal examination (palpable ovarian mass)
> - Genital examination (clitoromegaly)

following can be practiced for initiating evaluation for precocious puberty in girls <6 years with either breast development or pubic hair, girls <8 years with both breast development and pubic hair. For girls between 6 and 8 years, decision is individualized based on parent anxiety.

Precocious puberty can be central or peripheral depending upon underlying pathology (Box 1). In central precocious puberty, there is early maturation of hypothalamic–pituitary axis whereas peripheral precocious puberty is due to excess secretion of sex hormones from ovaries or adrenals or exogenous administration.

The approach to a child with precocious puberty involves the following considerations:
- Is the child below the threshold age warranting an evaluation for precocious puberty?
- Is it central, mediated through the hypothalamic–pituitary–gonadal axis or an autonomous peripheral origin?
- What is the cause of early sexual development? Whether it is attributable to androgen or estrogen excess?

Evaluation of a patient suspected to have precocious puberty begins with history and physical examination, which is helpful in determining the etiology of precocious puberty (Box 2).

HISTORY

The history of present illness includes the age of onset of initial pubertal changes, sequence and pace of pubertal events, evidence of linear growth acceleration. In centrally mediated or gonadotropin-dependent precocious puberty (GDPP), the changes of puberty are consonant and isosexual, i.e., they resemble the normal changes of puberty but at an early age due to premature activation of hypothalamic–pituitary–ovarian axis. While in peripherally mediated or gonadotropin-independent peripheral precocious puberty (GIPP), the changes are dissonant that is they do not follow the normal sequence of puberty. The changes may be isosexual or heterosexual depending upon the exposure to estrogens or androgens, respectively.

Presence of headaches, seizures, focal neurologic deficit, and visual disturbance is indicative of central nervous system (CNS) cause. Abdominal pain be suggestive of an ovarian cause namely complicated ovarian tumor or cyst. Any history of excessive mental or physical stress should be elicited.

Factors such as onset of puberty before 6 years of age, rapid pubertal progression, and associated symptoms of headache, seizures or focal neurological deficits suggest intracranial pathology.

Past History

Previous history of CNS disease or trauma and exposure to exogenous androgens or estrogens should be elicited.

Family History

Age of onset of initial pubertal events of the patient's parents and siblings is important.

Socioeconomic History

The geographical location, urban or rural living, and socioeconomic status have an influence on the timing of onset of puberty.

EXAMINATION

General Physical Examination

Measurements of height, weight, and height velocity (cm/year) can be a useful clue for early identification of precocious puberty as these girls display an early growth acceleration pattern compared to normal girls. Both malnutrition and moderate obesity have a bearing on the onset of puberty.

Dermatological examination to evaluate for the presence of café au lait spots as in McCune–Albright syndrome is carried out. Facies should be noted as facial dysmorphism is typically noted in McCune–Albright syndrome. Thyroid is examined for any enlargement. Any evidence of hirsutism is noted by Ferriman–Gallwey scoring.

Detailed pubertal staging SMR is assessed as objectively as possible (*see* Table 1). In girls, the diameter of glandular breast tissue is assessed by direct palpation. It includes compression with fingers to differentiate breast tissue from adipose tissue. The nipple-areolar complex should be measured. Accurate measurements are critical to determine whether further radiological or laboratory testing is necessary.

Systemic Examination

Neurological examination to detect any focal neurological deficit resulting from a CNS lesion is carried out and abdominal examination for any palpable ovarian mass is done. Ophthalmologic assessment is advisable to detect any visual field defects.

Examination of External Genitalia

Examination is done to determine whether the development of external genitalia is isosexual or heterosexual (ambiguous genitalia) indicating an excess of estrogens or androgens. Clitoromegaly should be checked as seen in cases of congenital adrenal hyperplasia or an underlying virilizing ovarian or adrenal tumor.

Fundus Examination

Ophthalmic examination is done to evaluate the fundus for presence or absence of papilledema indicative of increased intracranial pressure and visual fields.

INVESTIGATIONS

Investigations include laboratory tests and imaging.

Hormone Profile

Hormone profile is an important tool to identify the cause of precocious puberty. The various tests are as listed below:
- *Serum luteinizing hormone (LH)*: The basal levels of LH are raised in central precocious puberty. Recent studies have reported a role of morning urinary LH levels for diagnosis of central precocious puberty.[4] Urinary LH specially has a role in conditions where baseline LH levels are not confirmatory and there is a need for Gonadotropin-releasing hormone (GnRH) stimulation tests which is time consuming and requires multiple testing
- Follicle-stimulating hormone (FSH)
- Thyroid-stimulating hormone (TSH)
- GnRH stimulation test is required if the baseline testing does not yield a diagnostic picture. Especially, if the basal LH levels are low with a clinical suspicion of central precocious puberty, a GnRH stimulation test is considered
- Serum estradiol
- Serum testosterone
- Serum cortisol (drawn in the afternoon)
- Serum dehydroepiandrosterone (DHEA), DHEA sulfate (DHEA-S), and 17-hydroxyprogesterone
- Adrenocorticotropic hormone (ACTH) stimulation test
- Urinary steroid profile.

A systemic approach to a girl presenting with precocious puberty based on hormonal profile is described in Flowchart 1.

Ultrasound

Abdominal ultrasound is done to detect any ovarian or adrenal tumor. Pelvic ultrasound may be used to monitor pubertal progress in girls; uterine volume changes above 2 mL over a period of 1 year suggest progressive puberty. There is no difference in mean uterine volume from 2–7 years of age. From the age of 7 years, there is a slow, progressive increase in the size of the uterus, and this occurs in prepubertal girls in whom no secondary sexual features have, as yet, appeared. Unlike most organs in the body, which grow with the growth of the body, the uterus and external genitalia start to increase appreciably in size only at puberty. The fact that this also occurs in prepubertal girls may mean that uterine growth is the very first sign of puberty in girls, occurring even before breast development becomes visible making it an indirect indicator of precocious puberty.

Magnetic Resonance Imaging

Magnetic resonance imaging (MRI) brain is indicated in patients with suspected GDPP to detect hypothalamic lesions or other identifiable CNS causes. A routine MRI brain for all cases of precocious puberty is debatable, especially when the onset is after 6 years of age, BMI is more or there is a family history of precocity. In a recent meta-analysis, the prevalence of CNS lesions in cases of precocity before and after 6 years was 25% and 3%, respectively.[5] Evaluate for growth hormone deficiency if child has received cranial radiation. MRI abdomen and pelvis may be done in cases of peripheral precocity

Flowchart 1: Algorithm for clinical approach to a girl presenting with precocious puberty based on hormonal evaluation.

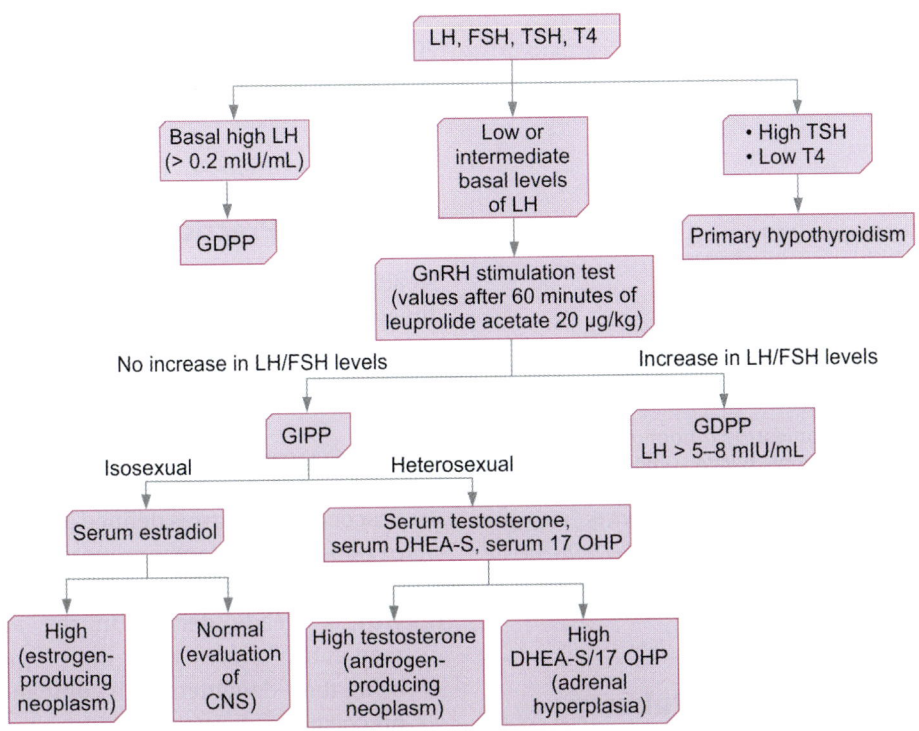

(CNS: central nervous system; DHEA-S: dehydroepiandrosterone sulfate; FSH: follicle-stimulating hormone; GDPP: gonadotropin-dependent precocious puberty; GIPP: gonadotropin-independent precocious puberty; GnRH: gonadotropin-releasing hormone; LH: luteinizing hormone; OHP: hydroxyprogesterone; TSH: thyroid-stimulating hormone; T4: thyroxine)

with suspicion of exogenous hormones from ovaries or adrenal tumors with or without virilization.

Bone Age

Bone age is indicated, especially in patients who have early secondary sexual findings confirmed by physical examination for assessment of skeletal maturation. The most used method is based on a single X-ray of the hand including the wrist and fingers. There is minimal radiation exposure and the bones in the X-ray are compared to the bones of a standard atlas, usually Greulich and Pyle.[6,7] A more complex method based on hand X-rays is the Tanner Whitehouse 2 ("TW2") method.[8] X-ray of the knee may also be used.

Further evaluation is warranted if the bone age is higher than chronological age or in patients with normal bone age, but clinical evidence of precocious puberty. If the patient has abnormal bone age, she is unlikely to have GDPP. If the clinical findings are consistent with incomplete precocious puberty, i.e., isolated premature thelarche or premature pubarche, and the bone age is normal, follow-up rather than further investigations is usually appropriate. Box 3 summarizes the investigations of a girl presenting with precocious puberty.

> **Box 3:** Investigations of a girl presenting with precocious puberty.
>
> *Investigations*
>
> - *Hormonal profile:*
>   S FSH, LH
>   TSH
>   Estradiol
>   Testosterone
>   DHEAS
>   17 hydroxy progesterone (17OHP)
>   – GnRH stimulation test
>   – ACTH suppression test
> - *Imaging:*
>   Ultrasound of abdomen and pelvis
>   MRI head
>   X-ray wrist and hand

(ACTH: adrenocorticotropic hormone; DHEA-S: dehydroepiandrosterone sulfate; GnRH: gonadotropin-releasing hormone; FSH: follicle-stimulating hormone; LH: luteinizing hormone; MRI: magnetic resonance imaging; OHP: hydroxyprogesterone; TSH: thyroid-stimulating hormone)

MANAGEMENT

Central Precocious Puberty

When to Treat

In case of central precocious puberty, treatment should be considered in young girls with progressive central precocious puberty before the age of 6 years with breast and pubic hair development, advanced bone age, and accelerated height velocity.

Goals of Treatment

Treatment is targeted to allow a child to grow to a normal adult height and to relieve the psychosocial stress levels.

Treatment

Sustained-release formulations of GnRH agonists (leuprolide acetate), 3.75 mg or 11.5 mg, can be used monthly or every 3 months.

Treatment Duration

Treatment is continued long enough to optimize final adult height, yet still allow progression of pubertal characteristics at an age that is concurrent with the individual's peers.

Peripheral Precocious Puberty

Treatment depends upon the cause. It is directed at blocking the production of and/or response to the excess sex steroids by surgery or drugs.

KEY POINTS

- Precocious puberty is defined as the onset of pubertal development more than 2 to 2.5 SD earlier than the average age.
- With a steady decline in the age at menarche, more and more parents bring their daughters with complaints of precocious puberty.
- It is important to identify those girls in whom detailed workup is indicated. Detailed history and examination are important tools to reach this decision and reassure others.
- Basal LH, FSH, estradiol, and testosterone are the baseline investigations for evaluating the type of precocious puberty whether central or peripheral. (Basal LH levels are elevated in central precocious puberty).
- If there is a clinical suspicion of central precious puberty not substantiated by a raised basal LH levels, GnRH stimulation test is indicated.
- MRI brain in indicated in girls with the onset of puberty at <6 years of age, rapidly progressing and features suggestive of CNS lesion such as headache, convulsions, and focal neurologic deficit.

REFERENCES

1. Marshall WA, Tanner JM. Variations in pattern of pubertal changes in girls. Arch Dis Child. 1969;44(235):291-303.
2. Herman-Giddens ME, Slora EJ, Wasserman RC, Bourdony CJ, Bhapkar MV, Koch GG, et al. Secondary sexual characteristics and menses in young girls seen in office practice: a study from the Pediatric Research in Office Settings Network. Pediatrics.1997;99(4):505-12.
3. Kaplowitz PB, Oberfield SE. Reexamination of the age limit for defining when puberty is precocious in girls in the United States: implications for evaluation and treatment. Drug and Therapeutics and Executive Committees of the Lawson Wilkins Pediatric Endocrine Society. Pediatrics.1999;104:936-41.
4. Lee DM, Chung IH. Morning basal luteinizing hormone, a good screening tool for diagnosing central precocious puberty. Ann Pediatr Endocrinol Metab. 2019;24(1):27-33.
5. Cantas-Orsdemir S, Garb JL, Allen HF. Prevalence of cranial MRI findings in girls with central precocious puberty: a systematic review and meta-analysis. J Pediatr Endocrinol Metab 2018;31(7):701-10.
6. Büken B, Safak AA, Yazici B, Büken E, Mayda AS.. "Is the assessment of bone age by the Greulich-Pyle method reliable at forensic age estimation for Turkish children?". Forensic Sci Int. 2007;173(2–3):146-53.
7. Greulich WW, Pyle SI. Radiographic Atlas of Skeletal Development of the Hand and Wrist, 2nd edition. Stanford, CA: Stanford University Press;1959.
8. Tanner JM, Whitehouse RH, Marshall WA, Healey MJR, Goldstein H. Assessment of Skeletal Maturity and Prediction of Adult Height (TW2 Method). New York: Academic Press; 1975.

SUGGESTED READING

1. Kaplowitz P, Bloch C; American Academy of Pediatrics. Evaluation and referral of children with signs of early puberty. Pediatrics. 2016; 137(1).
2. Sklar CA, Antal Z1, Chemaitilly W, Cohen LE, Follin C, Meacham LR, et al. Hypothalamic-pituitary and growth disorders in survivors of childhood cancer: An Endocrine Society Clinical Practice Guideline. J Clin Endocrinol Metab. 2018;103(8):2761-84.

45

Approach to a Girl Presenting with Delayed Puberty

K Aparna Sharma, Sadia Mansoor

INTRODUCTION

Absence or incomplete development of secondary sexual characteristics by an age at which 95% of girls of that culture have sexually matured is defined as delayed puberty. More objectively, a girl is said to have delayed puberty if there is lack of breast budding or thelarche by 13 years of age, or she has not attained menarche for 4 or more years since the onset of pubertal development.[1,2]

True puberty is heralded by breast development and reflects ovarian maturation. Generally, in 95% of healthy girls, changes of puberty complete within 4 years of initiation. Puberty is said to be "stalled" when it has initiated but not completed within 4 years of first sign of pubertal growth, i.e., thelarche. In girls, features of early sexual maturation such as pubic hair, axillary hair, and acne depict adrenal maturation (adrenarche) and are typically visible around 6 months after the onset of true puberty.

Delayed puberty can be hypergonadotropic or hypogonadotropic according to the circulating levels of the gonadotropins that is follicle-stimulating hormone (FSH) and luteinizing hormone (LH). Hypergonadotropic or primary hypogonadism is associated with gonadal failure or defects in the receptors on the gonadal cells whereas hypogonadotropic or secondary hypogonadism is associated with normal gonads, but hypothalamic or pituitary dysfunction. Hypothyroidism and hyperprolactinemia can also result in secondary hypogonadism.

DIFFERENTIAL DIAGNOSIS

The various causes of delayed puberty are tabulated in Box 1.

Box 1: Differential diagnosis of delayed puberty.

Causes of delayed puberty:
- Constitutional delay in puberty
- *Primary hypogonadism*: High follicle-stimulating hormone (FSH) and luteinizing hormone (LH):
  - *Congenital*: Chromosomal abnormalities, Turner's syndrome (45XO)
  - *Acquired*:
    » Autoimmune or post infection
    » Trauma or surgery on ovaries
    » Chemotherapy
    » Radiation therapy
- *Secondary hypogonadism*: Low to normal FSH and LH:
  - *Acquired*:
    » Tumors:
      ➢ Benign tumors and cysts of brain
      ➢ Craniopharyngiomas
      ➢ Germinomas, meningiomas, gliomas, astrocytomas
      ➢ Metastatic tumors (breast, lung, prostate)
    » *'Functional' gonadotropin deficiency*:
      ➢ Chronic systemic disease
      ➢ Acute illness
      ➢ Malnutrition
      ➢ Hypothyroidism, hyperprolactinemia, diabetes mellitus, Cushing's disease
      ➢ Anorexia nervosa, bulimia
    » *Infiltrative diseases*:
      ➢ Hemochromatosis
      ➢ Granulomatous diseases
      ➢ Histiocytosis
      ➢ Thalassemia

Contd...

Contd...

- » Head trauma
- » Pituitary apoplexy
- » *Drugs*: Marijuana
- Congenital:
  - » *Isolated gonadotropin-releasing hormone (GnRH) deficiency*:
    - ➢ Without anosmia
    - ➢ Kallmann syndrome
    - ➢ Associated with congenital adrenal hypoplasia
  - » *GnRH deficiency associated with mental retardation/obesity*:
    - ➢ Laurence-Moon-Biedl syndrome
    - ➢ Prader-Willi syndrome
  - » Idiopathic forms of multiple anterior pituitary hormone deficiencies
  - » Congenital malformations often associated with craniofacial anomalies
- Unclassified

The most common cause of delayed puberty is constitutional delay in puberty,[3] followed by functional hypogonadotropic hypogonadism and hypergonadotropic hypogonadism.

Because most patients with hypogonadotropic hypogonadism have in common, a functional defect in gonadotropin-releasing hormone (GnRH) secretion and/or its action; no single test except for observation overtime reliably distinguishes patients with constitutional delay of puberty that is those who will eventually progress spontaneously through puberty from patients with other causes of delayed puberty, particularly congenital GnRH deficiency. As a result, a complete history and physical examination should precede any biochemical testing or imaging studies.

HISTORY

The history is taken to find out whether pubertal development is totally absent or had started but "stalled." Patients with constitutional delay have delayed growth, adrenarche, and sexual development. It is associated with a slow growth velocity and delayed skeletal maturation.

Nutritional habits, intensity of exercise, prior medical illness, or use of certain medications may delay the onset or slow the tempo of puberty. Delay in sexual maturation and growth velocity often can be the first clinical signs of underlying metabolic disorders such as inflammatory bowel disease, hypothyroidism, diabetes mellitus, or psychosocial deprivation.

The presence of associated congenital abnormalities such as midline defects and skeletal abnormalities (cleft lip/palate, or scoliosis) suggests congenital GnRH deficiency. This deficiency particularly results from mutations in the fibroblast growth factor (FGF) signaling pathway with or without other hypothalamic defects.

Neurologic symptoms such as headache, visual disturbances, anosmia, dyskinesia, seizures, and intellectual disability (mental retardation) strongly suggest a central nervous system disorder.

A positive family history of either constitutional delay of puberty or congenital GnRH deficiency can be a useful clue. However, this finding is nonspecific and is common in both constitutional delay and idiopathic hypogonadotropic hypogonadism due to mutations in fibroblast growth factor receptor 1 (FGFR1), which is an autosomal dominant condition.

History of galactorrhea suggests hyperprolactinemia. Any history of trauma, chemotherapy, or radiotherapy is important. History of any psychological disorder or emotional stress should be elicited.

The presence of an abnormal sense of smell, anosmia, strongly suggests the existence of a genetic defect in genes such as *KAL1*, *FGF8*, *FGFR1*, *PROK2*, or *PROKR2*.

EXAMINATION

Examination essentially includes careful measurement of height, weight, arm span, and secondary sex characteristics. Both the standing height and the arm span should be measured. An arm span exceeding the height by >5 cm (i.e., eunuchoid body habitus) suggests delayed epiphyseal closure secondary to hypogonadism. The height should be plotted on growth charts that include normal growth patterns with centiles to place the current height in the proper developmental context and to allow comparison with both normal and subsequent bone age determination. The height velocity should be carefully documented for at least 6 months.

Secondary sexual characteristics should be staged according to the Tanner criteria, also called sexual maturity rating (SMR). The use of stage line diagrams (puberty nomograms) aids the identification of pubertal delay or arrest delay based on the onset as well as tempo of pubertal development.[4]

All girls with delayed puberty should be evaluated for features of Turner's syndrome that is low hair line, epicanthal folds, webbed neck, low-set ears, cubitus valgus, broad barrel-shaped chest with widely spaced nipples, high-arched palate, and hypoplastic finger and toenails.

The girl is assessed for presence of anosmia and color blindness.

INVESTIGATIONS

Hormonal Assessment

The hormonal evaluation should include serum LH, FSH, estradiol, prolactin, TSH, and free T3, T4.

Serum Luteinizing Hormone and Follicle-stimulating Hormone, Estradiol

It is done to distinguish between primary and secondary hypogonadism. FSH levels are most useful. Girls with raised FSH and LH levels and low estradiol levels are diagnosed as primary hypogonadism, whereas those with low FSH and LH and estradiol levels are diagnosed with secondary hypogonadism as in constitutional delay of puberty and congenital GnRH deficiency.

Ultrasensitive immunofluorometric assays for LH and FSH may eventually prove capable of distinguishing between the low gonadotropin levels of patients with constitutional delay versus the undetectable levels in GnRH-deficient patients; however, these assays have not yet been widely validated for the screening of true GnRH-deficient patients.

The GnRH stimulation testing is not recommended[5] because it does not help to distinguish between these disorders as there is a significant overlap of LH and FSH responses between these two groups of patients. In most patients, however, the distinction between congenital GnRH deficiency and constitutional delay of puberty can be resolved only with serial observations. In some patients, therapy may be initiated prior to determining the diagnosis.

Serum Prolactin

Serum prolactin should be obtained to detect hyperprolactinemia, which can present clinically as "stalled" puberty. An elevated serum prolactin level can result from a prolactinoma lactotroph adenoma or from any hypothalamic or pituitary disorder that interrupts hypothalamic inhibition of prolactin secretion. In the absence of obvious history of prolactin-raising medication, a magnetic resonance imaging (MRI) of head is indicated for evaluation of the hypothalamus and the pituitary region.

Thyroid Function Tests

Hypothyroidism delays puberty by yet unknown mechanisms. It is particularly important if growth velocity has suddenly slowed and the bone age is markedly delayed. An elevated serum concentration of thyroid-stimulating hormone (TSH) is the hallmark of primary hypothyroidism; however, the values are usually normal or low when hypothyroidism is a result of hypothalamic or pituitary disease. Serum free T4 or total T4 and free T4 index should be measured, if CNS disease is suspected.

General Tests

Further evaluation should be directed at the possibility of nutritional disorders, occult chronic illness such as chronic inflammatory bowel disease, celiac disease, or hepatic disorder that may affect the hypothalamic GnRH pulse generator and hormonal abnormalities.

These include complete blood count, erythrocyte sedimentation rate, renal and liver function tests, and IgA antibodies to transglutaminase (TG).

Other Tests

Serum Iron Studies

Evaluation of iron overload by estimation of serum ferritin and serum transferrin saturation should be done in patients with a history of multiple blood transfusions suggestive of thalassemia major or with unexplained cardiac or liver disease. Conditions such as juvenile hemochromatosis can lead to secondary hypogonadism and hence delayed puberty.

Karyotype

Karyotype should be performed in every patient with primary hypogonadism to evaluate the possibility of Turner's syndrome. Delayed puberty as an isolated finding is rare in these syndromes because almost all patients have other physical findings that are suggestive of this disease. Besides panel of genetic testing should be offered to patients with anosmia with other associated features such as neurosensory hearing loss, synkinesia, unilateral renal agenesis, skeletal abnormalities or midline defects as these patients often have isolated GnRH deficiency.

Imaging Studies

A conventional X-ray of the left hand and wrist to evaluate bone age may be obtained at the initial visit to assess skeletal maturation and repeated over time if needed. The baseline X-ray provides valuable information about the relationship between chronologic age and skeletal maturation, the potential for future skeletal growth, and allows a preliminary prediction of adult height. Patients with constitutional delay of puberty typically have bone ages of 12–13.5 years, but rarely progress beyond this age due to absence of pubertal levels of gonadal steroids required for epiphyseal closure (Flowchart 1).

Magnetic resonance imaging of head is warranted in girls with symptoms suggestive of neurologic involvement such as headaches, projectile vomiting, visual disturbances or presence of associated features such as midline defects and anosmia. Laboratory findings such as hyperprolactinemia, central hypothyroidism, and central adrenal insufficiency should also trigger need for MRI mostly to rule out any intracranial tumor or sometimes presence or absence of olfactory bulbs and tracts.

Section 2: Gynecology

Flowchart 1: Algorithm for clinical approach to a girl presenting with delayed puberty.

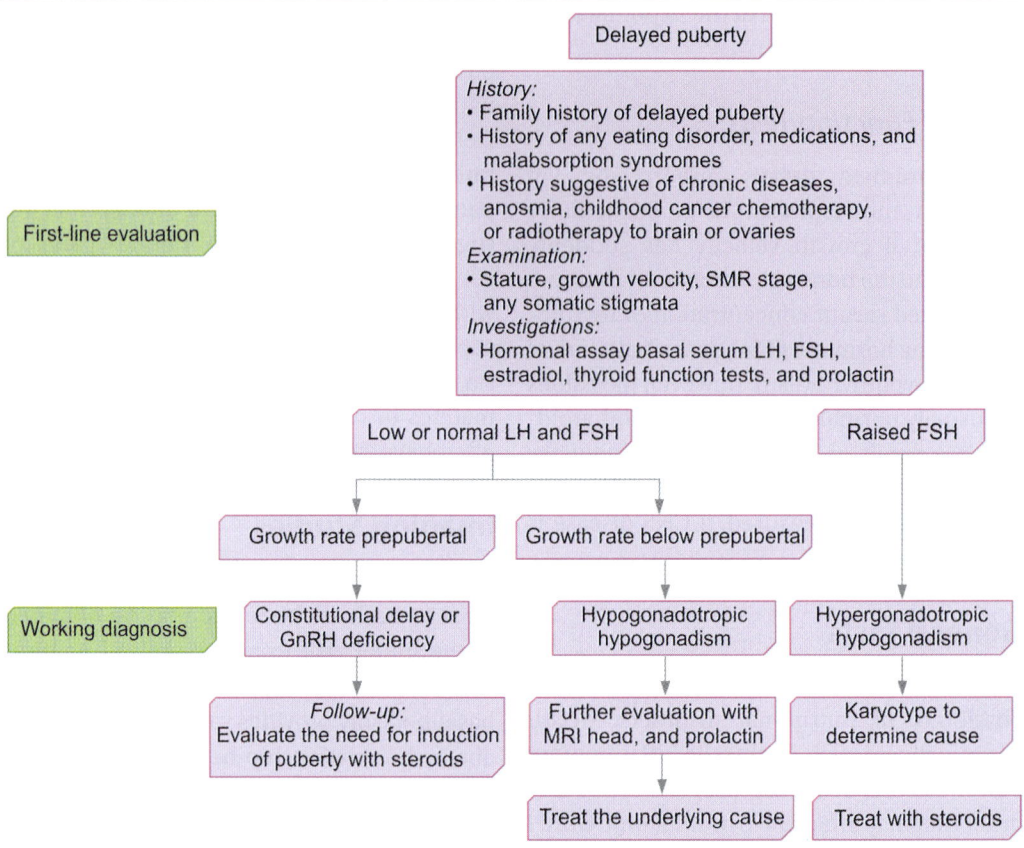

(LH: luteinizing hormone; FSH: follicle-stimulating hormone; MRI: magnetic resonance imaging; GnRH: gonadotropin releasing hormone; SMR: sexual maturity rating; TSH: thyroid stimulating hormone)

Pelvic ultrasonography may be performed in girls with delayed puberty to determine the presence or absence of a uterus. The uterus is absent in girls with androgen insensitivity and disorders of the Müllerian duct system. It is also performed when a mass is detected in lower abdomen on abdominal or pelvic or per rectal examination.

MANAGEMENT

The principles of management are:
- To induce the appearance of secondary sexual characteristics or the acceleration of growth to mitigate psychosocial difficulties associated with pubertal delay and short stature.
- To prevent harmful effects of estrogen insufficiency on bones, heart by prescribing hormonal therapy till the age of menopause in hypogonadism.
- To counsel regarding options for achieving pregnancy. Ovulation induction with gonadotropins along with luteal phase support for women with hypogonadotropic hypogonadism, and in vitro fertilization with donor oocyte in women with

hypergonadotropic hypogonadism or premature ovarian failure provided the uterus and semen analysis is normal.

Constitutional Delay

The treatment options include expectant observation or therapy with low-dose estrogen. If puberty has started, clinically or biochemically, and stature is not a major concern, expectant management is usually reasonable. Treatment may be indicated for psychosocial reasons. In these cases, estrogen may be started (ethinyl estradiol 2 μg or conjugated equine estrogen 0.625 mg daily for 6–12 months).

Permanent Hypogonadism

In girls with hypogonadotropic hypogonadism, initial sex-steroid therapy is the same as that for constitutional delay but doses are gradually increased to full adult replacement levels during a period of approximately 3 years. The treatment with estrogen needs to be combined with progestin for endometrial cycling. This is continued till the age of expected age of menopause.

In patients with a uterus, add in oral cyclical progesterone (e.g., norethisterone 5 mg or medroxyprogesterone acetate 5 mg) from day 14–25 of cycle, or change to a combined oral hormone replacement therapy (HRT) which includes cyclical progesterone at the onset of menstruation or when adult dose is reached even without onset of menstruation (Table 1).

Table 1: Suggested protocol for hormone replacement therapy (HRT).[5]

1st year	EE 2 μg
2nd year	EE 4 μg
2.5 year	EE 6 μg
3rd year	EE 8 μg
3.5 year	EE 10 μg
Adult dose	EE 20–30 μg

(EE: ethinyl estradiol)

KEY POINTS

- Delayed puberty is a condition, which generates immense anxiety both in the young girl and her parents.
- Delayed puberty is termed in girls who fail to develop any breast budding or thelarche by the age of 13 years, have not had menarche by 15 years or have not attained menarche 4 or more years since the onset of pubertal development.
- The most common cause of delayed puberty is constitutional delay in puberty.
- A thorough evaluation is desirable to categorize the type and cause and institute treatment at the earliest.
- Management involves expectant observation or therapy with low-dose sex steroids.
- The routine use of growth hormone, anabolic steroids, or aromatase inhibitors is not currently recommended.

REFERENCES

1. Childhood Growth Foundation. Girls four-in-one growth charts (Birth—20 years). UK Cross-sectional reference data:1996/1 (updated in 2002 for use with 5% and 95% thrive lines). South Sheilds, England: Harlow Printing Ltd.
2. Dye AM, Nelson GB, Diaz-Thomas A. Delayed puberty. Pediatr Ann. 2018;47(1): e16–22.
3. Abitbol L, Zborovski S, Palmert MR. Evaluation of delayed puberty: what diagnostic tests should be performed in the seemingly otherwise well adolescent? Arch Dis Child. 2016;101(8):767-71.
4. van Buuren S, Ooms JC. Stage line diagram: an age-conditional reference diagram for

tracking development. Stat Med. 2009;28: 1569-79.
5. Wei C, Crowne EC. Recent advances in the understanding and management of delayed puberty. Arch Dis Child. 2016;101(5): 481-8.

SUGGESTED READING

1. Carel JC, Eugster EA, Rogol A, Ghizzoni L, Palmert MR, Antoniazzi F, et al. Consensus statement on the use of gonadotropin-releasing hormone analogs in children. Pediatrics. 2009;123(4):e752-62.
2. Royal College of Obstetricians and Gynaecologists (RCOG) (2013). Scientific impact paper no. 40: Sex steroid treatment for pubertal induction and replacement in the adolescent girl. [online] Available from: https://www.rcog.org.uk/globalassets/documents/guidelines/scientific-impact-papers/sip_40.pdf. [Last accessed March, 2020].
3. Sklar CA, Antal Z, Chemaitilly W, Cohen LE, Follin C, Meacham LR, et al. Hypothalamic-pituitary and growth disorders in survivors of childhood cancer: An Endocrine Society Clinical Practice Guideline. J Clin Endocrinol Metab. 2018;103(8):2761-84.

46 Approach to a Woman Presenting with Breast Lump

Vishrut Narang

INTRODUCTION

A lump in the breast is a localized swelling that feels different from the surrounding breast tissue. It is the most common presentation of breast diseases. The lesion can be benign or malignant, so a thorough work-up is essential for reaching an early diagnosis and instituting timely treatment of breast pathology.

DIFFERENTIAL DIAGNOSIS

The differential diagnosis of lump in the breast is as given in Box 1.

HISTORY

History of Present Illness

In women presenting with a lump or swelling in the breast, the mode of onset, duration, and progress should be asked for. Short duration and rapid progression are suggestive of either breast cancer or benign conditions like hematoma or fat necrosis following trauma. An exception to the rate of growth is atrophic scirrhous carcinoma of breast, which is a slow-growing tumor. Any history of swelling in axilla should also be elicited.

History of associated mastalgia or pain in breast should be asked for as regards to its duration, type, timing, site, and relation to menstruation. It is important to note that lumps in early stages of breast cancer are usually painless and it is the benign lumps such as fibroadenosis, abscess, hematoma, fat necrosis, etc. that are painful.

Any associated history of discharge from the nipple is elicited especially with respect to its duration and the color. Breast discharge due to non-neoplastic causes is bilateral, clear, serous, or milky. Pathological discharge is nonlactational, spontaneous, persistent, and usually unilateral.

Any recent change in nipple such as retraction, deviation, destruction or displacement may suggest a possibility of carcinoma breast.

Other important points to be asked for, i.e., any history of trauma, which can cause hematoma or fat necrosis. History of weight loss and loss of appetite may be present in cases of carcinoma and tuberculosis. Pulmonary Koch's can lead to a retromammary abscess. Any history suggestive of metastasis in breast carcinoma is elicited. This includes any history of chest pain, breathlessness,

Box 1: Differential diagnosis of breast lump.
- Fibrocystic disease or aberration of normal development and involution
- Abscess or other benign swellings, e.g., galactocele
- Fibroadenoma
- Pseudolump, e.g., fat necrosis, lipoma, hematoma
- Duct ectasia
- Breast cancer
- Breast implant

hemoptysis for pulmonary metastasis, abdominal pain, jaundice and abdominal distension for liver metastasis, pain in back, shoulder or hip for bone metastasis and convulsions, loss of consciousness, vomiting, weakness of limbs, and visual disturbances for central nervous system (CNS) metastasis.

Past History

Conditions such as fibroadenosis, tuberculosis, and carcinoma may recur. Past history of any surgery or treatment should be asked for.

Personal History

Any history of smoking, alcoholism, dietary habits, and drug intake should be noted.

Menstrual and Obstetrical History

Carcinoma of breast and fibroadenosis are more common in unmarried and nulliparous women. Early menarche and late menopause are associated with cancer of breast. Usage of hormone replacement therapy should be asked for as it predisposes to breast cancer.

Family History

Carcinoma of breast may have a genetic predisposition and occur as a familial disease, so questions should be asked for any history of breast, endometrial or ovarian cancer in first-degree relatives (mothers, sisters, and daughters). It is important to know the age at which cancer occurred as it is usually of significance, if it occurred at a younger age, i.e., less than 50 years.

General Physical Examination

Pallor may be present in cases with chronic disease or carcinoma. Jaundice, edema feet, and clubbing are suggestive of liver failure secondary to liver metastasis. Lymphadenopathy, especially axillary lymph nodes, should be carefully examined for any enlargement and hardness.

Systemic Examination

Systemic examination is focused to look for the presence of any secondaries in chest, liver, ovaries or bones.

Per Abdomen Examination

Per abdomen examination is done to detect any hepatomegaly or any abdominopelvic lump suggestive of ovarian tumor.

Per Vaginal Examination

Per vaginal examination is done to look for the presence of any adnexal mass or masses due to ovarian enlargement like Krukenberg's tumor.

Per Rectal Examination

Per rectal examination should be done to look for any secondaries of carcinoma breast and stomach in the pouch of Douglas (Blumer's shelf).

Breast Examination

Breast examination is the most important examination and should be carried out in adequate light, maintaining privacy, and preferably with a female chaperone. Proper exposure should be done by asking the patient to strip till her waist.

Local examination of the breast is carried out in the following positions:
- Sitting position with arms by her side
- Semirecumbent position

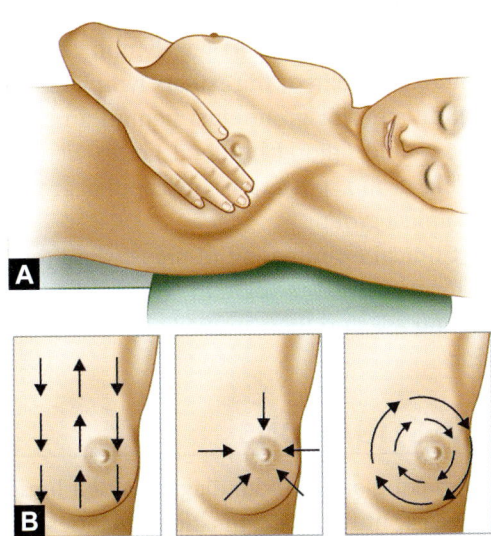

Figs. 1A and B: Breast self-examination. (A) Position for breast self-palpation; (B) Various schemes for self-palpation.

- *Bending forward position*: For better appreciation of retraction of nipples, if present
- *Lying down position*: Used mainly for breast self-examination (Figs. 1A and B).

Inspection

Breasts are checked for their position, size, shape, and any dimpling or puckering. Any ulcer or visible swelling should be described. Patient should be asked to raise her hands and one should look if breast is adherent to chest wall.

Skin over the breast should be checked for its color; it is red in inflammatory conditions, engorged veins, dimpling, retraction, puckering or peau d'orange appearance, nodules, and ulceration or fungation.

Nipples are inspected for their number, position, texture, any discharge or retraction. In carcinoma of breast, the nipple may be drawn toward the lump which is usually best observed when patient raises her hands and it is drawn away from the lump in fibroadenoma. Ulceration is observed in Paget's disease or eczema. Any discharge, if present, should be observed for its color. Blood-stained discharge from the nipple in association with lump breast points toward ductal carcinoma. As regards to retraction, if it is recent, it points toward carcinoma, whereas long-standing retraction may be present since puberty or in chronic inflammation. Physiological retraction is usually slit-like compared to circumferential in carcinoma. Retraction should be differentiated from nipple inversion, which may be present since birth and can be coaxed into normal by some sort of stimulation.

Next the areola is examined for its size, surface, and presence of any Montgomery tubercles as seen in pregnancy. The size is increased in large fibroadenomas and decreased in scirrhous carcinoma. The surface is looked for any cracks or eczema.

The surrounding arm, axilla, thorax, and supraclavicular fossa are inspected. The arm is observed for any edema due to lymphatic obstruction, cancer encuirasse, i.e., thickened skin with nodules like an armor coat. Axilla and supraclavicular fossa should be checked for any visible swelling consequent to enlarged lymph nodes.

After completing above steps, patient should be asked to raise her hands and the undersurface of breast should be inspected.

Palpation

Palpation should be done in various positions, sitting, semirecumbent, and lying down. Remember to palpate the normal breast first.

Palpation should be done with the flat of the hand, which is palmar surface of fingers. All quadrants of breast, axillary tail, nipple, and areola should be palpated. Normal breast has a lobular feeling with nodularity.

On detection of a lump, following characters of the lump should be noted; its location in the breast, temperature over the skin, any tenderness, its number, size, shape, consistency, margins, surface, and its fixity to underlying structures and skin. Carcinoma and fibroadenosis are more common in upper outer quadrant whereas fibroadenoma is more common in lower quadrants. Carcinoma is hard in consistency whereas fibroadenoma is firm and galactocele is cystic in consistency. Carcinoma has a granular or uneven surface whereas fibroadenoma is rounded with a smooth surface.

Fixity

Fixity of lump is assessed to skin, breast tissue, and underlying muscle and fascia. Fixity to skin can be either due to invasion of suspensory ligaments of breast alone or skin also. In case only suspensory ligaments are invaded, the skin can be moved to some distance over the lump after which puckering occurs; this is described as tethering whereas if the skin is also invaded, the lump is adherent to skin with visible puckering. Fixity of lump to breast tissue is assessed by holding the lump in one hand and breast tissue in other. Carcinoma is fixed to breast tissue whereas fibroadenoma is mobile in breast tissue.

Fixity to underlying muscle is checked by asking the patient to place her hand on her hip and press, and the anterior axillary fold is held to check if the muscle is taut. The lump is then moved in two directions, one parallel to and other perpendicular to the muscle fibers. Fixity to serratus anterior muscle is checked by asking the patient to push against the wall and moving the lump.

At the end, axillary lymph nodes and supra- and infraclavicular lymph nodes should be palpated. The axillary lymph nodes include anterior group; just behind anterior axillary fold, lateral humeral group, central medial group, posterior subscapular group, and apical group.

Clinical examination of breast should be performed every 3 years in women in their 20s and 30s and then annually after 40 years of age.

INVESTIGATIONS

For making an accurate diagnosis of a lump in breast, multiple diagnostic modalities are used. The most common approach is the triple assessment, which includes clinical examination, imaging, and tissue diagnosis.

Ultrasonography

Ultrasonography (USG) is mainly used to differentiate solid masses from cystic masses. It is also a useful adjunct to mammography. The characteristics of benign and malignant masses on ultrasound are given in Table 1.

Mammography

Mammography is X-ray imaging of breast and can be used for screening or diagnosis. It is the most reliable means to detect cancer even before a lump is palpable. The

Table 1: Ultrasound features of benign and malignant lumps of breast.

Benign masses	Malignant masses
Usually anechoic cystic	May be cystic or solid
Benign masses are round or ellipsoid in shape, hyperechoic or hypoechoic with smooth well-circumscribed margins	Malignant masses are irregular, hypoechoic with posterior acoustic shadowing, i.e., taller than wider (deeper)

Table 2: Findings on mammography for benign and malignant lesions.

Benign	Malignant
Macrocalcification (>5 mm) smooth margin, homogeneous	Microcalcification (<5 mm) well defined; stellate, speculated or comet-tail appearance
Low-density lesion	High-density lesion

mammographic findings of benign and malignant breast lesions are detailed in Table 2. Mammography is slightly less accurate in young females because of increased density of breast tissue. Mammography is recommended annually starting at the age of 40 till the woman is in good health. Patients with suspicious findings should be advised to undergo magnetic resonance imaging (MRI).

Tissue Diagnosis

Tissue diagnosis is done by two methods; fine needle aspiration (FNA) and core needle biopsy. Main use of FNA is to differentiate solid from cystic masses, which has been replaced by USG. FNA can give a diagnosis of carcinoma, but it cannot differentiate between noninvasive and invasive carcinoma for which core needle biopsy is preferred and definitive treatment plans are based upon it.

With the development of breast ultrasonography and breast MRI, both complementary to mammography, additional algorithms for diagnostic work-up and screening high-risk subgroups of women have emerged. A substantial part of breast imaging practices these days also involves breast interventional procedures, both percutaneous biopsies to obtain tissue diagnosis and localization procedures to guide surgical excision. Diffuse optical imaging of the breast is a noninvasive means of gathering metabolic information by using near-infrared tissue absorption of light to measure hemoglobin concentration.

Table 3: Management of breast lump.

Condition	Treatment
Fibroadenoma	• *Asymptomatic*: Conservative • *Symptomatic or sudden increase in size*: Surgical excision
Fibrocystic disease	Conservative

Cysts: Simple and complex	• *Simple cysts*: No intervention
	  – Aspiration culture and cytology, if infection/inflammation
	  – If persist after aspiration, US-guided core needle biopsy (CNB)
	• *Complex cysts*: Image-guided CNB

Galactocele	Repeated needle aspiration or surgical excision
Fat necrosis	Conservative
Breast abscess	Antibiotics, US-guided aspiration
• Breast cancer • Early stage	• Breast conserving surgery + radiation therapy (RT) or Mastectomy ± RT • Axillary L/N management
• Locally advanced	• Neoadjuvant chemotherapy + Surgery ± RT

(CNB: core needle biopsy; RT: radiation therapy; LN: lymph node; US: ultrasound)

Newer technologies such as tomosynthesis, optical breast imaging, and breast CT are topics of current research for improved detection and characterization of breast lesions.

MANAGEMENT

Management of a woman diagnosed with a breast lump depends upon the cause. Table 3 outlines the management principles of different conditions.

Flowchart 1: Algorithm for clinical approach to a woman presenting with breast lump.

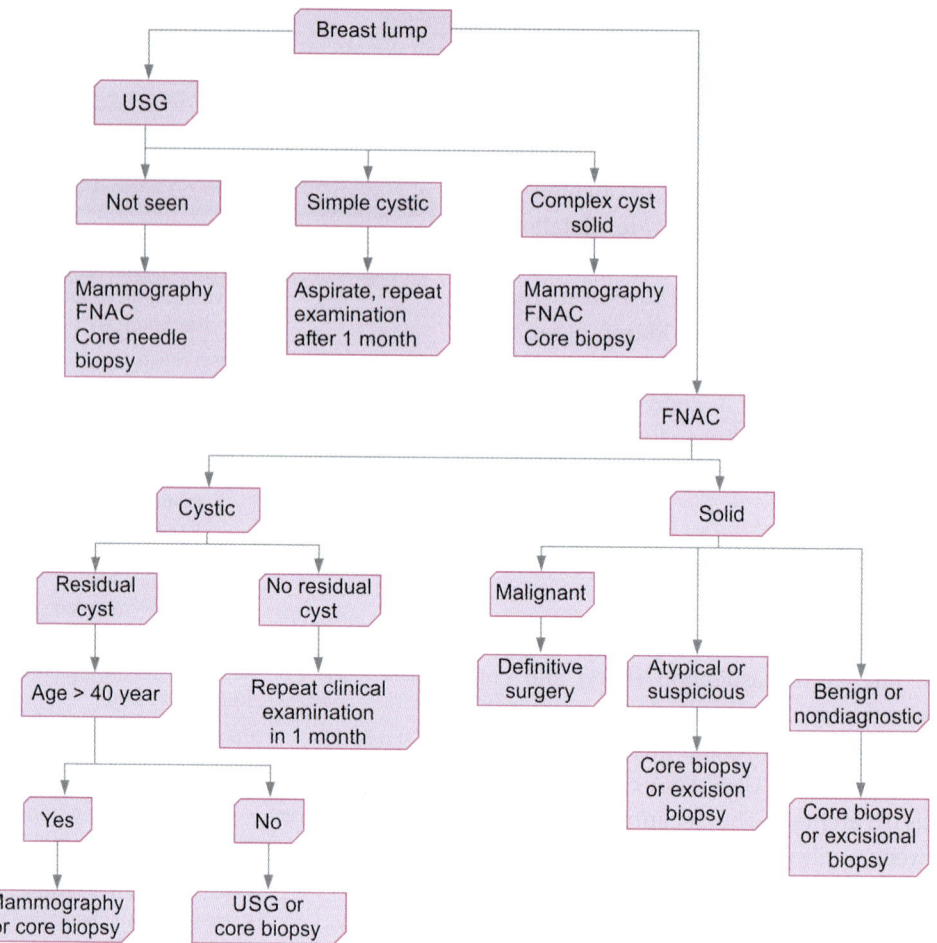

(FNAC: fine needle aspiration cytology; USG: ultrasonography)

KEY POINTS

- Lump in the breast is a common complaint among women.
- Any woman presenting with breast lump should be subjected to a detailed history and examination by the attending physician before being referred to a surgeon.
- The knowledge of the various conditions that can cause lump in the breast helps the clinician to reach a diagnosis and guide the patient accordingly.
- The diagnosis should be made by a combination of modalities. Triple assessment includes clinical examination, radiological imaging, i.e., USG, MRI, mammography, and tissue analysis which includes fine needle aspiration cytology (FNAC), core biopsy, excision biopsy, and image-guided biopsy (Flowchart 1).
- It is important to lay emphasis on monthly self-examination of breast and counsel the patient regarding the importance of mammography and clinical examination

after the age of 40 years for early detection of carcinoma breast.
- Newer techniques such as USG and MR imaging have become an integral part of current breast imaging practice.

SUGGESTED READING

1. Denduluri N, Chavez-MacGregor M, Telli ML, Eisen A, Graff SL, Hassett MJ, et al. Selection of optimal adjuvant chemotherapy and targeted therapy for early breast cancer: ASCO Clinical Practice guideline focused update. J Clin Oncol. 2018; 36(23): 2433-43.
2. Dimitrova N, Parkinson ZS, Bramesfeld A, Ulutürk A, Bocchi G, López-Alcalde J, et al. (2017). European guidelines for breast cancer screening and diagnosis-The European Breast Guidelines. [online] Available from: https://publications.jrc.ec.europa.eu/repository/bitstream/JRC104007/european%20breast%20guidelines%20report%20(online)%20(non-secured).pdf [Last accessed March, 2020].
3. Lyman GH, Somerfield MR, Bosserman LD, Perkins CL, Weaver DL, Giuliano AE. Sentinel Lymph Node Biopsy for Patients With Early-Stage Breast Cancer: American Society of Clinical Oncology Clinical Practice Guideline Update. J Clin Oncol. 2017;35(5): 561-4.
4. NICE (2018). Guideline on early and locally advanced breast cancer: Diagnosis and management. [online] Available from: https://www.nice.org.uk/guidance/ng101 [Last accessed March, 2020].

47. Approach to a Woman Presenting with Nipple Discharge

Laxmi Goel

INTRODUCTION

Nipple discharge is a common complaint among women. It is the third most frequent breast complaint after lumps and nipple pain.[1] Nipple discharge accounts for 7–10% of all breast symptoms. Majority of women with nipple discharge have benign etiology. Galactorrhea accounts for 20–25% of breast discharge.[1] Louie et al. found that 7–15% of women with nipple discharge have breast cancer.[2] But the risk increases to 60% in women with nipple discharge and coexisting lump.[3] Nipple discharge is a true direct drainage from the mammary ducts through nipple or nipple-areolar complex. Physiological discharge refers to milky discharge from bilateral breast related to mid-trimester abortion or childbirth. Galactorrhea is milky breast discharge unrelated to physiological discharge of breastfeeding 1 year after cessation of breastfeeding. It can also occur in nulliparous and postmenopausal women, and even in men. Pathological discharge is nonlactational, spontaneous, persistent, and unilateral, usually arising from one duct. It is important to evaluate every woman presenting with this complaint carefully.

DIFFERENTIAL DIAGNOSIS

The differential diagnosis of a woman presenting with discharge from nipple is as listed in Box 1.

Box 1: Differential diagnosis of nipple discharge.

Physiological condition:
- Breast or nipple stimulation
- Pregnancy and lactation
- Second trimester abortion
- Sexual stimulation

Secondary to chest wall conditions: Trauma, tumor and scars

Endocrinological abnormality:
- Thyroid disorders
- Hyperprolactinemia

Drugs:
- *Antihypertensives*: Labetalol, atenolol, reserpine, alpha-methyldopa, clonidine, and verapamil
- H_2 *blockers*: Ranitidine, cimetidine
- Metoclopramide
- Oral contraceptives
- *Antipsychotics*: Phenothiazines, haloperidol
- *Antidepressants*: Tricyclic

Neoplastic:
- Benign growths like papilloma, papillomatosis
- Breast cancer, intraductal cancer

Others:
- Periductal mastitis
- Mammary duct ectasia
- Fibrocystic disease of breast
- Cirrhosis of liver
- Chronic renal failure

There are a few conditions which do not cause discharge from the breast, but mimic it. These include Paget's disease of breast, eczema with discharge, and nipple adenoma. The differential diagnosis is based on the nature of discharge as shown in Flowchart 1.

Flowchart 1: Algorithm for differential diagnosis of woman presenting with nipple discharge based on nature of discharge.

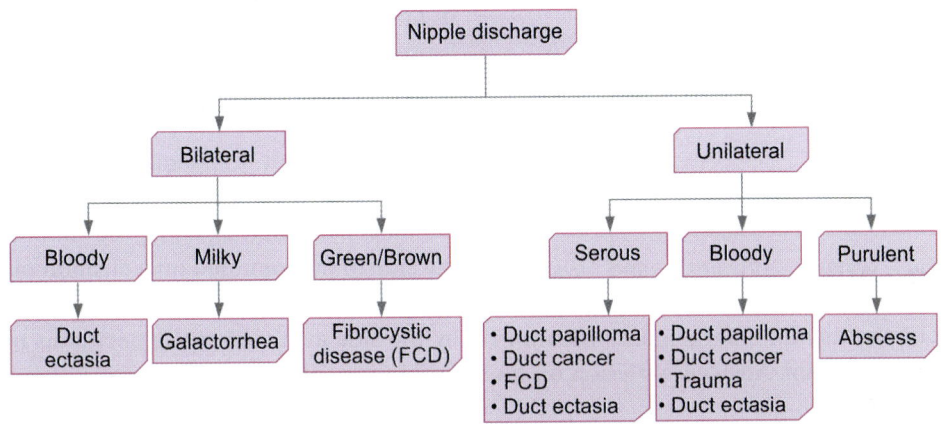

HISTORY

A detailed history should be sought from any woman presenting with breast discharge. The duration of complaint is important. History is aimed to determine whether the discharge is physiologic, pathologic or galactorrhea. It should be sought whether the discharge follows manipulation or is spontaneous, what is the color of the discharge? Is it clear serous, milky, yellow, green, pink, bloodstained, brown or black? Is it unilateral or bilateral? Is there any history of any drug intake? Breast discharge due to non-neoplastic causes is usually bilateral from multiple ducts and is clear, serous, milky or yellow in color. Breast discharge during pregnancy is bilateral and can be bloodstained due to rapid proliferation of breast tissue. This milky discharge is from multiple ducts in both the breasts. It is normal for 1–2 years after pregnancy.

Any history of associated lump in the breast, any pain, redness, change in shape of nipple or any lesion on skin, itching, and fever should be asked for. Any history of headaches, visual disturbance, vomiting suggestive of raised intracranial tension is important and may point toward some brain tumor. Any history of chest trauma or chest surgery should be asked for. Any history of prolonged illness or drug intake should be elicited.

Medical History

Any history of hypertension, psychiatric disorder, hypothyroidism, chronic liver or renal disease is asked.

Menstrual History

Menstrual history is important to know about any change in pattern of menstrual cycles as regards to cycle length and flow. In women with hyperprolactinemia, there can be menstrual disturbance in the form of amenorrhea, oligomenorrhea, and/or hypomenorrhea.

Obstetrical History

It is important to know if the woman is a nullipara or multipara. If she is multipara, the age of last childbirth and when did she stop feeding that baby. Sometimes, there can be galactorrhea associated with mid-trimester abortions. History of contraception should be elicited, as sometimes galactorrhea may be associated with use of oral contraceptive pills.

Family History

Any history of breast cancer in the family is important.

EXAMINATION

Routine general, physical, and systemic examination is carried out with special reference to any thyroid enlargement or features of hypothyroidism. Any scar or lesion on the chest is noted.

A thorough breast examination should be performed. Detailed inspection is the first part of examination and initially the patient should be sitting comfortably with her arms by the sides. The breasts are inspected to look for any retraction or eczema of the nipple, dimpling of the skin, redness, lumps, deformity or asymmetry.

Inspection is repeated after the patient is asked to raise her arms above her head (Fig. 1). It highlights any minor asymmetry, which is very common in between the breasts and makes minor skin tethering more obvious. The nipples are observed for any inversion and whether the patient can evert it. Long-standing "benign" nipple retraction is usually slit-like and easily everted.

The patient should now be examined lying down. The breasts cannot be palpated with the patient in standing position. In women with large pendulous breasts, examination is facilitated by lifting the shoulder of the side to be examined on a cushion placed behind it. Initially the arms of the woman are by the side as it relaxes the pectoralis major facilitating the detection of small lesions, but later raised above the head for examining the lateral part of breast and axillary tail.

The flat of the fingers is used to palpate the breast rather than the tips. Palpation is done with a circular motion of examining fingers, gradually increasing the pressure to perform superficial to deep palpation (Fig. 2). It is important to palpate the axillary tail and the nipple.

The patient should be asked to express the breast to demonstrate any nipple discharge. All quadrants should be palpated and compressed to find out the quadrant from which the drainage emanates (Figs. 3 and 4). The color of the fluid and the site of duct orifice

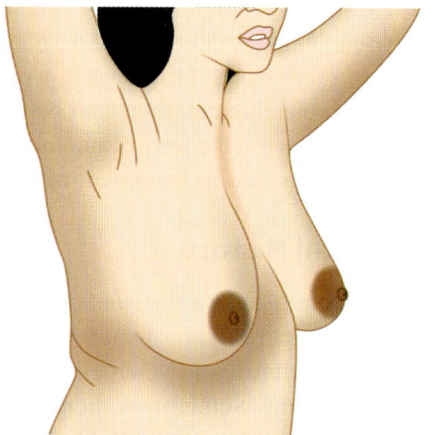

Fig. 1: Inspection of bilateral breasts with raised arms.

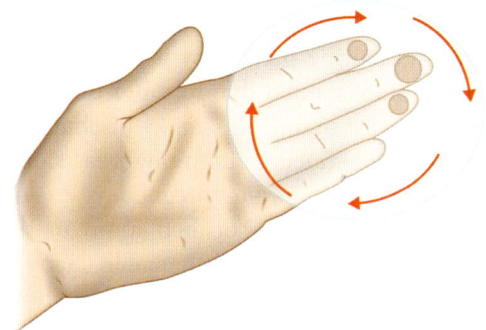

Fig. 2: Palpation of breast tissue with flat of hands in circular motion.

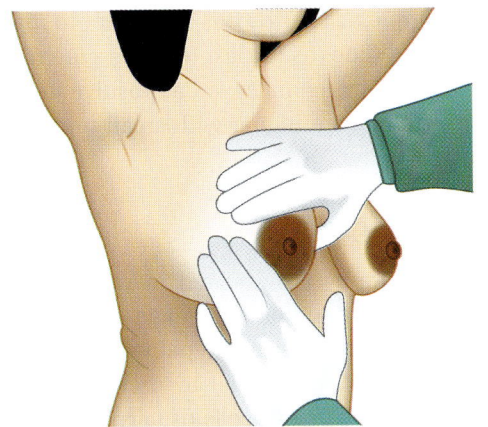

Fig. 3: Palpation to identify the trigger point.

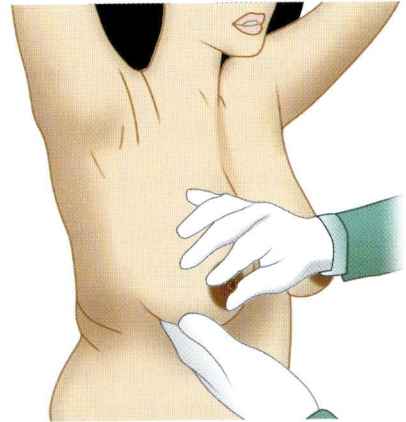

Fig. 4: Demonstrating discharge from nipple.

Table 1: Clinical approach to a woman presenting with nipple discharge.

Cause	Suggestive findings	Diagnostic approach
Benign breast disorders		
Intraductal papilloma (most common cause)	• Unilateral • Bloodstained or serosanguinous discharge	Evaluation as for breast lump
Mammary duct ectasia (second most common cause)	Unilateral or often bilateral bloodstained, serosanguinous, purulent, gray or milky discharge; common in perimenopausal women	Evaluation as for breast lump
Fibrocystic changes	• Lump, often rubbery and tender • Usually in premenopausal women; may have history of other lumps	Evaluation as for breast lump
Abscess or infection	Acute onset with pain, tenderness, induration, and/or erythema or a tender fluctuant lump; usually purulent discharge	Clinical evaluation, if discharge does not resolve with treatment, evaluation as for breast lump
Breast cancer		
Most often, intraductal carcinoma or invasive ductal carcinoma	Unilateral bloody discharge, may have palpable lump, skin changes or lymphadenopathy	If suspected, evaluation as for breast lump
Hyperprolactinemia		
Many causes	• Often bilateral, milky discharge with multiple ducts involved and no lumps; may be associated with menstrual irregularities or amenorrhea • If pituitary lesion is the cause, may have signs of central nervous system mass (visual field changes, headache) or other endocrinopathy	• Prolactin level, thyroid-stimulating hormone (TSH), review of drug use • If prolactin or TSH is elevated, magnetic resonance imaging of head

whether from one duct or more is noted. Use of a magnifying glass is helpful to inspect the duct openings.

It is important to identify any specific area of breast, on pressing which the discharge can be expressed. This is helpful in suspected intraductal lesions.

The clinical approach to a woman presenting with discharge from nipple(s) is summarized in Table 1.

INVESTIGATIONS

These are decided on the basis of history and examination.

Hormonal Assessment

Serum prolactin and thyroid function tests should be performed in all women with breast discharge especially in those without any palpable lump. If serum prolactin is raised above 100 ng/mL, pituitary adenoma should be ruled out by magnetic resonance imaging (MRI) and assessment of visual fields. It is important to note that transient and moderate elevation of prolactin levels is associated with breast stimulation, chest trauma or thoracotomy.

Mammography

Mammography is indicated in any woman with pathological nipple discharge. It is helpful in detection of occult lesions such as carcinoma, fibrocystic disease of breast, and fat necrosis.

Breast Ultrasonography

Breast ultrasonography is useful in evaluating the nature of the underlying lesion, i.e., whether cystic or solid; and its communication with the ductal system manifesting as discharge from the nipple.

Fine Needle Aspiration Biopsy

Fine needle aspiration biopsy is indicated in all palpable breast lumps. In case the tissue obtained is inadequate or the index of suspicion of malignancy is high, excisional biopsy is indicated.

Nipple Discharge Cytology

Nipple discharge cytology is done to detect for the presence of any malignant cells in the nipple discharge. It is important to make multiple slides as the last few drops are more cellular. The chances of a positive report on cytology are higher with small tumors in major ducts.

Galactography

Galactography is indicated in women with spontaneous, unilateral single-duct nipple discharge. The breast is palpated to identify the discharging duct by pressing on the breast tissue. Its orifice is usually bigger and slightly red compared to others. This is gently cannulated with a cannula or blunt needle usually up to the hub. A plastic catheter of a blunt sialography needle can be used to cannulate the duct. Under all aseptic conditions, 0.2–0.4 mL of undiluted water-soluble contrast is slowly injected through it. The injection is stopped if the patient has pain or burning. The catheter is secured on the nipple with paper tape. Subareolar magnification images in the craniocaudal and 90° lateral positions are obtained.

Compared to cytology and mammography, galactography is more sensitive in the detection of intraductal lesions. However, it cannot accurately differentiate between benign and malignant ductal tumors. Solitary lesions located in the central portion of breast are usually benign, whereas multiple lesions situated peripherally are more likely to be malignant. Ductographic findings such as distortion or displacement of ducts, deep-seated irregular filling defects, and intravasation of contrast are suggestive of ductal carcinoma, whereas smooth filling defects with ductal expansion are suggestive of a benign pathology like ductal papilloma. Complete obstruction to flow of contrast may be present with either benign or malignant lesions. The ducts are dilated with minimal branching in mammary duct ectasia.

Fiberoptic Ductoscopy

Fiberoptic ductoscopy is a useful investigation, which allows for direct visualization of the ducts. A directed biopsy from the lesion can be taken with the help of this instrument.

Magnetic Resonance Imaging

Bloody nipple discharge could be a predictor of breast cancer risk particularly in patients of more than 50 years. The mammography and breast ultrasonography are the imaging procedures to realize in first intention but they turn out useful only when they detect radiological abnormalities. Galactography has only a localizing value of possible ductal abnormalities. Thus, in the diagnostic investigation of a suspicious nipple discharge, breast MRI is recommended.[4,5]

MANAGEMENT

The treatment of the various conditions causing nipple discharge is listed in Table 2.

KEY POINTS

- Nipple discharge occurs from lactiferous ducts.
- Management depends on presence of underlying lump, presence of blood in discharge, and whether the discharge is from a single duct or multiple ducts.
- Cytology may reveal malignant cells, although negative results do not exclude carcinoma.
- A clear, serous discharge may be physiological or associated with duct papilloma or mammary dysplasia.
- Blood-stained discharge may be due to duct ectasia, duct papilloma or carcinoma.
- Black or green discharge is usually due to duct ectasia.

Table 2: Treatment of different conditions causing nipple discharge.

Condition	Treatment
Physiological	Reassurance
Drug-induced	Patient education and reassurance
Hyperprolactinemia	Treatment with cabergoline or bromocriptine
Duct papilloma	Duct excision surgery or lumpectomy in cases of DCIS
Abscess	Incision and drainage, antibiotics
Mammary duct ectasia	NSAIDs, antibiotics if mastitis
Fibrocystic disease	Hormonal therapy in form of OCPs
Breast cancer	Management as breast lump

(DCIS: ductal carcinoma in situ; NSAIDs: nonsteroidal anti-inflammatory drugs; OCP: oral contraceptive pills)

REFERENCES

1. Hussain AN, Policarpio C, Vincent MT. Evaluating nipple discharge Obstet Gynecol Surv. 2006;61(4):278-83.
2. Peña KS, Rosenfeld JA. Evaluation and treatment of galactorrhea. Am Fam Physician. 2001;63(9):1763-70.
3. Louie LD, Crowe JP, Dawson AE, Lee KB, Baynes DL, Dowdy T, et al. Identification of breast cancer in patients with pathologic nipple discharge: does ductoscopy predict malignancy? Am J Surg. 2006;192(4):530-3.
4. Leis HP Jr. Management of nipple discharge. World J Surg. 1989;13(6):736-42.
5. Ouldamer L, Kellal I, Legendre G, Ngô C, Chopier J, Body G. Management of breast nipple discharge: Recommendations. J Gynecol Obstet Biol Reprod. 2015;44(10):927-37.

SUGGESTED READING

1. Leitch M, Ashfaq R. Discharges and secretions of the nipple. In: Bland KI, Copeland EM, Klimberg VS, Gradishar WJ (Eds). The Breast: Comprehensive Management of Benign and Malignant Diseases, 5th edition. US: Elseviers; 2018.
2. Nipple discharge. In: Mansel R, Webster D, Sweetland H (Eds). Hughes, Mansel & Webster's Benign Disorders and Diseases of the Breast, 3rd edition. China: Saunders; 2009.

48. Approach to a Survivor of Sexual Assault

Monika Madaan

INTRODUCTION

Sexual violence is a global problem. It affects all age groups and can occur in a variety of settings. The World Health Organization (WHO) has defined sexual violence as "any sexual act, attempt to obtain a sexual act, unwanted sexual comments/advances and acts to traffic, or otherwise directed against a person's sexuality, using coercion, threats of harm, or physical force, by any person regardless of relationship to the victim in any setting, including but not limited to home and work." (WHO, 2003).

According to The Criminal Law Amendment Act (CLA) 2013, rape includes all forms of sexual violence—penetrative (oral, anal, and vaginal) including by objects/weapons/fingers and nonpenetrative (touching, fondling, stalking, etc.). All survivors/victims of sexual violence have the right to be treated by the public and private healthcare facilities. Failure to treat is now an offence under the law. The law further disallows any reference to past sexual practices of the survivor.

Sexual assault in the form of rape can have numerous short- and long-term health consequences for the survivor. This can result in both physical and psychological trauma. Physical trauma can be in the form of genital or nongenital injuries and psychological trauma can predispose the woman to an increased risk of depression, anxiety, social phobias, substance abuse, and suicidal tendencies. The incidence of rape trauma syndrome and post-traumatic stress disorder is significantly high in the survivors. Hence, there is a need for comprehensive and gender-sensitive health services. These women need to be managed with sensitivity and empathy. The attending physician should carefully document the history and examination findings and collect evidence to be produced in court to facilitate the conviction of the accused.

ASSESSMENT OF A SURVIVOR OF SEXUAL ASSAULT

Section 164 (A) of the Criminal Procedure Code lays down certain legal obligations of the health worker in cases of sexual violence. It states that examination of a case of rape shall be conducted by a registered medical practitioner (RMP) employed in a hospital run by the government or a local authority and in the absence of such a practitioner, by any other RMP without any delay.

The Criminal Law Amendment Act 2013, Section 357C CrPC says that both private and public health professionals are obligated to provide treatment. Denial of treatment of rape survivors is punishable under Section 166 B IPC with imprisonment for a term which may extend to 1 year with or without fine.

Whenever a survivor of sexual assault presents to the hospital, a detailed medical and forensic examination needs to be done at a place where there is optimal access to the full range of facilities required by the patient. There should be a separate room with adequate lighting, comfortable examination couch, all the equipment required for thorough examination and toilet facilities so that privacy is maintained and the patient feels secure. Readymade kits like the Sexual Assault Forensic Evidence Collection (SAFE) kit containing all the items required for collecting medicolegal evidence should be available (Figs. 1A to D). Every hospital must have a Standard Operating Procedure (SOP) for management of cases of sexual violence. The SOP must be printed and available to all the staff of the hospital.

It is important that all victims be treated with dignity and the healthcare providers should be empathetic and nonjudgmental, and have a close liaison with the law enforcement agencies, social service providers, rape crisis centers, and nongovernmental agencies. Ideally the medicolegal and the health services should be provided simultaneously, at the same place and by the same person. The foremost priority must be given to the health and welfare of the patient, and provision of medicolegal services assume a secondary place. Wherever possible, female doctors or nurses should be available and invasive physical examinations and interviews must be minimized. The police personnel should not be allowed in the examination room during consultation with the survivor. An ethical, compassionate, objective, and patient-centered care must be provided.

The components of a detailed medical and forensic examination of a sexual assault survivor are as given in Box 1.

CONSENT

Informed consent for conducting a detailed medical and forensic examination is must. It

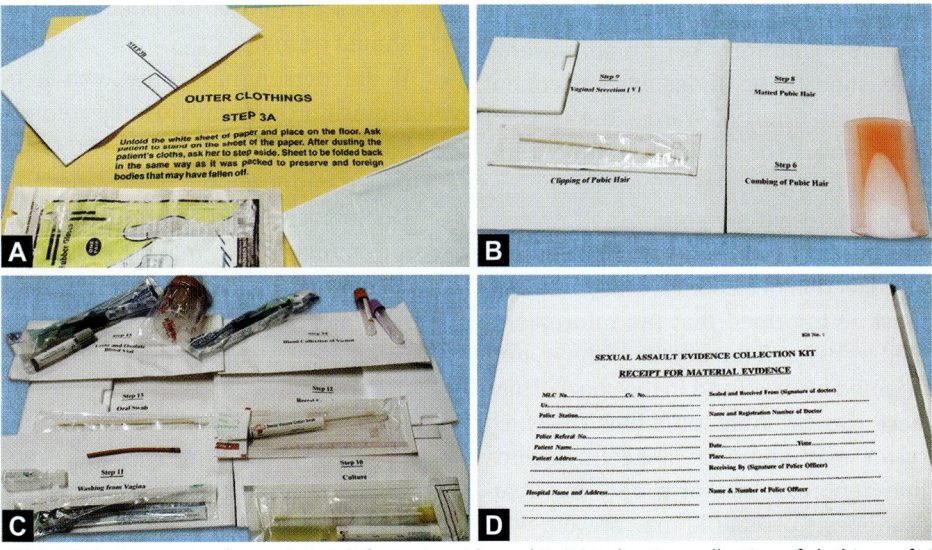

Figs. 1A to D: Components of sexual assault forensic evidence kit. (A) Indicating collection of clothings of victim; (B) Materials for collection of samples of pubic hair; (C) Materials for collection of various swabs; (D) Receipt for material evidence.

Box 1: Components of medical and forensic examination.

- Initial resuscitation/first-aid
- Informed consent
- Detailed history
- Thorough general physical and genital examination
- Recording and classifying injuries
- Collection of samples for medical purposes, if indicated
- Forensic specimens for medicolegal purposes
- Labeling, packaging, and handing over of forensic specimens
- Proper documentation and preparation of medicolegal report
- Any treatment, if required
- Follow-up care

should be signed by the patient herself or by the guardian if the victim is under 12 years of age, or unable to give consent due to mental and/or physical disability. The definition of guardian, according to the Hindu Minority and Guardianship Act, 1956, is a person in-charge of care of a minor or his/her property or both. It includes a natural guardian or a guardian appointed by the will of the minor's father/mother or a guardian appointed or declared by a court or a person empowered to act as such by or under any enactment relating to any Court of Wards. The consent form also needs to be signed by a witness and the examining doctor. The witness can be any major "disinterested" person.

The consent needs to be taken for examination, collection of evidence, and treatment. She must be informed that the information provided by her and the details of the examination would be produced in the court of law.

There can be three situations in which a survivor may approach a health facility. She may report on her own only for treatment for effects of assault, may present with a police requisition after police complaint or may come with a court directive. Following applies to each of these situations:

- In case a person has come directly to the hospital without the police requisition, the hospital is bound to provide treatment and conduct a medical examination with her consent. A police requisition is not needed here. If a survivor has come on her own without FIR (first information report), she may or may not want to lodge a complaint but requires a medical examination and treatment. In such cases, it is the duty of the doctor to inform the police as per law. However, neither court nor police can force the survivor to undergo medical examination. It has to be with the informed consent of the survivor/parent/guardian (depending on the age). Even in cases where the survivor does not want to pursue a police case, a medicolegal case (MLC) must be made and she must be informed that she has the right to refuse to file FIR. An informed refusal must be documented in such cases. At the time of MLC intimation being sent to the police, a clear note stating "informed refusal for police intimation" should be made.
- If the person has come with a police requisition or wishes to lodge a complaint later, the information about MLC no. and police station should be recorded.
- Doctors are legally bound to examine and provide treatment to survivors of sexual violence. The timely reporting, documentation, and collection of forensic evidence may assist the investigation of the crime.

HISTORY

A thorough history is a must for the medical and legal management of the case. This includes history of assault, gynecological history, and a general medical history.

> **Box 2:** History of assault.
>
> - Date, time, and location of the alleged assault
> - Identity number of assailants and their relationship to victim
> - Use of weapons, restraints, medications, drugs, or alcohol
> - Detailed account of violence inflicted
> - Damage or tearing of clothes
> - *Details of attempted or actual sexual activity*:
>   - Whether penetration was vaginal, oral, or anal
>   - Whether penetration was by penis, fingers, or any object
>   - Whether or not the body fluids (semen and saliva) were left in or on the victim
>   - Use of condoms or lubricants
> - Any subsequent activity that may alter the evidence such as change of clothes, bathing, wiping, douching, vomiting, micturition, defecation, and ingestion of food or drink
> - *Development of any subsequent symptoms such as*:
>   - Genital pain, itching, and bleeding
>   - Anal pain or bleeding
>   - Urinary problems
>   - Abdominal pain

History of the Assault

History of the assault includes the details, exact nature, and the events that followed rape (Box 2).

Gynecological History

Gynecological history includes menstrual, sexual, contraceptive, and obstetric history. If the survivor is menstruating at the time of examination, then a second examination is required on a later date in order to record the injuries clearly. In young girls, it is important to ask if menarche has been attained or not. If yes, then at what age, the pattern of menstrual cycle and the date of last menstrual period. The sexual history is important to know whether the woman was sexually active prior to this event and when did she have the last consensual sexual intercourse, whether it was with or without the use of condom or lubricants. Contraceptive history as regards the duration of use and type of contraceptive is to be elicited. Obstetric history includes the number of abortions and deliveries she has had and any associated complications. Any past history of sexually transmitted diseases (STDs) is noted.

General Medical History

General medical history includes history of any prolonged illness, treatment, hospitalization, or surgery in the past. It is important to note if the victim has any psychiatric illness at present or in the past. It is also significant to find out any history of easy bruising or any skin problems. History of any drug allergies should be recorded.

EXAMINATION

Examination must be conducted gently and thoroughly in a calm environment, ensuring privacy and explaining each step to the patient. Collection of samples is a very crucial step in the medicolegal examination of a rape victim so samples for forensic evidence are to be collected simultaneously during examination (Table 1).

General Physical Examination

General physical examination is important to note the patient's general appearance, and emotional and mental status. The vital signs—pulse, blood pressure, respiratory rate, and temperature are recorded. At least two marks of identification of the victim are noted. Left thumb impression is taken on the examination sheet. The victim is asked to stand on a clean sheet of white paper and undress herself. Any material that falls on the paper

Section 2: Gynecology

Table 1: Various samples and site and technique of sample collection.

Site	Material	Equipment	Technique
Clothing	Clothes	Paper bags	• Patient is asked to stand on a white sheet of paper and undress herself • Presence of stains such as semen, blood, and foreign material should be properly noted • If clothes are already changed then the survivor must be asked for the clothes that were worn at the time of assault and these must be preserved • Each piece of clothing is put in separate paper bag after air drying them, duly labeled and sealed
Debris collection	Dust, fiber, etc.	• Sterile toothpick stick • Forceps	• Pick up any debris or fiber with forceps or stick and put it in an envelope
Fingernail clippings or scrapings	Skin, blood, fibers, etc.	• Sterile toothpick or nail clipper • Cotton swab	• Toothpick is used to collect material from under the nails • Nails can also be clipped and placed in a sterile container • A swab can be collected
Hair: • Pubic hair combings • Pubic hair clippings • Matted pubic hair	Hair and semen	Hair and semen	• Pick up any debris or fiber with forceps or stick and put it in an envelope • Place a paper under the buttocks of the patient, comb the pubic hair, and collect loose hair in the same paper and seal in the envelope • Matted pubic hair can be clipped with scissors and separately sealed in an envelope
Vagina	Swab for semen, sexually transmitted organism	Sterile cotton swabs and tube	• Two swabs are taken from the vulva and vagina, depending on the history and examination only if there is a history of penetration • Two vaginal smears are to be prepared on the glass slide, air-dried and sent for seminal fluid/spermatozoa examination
Endocervix	Swab for semen, sexually transmitted organism	Sterile cotton swabs and tube	• Fluid and mucus is collected from the cervix and slide prepared. The swab is placed in the tube and sealed • Another swab is taken and stroked on a chocolate agar plate and swab is discarded
Vagina	Washings for semen or spermatozoa	Distilled water, syringe	• Vaginal washing is collected using a syringe and a small rubber catheter. 2–3 mL of saline is instilled in the vagina, fluid is aspirated and fluid-filled syringe is sent to FSL laboratory
Perianal area, anus-rectum	Swab for semen or spermatozoa	Cotton swabs (dry or moist) and slides	• Cotton swabs are used to collect the material • Swab sticks for collecting samples should be moistened with distilled water provided and air dried • Drying of swabs is mandatory as there may be degradation of evidence which can render it unusable

Contd...

Contd...

Site	Material	Equipment	Technique
Oral cavity	Swab for semen or spermatozoa	Cotton swabs	Oral swabs should be taken from the posterior parts of the buccal cavity, behind the last molars where the chances of finding any evidence are highest
	Blood	Tube	Blood is collected for DNA profile, toxicology screen, blood grouping, HIV, hepatitis B, and syphilis
	Urine	Appropriate container	Urine is collected for alcohol, toxicology screen, and pregnancy testing

(DNA: deoxyribonucleic acid; HIV: human immunodeficiency virus; FSL: forensic science laboratory)

and the clothes are preserved separately in tamper-evident bags provided in the kit.

The whole body is examined for any injuries and documented on a body chart. This includes forearms for defence injuries, inner surface of upper arms or axilla for bruising, fingernails for any damage, nose for bleeding, neck, breasts, trunk for any bruising or suction type injury from bites and legs, inner thighs, buttocks and back for any abrasions or lacerations. Complex injuries should be photographed as a part of medicolegal evidence.

Oral cavity is examined for any bleeding, discharge, tenderness, etc.

Abdominal Examination

Thorough palpation is carried out for any internal trauma and detecting any preexisting pregnancy.

Genital Examination

Genital examination must be performed after taking the patient into full confidence and in dorsal or lithotomy position. Samples are collected and clearly labeled and sealed in tamper-evident bags before being handed over to the police to be carried to the forensic laboratory (see Table 1).

Pubic hair are inspected for any debris or matting with blood or semen. Any debris is collected with forceps and pubic hair clipping and combing for any foreign hair are all collected separately. On examination of external genitalia the labia majora, labia minora, posterior fourchette, and perineum are inspected for any abrasions, bruising and/or swelling. The status of hymen is irrelevant because the hymen can be torn due to several reasons such as cycling, riding, or masturbation among other things. An intact hymen does not rule out sexual violence, and a torn hymen does not prove previous sexual intercourse. However, if hymen ruptured, the site, nature, extent of damage, and whether old or freshly ruptured is noted.

Internal examination is performed with the help of a speculum examination, except if the victim refuses or if she is not sexually active as in children and young girls. In these circumstances, blind vaginal swabs can be collected. Speculum examination is done to inspect the vaginal walls for any signs of injury, bleeding, or foreign body in the vagina. The vaginal swabs and washings are collected from posterior fornix and a swab from endocervical canal for sperms. Per vaginum examination must not be conducted for establishing sexual violence and the size of the vaginal introitus has no bearing in a case of sexual violence. Per vaginum examination can be done only in adult women when medically indicated. Sometimes in case of young children, examination under anesthesia is done to assess the damage to genital tract and repair the injuries.

Anal Examination

Anal examination is best performed in the left lateral position. The anal verge is examined for any bruises, lacerations, or abrasions. Perianal, anal, or rectal swab dry or wet as appropriate should be collected. A digital rectal examination is done, if there is any suspicion of foreign body in the anal canal. Proctoscopy should be done if there is severe anal pain, bleeding, or suspicion of a foreign body.

INVESTIGATIONS

The various forensic samples and the specimens are properly labeled, sealed, and kept in refrigerator under safe custody till they are handed over to the police constable to be taken to the central forensic laboratory.

Sample Collection for the Hospital Laboratory

The following samples are collected by doctor and sent to hospital laboratory:
- Urine for carrying out urine pregnancy test and its report should be documented.
- Blood sample for baseline human immunodeficiency virus (HIV), hepatitis B surface antigen (HBsAg), and venereal disease research laboratory (VDRL).
- Radiographs of wrist, elbow, shoulders, dental examination, etc., for age estimation, if needed.
- For any suspected fracture/injury, appropriate investigation for the relevant part of the body is advised.

Sample Collection for the Forensic Science Laboratory

All the samples listed in Table 1, except blood sample for HIV, HBsAg, and VDRL, will go to Forensic Science Laboratory (FSL). The following points are to be taken into consideration while taking samples:
- Which samples need to be collected would depend upon nature of assault, time lapsed between assault and examination, and if the person has bathed/washed herself since the assault. It would be determined after thorough evaluation of the case. For example, if the survivor is certain that there is no anal intercourse; anal swabs need not be taken.
- All evidence including swabs must be collected, if a woman reports within 96 hours (4 days) of the assault. However, the likelihood of finding evidence after 72 hours (3 days) is greatly reduced.
- The spermatozoa can be identified in the samples for 72 hours after the assault. So if a survivor has suffered the assault >3 days ago, it is better to send swabs for identifying semen and not spermatozoa.
- Evidence on the external body parts and on materials such as clothing can be collected even after 96 hours.

Certain investigations are not done as a routine, but performed only when indicated. These include colposcopy and/or toluidine blue for examining microtrauma and Wood's lamp examination for stains of semen, which appear fluorescent when seen with Wood's lamp. These areas should be moistened with sterile water and swabbed with cotton-tipped applicator or directly with moist cotton swab. Dental floss can be used for bite mark casting.

In India, the Delhi High Court passed a judgment in April 2009 laying down the guidelines to be followed by different agencies such

> **Box 3:** Contents of a sexual assault forensic evidence (SAFE) kit.
>
> - Detailed instructions for the examiner
> - Forms for documentation
> - Tube for blood sample
> - Urine sample container
> - Paper bags for clothing collection
> - Large sheet of paper for patient to undress over
> - Cotton swabs for biological evidence collection
> - Sterile water
> - Glass slides
> - Unwaxed dental floss
> - Wooden stick for fingernail scrapings
> - Envelopes or boxes for individual evidence samples
> - Labels

> **Box 4:** Label of evidence box.
>
> - Kit number
> - Name of the hospital and address
> - Hospital registration number and date
> - Police station with MLC number
> - Docket number of constable receiving the box
> - Name of the survivor with age and sex
> - Date, time and signature of doctor with seal including medical council registration number

as police, hospital, child welfare committees, Session Court, and Prosecutors to effectively tackle survivors of sexual assault. The court has directed all the hospitals to identify a dedicated place for examination of rape victims 'one stop center' and to use SAFE kits (Box 3) for collection of specimens. The SAFE kit consists of a set of items used by medical personnel for gathering and preserving physical evidence following a sexual assault.

Provisional Opinion and Handing over of Report

- After thorough evaluation of the survivor including detailed history and clinical examination, the doctor must document a provisional opinion and an inference in brief mentioning relevant aspects of the history of sexual violence, clinical findings, and samples which are sent for analysis to FSL.
- Each page of the report must be signed to avoid tampering. The total number of pages attached should be mentioned on the last page.
- The report should be signed, sealed, and handed over to the police with due acknowledgement.
- It is the responsibility of the examining doctor that all evidence is packed, sealed, stored, and handed over to the police. Box 4 shows the things to be mentioned while labeling the box.
- The report should be made in triplicate—one copy to be given to the police, one copy to be kept for hospital records, and one copy of all documents be given to the survivor as it is her right to have this information.

Treatment and Psychosocial Support

- All the survivors of sexual assault should be treated for their injuries, provided emergency contraception, and prophylaxis for STDs such as gonorrhea, syphilis, and chlamydial infection.
- Postexposure prophylaxis for HIV is prescribed after assessing the risk if a survivor reports within 72 hours of the assault. Hepatitis B and tetanus vaccinations are given depending upon the immunization status of the victim.
- At the completion of the medicolegal examination, the patient should be encouraged to ask questions and clarify doubts and should be provided moral support and reassurance. Importance

of maintaining hygiene, refraining from sexual intercourse for some time, signs and symptoms of STDs, and need to follow-up should be explained. It should be emphasized that the course of medications should be completed. A written documentation should be given to the patient regarding tests performed, treatment given, and follow-up visits at 2 days post assault (to note the delayed appearance of injuries) if needed and thereafter at 3 and 6 weeks.
- If needed, the patient can be referred for supportive care to rape crisis centers, nongovernmental organizations (NGOs), shelters or safe houses, HIV counseling centers, psychologist, or social service agencies.
- *Provision for medical termination of pregnancy (MTP)*: In women undergoing MTP resulting from an assault, following points needed to be taken care of:
  - The products of conception (POC) are collected as evidence and sent to FSL for establishing paternity. They are collected in a container and rinsed with normal saline.
  - A DNA kit needs to be arranged from the FSL by contacting the respective police station. The DNA kit is used to collect blood sample of the survivor. The form is duly filled by the doctor along with a photograph of the survivor.
  - DNA samples of the survivor and the POC must be handed over to the police immediately or stored at 4°C till handover occurs. The police also needs to transport the samples at 2–8°C.

The approach to a victim of sexual assault is outlined in Flowchart 1.

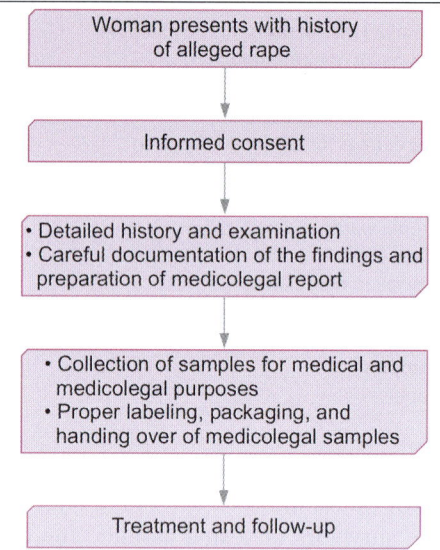

Flowchart 1: Algorithm for approach to a victim of sexual assault.

KEY POINTS

- Sexual assault in the form of rape is a challenging condition for the attending physician to handle.
- Sexual violence can have short- and long-term physical, psychological, and social impacts for the survivor.
- It is important that the attending physician is sensitive and sympathetic.
- The responsibility of correct record of history and examination findings and meticulous collection of evidence lies with the attending physician.
- The survivor should not only be treated for injuries but also be provided moral and psychological support.
- The survivor of sexual assault must be provided with accurate information about where they can receive services to address their immediate and longer-term needs (e.g., health, psychosocial, legal, economic, safety, and security).

SUGGESTED READING

1. Feeney NC. Medical examination of rape victim. The Merck Manuals. 2009.
2. Ministry of Health & Family Welfare, Government of India. (2014). Guidelines and Protocols: Medico-legal care for survivors of sexual violence. [online] Available from https://mohfw.gov.in/sites/default/files/953522324.pdf. [Last accessed March, 2020].
3. National Commission for Women. (2009). Guidelines to enable the authorities to effectively tackle sexual offences including incest and child sexual abuse offences. [online] Available from http://ncwapps.nic.in/PDFFILES/Delhi_High_Court_judgement_on_guidelines_for_dealing_rape_cases_by_various_authorities.pdf. [Last accessed March, 2020]
4. UNICEF_and_Department_of_Women_and_Child_Development, India. Manual for medical officers. Dealing with medico-legal case of victims of trafficking for commercial sexual exploitation and child sexual abuse. UNICEF. 2005.
5. World Health Organization. (2003). Guidelines for medico-legal care for victims of sexual violence. [online] Available from https://apps.who.int/iris/bitstream/handle/10665/42788/924154628X.pdf;jsessionid=5A28ACFE7DE3BF02BABD-236B4E81CB1C?sequence=1. [Last accessed March, 2020]. .

Section 3

General

- Minor Procedures in Gynecology
- Minor Procedures in Obstetrics
- Minor Procedures for Screening and Diagnosis of Cervical Cancer
- Obstetrical and Gynecological Instruments
- Endoscopic Equipment and Instruments
- Cardiotocography
- Forceps and Ventouse
- Contraception
- Medical Termination of Pregnancy and Sterilization
- Government Initiatives to Improve Maternal and Neonatal Health

49. Minor Procedures in Gynecology

*Kirti Kishore Sharma, Richa Aggarwal**

INTRODUCTION

There are several minor procedures in gynecology. The knowledge of indications, contraindications, prerequisites, details of the procedure, complications, interpretation of results, and follow-up is essential for the successful performance of the procedures. This chapter systematically describes some common office procedures as listed in Box 1.

ENDOMETRIAL BIOPSY

Endometrial biopsy is a diagnostic procedure performed for the evaluation of the endometrium. The conventional form was popularized by the famous gynecologist Howard Kelly in 1920s.[1] The procedure has undergone various modifications and today a variety of instruments are available, which scrape, curette, and aspirate the endometrium for its examination. Endometrial sampling can be done as an outpatient procedure by endometrial aspiration using Pipelle endosampler or Karman cannula or endometrial biopsy by Novak endometrial biopsy curette, or as an inpatient or a day care procedure by dilatation and curettage (Figs. 1 and 2). Patients in whom the size of the uterus is not made out or the cervix is not accessible as in obese or postmenopausal women or women with previous cesarean section (CS) where the cervix is pulled up outpatient endo-aspiration should not be attempted. These patients are offered inpatient procedure under anesthesia.

Box 1: Minor procedures in gynecology.
- Endometrial biopsy
- Hysterosalpingography
- Hysteroscopy
- Culdocentesis and colpotomy
- Wet smear test

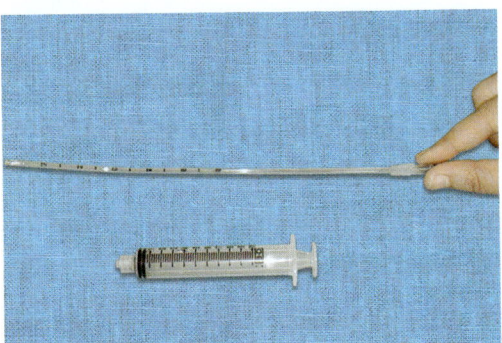

Fig. 1: Pipelle endometrial biopsy sampler.

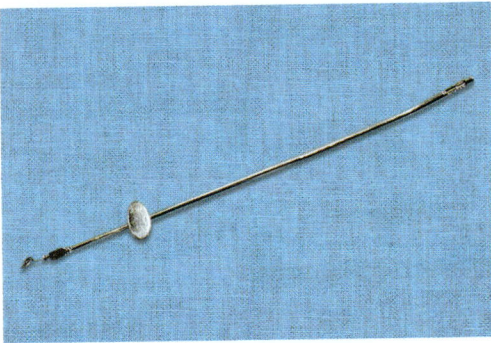

Fig. 2: Endometrial curette.

Indications and Contraindications

The indications and contraindications are as given in Table 1.

Preprocedure Considerations

It is usually done in the premenstrual phase, except if a perimenopausal woman has continuous bleeding and the endometrium is documented to be thick usually ≥7 mm on ultrasonography.

The patient should be advised to use protection either through barrier contraceptive or abstinence during the cycle in which she is planned for endometrial biopsy, as there is a risk of disrupting early pregnancy when done in premenstrual phase. An informed consent of the patient should be taken.

Timing of Procedure

The procedure is performed in the premenstrual phase to ensure the presence of adequate endometrial tissue and to know whether the woman has ovulatory cycles or not. The pattern in the premenstrual phase is secretory in ovulatory cycles (Fig. 3) under the influence of progesterone secreted from corpus luteum whereas it is proliferative in anovulatory cycles (Fig. 4). In postmenstrual phase, the pattern will always be proliferative, irrespective of whether the cycles are ovulatory or anovulatory.

In case of irregular menstrual cycles, endometrial biopsy should be performed after 3 weeks of last menstrual cycle to allow for regeneration of the endometrium or within 6–8 hours of onset of menses. Endometrial sampling for infertility for documentation of ovulation is no longer advocated as other noninvasive methods, such as serial ultrasound for follicular monitoring and day 21 serum progesterone levels, are available. However, it is still performed to rule out endometrial tuberculosis in some centers where prevalence of tuberculosis is high. In these cases, sampling is done in the premenstrual phase and sample is collected from the cornual ends due to its proximity to the fallopian tubes. This gives the pathologist the best chance to detect the giant cells and the tubercles (Fig. 5). The length of the cycle and the date of the last menstrual period (LMP) should be recorded for correct interpretation of histopathological report.

Table 1: Indications and contraindications of endometrial biopsy.

Indications	Contraindications
• Abnormal uterine bleeding: To know the pattern of endometrium whether proliferative or secretory and to rule out endometrial hyperplasia/carcinoma • *Infertility*: To rule out endometrial tuberculosis • *Suspected genital tuberculosis*: Hypomenorrhea, amenorrhea, and infrequently menorrhagia	• Pelvic infection • Suspected pregnancy • Active uterine bleeding (relative contraindication)

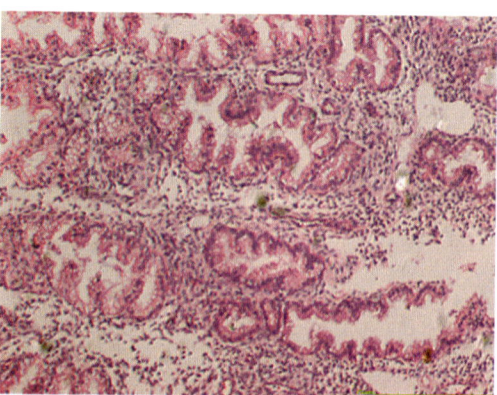

Fig. 3: Secretory phase.

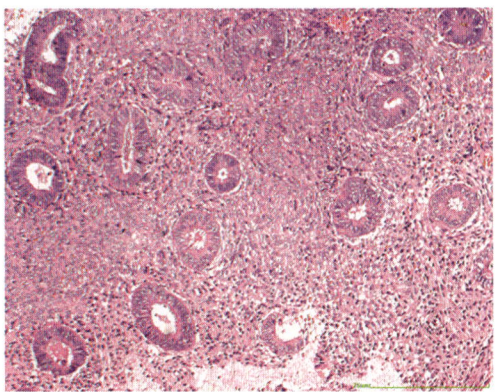
Fig. 4: Proliferative phase.

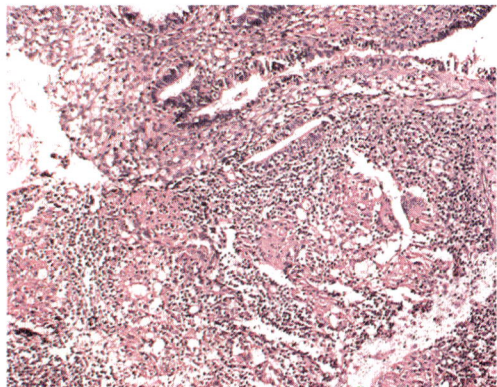
Fig. 5: Endometrial biopsy showing granulomas.

Pretreatment with Analgesics

The woman can be administered tablet paracetamol 650 mg orally, or a nonsteroidal anti-inflammatory agent ibuprofen 400 mg, or naproxen 750 mg half an hour before procedure to reduce procedure-related pain.

Procedure

The patient is asked to lie in the dorsal position. Under strict aseptic precautions, bimanual examination is performed to assess the position and size of the uterus. The cervix is exposed by retracting the posterior vaginal wall with Sims' speculum and anterior vaginal wall with anterior vaginal wall retractor. The anterior lip of the cervix is held with vulsellum, tenaculum, or long-Allis forceps. The cervix is cleaned with povidone–iodine solution. An endometrial biopsy sampler, Pipelle or a Karman cannula, is inserted into the endometrial cavity. Two or three endometrial stripes are removed for evaluation. For detection of ovulation, only one stripe may be enough; however, in cases of abnormal uterine bleeding or suspected endometritis, multiple areas of the endometrium must be sampled. All four walls are sampled, one strip each from anterior, posterior, and lateral walls. When Karman cannula or the Pipelle endosampler is used, a 20 cc syringe may be attached to the cannula to create negative pressure. This will result in a greater volume of endometrium being aspirated. The tissue is then placed in 8–10% formalin for histopathological examination and in saline for culture of microorganisms or acid-fast bacilli (AFB).

Cervical stenosis or spasm, or an acutely anteverted or retroverted cochleate uterus may make the navigation of cannula difficult. In these cases, applying a gentle traction on the cervix may straighten the cervicouterine axis and facilitate the entry of biopsy cannula. Otherwise analgesia or paracervical block with 1% lignocaine may be used. The uterine sound is negotiated to confirm the position and size of the uterus followed by a cannula. Pretreatment with tablet misoprostol 200–400 μg vaginally 2–4 hours before endometrial biopsy may be useful in women with failure to obtain sample or else it may be carried out under ultrasound or hysteroscopic guidance. Sometimes doing it on a semi full bladder is helpful.

Box 2: Complications of endometrial biopsy.
- Failure to obtain sample due to cervical stenosis, spasm, or cochleate uterus
- Uterine perforation: One or two cases per 1,000 procedures
- Postprocedure infection
- *Bleeding*: Rare
- Severe vasovagal reflex*

*Can be prevented by premedicating with nonsteroidal anti-inflammatory drugs (NSAIDs).

Table 2: Indications and contraindications of hysterosalpingography.

Indications	Contraindications
• Infertility	• Acute pelvic infection
• Congenital uterine defects, i.e., Müllerian duct anomalies	• Active uterine bleeding
• Acquired uterine defects, i.e., submucosal fibroid	• Pregnancy
• Asherman's syndrome	• Iodine allergy
• Cervical incompetence	
• Preoperative assessment for tubal recanalization	

Complications

The complications of the procedure are as given in Box 2.

HYSTEROSALPINGOGRAPHY

Hysterosalpingography (HSG) is a radiographic imaging technique, used primarily for the evaluation of tubal factor in infertility. The procedure is used to evaluate the endocervical canal, endometrial cavity, lumen and the patency of the fallopian tubes by injecting radiopaque contrast medium through the cervical canal. Initially, oil-based dyes were used, which have been replaced by water-soluble dyes. Today, despite the advent of laparohysteroscopy for evaluation of the uterine cavity and fallopian tubes, HSG remains an important primary investigation of choice for evaluation of tubal factor in women with infertility.

Indications and Contraindications

The indications and contraindications of HSG are as listed in Table 2.

Timing of Procedure

The procedure is carried out postmenstrual in the follicular phase of the cycle between cycle days 5 and 10. This avoids interference from intrauterine bleeding and clots, prevents the risk of woman being pregnant, and exposure of the fertilized ovum to irradiation and flushing it from the fallopian tube. It is advisable that the patient should be dry for 2–3 days after menstruation to prevent intravasation of dye in open sinuses and flushing of endometrial tissue into the peritoneal cavity.

Preprocedure Considerations

Treatment with Antibiotics

Prophylactic antibiotics are usually not prescribed routinely, except in women with a history of pelvic inflammatory disease or those with dilated tubes or findings suggestive of peritubal adhesions on HSG. Doxycycline 100 mg twice a day for 5 days may be prescribed.

Pretreatment with Analgesics

Pretreatment with analgesics such as acetaminophen 650 mg orally or nonsteroidal anti-inflammatory drugs (NSAIDs), e.g., ibuprofen 400 mg or naproxen 750 mg 30–60 minutes before the procedure is helpful to decrease the discomfort associated with the procedure.

In areas where the prevalence of tuberculosis is high, endometrial tuberculosis is ruled out by endometrial biopsy or menstrual blood for AFB smear and culture prior to HSG to prevent the risk of dissemination in women where HSG is done for infertility. It is important to note that endometrial biopsy or menstrual blood examination for ruling out tuberculosis is not required in women undergoing HSG for uterine anomalies, cervical incompetence, or preoperative assessment for tubal recanalization.

Procedure

The patient is given a prior appointment at an appropriate date according to her date of LMP, the procedure is explained, and consent is taken. On the day of the procedure, the patient is given oral or parenteral analgesic 30–60 minutes before the procedure. The instrument tray is checked (Fig. 6). With the patient in dorsal or lithotomy position, under all aseptic conditions, a per speculum and per vaginum examination is done to rule out genital tract infection. The posterior vaginal wall is retracted using a Sims' speculum, and cervix and vagina are visualized and cleaned with povidone–iodine swab. The cervix is held with vulsellum or a long Allis forceps.

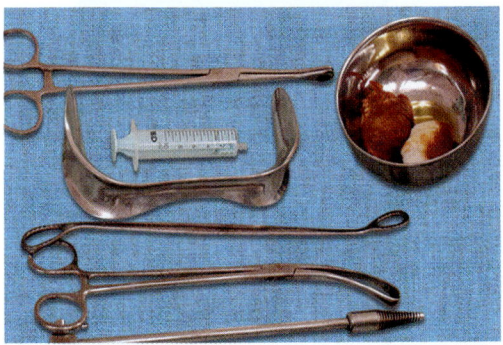

Fig. 6: Tray with instruments for hysterosalpingography.

A Leech-Wilkinson cannula, Collin's cannula, acorn cannula, a pediatric Foley catheter with a stent, or designated injection catheter is introduced in the cervix. While using the Leech-Wilkinson or Collin's cannula, care is taken not to screw the cannula too far in the cervix as it can then get obstructed by the anterior or posterior walls of the uterus in a posterior or anterior cochleate uterus, respectively. Before fixing the cannula to the cervix, air from the cannula is displaced by flushing it with a small amount of dye to avoid the displaced air bubbles from blocking the cornual ends of the tubes, while pushing in the dye and resulting in a false-positive result. If a Foley catheter is used, it should be ensured that the portion of the catheter with the bulb is beyond the internal os in the uterine cavity; otherwise the catheter will slip out when the bulb is distended with saline. The Foley bulb is inflated with 3 cc of saline and pulled down, to obstruct the internal os. A 20 mL syringe with water-soluble radiopaque dye is fixed to the cannula.

The Sims' speculum is then removed; traction applied on the vulsellum to straighten the cervicouterine axis and contrast medium is injected slowly. Slow injection is important as a rapid injection can cause discomfort, tubal spasm, and back flow. Once the uterine cavity is delineated on fluoroscopy, a still image is obtained and dye is again slowly pushed to visualize the Fallopian tubes and the spill. Usually not more than 10–15 mL of media is required as the capacity of uterine cavity is 3–5 mL; 1–2 mL is required to outline each tube and another 1–2 mL is required for the spill. In case there is bilateral cornual block, an antispasmodic drug-like injection Buscopan may be administered and the procedure is repeated. Usually, only three basic films are required. A scout film to compare with, one film to document the uterine contour and tubal patency, and a postevaluation film to detect any areas of contrast loculation due to peritubal adhesions.

On an average, HSG is performed in 10 minutes, which involves approximately 90 seconds of fluoroscopic time and has an average radiation exposure of 1–2 rads. The choice of media available is between oil-soluble media or water-soluble media. There are no proven merits of one over the other and either choice is appropriate. Arguments against oil-soluble media are that, it is too viscous to reveal internal tubal architecture, disperses poorly in the pelvis, and has significant risks such as granulomatous reactions, intravasation, and embolism. Those in favor cite studies that reveal increased pregnancy rates in women following HSG with oil-soluble media as against those in whom water-soluble media has been used.[2] Compared to laparoscopy, which is the gold standard method for evaluating tubal factor, HSG has only moderate sensitivity of 65%, i.e., the ability to detect patent tubes when true and a high specificity of 83%, i.e., the ability to detect blocked tubes when true and can help decide whether laparoscopy is needed before beginning the treatment for infertility.[3]

Interpretation of the Hysterosalpingography

Normal HSG shows a triangular endometrial cavity. The contour of the endometrium is usually smooth. Both the Fallopian tubes are outlined and show a free spill. The mucosal pattern can be appreciated in the ampullary part as some black shadows (Fig. 7).

The HSG may reveal unilateral or bilateral tubal occlusion, which may be proximal, midsegmental, or distal. Hydrosalpinx appears like a distended retort-shaped tube (Fig. 8). It may also reveal uterine anomalies like a septate or arcuate uterus (Fig. 9); some intrauterine filling defects as seen in submucosal fibroid, and intrauterine adhesions. Sometimes artifacts may be confused with filling defects. Loculated spill may occur in women with peritubal adhesions due to prior pelvic inflammatory disease or tuberculosis (Fig. 10). The margins of the uterine cavity may be irregular in cases of chronic endometritis. An irregular, contracted cavity with irregular margins and marked intravasation of dye is suggestive of endometrial tuberculosis (Fig. 11).

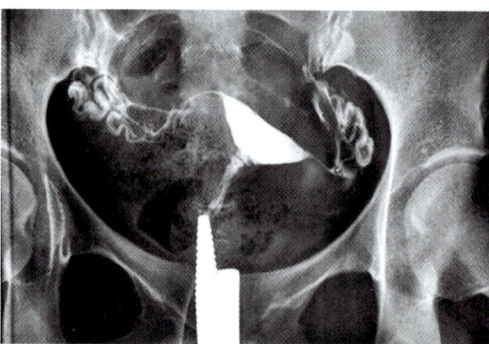

Fig. 7: Normal hysterosalpingogram.

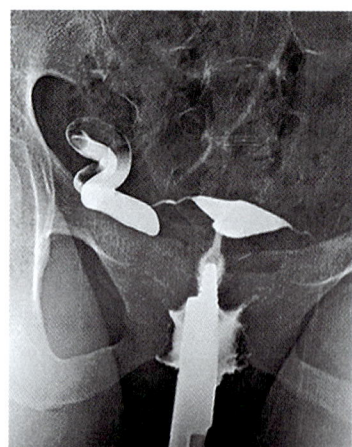

Fig. 8: Hysterosalpingogram showing right-sided hydrosalpinx and left-sided isthmic block.

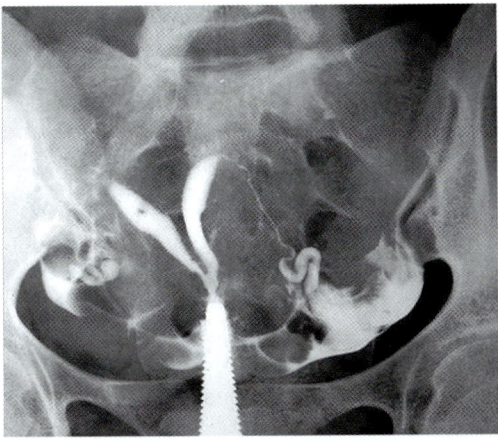

Fig. 9: Hysterosalpingogram showing bicornuate uterus with a single cervix.

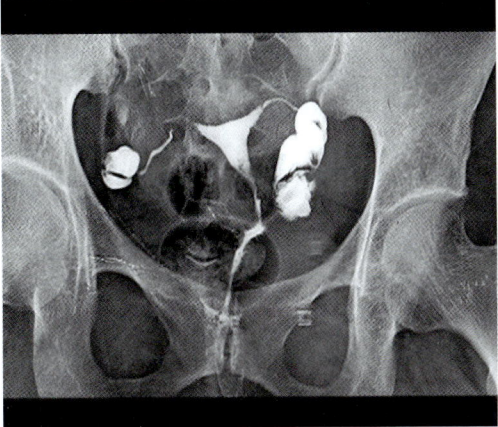

Fig. 10: Hysterosalpingogram with bilateral hydrosalpinx and left-sided loculated spill.

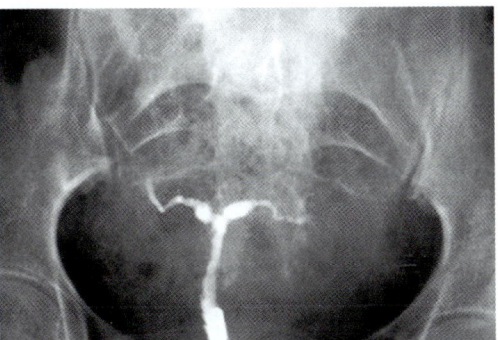

Fig. 11: Hysterosalpingogram showing irregular contracted uterine cavity.

Complications

The complications are uncommon and are listed in Box 3.

Postprocedure Advice and Follow-up

The patient may be prescribed an antibiotic doxycycline 100 mg twice a day for 3–5 days if indicated and a pain killer as per need. She is asked to come for follow-up after 2 weeks for a pelvic examination to rule out pelvic infection or earlier if she has any symptoms

> **Box 3:** Complications of hysterosalpingography.
> - Pelvic infection
> - Vasovagal reaction
> - Allergic reaction to contrast
> - Intravasation
> - Embolism
> - Granuloma formation
>
> *Note*: Last two complications are seen with oil-based contrast agents only.

suggestive of pelvic infection such as pain in lower abdomen or discharge per vaginal. If tubes are patent, the couple is advised to have midcycle contact as the chances of conception may increase after HSG. There is no need to abstain.

HYSTEROSCOPY

Hysteroscopy is a procedure performed to directly visualize the cervical canal and uterine cavity. The procedure was first performed on a living patient by Pantaleoni in 1869 using the hysteroscope developed by Desormeaux in 1865.[4] It took a century of further development in technique, optical instrumentation, and advances in distension media to enable Hamou in 1979[4] to use the contact microhysteroscope with the panoramic view.

Today, hysteroscopy is considered as the gold standard for visualizing the cervical canal and uterine cavity and taking a directed endometrial biopsy. We can now perform office hysteroscopy both diagnostic and therapeutic with minimum discomfort to the patient and promising results. Office hysteroscopy refers to performance of hysteroscopy, either diagnostic or operative, on an outpatient basis in the absence of or minimal use of anesthesia.

Indications

With the development in technology and increasing popularity of "see and treat" approach, the indications of office hysteroscopy are ever increasing, and several diagnostic and operative procedures can be carried out in one setting. The decision must be individualized depending on available technology, associated complications, patient demands, and technical expertise of the clinician. Table 3 gives the indications of office hysteroscopy.

Contraindications

The contraindications of hysteroscopy are listed in Box 4.

Preparation

A detailed history and examination should be coupled with relevant investigations before the decision for hysteroscopy. A "see and treat" possibility must be explained to the patient with the need to switch from a diagnostic to operative approach, if required. Informed consent should be taken and need for anesthesia should be assessed. Menstrual history including date of LMP should be enquired for and the procedure is best performed in the postmenstrual proliferative phase of the cycle.

To avoid discomfort to the patient, 650 mg of acetaminophen or 500 mg of naproxen or 400 mg of ibuprofen can be given oral preoperatively about an hour before the procedure. Some surgeons advocate the use of prostaglandin E1 (PGE1) tablets by vaginal route in the dose of 200–400 μg 12–24 hours before the procedure to facilitate atraumatic entry of the hysteroscope in the cervix.

For details of hysteroscopic equipment, and instruments refer to Chapter 53 on Endoscopic Equipment and Instruments.

Box 4: Contraindications of hysteroscopy.
- Viable intrauterine pregnancy
- Active pelvic infection
- Known cervical or uterine cancer
- Excessive uterine bleeding

Table 3: Indications of hysteroscopy.

Diagnostic hysteroscopy	Operative hysteroscopy
• Abnormal uterine bleeding (AUB) • *Infertility/subfertility*: In selected cases with abnormal ultrasonogram or hysterosalpingogram • Unexplained infertility • Recurrent spontaneous abortions • Evaluation of suspected Müllerian abnormalities • Chronic pelvic pain • Evaluation of the tubocornual block • Postabortal or postpartum for any retained products	• Hysteroscopy-directed biopsy • Resection of submucous myoma • Removal of endometrial polyp • Excision of uterine septum • Endometrial ablation for AUB • Removal of foreign body and misplaced intrauterine device • Adhesiolysis of uterine synechiae • Tubal cannulation for isolated proximal tubal obstruction • Hysteroscopic sterilization

Procedure

Method

With the patient in dorsal or lithotomy position, the vaginal walls are either retracted using the preferred speculum, or a vaginoscopic no-touch technique may be employed. Paracervical block is given with 1% lignocaine, if cervical dilatation is required. The hysteroscope is introduced into the cervical canal gently and the cervical canal is examined. In office hysteroscopy, smallest possible diameter of hysteroscope is used to avoid routine cervical dilatation to minimize trauma to endocervix and endometrium. Appropriate choice of distension medium should be made according to the procedure. For diagnostic procedures, gaseous or low-viscosity media can be chosen and if use of monopolar cautery is contemplated, then nonconducting medium like glycine 1.5% should be opted for. Normal saline can be used if bipolar energy source is used. Intrauterine pressures of 40–50 mm Hg for diagnostic and 70–80 mm Hg for operative purposes should be maintained.

The internal os is visualized and a panoramic view of the endometrial cavity is taken (Fig. 12). The tip of instrument is placed 1–1.5 cm from fundus and a view of the whole cavity and tubal ostia can be gained. With a 30° telescope, the light cable is used to rotate the telescope along its axis. Look for intrauterine lesion such as polyps or myomas. Myomas would appear as smooth rounded masses covered by a network of thin, fragile vessels (Figs. 13 and 14). The uterine septum will appear as a avascular blanched structure hindering the visualization of fundus and bilateral cornu in a single field.

The pathologies that may be detected on hysteroscopy and interventions indicated for the same are tabulated in Table 4.

Complications

Complications with hysteroscopy are rare but can be life threatening. The complications are

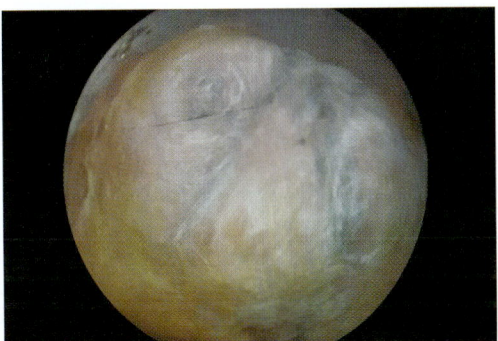

Fig. 13: Hysteroscopic view of a submucous fibroid.

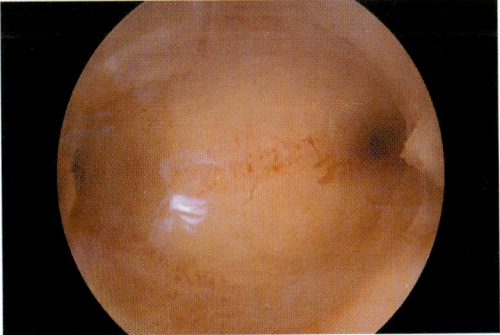

Fig. 12: Normal panoramic view of uterine cavity on hysteroscopy.

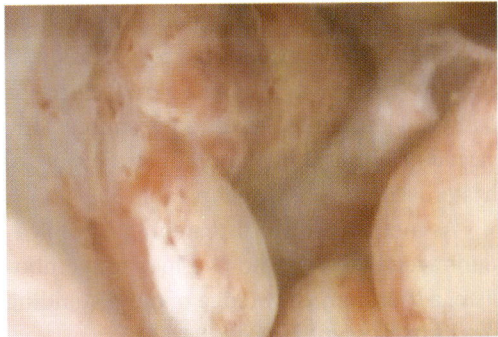

Fig. 14: Hysteroscopic view of multiple submucous myomas.

Table 4: Pathologies detected on hysteroscopy and the interventions indicated.

Diagnosis	Prerequisites for operative intervention	Methods	Practice points
Polyp		• The pedicle can be cut with scissors using a liquid or gaseous medium • The pedicle can be excised, or the polyp can be resected if sessile using loop electrode in liquid medium	Remove en bloc or in fragments Use of ball electrode for control of bleeding from base
Submucous myoma	• Uterus is normal or bulky in size • Size of myoma ≤3 cm (can be bigger depending upon skill of surgeon) • Intramural extension is less than 50%	• Needle or loop electrode to cut pedicle • Resection with a resectoscope	• Preoperative treatment with GnRH analogs may be useful • Can be done as a two-stage procedure
Uterine septum	• Associated with recurrent abortion or unexplained infertility or infertility with failed IVF	• Resection should be done from below upward using scissors if septum is thin or a Colin's knife resectoscope electrode	• Appearance of bleeding indicates resection is complete • Bilateral cornual ends are visualized in the same view
Endometrial ablation	• Abnormal uterine bleeding with failed medical management and premalignant and malignant lesions have been ruled out	• Resection using loop • Roller ball coagulation • Laser ablation	• Preoperative treatment with GnRH analogs may be done to make the endometrium thin
Intrauterine adhesions/ synechiae	• Adhesions leading to amenorrhea, infertility, or chronic pelvic pain • Treatment for specific condition, e.g., tuberculosis before surgical procedure	• Using scissors or monopolar cautery, the flimsy and central adhesions to be cut first following the flow of media followed by the marginal, dense adhesions from below upward	• Laparoscopy may be needed if dense adhesions are present • Postoperative IUCD or estrogen may be needed

(IVF: in vitro fertilization; GnRH: gonadotropin-releasing hormone; IUCD: intrauterine contraceptive device)

lesser with diagnostic procedures compared to operative procedures. Electrosurgical injuries are lesser with bipolar energy source as compared to unipolar energy source. The various complications and adverse events of hysteroscopy are as listed in Table 5.

As most of the life-threatening complications are related to fluid overload and embolism, a thorough knowledge of the distending medium is essential.

The distension media are the agents, which convert the potential space in the uterine cavity into a real space for aiding the visualization of the uterine walls and carrying out interventions. The various types of distending media are as described below.

Gaseous

Carbon dioxide is ideal for office hysteroscopy. Flow rate should not exceed 100 mL/min and the pressure should be adjusted below 150 mm Hg. Trendelenburg position should be avoided with this medium. The advantages include neatness as spillage

Table 5: Complications and adverse events of hysteroscopy.

Complications	Remarks
Uterine perforation	• Most common complication (0.1–1%) • Suspected when instrument passes beyond the depth of fundus, loss of visualization, sudden increase in fluid deficit, and visualization of omentum or bowel
Cervical trauma	• Common in women with cervical stenosis
Urinary tract or bowel injury	• Usually in association with uterine perforation and use of electrical current
Fluid overload and dyselectrolytemia	• Rare complication occurs when fluid deficit with electrolyte-poor media (glycine) is >1,000 mL and with electrolyte-containing media (normal saline) is >2,500 mL. The patient can have difficulty in breathing confusion or coma. • Serum Na^+ and K^+ need to be monitored
Embolism	• CO_2 or air embolism can cause cardiovascular collapse and is a life-threatening complication. Care is taken to remove all air bubbles in the inflow tubing before starting the procedure
Hemorrhage	• Potential sites are operative site, uterine perforation and cervical laceration. Cervical laceration can be sutured, operative site hemostasis can be achieved with ball cautery or with an intrauterine Foley's catheter bulb inflated with 15–30 mL saline
Electrosurgical Injury	• Local from active electrode or remote from diversion of current • Avoided by always moving the electrode once it is activated
Infection	• Endomyometritis • Peritonitis
Late complications	• Intrauterine adhesions (synechiae) • Pregnancy-related complications Uterine rupture, placenta accreta/increta

cannot occur and it allows entry evaluation of the endocervical canal. The disadvantages are that it cannot be used for operative work as it cannot flush the cavity of debris; it is further unsuitable for use if bleeding is present, as it mixes with blood very easily and obscures vision. The potential risk of gas embolism exists with CO_2 as the distention medium.

Liquid

These are available as low-viscosity or high-viscosity media.

Low-viscosity distension media: Normal saline, 0.9% sodium chloride solution, has the advantage of being isotonic and hence decreased chances of hemolysis in case of intravasation. It can be combined with use of neodymium-doped yttrium aluminum garnet (Nd:YAG) laser, potassium-titanyl-phosphate (KTP) laser, mechanical devices such as scissors and graspers, bipolar electrodes and hence can be used for operative hysteroscopy. The disadvantages include the need to maintain constant infusion and high flow rates for distension as it leaks out of the uterus easily. Large volumes may be needed in case of operative hysteroscopy. It mixes with blood easily, hence making high flow rates paramount. Monopolar electrodes cannot be used with saline medium as it is a good conductor of current. With electrolyte media, the procedure should be stopped if the fluid deficit reaches 2.5 L.

Glycine 1.5%, sorbitol 3%, and mannitol 5% are low-viscosity, nonconducting fluids. Their main advantage over saline is that they can be used with monopolar cautery. The disadvantages are, however, significant. Glycine can cause acute hyponatremia, if there is vascular absorption. Hence, volume absorbed must be calculated every 15 minutes by maintaining an inflow-outflow chart. If absorbed fluid exceeds 500 mL, serum electrolytes should be measured, and the procedure should be stopped if fluid deficit exceeds 1 L with nonelectrolyte medium. When delivered at high pressure, glycine can cause disturbance in oxygenation and coagulation, and lead to elevated ammonia levels. Usually an infusion pressure of 70-80 mm Hg is adequate. Excessive sorbitol can cause hyperglycemia.

High-viscosity distension media: Hyskon (32% dextran-70 in 10% dextrose) is a colorless, viscid solution. It is immiscible with blood and provides very good visualization even with bleeding. The disadvantages are however, several; it tends to caramelize on instruments, can cause anaphylactoid reactions, fluid overload, electrolyte disturbances, pulmonary edema, and bleeding diathesis, hence not used commonly.

CULDOCENTESIS AND COLPOTOMY

Culdocentesis is defined as aspiration of fluid from cul-de-sac, i.e., pouch of Douglas (POD), with a needle puncturing the vaginal wall in between the uterosacral ligaments. It is a diagnostic procedure, which is indicated when fluid aspirated from the rectouterine pouch will help confirm a clinical diagnosis.

Colpotomy is giving an incision in a mass bulging in cul-de-sac through the posterior fornix to drain pus in women with a midline pelvic abscess dissecting in the rectovaginal septum.

In present day practice, owing to the advent of effective diagnostic tools, the use of culdocentesis is limited to emergency situations when ultrasound is not available or the patient is hemodynamically unstable. Culdocentesis is the fastest diagnostic modality available.

Indications and Contraindications

The indications and contraindications of culdocentesis are as shown in Table 6.

Procedure

Before proceeding with culdocentesis, a written informed consent is taken from the patient, even if the procedure is being carried out in emergency. The patient is made to lie in dorsal or lithotomy position on the examination table with adequate exposure and lighting.

A bimanual pelvic examination is carried out before performing the procedure. The posterior vaginal wall is retracted by a vaginal

Table 6: Indications and contraindications of culdocentesis.

Indications	Contraindications
• Suspected hemoperitoneum due to ruptured ectopic pregnancy or ruptured corpus luteum cyst • Pelvic abscess secondary to pelvic inflammatory disease, ruptured tubo-ovarian (TO) abscess, uterine perforation, or puerperal sepsis • Prior to colpotomy for pelvic abscess	• Uncooperative patient • Immobile retroverted uterus • Coagulopathies

speculum such as Cusco's or Sims' speculum. The posterior lip of cervix is held with a tenaculum, vulsellum, or a long Allis forceps. The cervix is pulled anteriorly by applying traction to the tenaculum to stretch the posterior vaginal wall between the blade of the speculum and its attachment to the cervix and stabilize it for aspiration. An 18-gauge spinal needle with a 20 mL syringe is used for the aspiration. The needle is then advanced along the lower blade of the speculum. It is inserted at approximately 1.0–1.5 cm lower than the point at which the vagina is attached to the cervix in the midline. Insert it to a depth of 2–2.5 cm. A gentle suction is applied, while stabilizing the needle. The needle is then slowly drawn out while maintaining the suction. The blood or fluid may be obtained immediately or while withdrawing the needle. The syringe may be filled with 2–3 mL of normal saline (non-bacteriostatic) prior to the procedure. The fluid may be used to confirm entry and to dislodge any plugs, which may have formed on puncture. The procedure may be repeated in case of a negative tap with slight manipulation of the needle tip, but excessive depth or lateral movement should be avoided.

Interpretation of Results

Depending upon the nature of fluid aspirated, the result of culdocentesis is interpreted as shown in Table 7.

Complications

Culdocentesis is a very safe procedure, but complications have been reported. These include rupture of tubo-ovarian mass, intestinal perforation, and bleeding in case of a woman with coagulopathy. Thus, culdocentesis retains a minor, but important role in present-day practice.

Table 7: Interpretation of results of culdocentesis.

Nature of aspirated fluid	Differential diagnosis
Clear, serous, straw colored (usually only a few mL)	Normal peritoneal fluid
Large amount of clear fluid	• Ruptured or large ovarian cyst • Ascites • Ovarian, tubal, or peritoneal carcinoma

Turbid serous fluid: Exudate with polymorphonuclear leukocytes	• *Pelvic inflammatory disease*:
	  – Gonococcal salpingitis
	  – Chronic salpingitis

Purulent fluid	• Pelvic abscess • Ruptured tubo-ovarian abscess • Ruptured appendicular abscess • Diverticulitis with perforation
Bright red blood	• Acute ruptured ectopic • Bleeding corpus luteum • *Intra-abdominal injury*: Rupture of liver, spleen, and other organs • Ruptured aortic aneurysm
Old, brown and non-clotting blood	• Endometrioma • Old or chronic ectopic pregnancy • Old intra-abdominal injury (e.g., delayed splenic rupture)
Oily, sebaceous fluid	Benign teratoma

Colpotomy

The procedure for colpotomy is essentially the same as culdocentesis but is done under anesthesia, regional or general. Here a wide-bore needle is introduced at the site of maximum bulge in POD. After pus is aspirated on culdocentesis, a stab incision is given at the same point to drain the pus. A finger is introduced to break the loculi and a wide-bore drain Malecot's catheter is left in the opening and fixed to the incision site. It is connected to a bag. The pus is sent for culture sensitivity.

This procedure is useful in cases of septic abortion or pelvic inflammatory disease where the pelvic abscess is localized and walled off the abdomen. The upper abdomen is normal. These women may have rectal symptoms such as increased frequency of defecation and on per rectal examination there may be a bulge felt through the anterior wall of rectum.

There is a risk of rectal injury if the abscess is not midline and dissecting into the rectovaginal septum.

VAGINAL WET MOUNT

A vaginal wet mount is also called vaginal smear, wet smear, or wet prep. It is a quick and easy outpatient investigation and should be routinely carried out to obtain information on vaginal infections.

Indication

A vaginal wet smear is indicated in women presenting with complaints of excessive or malodorous vaginal discharge and/or vulvar itching. It is used to diagnose vulvovaginal candidiasis, trichomoniasis, and/or bacterial vaginosis.

Prerequisites

Avoid vaginal douching, vaginal pessaries, and use of tampon for 2–3 days before the test. Sexual intercourse should be avoided for 24 hours before the test as it can affect the vaginal pH.

Procedure

Patient is made to lie in dorsal position. Posterior vaginal wall is retracted with Sims' speculum followed by retraction of the anterior vaginal wall with an anterior vaginal wall retractor. The discharge collected on the blade of speculum is placed directly on a slide and a wet mount is prepared by adding a drop of saline and covering it with a cover slip. It is examined under a microscope first under 10X and then with 40X magnification.

Additional information can be obtained from another wet mount prepared by suspending vaginal secretions in a drop of 10% potassium hydroxide (KOH) placed on a slide. In case of bacterial vaginosis, a strong fishy odor is emitted on adding a few drops of a KOH solution to the sample of the vaginal discharge before placing a cover slip. This is known as whiff test. The interpretation of the wet smear is described in Table 8. The pH of the discharge can be assessed and if it is >4.5 it is likely to be bacterial vaginosis or trichomonas vaginalis.

Complications

The test is without any risks. Minor bleeding or some discomfort may occur to the patient otherwise.

KEY POINTS

- Any procedure, whether minor or major, is fraught with complications.
- Proper selection of patients prior to any minor procedure is important.
- It is important that there should be a valid indication, appropriate timing, and no contraindication to the procedure.
- An informed consent and preprocedure counseling before every procedure is mandatory.
- The knowledge of the potential complications with various procedures, preventive measures, and early diagnosis is important for the safety of the patients.

Table 8: Interpretation of wet smear examination.

Wet smear examination	Normal vaginal secretions	Abnormal vaginal secretions
Gross examination	Small in amount, nonfoul smelling, white in color, floccular in consistency, usually located in posterior fornix	• *Bacterial infection:* Mucopurulent • *Candidiasis:* White, lumpy discharge resembling cottage cheese • *Trichomoniasis:* Foul smelling, yellow-green, foamy discharge • *Bacterial vaginosis:* Thin, gray-white vaginal discharge with a strong fishy odor
Microscopic examination	Superficial epithelial cells with few white blood cells	• *Bacterial infection:* Abundant white blood cells present • *Candidiasis:* Yeast cells and hyphae on potassium hydroxide (KOH) solution wet mount (Fig. 15) • *Trichomoniasis:* Motile trichomonads and increased leukocytes (Fig. 16) • *Bacterial vaginosis:* Clue cells* and few leucocytes
Vaginal pH	3.8–4.2	• *Bacterial infection:* >4.5 • *Candidiasis:* <4.5 • *Trichomoniasis:* >4.5 • *Bacterial vaginosis:* >4.5
KOH "whiff test"	Absent	• *Bacterial infection:* Absent • *Candidiasis:* Absent • *Trichomoniasis:* May be present • *Bacterial vaginosis:* Present

*Clue cells are superficial vaginal epithelial cells with adherent bacteria, usually Gardnerella vaginalis, which obliterates the crisp cell border when examined microscopically.

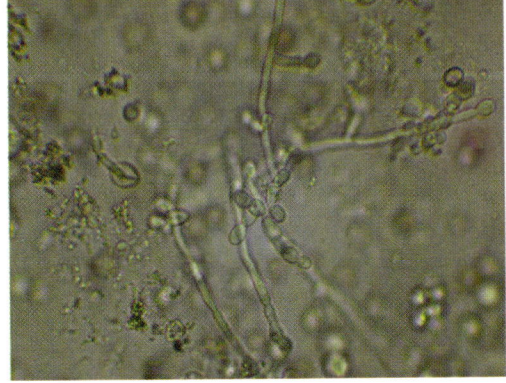

Fig. 15: Yeast mycelia seen on potassium hydroxide mount.

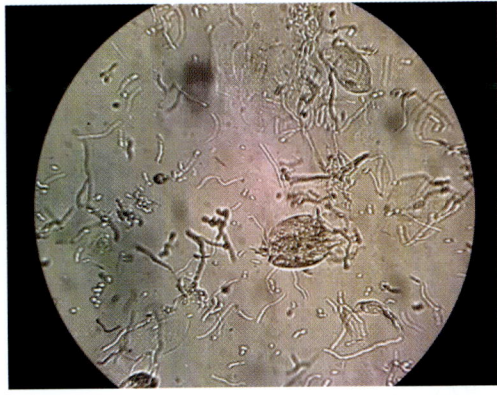

Fig. 16: *Trichomonas vaginalis* in saline smear.

REFERENCES

1. Katz VL, Lentz C, Lobo RA, Gershenson DM. Comprehensive Gynecology, 5th edition. Chicago: Mosby; 2007.
2. Watson A, Vandekerckhove P, Lilford R, Vail A, Brosens I, Hughes E. A meta-analysis of the therapeutic role of soluble contrast media in hysterosalpingography: a surprising result? Fertil Steril. 1994;61(3):470-7.
3. Swart P, Mol BW, van der Veen F, van Beurden M, Redekop WK, Bossuyt PM. The accuracy of hysterosalpingography in the diagnosis of tubal pathology: a meta-analysis. Fertil Steril. 1995;64(3):486-91.
4. Mettler L, Scholfmanyer T, Ruther D, Alkatout I. Practical Manual for Hysteroscopic Gynaecological Surgery, 2nd edition. New Delhi: Jaypee Brothers Medical Publishers (P) Ltd; 2013.

SUGGESTED READING

1. ACOG Technology Assessment No. 13: Hysteroscopy. Obstet Gynecol. 2018;131(5):e151-6.
2. Practice Committee of the American Society for Reproductive Medicine. Diagnostic evaluation of the infertile female: A committee opinion. Fertil Steril. 2015;103(6):e44-50.
3. Royal College of Obstetricians and Gynaecologists (RCOG) (2011). Hysteroscopy, Best Practice in Outpatient (Green-top Guideline No. 59) [online] Available from https://www.rcog.org.uk/en/guidelines-research-services/guidelines/gtg59/. [Last accessed March, 2020].

50. Minor Procedures in Obstetrics

Nishtha Jaiswal

INTRODUCTION

There are several minor procedures in obstetrics. This chapter systematically describes some common procedures as listed in Box 1. The indications, contraindications, timing of procedures, surgical steps of procedure, and their complications have been described briefly.

Box 1: Minor procedures in obstetrics.
- Amniotomy
- Pudendal block
- Perineal infiltration
- Episiotomy
- Obstetric anal sphincter injury
- Cervical tear
- Vaginal tear

AMNIOTOMY

Amniotomy, also known as artificial rupture of membranes (ARM), is the intentional rupture of the amniotic sac. Typically, the amniotic membranes will spontaneously rupture, releasing the amniotic fluid either before or during the onset of spontaneous labor.[1-3]

Indications

Induction or Augmentation of Labor

Artificial rupture of membranes can be used to induce or augment labor. The main disadvantage of amniotomy used alone for labor induction is the unpredictable and long interval between ARM and onset of labor. The American College of Obstetricians and Gynecologists (2013a)[4] recommends the use of amniotomy to enhance progress in active labor, but with a possible increase in the risk of infection and maternal fever.

For Internal Fetal Monitoring for Direct Assessment of Fetal Status

Monitoring of the fetal heart rate as well as uterine activity can be easily obtained via external monitoring systems. However, in certain circumstances, more direct evaluation of the fetal heart rate or uterine activity is required during labor. The amniotic membranes present a physical barrier to this form of monitoring, and membranes must be ruptured to place a fetal scalp electrode or intrauterine pressure catheter.[5,6]

Qualitative Assessment of the Amniotic Fluid

Artificial rupture of membranes helps in identification of thick meconium, which may be dangerous to the fetus if aspirated. The viscosity of meconium signifies the lack of liquor and thus oligohydramnios. The amniotic fluid may be blood stained in women with placental abruption.

Contraindications

Artificial rupture of membranes should not be undertaken in the case of:
- Malpresentation
- Free head
- Vasa previa.

Preprocedure Assessment and Surgical Technique

Amniotomy is easily performed with the use of especially designed instruments intended to grab and tear the amniotic membrane. The commonly used devices are:
- Kocher's clamp
- Rod with a hook on the end
- Finger cot with a hook on the end of the cot.

With either device, a per-vaginal examination is indicated to assess the cervical dilation, confirmation of the presenting part which should be a vertex, and the station of head is assessed. One must ensure that the presenting part is the fetal head and that fetal head is well engaged in the pelvis.[7,8]

During amniotomy, to minimize the risk of cord prolapse, dislodgement of the fetal head is avoided. The head is fixed by fundal or suprapubic pressure. If the vertex is not well applied to the lower uterine segment, a gradual drainage of amniotic fluid can be done by a needle. Following ARM, we should not immediately remove hand from vagina because it is at this point that the highest risk of cord prolapse can occur. Because of the risk of cord prolapse or abruption, the fetal heart rate must be assessed before and immediately after amniotomy.

Complications of Amniotomy

- *Cord prolapse*: The most common complication of ARM is umbilical cord prolapse. This occurs after rupture if ARM is performed when the head is not engaged in the maternal pelvis. This will allow the fetal head to compress the part of umbilical cord preceding the head, leading to fetal bradycardia and necessitating emergency cesarean section.[9]
- *Chorioamnionitis*: Rupture of membranes eliminate the primary barrier between the fetus and the polymicrobial environment of the vagina. If performed too early in the labor, there can be an increased risk of intrapartum chorioamnionitis.
- *Fetal injury*: Iatrogenic injury to fetal scalp is a rare complication.
- *Placental abruption*: Abruption due to sudden decompression of uterus as in hydramnios.

PUDENDAL BLOCK

Pain with vaginal delivery arises from stimuli from the lower genital tract. These are transmitted primarily through the pudendal nerve, the peripheral branches of which provide sensory innervation to the perineum, anus, vulva, and clitoris. The pudendal nerve passes beneath the posterior surface of the sacrospinous ligament just as the ligament attaches to the ischial spine. Thus, when injecting local anesthetic for a pudendal nerve block, the ischial spine serves an identifiable landmark.

Indication

The pudendal nerve block is a relatively safe and simple method of providing pain relief during labor and/or delivery.

Contraindication

Allergy to lidocaine and other local anesthetic.

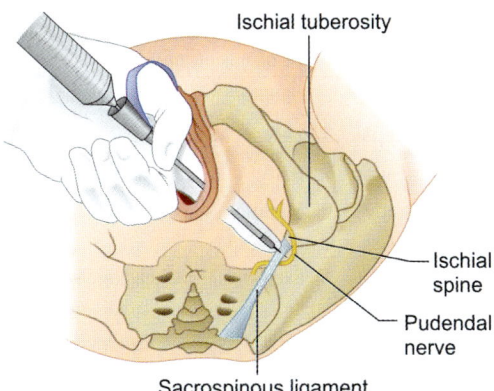

Fig. 1: Pudendal block (transvaginal technique showing the needle extended beyond the needle guard and passing through the sacrospinous ligament to reach the pudendal nerve).

Technique[10]

As shown in Figure 1, a tubular introducer is used to sheath and guide a 15 cm 22-gauge needle into position over the pudendal nerve. The end of the introducer is placed against the vaginal mucosa just beneath the tip of the ischial spine.

The introducer allows 1.0–1.5 cm of needle to protrude beyond its tip, and the needle is pushed beyond the introducer tip into the mucosa. A mucosal wheal is made with 1 mL of 1% lidocaine solution. To guard against intravascular infusion, aspiration is attempted before this and all subsequent injections. The needle is then advanced until it touches the sacrospinous ligament, which is infiltrated with 3 mL of lidocaine. The needle is advanced further through the ligament. As it pierces the loose areolar tissue behind the ligament, the resistance of the plunger decreases. Another 3 mL of solution is injected into this region. Next, the needle is withdrawn into the introducer, which is moved to just above the ischial spine. The needle is inserted through the mucosa and 3 more mL is deposited. The procedure is then repeated on the other side.

If delivery occurs before the pudendal block becomes effective and an episiotomy is indicated, then the fourchette, perineum, and adjacent vagina can be infiltrated with 5–10 mL of 1% lidocaine solution directly at the planned episiotomy site. By the time of repair, the pudendal block usually has become effective.

Complications

The complications are infrequent and include the following:
- Intravascular injection of a local anesthetic agent may cause serious systemic toxicity.
- Hematoma formation from perforation of a blood vessel is most likely when there is a coagulopathy.[11]
- Rarely, severe infection may originate at the injection site.

EPISIOTOMY

Episiotomy is a planned incision given over the perineum and posterior vaginal wall to aid in vaginal delivery. This incision may be made in the midline, creating a median or midline episiotomy. It may also begin on the midline and directed laterally and downward away from the rectum, termed a mediolateral episiotomy (Fig. 2).

Indications

The American College of Obstetricians and Gynecologists (2016b)[4] has concluded that restricted use of episiotomy is preferred to routine use. It should be applied selectively for appropriate indications such as:
- Rigid perineum and markedly short perineal length
- *Anticipation of significant perineal and rectal trauma*: Shoulder dystocia, breech

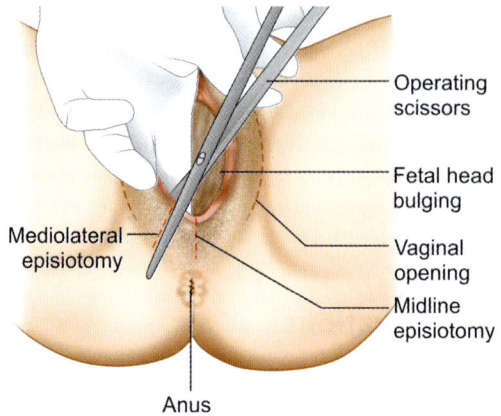

Fig. 2: Episiotomy incision.

Table 1: Midline versus mediolateral episiotomy.

Characteristic	Type of episiotomy	
	Midline	Mediolateral
Surgical repair	Easy	More difficult
Faulty healing	Rare	More common
Postoperative pain	Minimal	Common
Anatomical results	Excellent	Occasionally faulty
Blood loss	Less	More
Dyspareunia	Rare	Occasional
Extensions	Common	Uncommon

delivery, fetal macrosomia, and persistent occiput posterior positions
- Operative vaginal deliveries (Mediolateral episiotomy preferred)
- Previous perineal surgeries.

Timing of Procedure

If performed early, unnecessary bleeding from the episiotomy site may result during the interval between incision and delivery. If it is performed too late, lacerations will not be prevented. Typically, episiotomy is performed at the crowning of fetal head that is when the head stretches the vulva and does not recede in between the contractions. In forceps delivery, episiotomy is usually performed after application of the blades. The cut should be done at the height of a uterine contraction, when the tissues are stretched the most and the pressure of the presenting part will lead to lesser blood loss from episiotomy site.[12]

Procedure

For midline episiotomy, fingers are inserted between the crowning head and the perineum. The scissors are positioned at 6 o'clock position on the vaginal opening and directed posteriorly (Fig. 2). The incision length varies from 2 to 3 cm depending on perineal length and degree of tissue thinning. The incision should stop well before reaching the external anal sphincter. With mediolateral episiotomy, scissors are positioned at 7 o'clock or at 5 o'clock, and the incision is extended 3–4 cm toward the ipsilateral ischial tuberosity. The mediolateral technique is recommended, with careful attention to ensure that the angle is 60° away from the midline when the perineum is distended.[13]

Differences between the two types of episiotomies are summarized in Table 1.

Repair of Episiotomy

Episiotomy is a second-degree perineal tear involving vaginal mucosa, underlying perineal muscles, and perineal skin. Hemostasis and anatomical restoration without excessive suturing is the key to successful repair.

Suture Materials for Repair

The suture material commonly used is polyglycolic acid suture (synthetic) or 2-0 chromic catgut (natural). Polyglycolic/polyglactin sutures are preferred over chromic catgut as they have superior tensile strength, non-allergenic properties, and are associated with a lower rate of infectious complication. A decrease in postsurgical pain and lower risk of wound dehiscence are the major advantages of synthetic materials.[14,15] Closures with delayed absorbable synthetic sutures require suture removal on day 7/8 of repair after healing of wound as it can cause pain or dyspareunia. This disadvantage may be reduced using a rapidly absorbed polyglactin 910.[16,17] A tapering or round bodied needle should be used, as a cutting needle is more traumatic and causes more bleeding. A curved needle is preferred over a straight needle.

Technique of Repair

- Good light is essential
- Position the woman in dorsal or lithotomy position with buttocks at the edge of table
- Clean the perineum with antiseptic solution
- Anesthetize the perineum early to provide enough time for effect: 10 mL of 0.5% or 5 mL of 1% lidocaine solution should be used to infiltrate beneath the skin of the perineum, beneath the vaginal mucosa, and deeply into the perineal muscle. Insert the needle along the planned incision site or on each side of the vaginal tear and slowly inject the lignocaine solution after withdrawing the needle to ensure that it is not in a blood vessel
- A tampon may be inserted into the upper vagina to absorb any blood from the uterus if it interferes with repair, thereby ensuring a clear suturing field. Do not forget to remove this at the end of the procedure.

Repair of the Perineal Muscle Layer

- Approximate the perineal muscles using an interrupted 2-0 suture
- Attempt to identify and ligate any bleeding blood vessel
- It is important that any potential dead space is obliterated, as this can later lead to hematoma formation.

Repair of the Vaginal Mucosa

- Repair the vaginal mucosa using a continuous 2-0 suture
- Ensure that the first suture is placed above the apex of episiotomy incision
- Continue the suture to the level of the vaginal opening till the level of hymen.

Repair of the Skin

- Repair the perineal skin using either an interrupted or subcuticular 2-0 suture
- Start at the level of the vaginal opening
- Ensure that the sutures are not placed too tightly.

At the end of procedure, rectal examination should be performed in all cases especially those with a deep episiotomy to ensure that no sutures have been placed in the rectum. If suture material is felt in the rectum, the repair is reopened and rectal sutures removed and repeat repair is done.[13]

Complications

Immediate Complications

- Extension of the incision to rectum, more likely in median episiotomies
- Vulvar hematoma.

Delayed Complications

- Infection
- Wound dehiscence.

Remote Complications

- Dyspareunia
- Scar endometriosis.

OBSTETRIC ANAL SPHINCTER INJURIES[13]

Obstetric anal sphincter injuries (OASIS) is unfortunately a common event associated with vaginal delivery. If these third- and fourth-degree perineal tears are not recognized and managed appropriately, these women are at high risk for developing several significant long-term complications including fecal incontinence, perineal pain, and dyspareunia.

Risk factors for sphincter injury include:
- Instrumental vaginal delivery
- Episiotomy
- Fetal macrosomia
- Shoulder dystocia
- Prolonged second stage
- Occipitoposterior positions
- Increasing maternal age
- Previous perineal injuries.

Diagnosis

- It may be obvious on inspection as no perineal tissue can be seen between the vaginal and anal opening.
- In incomplete tears, insert an index finger into anus and ask the woman to squeeze and contract anal sphincter and any loss of tone will suggest an underlying sphincter defect.
- Inspection at squeeze may reveal retraction of separated ends of a torn sphincter.
- Muscle bulk of sphincter should also be palpated between the thumb and index finger in a pill-rolling motion with the index finger in the rectum and the thumb in the vagina. This will help to detect any loss of sphincter bulk.

Anorectal Anatomy and Classification of Perineal Tears

Anal canal starts below the anorectal junction-puborectalis. The anal sphincter comprises:

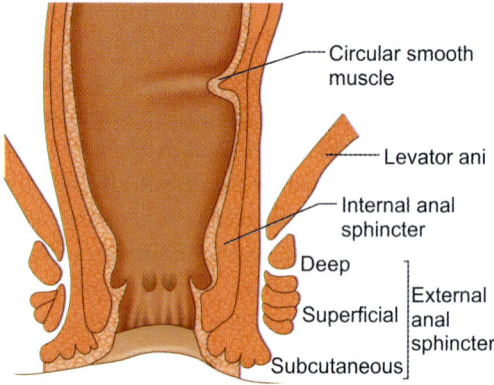

Fig. 3: Anatomy of anal sphincter.

Internal anal sphincter (IAS) (Fig. 3):
- Terminal thickened portion of the smooth circular muscle of GIT
- Autonomic control
- Contributes 85% of resting pressure of anal canal
- Critical to maintaining continence
- If damaged, it results in passive soiling and/or flatal incontinence.

External anal sphincter (EAS) (Fig. 3): It has three parts—(1) subcutaneous, (2) superficial, and (3) deep:
- It is a striated muscle (voluntary)
- Provides squeeze pressure for maintaining anal continence
- Innervated by pudendal nerve
- If damaged, can result in fecal incontinence.

The classification of perineal tears[18] is as follows:
- *First degree*: Injury to perineal skin and/or vaginal mucosa.
- *Second-degree tear*: Injury to perineum involving perineal muscles but not involving the anal sphincter.
- *Third-degree tear*: Injury to perineum involving the anal sphincter complex:
  - *Grade 3a tear*: Less than 50% of EAS thickness torn.

- *Grade 3b tear*: More than 50% of EAS thickness torn.
- *Grade 3c tear*: Both EAS and IAS torn.
- *Fourth-degree tear*: Injury to perineum involving the anal sphincter complex (EAS and IAS) and anorectal mucosa.

Repair of Third- and Fourth-Degree Perineal Tears

General Principles

- *Standard practice*: Repair immediately after delivery
- Adequate analgesia is ensured by local anesthesia or regional block or GA
- Repair must be done preferably in OT
- Complete relaxation of the anesthetized anal sphincter complex facilitates bringing torn ends of the sphincter together without tension
- Good lighting, appropriate instruments
- Figure of eight sutures should be avoided because they are hemostatic in nature and may cause tissue ischemia
- The burying of surgical knots beneath the superficial perineal muscles is recommended to minimize the risk of knot and suture migration to the skin.

Technique

Repair of the torn anal mucosa: The torn anorectal mucosa should be repaired with sutures using either the continuous or interrupted technique. Interrupted sutures with the knot tied within the anal canal using absorbable polyglactin (3-0) suture.

Internal sphincter:
- Should be repaired separately
- Only end-to-end repair
- Interrupted mattress suture 2-0 polyglactin 910.

External sphincter:
- *Overlap or end-to-end repair (Figs. 4 and 5)*: For repair of a full thickness EAS tear, either an overlapping or an end-to-end method can be used. For partial thickness (all 3a and some 3b tears), an end-to-end technique should be used.
- Monofilament delayed absorbable suture-3-0 polydioxanone sulfate (PDS) or 2-0 polyglactin 910.

Postrepair Management

- Use of prophylactic broad-spectrum antibiotics is recommended. It prevents postoperative wound infection and

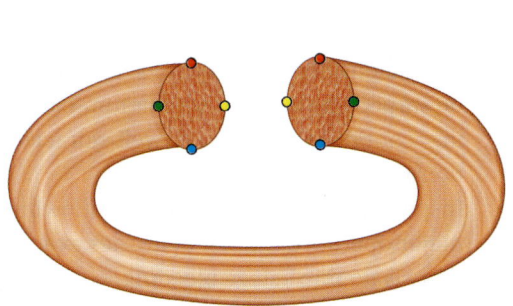

Fig. 4: End-to-end repair.

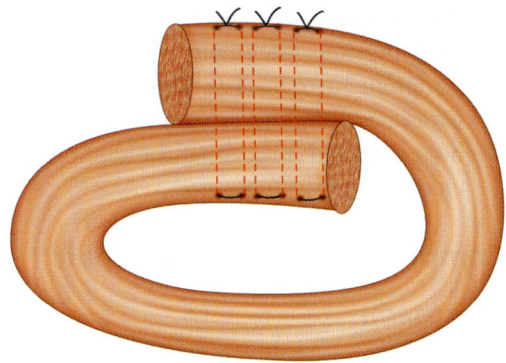

Fig. 5: Overlapping repair.

dehiscence as it is a clean contaminated wound.

Injection cefuroxime 750 mg IV every 12 hours plus injection metrogyl 500 mg IV every 8 hours for 24 hours followed by oral cefuroxime 500 mg twice a day plus metrogyl 400 mg twice a day for 5 days; Alternative regime is injection clindamycin 600 mg IV every 6 hours for 24 hours followed by oral clindamycin for 5 days.

WHO and SOGC recommend single dose second- or third-generation cephalosporin, cefotetan, and cefoxitin.[19]

- Stool softener laxatives for 7–10 days postpartum.
- Bulking agents should not be given routinely with laxatives.
- Perineal floor physiotherapy advised at discharge.
- Follow-up visit at 6 weeks and 12 weeks postpartum.

Future Deliveries

- All women who sustained OASIS in a previous pregnancy should be counseled about the mode of delivery and clear documentation is a must.
- The role of prophylactic episiotomy in subsequent pregnancies is not known and therefore it should only be performed if clinically indicated.
- All women who have sustained OASIS in a previous pregnancy and who are symptomatic or have abnormal endoanal ultrasonography and/or manometry should be counseled regarding the option of elective cesarean delivery.

Complications of OASIS Repair

Short-term

- Wound hematoma
- Wound breakdown
- Abscess formation
- Anal incontinence.

Long-term

- Anal incontinence
- Rectovaginal fistulas.

Unfortunately, normal function is not always ensured even with correct and complete surgical repair. Some women may experience continuing fecal incontinence caused by injury to the innervation of the pelvic floor musculature.[20]

CERVICAL AND VAGINAL LACERATIONS/TEARS

According to the American College of Obstetricians and Gynecologists (2016b),[4] up to 80% of women sustain some type of laceration at vaginal delivery. Superficial lacerations of the cervix can be seen on close inspection in more than half of all vaginal deliveries. In general, cervical lacerations of 1 and even 2 cm are not repaired unless they are bleeding. Such tears heal rapidly and when healed they result in the irregular, sometimes stellate appearance of the external cervical os that indicates previous delivery. Rarely, the cervix may be entirely or partially avulsed from the vagina and is referred to as colporrhexis.

Diagnosis and Exploration[21]

- Lacerations of the cervix or vagina should be suspected when the postpartum bleeding continues despite a well-retracted uterus.
- Inspect the cervix routinely following major operative vaginal deliveries even if there is no third-stage bleeding.
- Adequate exposure and visual inspection are best possible when an assistant

applies firm downward pressure on the uterus while the operator exerts traction on the lips of the cervix with ring forceps. A second assistant can provide help in better exposure by retracting vaginal walls with right-angle vaginal wall retractors.
- For optimum suturing, the operator uses three sponge holding forceps to evaluate the entire circumference of the cervix and expose the tears. These are most often found at 3 and 9 o'clock and are parallel with the axis of the cervix.

Repair[21]

- While cervical lacerations are repaired, associated vaginal lacerations may be tamponade with gauze packs to stop bleeding.
- Because hemorrhage usually comes from the upper angle of the tear from the descending cervical artery or its branch, the first suture using absorbable material is placed above the angle.
- Subsequently, either interrupted or continuous locking sutures are placed using absorbable suture (1-0 Vicryl or catgut) on a tapered needle (Fig. 6).
- Vaginal lacerations should be closed with the same type of suture, starting from the cranial end.

Special precautions in cervical tears with apex beyond vaginal vault:
- If the upper end of the tear cannot be seen, the uterus should be explored manually to evaluate the extent of the laceration.
- While repairing, the first suture is placed as high as possible and then traction is applied to place another suture above it. It is continued till the operator reaches above the apex of the tear.
- A laparotomy is indicated when the tear extends to the peritoneal cavity or to the parametrium leading to hemorrhage or a broad ligament hematoma. In these cases, the uterine artery or its branches may be torn.[22]

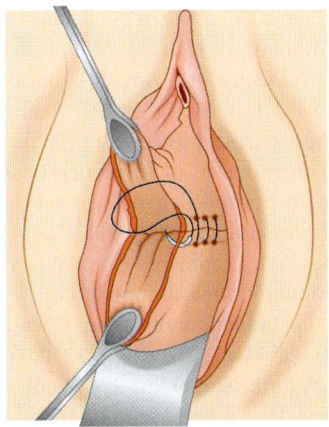

Fig. 6: Repair of cervical laceration with appropriate surgical exposure. Continuous or interrupted absorbable sutures are placed beginning at the upper angle of the laceration.

REFERENCES

1. ACOG Committee Opinion No. 766: Approaches to Limit Intervention During Labor and Birth. Obstet Gynecol. 2019;133(2): e164-73.
2. Worthley M, Kelsberg G, Safranek S. Does amniotomy shorten spontaneous labor or improve outcomes? J Fam Pract. 2018; 67(12):787-8.
3. Seikku L, Stefanovic V, Rahkonen P, Teramo K, Paavonen J, Tikkanen M, et al. Amniotic fluid and umbilical cord serum erythropoietin in term and prolonged pregnancies. Eur J Obstet Gynecol Reprod Biol. 2019;233:1-5.
4. American College of Obstetricians and Gynecologists (2016). Prevention and management of obstetric lacerations at vaginal delivery. Practice Bulletin No. 165.
5. Pasko DN, Miller KM, Jauk VC, Subramaniam A. Pregnancy outcomes after early amniotomy among Class III obese gravidas undergoing induction of labor. Am J Perinatol. 2019;36(5):449-54.

6. Penfield CA, Wing DA. Labor induction techniques: Which is the best? Obstet Gynecol Clin North Am. 2017;44(4):567-82.
7. Côrtes CT, Oliveira SMJV, Santos RCSD, Francisco AA, Riesco MLG, Shimoda GT. Implementation of evidence-based practices in normal delivery care. Rev Lat Am Enfermagem. 2018;26:e2988.
8. Abbas AM. Comments on manuscript: early amniotomy after dinoprostone insert used for the induction of labor. J Matern Fetal Neonatal Med. 2019;32(13):2270.
9. Ruamsap K, Panichkul P. The effect of early versus late amniotomy on the course of labor. J Med Assoc Thai. 2017;100(2):125-32.
10. American College Of Obstetricians and Gynecologists (2017). Obstetric analgesia and anesthesia. Practice Bulletin 177.
11. Lee LA, Posner KL, Domino KB, Caplan RA, Cheney FW. Injuries associated with regional anesthesia in the 1980s and 1990s: a closed claims analysis. Anesthesiology. 2004;101(1):143-52.
12. National Institute for Health and Clinical Excellence (2014). Intrapartum care for healthy women and babies: Clinical guideline [CG190]. [online] Available from https://www.nice.org.uk/guidance/cg190 [Last accessed March, 2020].
13. RCOG (2015). The Management of Third and Fourth degree perineal tears. Green-top Guideline No. 29. [online] Available from https://www.rcog.org.uk/globalassets/documents/guidelines/gtg-29.pdf [Last accessed March, 2020].
14. Jallad K, Steele SE, Barber MD. Breakdown of perineal laceration repair after vaginal delivery: a case-control study. Female Pelvic Med Reconstr Surg. 2016;22(4):276.
15. Kettle C, Dowswell T, Ismail KM. Absorbable suture materials for primary repair of episiotomy and second degree tears. Cochrane Database Syst Rev. 2010;(6):CD000006.
16. Bharathi A, Reddy DB, Kote GS. A prospective randomized comparative study of vicryl rapide versus chromic catgut for episiotomy repair. J Clin Diagn Res. 2013;7(2):326-30.
17. Leroux N, Bujold E. Impact of chromic catgut versus polyglactin 910 versus fast-absorbing polyglactin 910 sutures for perineal repair: a randomized, controlled trial. Am J Obstet Gynecol. 2006;194(6):1585-90.
18. Sultan AH. Obstetric perineal injury and anal incontinence. Clin Risk. 1999;5:193-6.
19. Buppasiri P, Lumbiganon P, Thinkhamrop J, Thinkhamrop B. Antibiotic prophylaxis for third- and fourth-degree perineal tear during vaginal birth. Cochrane Database Syst Rev. 2014;(10):CD005125.
20. Roberts PL, Coller JA, Schoetz DJ, Veidenheimer MC. Manometric assessment of patients with obstetric injuries and fecal incontinence. Dis Colon Rectum. 1990;33(1):16-20.
21. Obstetrical hemorrhage. In: Leveno KJ, Spong CY, Dashe JS, Casey BM, Hoffman BL, Cunningham FG, Bloom SL (Eds). Williams Obstetrics, 25th edition. US: McGraw-Hill Education; 2018. pp. 1686-7.
22. Rafi J, Muppala H. Retroperitoneal haematomas in obstetrics: literature review. Arch Gynecol Obstet. 2010;281(3):435.

51 Minor Procedures for Screening and Diagnosis of Cervical Cancer

Tahmina S

INTRODUCTION

Cervical cancer is the most commonly diagnosed cancer among women and the fourth most common cause of cancer deaths worldwide, with an estimated 570,000 cases and 311,000 deaths in 2018. Low- and middle-income countries account for 90% of the total mortality from cervical cancer. In India, cervical cancer is the second most common cancer among women and the second most common cause of cancer deaths, after breast cancer.[1,2]

The primary risk factor most strongly associated with the occurrence of cervical cancer is infection with certain high-risk strains of Human Papilloma Virus (HPV), a common sexually transmitted virus. It is estimated that about 5% of Indian women harbor cervical HPV16/18 infection, and 83.2% of invasive cervical cancers are attributed to HPV 16 or 18.[3] Most HPV infections resolve spontaneously, but persistent HPV infection can lead to cancer. Precancerous lesions caused by HPV progress to invasive cancer in about 10–20 years. Cervical cancer is thus largely preventable through detection of these precancerous lesions. The cure rate for cervical cancer is closely related to the stage of disease at diagnosis and the availability of treatment. Cervical cancer, if left untreated, is almost always fatal.

The World Health Organization (WHO) concluded that an effective program with screening at least once in the age group of 30–49 years with the "screen-and-treat" or "screen, diagnose, and treat" approaches is important in preventing the development of cancer or to treat cancer at an early stage.[4]

PROCEDURES FOR SCREENING OF CERVICAL CANCER

Three modalities are used in screening for cervical carcinoma (Box 1).

Cytology

Conventional Pap Smear

The Papanicolaou test, also called Pap smear, Pap test, or cervical smear, is used as a screening test to detect premalignant and malignant lesions in the ectocervix. It may also detect infections and abnormalities in the endocervix and endometrium. Named after its inventor, Dr George Nicholas

---

Box 1: Modalities for cervical cancer screening.

- *Cytology*:
  - Conventional Pap smear and liquid-based smear
- HPV DNA test
- *Visual inspection*:
  - With acetic acid (VIA)
  - With Lugol's iodine (VILI)

(HPV DNA: human papilloma virus deoxyribonucleic acid)

Papanicolaou, Pap smear is the most successful cancer screening technique till date, having reduced the incidence of cervical cancer and mortality in various parts of the world. It involves microscopic examination of cells removed from the surface of cervix, especially the transformation zone, where most cancerous lesions arise. A positive Pap smear test indicates the presence of precancerous cells or cancer cells of the cervix but is not enough to make a definitive diagnosis of cervical cancer. Further tests such as colposcopy and biopsy are required to confirm the diagnosis.

The USPSTF (United States Preventive Services Task Force) have recently updated their consensus guidelines regarding screening for cervical cancer in 2018.[5] They recommend screening for cervical cancer every 3 years with cytology alone for women aged 21–29 years, with cytology alone every 3 years, or high-risk HPV DNA testing alone or co-testing with cytology every 5 years in women between 30 and 65 years of age. Women younger than 21 years and older than 65 years with adequate prior screening, and women who have had a hysterectomy, need not be screened for cervical cancer. These recommendations are not applicable to women who are HIV positive, are immunosuppressed, were exposed to diethylstilbestrol (DES) in utero, or have been treated for cervical intraepithelial neoplasia 2 or 3 (CIN 2 or 3) or cervical cancer.

Routine cervical cytology testing should be discontinued in women who have had a total hysterectomy for benign conditions, if there is no history of CIN2 or CIN3. Screening should be discontinued at 65 years for women who have been adequately screened previously, where adequate screening is defined as three consecutive negative cytology results or two consecutive negative co-testing results within 10 years before stopping screening, with the most recent test within 5 years.[6] Women who have been vaccinated against HPV should follow the same screening guidelines as unvaccinated women since the vaccines do not protect against all high-risk HPV types.

Requirements for conventional Pap smear: Instruments (Fig. 1) and materials required for collecting a conventional Pap smear are listed in Box 2.

Procedure: After explaining the procedure to the woman and obtaining verbal informed consent for the test, the woman is asked to lie

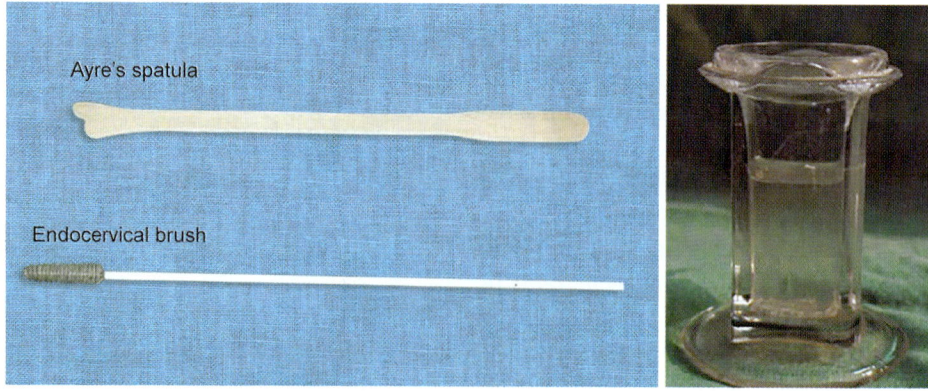

Fig. 1: Devices used for Pap smear and Coplin jar.

> **Box 2:** Requirements for conventional Pap smear.
> - Light source to examine the cervix
> - Examination table
> - Disposable examination gloves
> - Cusco's speculum
> - An extended-tip wooden or plastic spatula (Ayre's spatula)
> - A labeled glass slide
> - *Fixative solution*: Cytofix spray or Coplin jar containing 95% ethyl alcohol

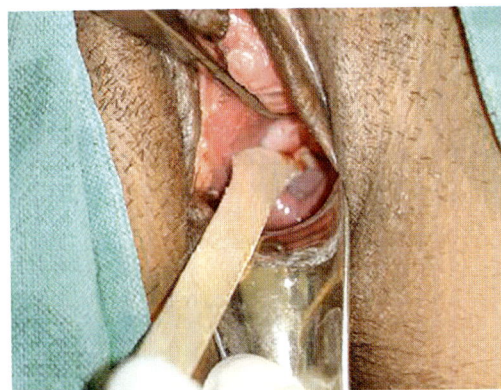

Fig. 2: Taking Pap smear with Ayre's spatula.

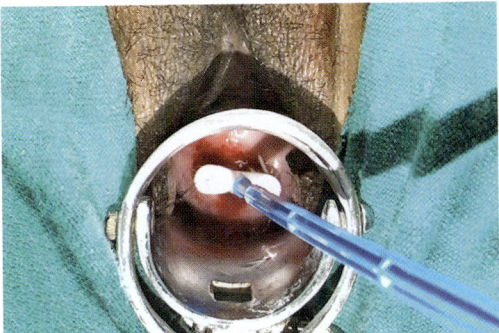

Fig. 3: Taking Pap smear and endocervical smear with cytobrush.

Table 1: Advantages and disadvantages of Pap smear.	
Advantages	Disadvantages/Limitations
• Simple procedure • Short learning curve • Takes less than 5 minutes • Not painful • Can be done in outpatient department (OPD)	• Does not test for the cause of cervical cancer • There is subjectivity and variability • Sampling errors • Nonprognostic • Follow-up dependent on patient compliance

on the examination table in a dorsal position with legs flexed at the hips and knees and buttocks at the edge of the table:

- A Cusco's speculum is inserted into the vagina and cervix is visualized.
- An Ayre's spatula (Fig. 2) is placed at the external cervical os with the long tip of the spatula into the cervical canal and is rotated through 360° once to obtain a sample of cells from the ectocervix.
- In perimenopausal and postmenopausal women, the sample is collected with an endocervical brush as the transformation zone recedes into the endocervical canal (Fig. 3).
- The material is immediately spread on a clean glass slide to make a smear.
- The slide is then immediately fixed, either by a spray fixative, or the slide is immersed in a Coplin jar containing 95% ethanol for at least 5 minutes.
- The speculum is gently closed and removed from the vagina.
- The slide is then sent to the laboratory where it is stained using the Pap technique. The pathologist then examines the slide using a light microscope and reports the results using the Bethesda classification. Presence of endocervical cells in the slide is a proof of a well-prepared Pap smear. The Pap test should not be done when there is acute inflammation or the woman is menstruating.

Advantages and disadvantages of Pap test are detailed in Table 1.

Box 3: Reporting of Pap smear Bethesda system.[8]

- *Negative for intraepithelial lesion or malignancy*:
  - *Infection with organisms:*
    » Trichomonas vaginalis
    » Fungal organisms morphologically consistent with *Candida species*
    » Shift in flora suggestive of bacterial vaginosis
    » Bacteria morphologically consistent with *Actinomyces species*
    » Cellular changes consistent with herpes simplex virus
  - *Other nonneoplastic findings such as*:
    » Reactive cellular changes associated with inflammation
    » Radiation effect
    » Intrauterine contraceptive device
    » Glandular cells status post-hysterectomy
    » Atrophy
- *Epithelial cell abnormality*:
  - *Squamous cells*:
    » Atypical squamous cell (ASC) of undetermined significance (ASC-US) cannot exclude high-grade lesion (ASC-H)
    » Low-grade squamous intraepithelial lesion (LSIL) (Fig. 4)
    » High-grade squamous intraepithelial lesion (HSIL) (Fig. 5)
    » Squamous cell carcinoma (Fig. 6)
  - *Glandular cells*:
    » Atypical glandular cells (AGC) (specify endocervical, endometrial, or not specified) of undetermined significance (AGUS)
    » AGC favor neoplasia (specify endocervical or not specified)
    » Endocervical adenocarcinoma in situ (AIS)
    » Adenocarcinoma

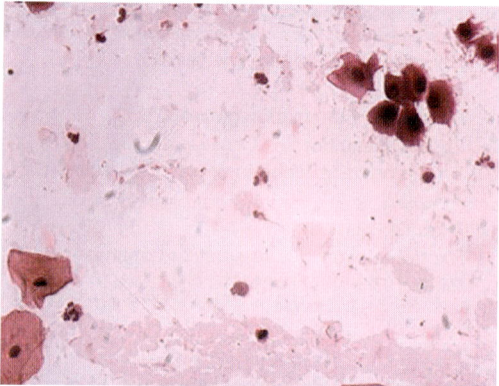

Fig. 4: Abnormal Pap smear showing low-grade squamous intraepithelial lesion.

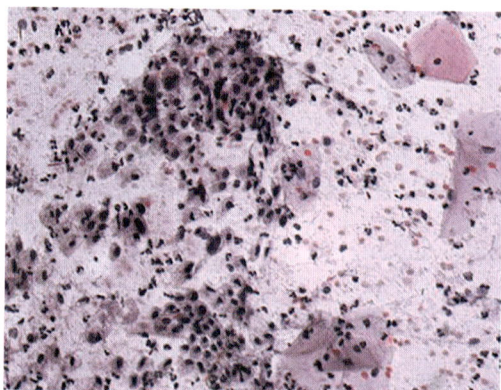

Fig. 5: Abnormal Pap smear showing high-grade squamous intraepithelial lesion.

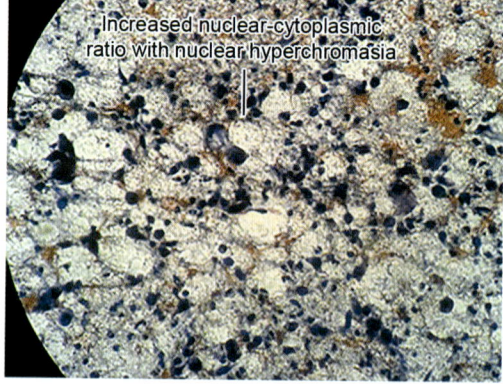

Fig. 6: Abnormal Pap smear (squamous cell carcinoma).

Reporting of Pap smear: Sensitivity and specificity of a single Pap test is 50–70% and 96.8%, respectively.[7] Pap smear is reported according to the Bethesda system (Box 3).

Follow-up: If the Pap test is normal (Fig. 7), the woman is advised to repeat Pap test within 3 years. In women with an abnormal Pap smear, additional tests (Table 2) are required to confirm the diagnosis and determine further management.

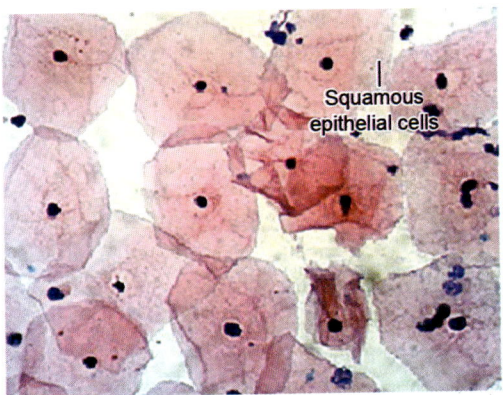

Fig. 7: Normal Pap smear.

Table 3: Advantages and disadvantages of liquid-based cytology.

Advantages	Disadvantages
• Fewer false negatives • Fewer unsatisfactory smears • More sensitive and specific than conventional Pap • Material collected can also be tested for human papilloma virus deoxyribonucleic acid (HPV DNA)	• Costlier • Needs specially trained staff

Table 2: Proposed actions in women with abnormal Pap smear.

Abnormal Pap	Action to be taken
Cervical growth	Take punch biopsy
Normal looking cervix	Colposcopy-directed biopsy *If colposcopy not available*: • Schiller's test • Blind four quadrant biopsy • Loop electrosurgical excision procedure (LEEP) biopsy

Liquid-based Cytology

Liquid-based cytology (LBC), introduced in the mid-1990s, involves sampling of the transformation zone with an Ayre's spatula or brush (as in conventional Pap smear), which is then transferred to a preservative solution by leaving the sampling device in it or rinsing it in the solution. The sample is centrifuged in the laboratory and a slide is prepared. LBC can be performed even during menses, although if bleeding is excessive, cervical cells can be obscured by endometrial cells. LBC is more expensive than conventional cytology and laboratory staff needs to be specially trained. However, it has some advantages over conventional methods (Table 3).

Human Papilloma Virus Deoxyribonucleic Acid Test

Human papilloma virus deoxyribonucleic acid (HPV DNA) test is another method for cervical cancer screening. HPV infections are frequent in young women less than 30 years and often resolve spontaneously, making the test less useful in younger women. It is indicated in women aged 30–65 years and a positive test indicates persistent infection in these women. One tenth of all infections become persistent, defined by presence of the same type-specific HPV DNA on repeated sampling after 6–12 months and these women can develop cervical precancerous lesions.

The preparation and materials required for taking the sample are the same as for a Pap smear. A swab or small brush is used to collect vaginal or cervical smears. The specimen is placed in a container with a preservative solution, transported to a laboratory, where it is processed and tested for high-risk HPV DNA. Sophisticated and expensive laboratory equipment is required for HPV DNA-based tests. The material collected for LBC test can also be used to test for HPV DNA.

When cytology (conventional or liquid based) and HPV DNA testing are done at the same time, it is called co-testing or HPV co-test. The main advantage of co-testing is that it allows extension of the screening interval from 3 years with cytology alone to 5 years with co-testing for women aged 30–65 years.

HPV DNA test alone is not a reliable and practical primary screening test. It has been studied as an alternative to cervical cytology testing and its role has been established in triage of Pap smears with ASCUS (atypical squamous cells of undetermined significance) and follow-up after treatment. The hybrid capture 2 assay and polymerase chain reactions (PCR) are the amplification tests used to detect HPV DNA. HPV infections mostly do not cause any serious consequences and the transient nature of HPV infection results in a low specificity in clinical practice.

It is mainly used in addition to cytology to assess the need for colposcopy in women with borderline Pap results. A combination of cytology and HPV testing has very high sensitivity and negative predictive value approaching 100% but performing the two tests together is expensive. The negative predictive value of HPV testing alone approaches 100%.[9] HPV testing is currently not recommended for use as a standalone test in screening for cervical cancer, since its specificity in identification of cancer is low.[6,9]

Advantages and disadvantages of HPV testing for cervical cancer screening are given in Table 4.

Visual Inspection

Visual inspection has been evaluated as a substitute to cytology in screening for cervical cancer. In this method, abnormalities of the cervix are identified by naked eye examination after application of dilute acetic acid or Lugol's iodine. This is an inexpensive technique and can be performed with minimal training in low-resource settings.

Visual Inspection with Acetic Acid

Principle: Application of 3–5% acetic acid causes swelling of the cervical epithelial tissue, dehydration of the cells, and a reversible coagulation of the cellular proteins which obscures the color of the underlying stroma. Normal squamous epithelium has a sparsely nucleated superficial cell layer and undergoes little coagulation. The deeper cells contain more nuclear protein, but the acetic acid does not reach these layers. Hence, normal cervical epithelium appears pink suggestive of a negative or normal result (Table 5 and Fig. 8).

Table 4: Advantages and disadvantages of HPV testing.

Advantages	Disadvantages
• Prolongs screening interval • Reduces the number of colposcopies in women with equivocal Pap results	• Expensive test, not useful in low-resource settings • Requires well-equipped laboratory • Requires highly trained technicians

Table 5: Interpretation of results of visual inspection with acetic acid (VIA).

VIA category	Clinical findings
Test negative	No acetowhite lesions or faint acetowhite lesions; polyp, cervicitis, inflammation, and nabothian cysts
Test positive	Sharp, distinct, well-defined, dense opaque, dull or oyster white acetowhite areas with or without raised margins touching the squamocolumnar junction (SCJ); CIN, leukoplakia, and warts
Suspicious for cancer	Clinically visible ulcerative, cauliflower-like growth or ulcer, bleeding on touch

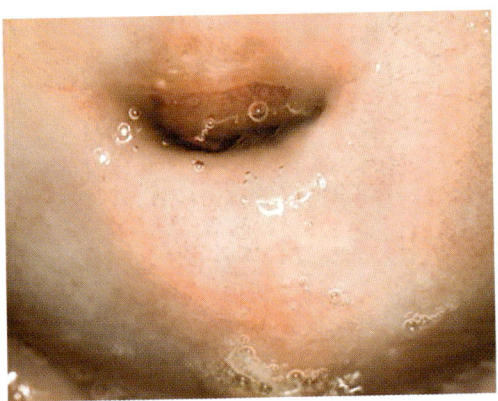 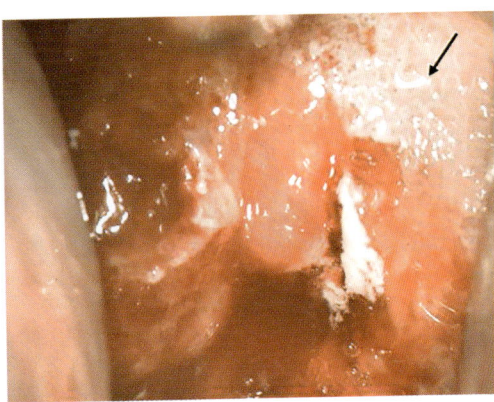

Fig. 8: Visual inspection with acetic acid acetowhite negative (normal result).

Fig. 9: Visual inspection with acetic acid acetowhite positive (abnormal result).

Areas with increased nuclear activity and DNA content as in CIN undergo maximal coagulation and appear white obliterating the subepithelial vessel pattern and show remarkable white color change or acetowhitening suggestive of a positive or abnormal result (Fig. 9).

In low-grade CIN, appearance of the acetowhitening is delayed and less intense due to the smaller amount of nuclear protein compared to high-grade CIN or preclinical invasive cancer, which appears densely white and opaque immediately due to higher concentration of abnormal nuclear protein content and the presence of dysplastic cells in the superficial epithelial layers.

The acetowhite appearance is also seen in other conditions such as immature squamous metaplasia in regenerating epithelium, leukoplakia, and condyloma, where there is an increase in nuclear protein content. With squamous metaplasia, the acetowhitening is pale, thin, and patchily distributed with ill-defined margins, in contrast with the acetowhitening associated with CIN and early invasive cancer, which is dense, thick, and opaque with well-defined margins.

The acetowhitening associated with immature metaplasia and inflammation usually disappears within 30–60 seconds, whereas those associated with CIN and invasive cancer appear quickly, persist for more than a minute and reverse slowly. Acetowhitening also occurs in the vagina, external anogenital skin, and anal mucosa. Invasive cancer may or may not be acetowhite, but has other distinguishing features that can be recognized at colposcopy.

The sensitivity of VIA for detection of precancer and cancer is reported to be 31–79% and specificity ranges from 87–94%.[10,11]

Visual Inspection with Lugol's Iodine

Principle: Lugol's iodine is glycophillic and hence, glycogen-containing tissue stains mahogany brown or black. Glycogen-poor tissues do not take up iodine and appear mustard-yellow or saffron-colored. Normal squamous epithelium and areas of squamous metaplasia are glycogen rich, whereas columnar epithelium, areas of CIN and invasive cancer, leukoplakia (hyperkeratosis) and condylomata are glycogen-poor areas (Fig. 10).

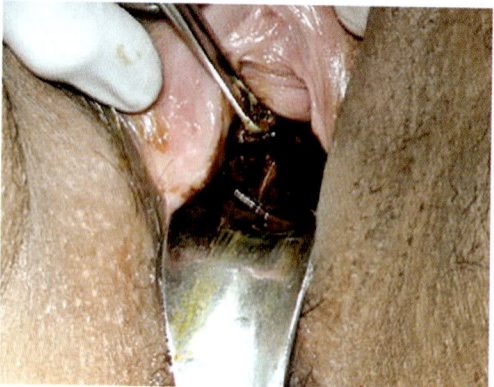

Fig. 10: Visual inspection with Lugol's iodine (VILI) test is negative, normal well-stained cervix.

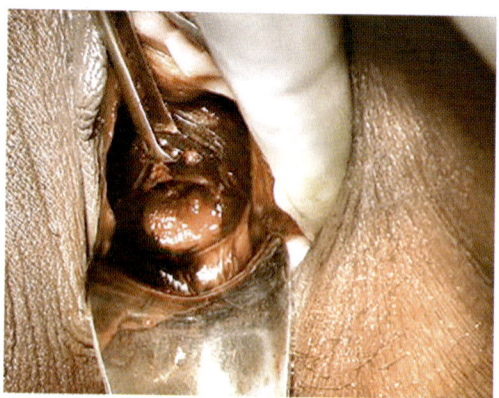

Fig. 11: Visual inspection with Lugol's iodine (VILI) test is positive unstained suspicious area on posterior lip of cervix and posterior vaginal wall.

Therefore, on applying Lugol's iodine to the cervix, precancerous and cancerous lesions appear well-defined, thick mustard or saffron-yellow in color, squamous epithelium stains brown or black, and columnar epithelium does not stain (Fig. 11). The sensitivity of visual inspection with Lugol's iodine (VILI) is higher than that of VIA. It can detect up to 92% of women with precancer or cancer.

Materials and instruments required: The materials and instruments required for carrying out visual inspection with iodine and acetic acid are as listed in Box 4.

Procedure of VIA and VILI:
- After explaining the procedure to the woman and obtaining an informed consent for the test, the woman is made to lie on the examination table in dorsal position with legs flexed at the hips and knees, and buttocks at the edge of the table.
- A Cusco's speculum is inserted into the vagina and cervix is visualized. The cervix is inspected for any abnormalities or any white areas, discharge, blood, or mucus from the cervix is removed using a moist cotton swab.

Box 4: Requirements for visual inspection of cervix: VIA and VILI.

- Light source to examine the cervix
- Examination table
- Disposable examination gloves
- Self-retaining bivalve speculum
- Cotton-tipped swabs
- Dilute acetic acid solution (3–5%) prepared by mixing 3–5 mL of glacial acetic acid in 95–97 mL of distilled water
- Lugol's iodine solution, prepared by dissolving 10 g potassium iodide in 100 mL of distilled water and slowly adding 5 g iodine crystals to it; the solution is filtered and stored in a tightly closed brown bottle

(VIA: visual inspection with acetic acid; VILI: visual inspection with Lugol's iodine)

- The squamocolumnar junction (SCJ) is identified and 3–5% acetic acid is applied to the cervix; after a minute, changes in the appearance of the cervix are observed.
- Areas of raised and thickened white plaques or acetowhite epithelium, if any, are noted.
- After removing any remaining acetic acid with a fresh cotton swab, Lugol's iodine is applied and color changes are looked for; any saffron-yellow colored areas

are noted; fresh swab is used to remove any remaining iodine solution from the speculum or vagina.
- The speculum is closed and gently removed.
- The observations are recorded and any abnormal findings are mapped on a diagram.

If the test is negative, the woman should have another test in three years. But, if the test is positive or cancer is suspected, the woman should be referred for colposcopy, biopsy, and further management accordingly.

The WHO now recommends VIA as an acceptable screening method along with cytology and HPV testing. However, it does not recommend visual screening methods for postmenopausal women since the transformation zone in postmenopausal women recedes inside the endocervical canal and is not visible on speculum examination.[4]

Advantages and disadvantages: Since these methods do not rely on laboratory services, they are promising alternatives to cytology in low-resource settings. The advantages and disadvantages of VIA and VILI are as tabulated in Table 6.

PROCEDURES FOR DIAGNOSIS OF CERVICAL CANCER

The various diagnostic procedures for confirmation of diagnosis of CIN or cervical cancer include colposcopy and cervical biopsy, which are discussed in the following section.

Colposcopy

Colposcopy is a procedure to examine the vulva, vagina, and cervix under illumination and magnification. It requires considerable training and expertise as compared to Pap smear. Colposcopy facilitates visualization of the entire transformation zone, identification of abnormalities and taking targeted biopsies from suspected areas for definitive histopathological diagnosis. Presently, Pap smear, VIA, and VILI are being used primarily as screening tests and colposcopy is usually done to examine the cervix either when a Pap smear report or other screening test is abnormal, or when the cervix looks abnormal during per speculum examination. It is used as a diagnostic tool for patients with a positive screening test.

The procedure is done using a colposcope (Fig. 12), which is a low-power microscope used for magnified visual examination. Low magnification (6x) is used to obtain a general impression of the surface architecture. Medium (8x–15x) and high (15x–25x) magnification is used to evaluate the vagina and cervix. Increase in magnification is indirectly proportional to the field of view and illumination levels. Higher powers are most useful in recognition of certain vascular patterns that may suggest the presence of more advanced precancerous or cancerous lesions.

Table 6: Advantages and disadvantages of visual inspection with acetic acid (VIA) and visual inspection with Lugol's iodine (VILI).

Advantages	Disadvantages
• Relatively simple procedure with a short learning curve	• High false-positive cases resulting in over diagnosis, and unnecessary anxiety
• No laboratory equipment or technician needed	• Not accurate in postmenopausal women as transformation zone recedes in the cervical canal
• Can be performed on outpatient basis	
• Short procedure and causes no pain	• Permanent record of the test is not available for subsequent review
• Results are available immediately, reducing loss to follow-up	
• Cheaper compared to other screening techniques	• Performance in periodic screening has not been assessed

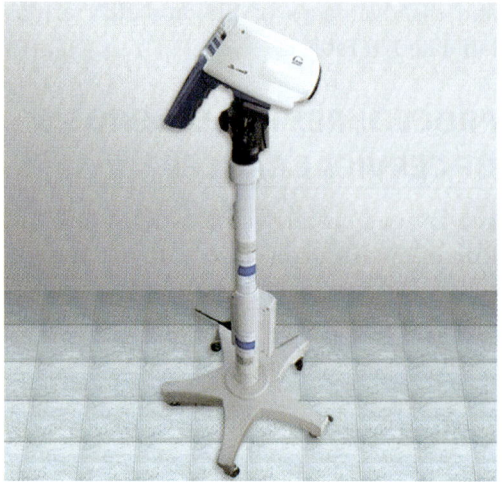

Fig. 12: Colposcope.

Table 7: Pattern of acetowhitening in various cervical lesions.

Conditions	Nature of acetowhitening
• Immature squamous metaplasia • Congenital transformation zone • Regenerating epithelium	• Grade 1 • Less pale, thin, and patchily distributed without well-defined margins; disappears within 30–60 seconds
• Leukoplakia • Condyloma • Cervical intraepithelial neoplasia (CIN) • Preclinical early invasive cancer	• Grade 2 or 3 • More dense, thick, and opaque with well-demarcated margins; appears quickly, persists for >1 minute and reverses slowly

A hand-held, low-cost, portable colposcope (Gynocular) is also available, which is as accurate in diagnosing cervical lesions as a stationary colposcope.[12]

Principle

Colposcopic appearance of the cervix depends on the degree of absorption and reflection of white light by the cervix. The interface between the surface and the underlying vascular stroma consists of cells with variable amounts of nuclei and cytoplasm. Changes in the cell microanatomy and microvascular growth pattern, related to different normal and abnormal cervical environments determine the color and vascular appearance of the cervix on colposcopy.

The main components of colposcopic assessment include examination of the cervical epithelium, after successive application of normal saline, 3–5% diluted acetic acid, and Lugol's iodine. The application of normal saline is useful in studying the subepithelial vascular architectural in detail and is done as the first step, since the vascular pattern of the cervix may be obscured after application of acetic acid and iodine solutions. Blue or green filtered light is used to facilitate visualization of blood vessels inside an acetowhite area. Normal capillaries are slender and show fine uniform branching whereas abnormal capillaries are thick, irregular with a bizarre pattern and appear as red spots due to thickened capillaries seen end on or a mosaic pattern.

Application of 3–5% acetic acid causes reversible coagulation of the nuclear proteins and cytokeratins visible as acetowhite areas. The degree of acetowhitening depends upon the amount of nuclear proteins and cytokeratins present in the epithelium. The details are as described under the section visual inspection. CIN, vaginal intraepithelial neoplasia (VAIN), vulvar intraepithelial neoplasia (VIN) and anal intraepithelial neoplasia (AIN) are some precancerous lesions that appear white after application of acetic acid. Acetowhitening may last for 2–4 minutes in the case of high-grade lesions and invasive cancer.

The nature of acetowhitening with respect to the nature of cervical lesion is as described in Table 7.

Application of Schiller's or Lugol's iodine causes mahogany brown or black staining of normal squamous epithelium due to their glycogen-rich content. It is especially useful when abnormal tissue cannot be visualized satisfactorily using acetic acid alone and to better define the limits of the transformation zone and lesions. The details are as described under the section visual inspection.

The colposcopic findings must be documented carefully, including diagrammatic representation of the colposcopic appearance indicating the abnormal areas, immediately after the examination. The clinical findings are also recorded simultaneously. It is essential to visualize the complete transformation zone (TZ) and margins of the lesion for a satisfactory colposcopic examination. It is inadequate or unsatisfactory if either the TZ or the lesion is not completely visualized as is common in postmenopausal women where the TZ recedes in the cervical canal (Figs. 13 and 14).

Indications

Colposcopy is used to visually evaluate lesions, to define their extent, to identify abnormal areas for a guided biopsy, assist in treatment with cryotherapy or loop electrosurgical excision procedure (LEEP).

The indications of colposcopy are listed in Box 5.

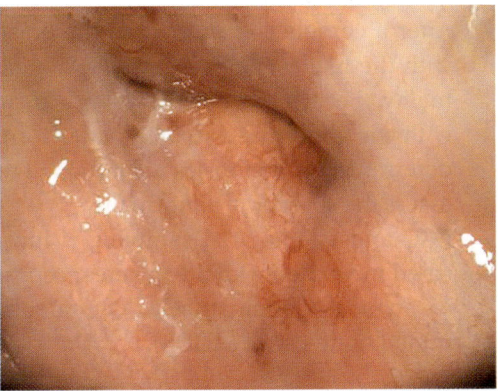

Fig. 13: Incomplete visualization of transformation zone on colposcopy.

Box 5: Indications of colposcopy.

- Women with unhealthy cervix
- Women with abnormal cytology, persistent inflammatory smear, atypical squamous cells of undetermined significance (ASCUS), cervical intraepithelial neoplasia 2 (CIN2) or CIN 3
- Women with a history of diethylstilbestrol (DES) exposure in utero
- Unexplained persistent cervicovaginal discharge
- Unexplained abnormal lower genital tract bleeding
- History of lower genital tract neoplasia (cervical, vaginal, and vulvar)
- Posttreatment surveillance

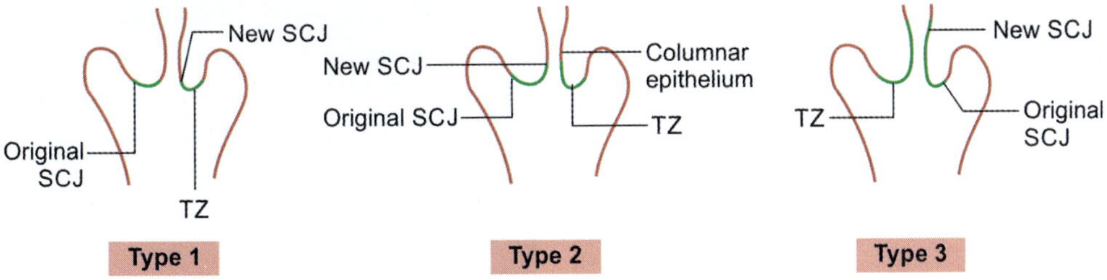

Fig. 14: Types of transformation zone (TZ). Type 1: Ectocervical; entire TZ visible. Type 2: Endocervical component but is still fully visible. Type 3: Endocervical component, and the upper limit is not fully visible; entire TZ not visible. (SCJ: squamocolumnar junction)

Procedure

- A written informed consent is taken after explaining the procedure to the patient.
- With the woman in a dorsal lithotomy position or dorsal position and buttocks at the edge of the table, the perineum and vulva are inspected.
- The widest possible self-retaining speculum that can be comfortably inserted into the vagina is used for optimal visualization of the cervix. Vaginal side walls can be retracted using retractors or a latex condom can be used on the speculum, the tip of which is cut open with scissors. Any obvious areas of abnormality such as ectropion, polyp, nabothian follicles, congenital transformation zone, atrophy, inflammation and infection, leukoplakia (hyperkeratosis), condylomata, ulcer, growth and any obvious lesions in the vaginal fornices are noted.
- Using a syringe, a gentle lavage of the cervix and vaginal walls is done with normal saline to remove mucus and debris.
- The cervix is inspected and the transformation zone or SCJ is identified. This is the anatomical zone where CIN and invasive cervical carcinoma arise and hence is the area of focus during examination. If the entire SCJ is not visible, the colposcopic procedure is termed inadequate or unsatisfactory and an endocervical curettage (ECC) should be done.
- The cervix is inspected with a green filter and 15x magnification, noting any abnormal vascular pattern.
- Using a cotton applicator or cotton swabs, 3–5% acetic acid is applied on the cervix. After 1–2 minutes, areas of acetowhitening are noted with special attention to abnormalities close to the SCJ (Fig. 15).
- Next, Lugol's iodine solution is applied and cervix visualized (Fig. 16).
- The findings of colposcopic examination are recorded immediately.
- After a complete examination, the areas with the highest degree of visible abnormality, i.e. acetowhite areas and areas with an abnormal vascular pattern are determined and biopsies are obtained to assess the severity of abnormality.
- ECC and endometrial sampling is indicated in women with a Pap smear report of atypical glandular cells of undetermined significance (AGUS).

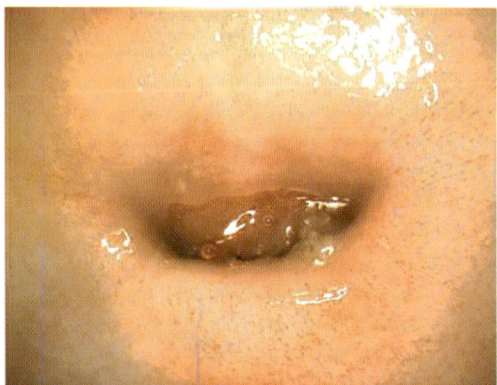

Fig. 15: Normal cervix on colposcopy after application of acetic acid.

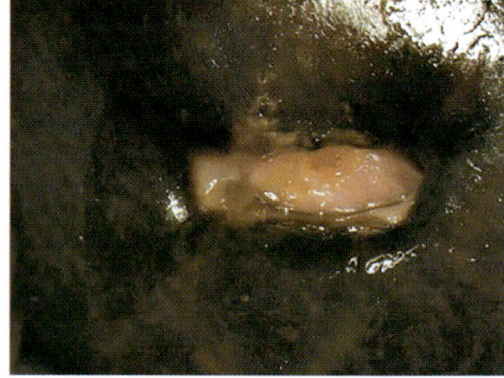

Fig. 16: Normal cervix on colposcopy after application of Lugol's iodine.

Follow-up Advice

At the end of the procedure, the patient should be advised to observe abstinence till the discharge or bleeding per vaginum ceases. She is apprised of the danger signals such as active bleeding per vaginum, pain in lower abdomen, purulent discharge per vaginum, or fever necessitating a visit to the hospital. She is asked to report for follow-up after 2–3 weeks for review with histopathological report for further advice and management.

Interpretation

It is important to be aware of and appreciate the colposcopic features of the normal cervix (Table 8). This provides the basis for appreciating abnormal colposcopic findings.

Nearly all cervical neoplasia, both squamous and columnar, develop within the transformation zone, usually adjacent to the new SCJ.[13] Colposcopically, the proximal end of the transformation zone, the new SCJ is at the junction of the squamous epithelium with the columnar epithelium and the distal end or old SCJ is determined by an imaginary line drawn linking the most distal gland openings and/or nabothian follicles seen around the external os. The skill to trace the whole new SCJ decides the adequacy of the colposcopic examination. For aiding complete visualization of SCJ; tip of a cotton swab stick, opening the blades of the vaginal speculum widely, use of the tips of a long dissection forceps or an endocervical speculum may be used.

Vasculature

For the examination of vasculature, the cervix is cleaned with normal saline and visualized under higher magnification using a green or blue filter to enhance the contrast of the vessels.

The regular structure and fine branching of vessels is a normal finding. It is important to note that abnormal vascular features such as punctation, mosaic pattern, and atypical vessels are significant only if these are seen in a background of acetowhite areas.

The grade of CIN can be judged by the nature of vascular changes. Low-grade CIN is associated with fine punctation and/or fine mosaics, whereas high-grade CIN is associated with coarse punctation and/or coarse mosaics in acetowhite areas. Vessels exhibiting punctation and mosaic are more obvious than the normal stromal vessels because these vessels penetrate into the epithelium and are thus closer to the surface (Table 9).

Table 8: Normal findings on colposcopic examination of cervix.

Type of epithelium	Appearance after application of normal saline solution	Appearance after application of acetic acid	Appearance after application of Lugol's iodine
Squamous epithelium	Smooth translucent pink	Dull and pale	Mahogany brown or black
Metaplastic squamous epithelium	Light pink or whitish pink	Patchily distributed pale cluster or sheet-like areas or glassy areas, pinkish-white finger or tongue-like membranes pointing toward the external os with crypt or gland openings	*Mature squamous epithelium*: Mahogany brown or black *Immature squamous epithelium*: No staining or partial staining
Columnar epithelium	Dark pink /red with a villous appearance	Pale acetowhitening of the villi resembling a grape-like appearance	No staining

Table 9: Cervical lesions and vascular patterns on colposcopy.	
Nature of epithelium	Vascular pattern
Native or original squamous epithelium	• Reticular (network) capillaries • Hairpin-shaped capillaries
Inflammation of the cervix e.g. Trichomoniasis	Staghorn-like capillaries; focal round patches of dilated capillaries- "strawberry-spots"
Immature metaplastic squamous epithelium nearer the new squamocolumnar junction	Large branching surface vessels with three recognizable basic patterns: • Tree like branching • Those overlying nabothian cysts • Long vessels that run parallel to one another
Columnar epithelium	• Terminal capillary networks • Large, deep branching vessels may be seen in some cases
Leukoplakia/hyperkeratosis	Vasculature beneath such a thick area cannot be assessed
• Low-grade (CIN 1) lesions • High-grade (CIN 2, CIN 3) lesions and early preclinical invasive cancer	• Fine punctation, fine mosaic blood vessel patterns • Coarse punctation, coarse mosaic blood vessel pattern

Box 6: Description of various colposcopic findings for reporting.

Normal colposcopic findings:
- Original squamous epithelium
- Columnar epithelium
- Normal transformation zone

Abnormal colposcopic findings:
- Within transformation zone
- Outside transformation zone (ectocervix and vagina):
  - Acetowhite epithelium
  - Flat
  - Micropapillary or microconvoluted
  - Punctation—fine/coarse
  - Mosaic—fine/coarse
  - Leukoplakia
  - Iodine-negative epithelium
  - Atypical vessels

Colposcopically suspect invasive carcinoma

Unsatisfactory colposcopy:
- Squamocolumnar junction not visible
- Severe inflammation or severe atrophy
- Cervix not visible

Miscellaneous findings:
- Nonacetowhite micropapillary surface
- Exophytic condyloma
- Inflammation
- Atrophy
- Ulcer, others

Documentation of Colposcopic Findings[13]

The findings observed on colposcopic examination should be systematically documented pictorially for future reference and comparison. The various terms used for reporting the colposcopic findings are described in Box 6.

Several colposcopic grading systems that quantify various colposcopic signs have been developed to improve accuracy. The most used is the Reid Colposcopic Index (RCI), which has a good histologic correlation. The RCI is based upon four colposcopic lesion features: Peripheral margin, color, vascular patterns, and Lugol's staining. Each category is scored from 0 to 2 and the sum provides a numeric index which correlates with histology.[14] More recently, the Swede score has been used which is based upon the lesion size, margins/surface of the lesion, vascularity, acetic acid uptake and iodine staining. Each category is scored from 0 to 2 and a score of ≥5 is predictive of a high-grade cervical lesion. The Swede score is found to have a strong positive correlation with the RCI.[15-17]

Complications

Colposcopy is a relatively safe procedure. Complications may include burning sensation with application of acetic acid or Lugol's iodine, bleeding and infection of the biopsy site.

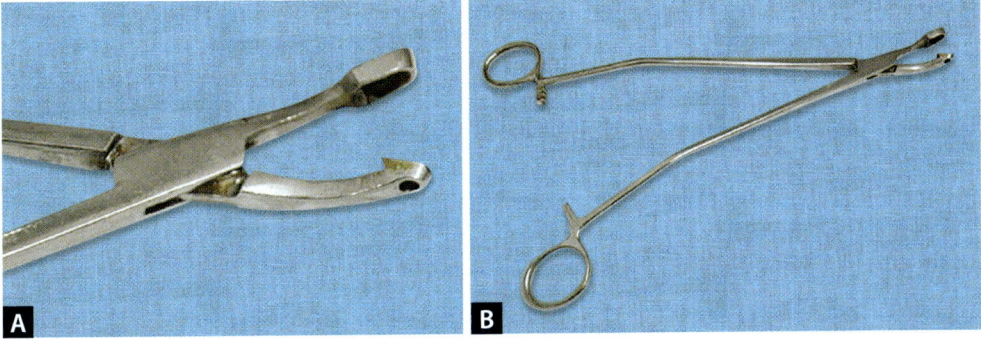

Figs. 17 A and B: Cervical punch biopsy forceps. (A) Magnified view of the blades; (B) Full view.

Cervical Biopsy

Colposcopy-guided cervical biopsy is the "gold standard" for diagnosing cervical abnormalities following an abnormal cytology. Cervical biopsy involves taking a small tissue sample from the abnormal areas of the cervix identified on colposcopy, VIA, or VILI for histopathological diagnosis. It can be taken using a cervical punch biopsy forceps, knife, or electric loop (Figs. 17A and B). The entire SCJ must be visible to allow for adequate assessment of the degree of abnormality and accurate identification of areas to be biopsied. If the SCJ or the transformation zone is partially or entirely inside the cervical canal, an ECC should be done to obtain a sample for histopathological examination.

Biopsy may cause mild discomfort or cramping. A paracervical block may be used to diminish patient discomfort, particularly if multiple biopsies are taken.

Procedure

- After obtaining a written informed consent for the procedure, colposcopy is carried out and abnormal areas on colposcopy are mapped. Lugol's solution (Schiller's test) may be used for clear demarcation of suspicious target areas.
- Posterior areas may be biopsied first to avoid blood dripping over future biopsy sites. Adequate tissue should be removed from the most abnormal area and a depth of 3 mm is mostly enough. It is not necessary to include normal appearing tissue with biopsy samples.
- In case of biopsy from a growth, biopsy from edge of lesion is preferred to avoid central necrosis.
- Tissues obtained are placed in labeled bottles containing 10% formalin and sent to the laboratory for histopathological examination.
- After the biopsy has been obtained, the site of the target area which has been biopsied, is indicated on the diagram of cervix in the reporting form.
- If necessary, an ECC is performed.
- Bleeding is usually minimal. If active bleeding is present, Monsel's paste or silver nitrate is applied to the bleeding areas on the surface of the cervix with cotton swabs to control bleeding. Monsel's solution and silver nitrate interfere with interpretation of biopsy specimen, so these substances should not be applied until all biopsies have been taken. Hemostasis can be achieved by applying pressure, ball cautery, or taking a stitch.

Postprocedure Advice

- No douching, intercourse, or tampons until spotting subsides
- Patients are instructed to return in case of foul vaginal odor or discharge, pelvic pain, or fever.
- Follow-up is advised in 1–3 weeks' time with the histopathological report for discussion regarding further management.

Using a sharp instrument for taking biopsies causes less pain. Sterilization by autoclaving can prematurely dull the sharp edges of biopsy forceps. Less-damaging sterilization methods include chemical sterilization, i.e., soaking in glutaraldehyde or sterilization with gas, are preferred.

Endocervical Curettage

Endocervical curettage is a simple procedure, in which some of the surface cells are gently scraped from the cervical canal with a cytobrush or curette and sent to laboratory for examination. Usually endocervical brushing is followed by endocervical curettage.

Indications for Endocervical Curettage

Endocervical curettage should be performed in the following circumstances:

- *If patient has a positive Pap smear, but no abnormality is detected on colposcopy*: There may be a precancerous lesion or cancer hidden inside the cervical canal, which can be detected by examining tissue obtained by curettage.
- *Pap smear showing a glandular lesion such as AGUS*: These usually arise from the columnar epithelium inside the canal or endometrium. In this case, endocervical and endometrial curettages are performed regardless of the colposcopic findings.
- *Unsatisfactory colposcopy*:
  - The ECC should not be done on pregnant patients due to the risk of excessive bleeding, which may be difficult to control. The risk of biopsy should always be weighed against the risk of missing an early invasive cancer. Noninvasive lesions may be evaluated postpartum.
  - The yield of an ECC is very low in inexperienced hands, so a negative ECC may not always be an evidence of absence of endocervical neoplasia.

Cone Biopsy/Cervical Conization

Cone biopsy involves removal of a cone-shaped tissue around external os including the whole SCJ. The cone can be a short cone with a broad base usually done in women of reproductive age group or a long cone with a narrow base done in postmenopausal women where the squamocolumnar junction recedes in the endocervical canal. The risk of hemorrhage is more with a long cone but is indicated when acetowhite lesion extends into the cervical canal. It can be taken with a scalpel (cold knife), LEEP, or large loop exclsion of transformation zone (LLETZ). Inadequate colposcopy with cytologic evidence of dysplasia frequently requires cervical cone biopsy for further workup. The indications of cone biopsy are as listed in Box 7.

Box 7: Indications of cone biopsy.

- Disparity between cytology and Pap smear
- Repeated abnormal cytology
- Inconclusive finding on ECC
- Lesions extending into cervical canal
- Unsatisfactory colposcopy
- Cervical intraepithelial neoplasia 3 (CIN 3) on colposcopically directed biopsy

Cold Knife Conization

Cold knife conization is the removal of a cone-shaped area around the external os with a knife under general or regional anesthesia including portions of the ectocervix and endocervix. It is used as a diagnostic test in lesions suspicious for microinvasive cancer, endocervical glandular neoplasia, abnormal endocervical curettage, and where LEEP is not possible.

The extent of the conization will depend on the size of the lesion and the likelihood of finding invasive cancer. The tissue obtained is sent for histopathologic diagnosis and to see if the margins of the cone are free of pathology indicating complete removal of abnormal tissue. The procedure should not be done in presence of infection, pregnancy, puerperium, and invasive cancer.

Procedure:
- After obtaining written informed consent, patient is placed in dorsal lithotomy position under anesthesia.
- Cervical canal is sounded to determine its length and position of internal os.
- A preconization cerclage or bilateral occlusion of descending cervical artery can be done using an absorbable suture chromic catgut or polyglycolic acid, to reduce bleeding.
- Conization is performed with a number 11 blade, pointing it toward the planned apex of the cone; posterior part of the cone is cut first to avoid blood obscuring the field.
- The entire transformation zone is included in the incision all around the external os on the ectocervix.
- Apex of the cone should end 1 cm below the internal os if the lesion does not extend into deep endocervical region, the excised cone is then sent for histopathologic examination. The 12 o'clock position should be marked in the cone for orientation.

Table 10: Advantages and disadvantages of cold knife conization.

Advantages	Disadvantages
Provides good specimen for histopathologic examination	More bleeding compared to other methods of conization
Tissue margins are well-preserved for histopathological examination	May result in cervical stenosis or incompetent os with associated complications such as hematometra, cervical dystocia, and precipitate or preterm labor
	Can be performed only by providers with surgical skills in a well-equipped surgical facility

- Bleeding after the procedure can be controlled by coagulation or by applying hemostatic sutures.
- Generalized oozing can be controlled by tight vaginal packing with sterile gauze or using Monsel's solution.

The advantages and disadvantages of cold knife conization are given in Table 10.

Complications: Hemorrhage is the most common complication; it can occur immediately (primary hemorrhage) or up to 14 days after the procedure (secondary hemorrhage). Secondary hemorrhage is usually related to infection and, should be managed with hemostatic drugs such as tranexamic acid 1 g every 4–6 hours and antibiotics.

Loop Electrosurgical Excision Procedure

Loop electrosurgical excision procedure, also called large loop excision of transformation zone (LLETZ), involves the removal of either the cervical lesion or the entire transformation zone using a thin, heated stainless steel or tungsten wire loop electrosurgically (Fig. 18).

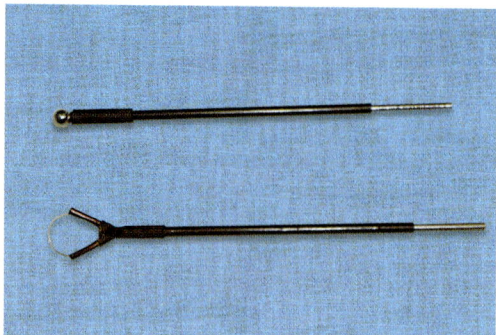

Fig. 18: Loop and ball electrodes for loop electrosurgical excision procedure (LEEP).

It can be performed for removal of lesions extending <1 cm into the endocervical canal where it aims to remove both the lesion and the entire transformation zone. The tissue removed can be sent for histopathological examination, to assess the nature of the lesion. It is successful in eradicating precancer in >90% of cases. Persistent lesion at 6 or 12 months follow-up is termed as treatment failure and is seen in <10% of women.

The LEEP should not be performed in following cases:
- When there is a suspicion of invasive cancer or glandular dysplasia or in any lesion extending >1 cm into the endocervical canal, or whose distal or upper extent is not visible. These lesions are preferably treated by cold knife conization.
- Cervical infection or pelvic inflammatory disease (PID) until it is treated or resolved.
- During pregnancy or within 12 weeks of childbirth.

Procedure:
- After obtaining written informed consent, patient is placed in dorsal lithotomy position under local anesthesia. A vasoconstrictor agent such as epinephrine is used along with lidocaine, to reduce blood loss.
- A grounding pad is placed.

Table 11: The advantages and disadvantages of LEEP or LLETZ.

Advantages	Disadvantages
Can be performed under local anesthesia on an outpatient basis	Requires specialized equipment like an electrosurgical unit
Blood loss less compared to cold knife conization/laser conization	Risk of electrical burns
Treatment as well as histopathological diagnosis of the lesion is possible	Requires trained personnel
	Can be done only in a well-equipped surgical facility, where complications, such as hemorrhage, can be managed

(LEEP: loop electrosurgical excision procedure; LLETZ: large loop excision of transformation zone)

- An insulated speculum is used to prevent electric shock.
- Loop size should be appropriate to remove the entire transformation zone.
- Tissue is ablated to a depth of 1 cm in the first pass, with the loop directed in a transverse or anteroposterior direction.
- Bleeding after the procedure can be controlled by roller ball coagulation or by applying Monsel's solution.

The advantages and disadvantages of LEEP or LLETZ are listed in Table 11.

Laser Conization

Conization can be done using laser, which can be excisional or by vaporization. The excisional method provides tissue for histopathological diagnosis, while vaporization only destroys tissue and no material is available for histopathology. Carbon dioxide laser is applied using a colposcopic micromanipulator.

Table 12: Advantages and disadvantages of laser conization.

Advantages	Disadvantages
Precise marking of ectocervical margins can be done	Margins of tissue may be burnt, interfering with histopathological reporting
	High cost
	Requires trained personnel
	Requires specialized equipment
	Requires a well-equipped facility

Procedure:
- After obtaining written informed consent, patient is placed in dorsal lithotomy position under anesthesia.
- A preconization cerclage can be placed or a vasoconstrictor agent such as epinephrine or dilute vasopressin can be injected, to reduce blood loss.
- Exocervical margins are outlined with 0.5–1 mm dots, using laser energy at low power (20–50 W).
- A laser incision is then performed and extended to a depth of 3–5 mm. Tissue obtained is then sent for histopathologic examination.
- Bleeding can be controlled by laser coagulation or diathermy.

The advantages and disadvantages of laser conization are as listed in Table 12.

Post conization, cervix heals in 6 weeks. Abstinence should be advised for at least 6 weeks to prevent bleeding and infection.

KEY POINTS

- The magnitude of problem of carcinoma cervix in developing countries necessitates offering universal screening of all sexually active women.
- Basic components of cervical cancer control include screening, early diagnosis, and treatment for precancerous lesions and early invasive cancer.
- The WHO recommends cytology, HPV testing, visual inspection with acetic acid (VIA), loop electrosurgical excision procedure (LEEP), and cold knife conization for screen-and-treat strategies for precancerous lesions of cervix.
- Cytology has been the mainstay of secondary prevention of cervical cancer.
- A positive Pap smear test alone is insufficient for the diagnosis of cervical cancer additional tests such as colposcopy and cervical biopsy are required to confirm the diagnosis.
- Pap smear screening is also recommended for those who have been vaccinated against HPV. LBC is more sensitive than Pap test with higher sensitivity and specificity.
- HPV testing is most useful when done in addition to a cytological test, in women aged 30–65 years. No benefit from HPV DNA-based screening before 30 years of age.
- The most important use of HPV DNA testing is for triaging women with a Pap result of ASC-US for colposcopy.
- Visual inspection techniques VIA and VILI are inexpensive, can be performed with significantly less training, and are useful in low-resource settings.
- Women who are positive for VIA, VILI may be referred for colposcopy and biopsy to rule out underlying high-grade CIN and invasive cancer.
- Colposcopy is the examination of cellular patterns in the epithelial layer and surrounding blood vessels of the cervix, vagina, and vulva under magnification, after application of normal saline, 3–5% dilute acetic acid, and Lugol's iodine solution in successive steps. It helps in identifying suspicious areas for biopsy.

- The area of interest is the transformation zone and if the SCJ is not visualized in its entire circumference, the colposcopic procedure is termed inadequate or unsatisfactory.
- Cervical biopsy, endocervical curettage, and conization are procedures which are used to obtain a definite histopathological diagnosis.
- The choice of procedure depends upon the type of lesion, its site and extent, and the availability of appropriate expertise and equipment.
- Conization may be done using a scalpel, laser, or LEEP.
- Conization may serve as a therapeutic measure in some cases.

REFERENCES

1. Bray F, Ferlay J, Soerjomataram I, Siegel RL, Torre LA, Jemal A. Global cancer statistics 2018: GLOBOCAN estimates of incidence and mortality worldwide for 36 cancers in 185 countries. CA Cancer J Clin. 2018;68(6): 394-424.
2. World Health Organization. Cervical cancer. [online] Available from https://www.who.int/cancer/prevention/diagnosis-screening/cervical-cancer/en/. [Last accessed February, 2020].
3. ICO/IARC Information Centre on HPV and Cancer. (2019). India: Human papillomavirus and related cancers, Fact Sheet 2018. [online] Available from https://hpvcentre.net/statistics/reports/IND_FS.pdf. [Last accessed February, 2020].
4. World Health Organization (2014). Comprehensive cervical cancer control: a guide to essential practice, 2nd edition. [online] Available from https://apps.who.int/iris/bitstream/handle/10665/144785/9789241548953_ eng.pdf;jsessionid= DFD61C32D78CBD8E4DEED27205 B43D32?sequence=1. [Last accessed February, 2020].
5. Curry SJ, Krist AH, Owens DK, Barry MJ, Caughey AB, Davidson KW, et al. Screening for Cervical Cancer: US Preventive Services Task Force Recommendation Statement. JAMA. 201821;320(7):674-86.
6. Saslow D, Solomon D, Lawson HW, Killackey M, Kulasingam SL, Cain J, et al. American Cancer Society, American Society for Colposcopy and Cervical Pathology, and American Society for Clinical Pathology screening guidelines for the prevention and early detection of cervical cancer. CA Cancer J Clin. 2012;62(3):147-72.
7. Sawaya GF, Sung H-Y, Kinney W, Kearney KA, Miller MG, Hiatt RA. Cervical cancer after multiple negative cytologic tests in long-term members of a prepaid health plan. Acta Cytol. 2005;49(4):391-7.
8. Solomon D, Davey D, Kurman R, Moriarty A, O'Connor D, Prey M, et al. The 2001 Bethesda System: terminology for reporting results of cervical cytology. JAMA. 200224; 287(16):2114-9.
9. Koliopoulos G, Nyaga VN, Santesso N, Bryant A, Martin-Hirsch PP, Mustafa RA, et al. Cytology versus HPV testing for cervical cancer screening in the general population. Cochrane Database Syst Rev. 2017;8:CD008587.
10. Basu P, Mittal S, Banerjee D, Singh P, Panda C, Dutta S, et al. Diagnostic accuracy of VIA and HPV detection as primary and sequential screening tests in a cervical cancer screening demonstration project in India. Int J Cancer. 2015;137(4):859-67.
11. Singla S, Mathur S, Kriplani A, Agarwal N, Garg P, Bhatla N. Single visit approach for management of cervical intraepithelial neoplasia by visual inspection & loop electrosurgical excision procedure. Indian J Med Res. 2012;135(5):614-20.
12. Nessa A, Wistrand C, Begum SA, Thuresson M, Shemer I, Thorsell M, et al. Evaluation of stationary colposcope and the Gynocular, by the Swede score systematic colposcopic system in VIA positive women: a crossover randomized trial. Int J Gynecol Cancer 2014; 24(2):339-45.
13. Sellors JW, Sankarnarayanan R. Colposcopy and treatment of cervical intraepithelial neoplasia a beginner's manual. Geneva: World Health Organization; 2003.

14. Reid R, Scalzi P. Genital warts and cervical cancer. VII. An improved colposcopic index for differentiating benign papillomaviral infections from high-grade cervical intraepithelial neoplasia. Am J Obstet Gynecol. 198515;153(6):611-8.
15. Ranga R, Rai S, Kumari A, Mathur S, Kriplani A, Mahey R, et al. A Comparison of the strength of association of reid colposcopic index and swede score with cervical histology. J Low Genit Tract Dis. 2017;21(1):55-8.
16. Taghavi K, Banerjee D, Mandal R, Kallner HK, Thorsell M, Friis T, et al. Colposcopy telemedicine: live versus static swede score and accuracy in detecting CIN2+, a cross-sectional pilot study. BMC Women's Health. 2018;18(1):89.
17. Kushwah S, Kushwah B. Correlation of two colposcopic indices for predicting premalignant lesions of cervix. J Midlife Health. 2017;8(3):118-23.

SUGGESTED READING

1. FOGSI Gynaecologic Oncology Committee. (2018). FOGSI GCPR on screening and treatment of preinvasive lesions of cervix and HPV vaccination. [online] Available from https://www.fogsi.org/wp-content/uploads/2018/01/fogsi-gcpr-smplc-cervix-hpv-vaccination-document-2017-2018-final.pdf. [Last accessed February, 2020].
2. Screening & Immunisations Team, NHS Digital. Cervical Screening Programme 2017-18. [online] Available from https://digital.nhs.uk/data-and-information/publications/statistical/cervical-screening-programme/england---2017-18. [Last accessed February, 2020].
3. Smith RA, Andrews K, Brooks D, DeSantis CE, Fedewa SA, Lortet-Tieulent J, et al. Cancer screening in the United States, 2016: A review of current American Cancer Society guidelines and current issues in cancer screening. CA Cancer J Clin. 2016;66(2):96-114.

52. Obstetrical and Gynecological Instruments

Archana Kumari

INTRODUCTION

Instruments form an important tool of examination and management of every patient. Use of the right instrument at the right place makes the procedure easy. Hence the knowledge of various instruments used in obstetrics and gynecology as regard to their identification, technique, and indications for use, advantages, disadvantages, and complications is essential for all students.

Before proceeding to any examination or procedure, it is a good habit to check the trolley for availability of all instruments required for the proposed procedure and other requirements like drapes, chemicals for part preparation or otherwise, vials for collection of samples, etc. It is also important to know about how to maintain asepsis. This chapter describes the commonly used instruments in obstetric and gynecological practice. The various instruments have been described in an alphabetical order.

ABDOMINAL RETRACTORS

Doyen Retractor

Doyen retractor has a sturdy handle with a broad blade with uniform curvature (Fig. 1A). The broad retracting surface achieves good retraction as well as reduces blood loss from cut edges by compression. This is used for suprapubic retraction of abdominal wall after opening the parietal peritoneum. It also retracts the bladder once the uterovesical (UV) fold of peritoneum is opened.

Indications

Doyen retractor is used in:
- Cesarean section (CS)
- Abdominal hysterectomy
- Laparotomy for ruptured ectopic pregnancy
- Exploratory laparotomy for adnexal masses
- Abdominal sling surgeries for uterine prolapse
- Abdominal surgeries for repair of stress urinary incontinence.

Disadvantage

Doyen retractor is not very deep, so not preferred in gynecological surgeries carried out deep in the pelvis.

Morris Retractor

Morris retractor has a firm handle and a broad blade at right angles (Fig. 1B). It is not curved and is available in different sizes depending on the length and width of the blades. The uses of Morris retractor are the same as that of Doyen retractor.

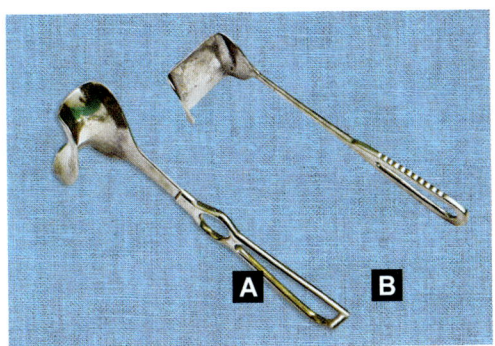

Figs. 1A and B: Abdominal retractors. (A) Doyen retractor; (B) Morris retractor.

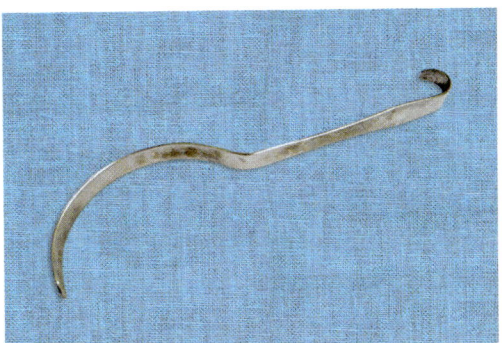

Fig. 2: Deaver retractor.

Deaver Retractor

Deaver is a long strip of stainless steel, which is bent into the shape of retractor (Fig. 2). It is available in three sizes—small, medium, and large. Its length and curvature make it ideal for retracting, while operating in depth. However, it is not good for retracting the abdominal incision. During retraction, the blade of the retractor is covered with a mop or veil so that it does not damage the structures retracted.

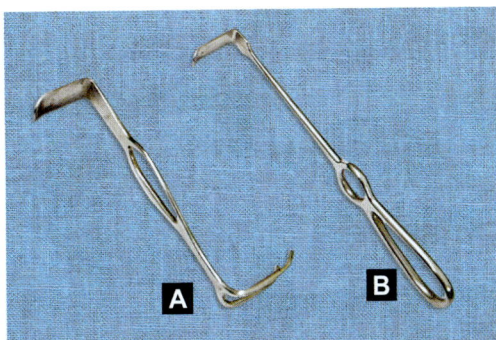

Figs. 3A and B: Abdominal retractors. (A) Czerny's; (B) Small right-angled retractor.

Indications

For retraction of sides of the incision and intraperitoneal structures during operations on the posterior abdominal wall, e.g., ligation of internal iliac artery, Shirodkar sling operation, retraction of bladder during abdominal hysterectomy.

Czerny's

Journey retractor is a retractor with a small right-angled blade on one side and two right-angled hooks on the other side. It is usually used, while opening or closing the abdomen and while doing mini laparotomy or postpartum tubal ligation (Fig. 3A).

Right-angled Retractor

Right-angled retractor is like a Journey retractor with small right-angled blade on one end but does not have any hooks on the other end (Fig. 3B). Instead, it has a handle on the other end. The indications are also same as Journey retractor.

ALLIS FORCEPS

Allis forceps is made of stainless steel and available in two sizes, 12 cm and 17.5 cm in length. The blades are curved inward and have 4 in 5 or 5 in 6 fine teeth, and a ratchet lock on the handles (Fig. 4). It is used to hold tough structures like rectus sheath, vaginal

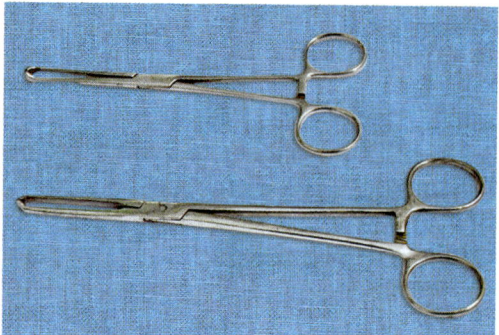

Fig. 4: Allis forceps.

edges during hysterectomy and does cause tissue damage. Some atraumatic Allis forceps are also available with double row of atraumatic teeth.

Indications

The indications are listed in Table 1.

ANEURYSM NEEDLE

Aneurysm needle is a blunt-tipped needle on a long handle with a subterminal eye

Table 1: Indications for use of Allis forceps.	
Obstetrical	*Gynecological*
To hold the rectus sheath during dissecting it from the underlying rectus muscle and while suturing it	*To hold the cut edges of vagina*: • In abdominal hysterectomy after opening the vagina and removing the specimen • In vaginal hysterectomy during closure of vault of vagina • In anterior and posterior repairs for dissection of vaginal mucosal flaps from underlying bladder and rectum, respectively • Excision of vaginal wall cyst • Enterocele repair • During sacrospinous fixation in vault prolapse
To hold the torn ends of external anal sphincter, while repairing third- and fourth-degree perineal tears	*To hold the cervix*: • Instead of a vulsellum • In abdominal hysterectomy to draw the cervix up after opening the vault of vagina
To hold the cut edges of the lower uterine segment during cesarean section when Green Armytage forceps is not available	*To hold the uterus*: • In abdominal hysterectomy, hold the fundus to give traction on and to manipulate the position of the uterus, while clamping the pedicles • In vaginal hysterectomy to pull down the uterus after ligating the uterine vessels to clamp fundal structures • In myomectomy to hold the cut edges of the capsule and facilitate enucleation of the myoma • In metroplasty to hold the cut edges of the uterus during suturing
To hold the tubes for ligation when Babcock is not available	*Other indications*: • To take vulvar biopsy • To take lymph node biopsy • To avulse a cervical polyp

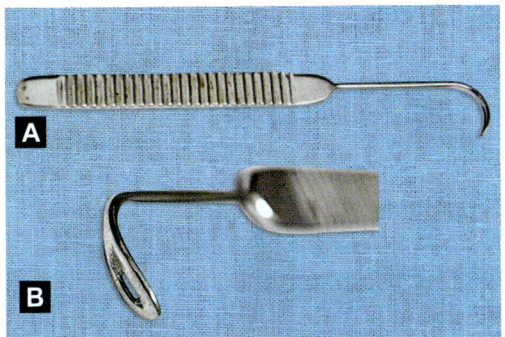

Figs. 5A and B: Aneurysm needle. (A) Curved needle on handle; (B) Subterminal eye and blunt tip.

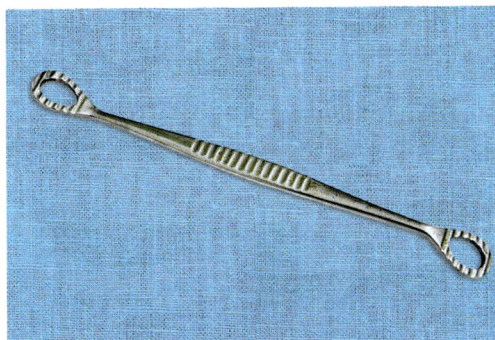

Fig. 6: Anterior vaginal wall retractor.

(Figs. 5A and B). It is used for ligating vessels such as internal iliac ligation and uterine artery.

ANTERIOR VAGINAL WALL RETRACTOR

Anterior vaginal wall retractor is a long instrument with spoon-shaped ends. It has transverse serrations on either surface to provide friction against rugosities of vaginal mucosa and aid in effective retraction. The broad ends make an angle of 15° with the shaft and are angled in opposite directions to facilitate retraction without blocking the view (Fig. 6).

Indications

Anterior vaginal wall retractor is used in conjunction with the Sims speculum for the retraction of anterior vaginal wall to expose the cervix.

ARTERY FORCEPS

Artery forceps are primarily used as hemostatic forceps to grasp the vessels and allow ligation or cauterization of those vessels (Figs. 7A and B). They vary in size depending on the caliber of the vessels to be caught. They are

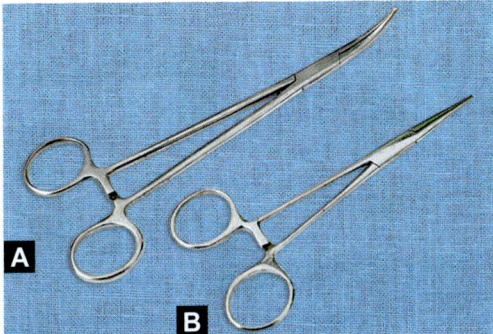

Figs. 7A and B: Artery forceps. (A) Curved artery forceps; (B) Mosquito forceps.

usually available as straight or curved artery forceps. The curve allows easier placement of ligatures around forceps. The mosquito forceps are the small artery forceps with fine tips and are usually 5–7 inches long. They can be used to grasp tissue, suture, and other prosthetic material, but as they are crushing forceps, they can damage delicate structures.

AYRE'S SPATULA

Ayre's spatula is made of wood or plastic. It is 15–17 cm long and has two ends. One end is 3 mm broad and 2 cm long. The other end has two projections; one of them projecting beyond the other (Fig. 8). The wooden spatula

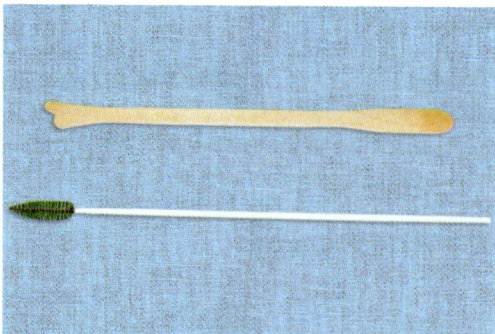

Fig. 8: Ayre's spatula and endocervical brush.

is better than the plastic spatula as more cells stick to the rough surface of wooden spatula compared to smooth plastic spatula.

Indications

Ayre's spatula is used for collection of the following:
- Superficial cervical biopsy (Pap smear) for cervical cancer screening
- Vault smear in posthysterectomy women
- Lateral vaginal wall smear for cytohormonal studies
- Buccal smear for Barr body count.

Technique of Use

For collecting a cervical smear, the projected end of the spatula is introduced into the external os and the shorter end rests on portio vaginalis. It is rotated through 360° to collect the cervical cells from the squamocolumnar junction. In postmenopausal women, the squamocolumnar junction recedes into the cervical canal and cannot be accessed by the Ayre's spatula. In these cases, an endocervical brush is used for sampling the transformation zone. Whereas for the vault smear in post-hysterectomy women and lateral vaginal wall smear, the broad flat end of the Ayre's spatula is used.

BLADDER CATHETERS

Foley Catheter

Foley catheter is a self-retaining urinary catheter made up of latex, which is sterilized by exposure to gamma irradiation. The catheter has a bulb at the end which passes into the urethra. It can be distended with saline to make the catheter self-retaining. The other end has two channels, one connects the catheter to the urine collecting bag and through the other, saline can be pushed to inflate the bulb and removed to deflate the bulb (Figs. 9A to C). The capacity of the bulb is 30–50 mL, however distension of the bulb by 5–10 mL saline is enough to make it self-retaining. The capacity of bulb is only 3 mL for pediatric Foley catheter. Pediatric Foley catheter usually has a stent in it, which can be removed after insertion (Figs. 10A and B). Special silicone-coated catheters are also available, which are better tolerated by the patient and can be kept in the bladder for longer duration of up to 3 weeks. The catheters are available in various sizes ranging from 6 to 18 Fr (1 Fr = 0.33 mm). In adult women, the size of Foley catheter used is 14 or 16 Fr.

Indications

The Foley catheter is used both in obstetrics and gynecology and the indications are as listed in Table 2.

Female Metal Catheter

Female metal catheter is a stainless steel curved blunt-tipped catheter approximately 15 cm (6 inch) in length and with a hole about an inch away from its tip for drainage of urine. Usually a 14 Fr catheter is used (Fig. 11).

Chapter 52: Obstetrical and Gynecological Instruments

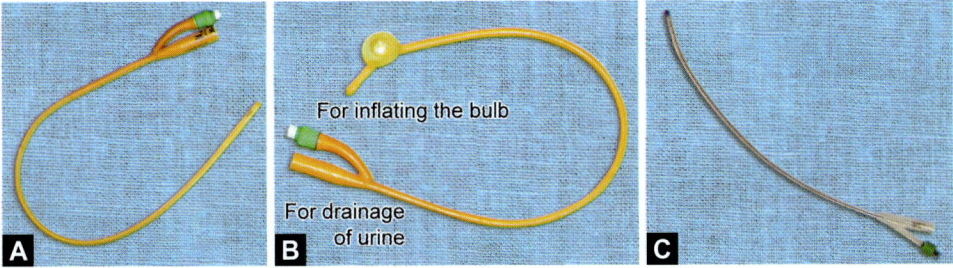

Figs. 9A to C: Adult Foley catheter. (A) Without inflated bulb; (B) With inflated bulb; (C) Silicon catheter.

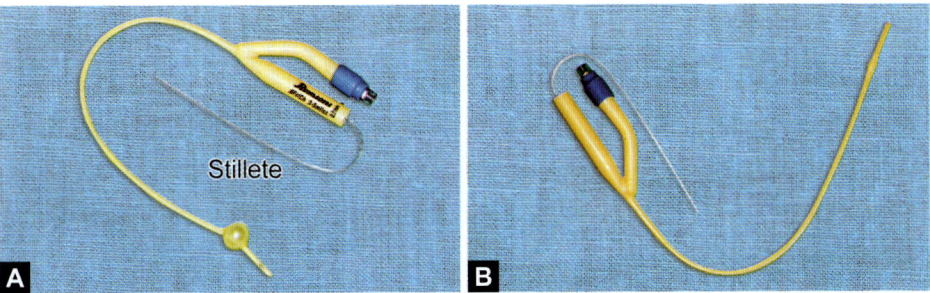

Figs. 10A and B: Pediatric Foley catheter. (A) With inflated bulb; (B) Without inflated bulb.

Table 2: Indications for use of Foley catheter.

Obstetrics	Gynecology

• During cesarean section for short-term drainage of urine
• In patients with obstructed labor for long-term drainage of 2–3 weeks to prevent ischemic necrosis and development of VVF
• Retroverted gravid uterus with retention of urine
• For ripening of cervix during induction of labor with Foley catheter No. 20 with bulb distended with 50 mL saline
• Induction of second trimester abortion by extraovular administration of ethacridine lactate
• *Cord prolapse*: To fill the bladder with 500 mL saline to displace the presenting part and prevent cord compression
• Monitor urine output in obstetrical conditions like severe pre-eclampsia, eclampsia, placental abruption, hemorrhagic or septic shock
• Atonic PPH for balloon tamponade of uterine cavity
• Amnioinfusion
	• *Prolonged bladder drainage following gynecological operations*:
	  – Anterior colporrhaphy: 2–3 days
	  – Kelly plication for SUI: 5 days
	  – Repair of bladder injury: 7–10 days
	  – VVF repair: 14–21 days
	  – McIndoe vaginoplasty: 7–15 days
	  – Wertheim's operation: 15 days
	• *Hysterosalpingography*: Pediatric Foley catheter No. 8 or 10 Fr is used
	• During cystoscopy in case of big VVF to occlude the fistulous opening by passing catheter through fistulous opening vaginally and inflating the bulb to prevent escape of fluid, while distending the bladder during cystoscopy
	• During repair of VVF placed behind pubic symphysis, to increase the accessibility of VVF by applying traction on the inflated catheter bulb passed through the fistulous opening into the bladder
	• During Kelly's repair for SUI to identify bladder neck
	• During Burch colposuspension for SUI
	• In Asherman's syndrome, to prevent the reformation of adhesions after hysteroscopic lysis, the bulb is inflated with 2–3 mL of saline and left in uterine cavity for a week
	• Saline sonohysterosalpingography
	• To control intrauterine bleeding with balloon tamponade after hysteroscopic surgery such as division of uterine septum, resection of submucous myoma
	• As a tourniquet in myomectomy as an alternative to myomectomy clamp

(VVF: vesicovaginal fistula; PPH: postpartum hemorrhage; SUI: stress urinary incontinence)

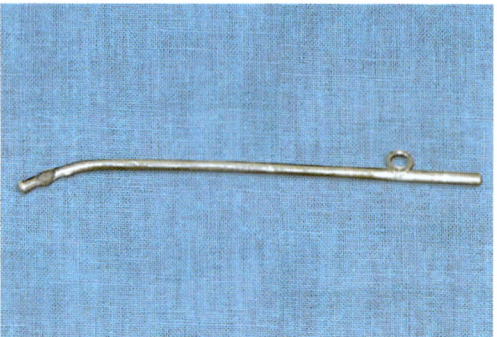

Fig. 11: Female metal catheter.

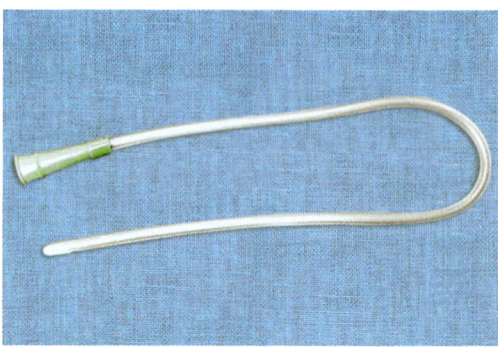

Fig. 12: Plain disposable catheter.

Indications

- To empty the bladder prior to gynecological vaginal operations in order to minimize injury to the bladder.
- *To differentiate Gartner's cyst from cystocele*: The metal catheter tip introduced per urethra fails to come underneath the vaginal mucosa in case of Gartner's cyst. The other differences between the Gartner's cyst and the cystocele are that in the Gartner's cyst, the rugosities of the overlying vaginal mucosa are lost, and margins are well-defined. It is not reducible and there is no cough impulse on coughing.

Plain Disposable Catheter

The plain disposable catheters are also available in various sizes (Fig. 12). They are made of polyvinyl chloride (PVC) and are not self-retaining.

Indications

- To empty the bladder in retention of urine
- To empty the bladder in a pregnant woman in labor
- As a tourniquet in myomectomy operation as an alternative to myomectomy clamp.

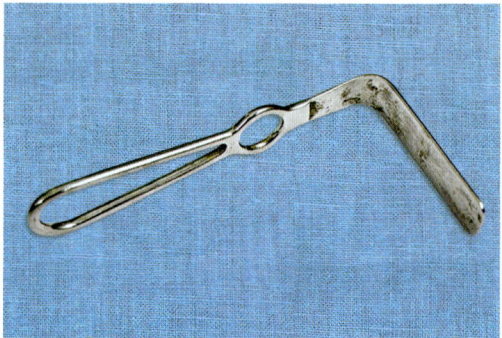

Fig. 13: Landon vaginal retractor.

Landon Vaginal Retractor

Landon vaginal retractor is a L-shaped blade, which is 2 cm wide. The handle has a fenestration in its center for the thumb. The blade is narrow and flat, occupying very little space (Fig. 13). Hence, it is ideal for vaginal operations where space is limited.

Indications

The Landon vaginal retractor is used to retract the bladder away from the cervix during vaginal hysterectomy. As the ureters are also retracted away along with the bladder base, hence it protects them from accidental injury during operation.

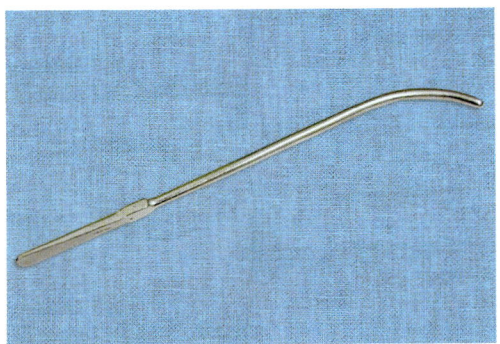

Fig. 14: Bladder sound.

Bladder Sound

Bladder sound is a 25 cm long instrument made of stainless steel with a long rod-shaped, blunt-tipped sounding portion, which is curved in its terminal 5 cm (Fig. 14). It needs to be differentiated from uterine sound. Unlike uterine sound, it is not graduated, does not have an angulation and olive tip of uterine sound.

Indications

- *During vaginal hysterectomy*: To define the limits of bladder in the anterior vaginal wall
- *To diagnose and differentiate suburethral cyst from urethral diverticulum*: The tip of sound cannot enter the suburethral cyst
- For urethral dilatation
- To sound the urinary bladder for foreign body namely stone, perforated intrauterine contraceptive device (IUCD).

Bonney's Myomectomy Clamp

Bonney's myomectomy clamp is an instrument, which has two pairs of finger grips proximal and distal, with a ratchet lock on the handle near the proximal finger grip. The blades are at an angle of 120° with the handles. There are two overlapping transverse bars attached to the blades, one on each. The blades distal to transverse bars are covered with rubber caps. This instrument is used for temporary compression of uterine blood vessels and to decrease intraoperative blood loss during myomectomy. The distal finger grips are used while application of the instrument because the blades can be opened widely with the finger in distal finger grips. The proximal finger grips are used for tightening the lock as well as releasing it because they offer greater degree of mechanical advantage than the distal ones.

Technique of Using the Instrument

The instrument is placed at the level of internal os with the concavity fitting into the convexity of the symphysis pubis. The round ligaments of both sides are included inside the clamp to prevent slipping of the instrument and preventing the uterus from falling back. Thus, the space between the blades distal to transverse bars includes the uterus just above the cervix and both the round ligaments. The transverse bars thus prevent the round ligaments from slipping. In case the operative time is prolonged, the clamps must be released every 20 minutes for 10 minutes to prevent uterus from anoxia and acute vasodilation and hypotension due to sudden release of histamine-like substance into the circulation.

A red rubber or Foley catheter can be used instead of Bonney's myomectomy clamp as a tourniquet around the isthmus for decreasing the blood supply to uterus. In addition to control the blood supply through the ovarian vessels, sponge-holding forceps may be applied over each infundibulopelvic ligament during operation. The clamp is removed after suturing the myoma beds, but before

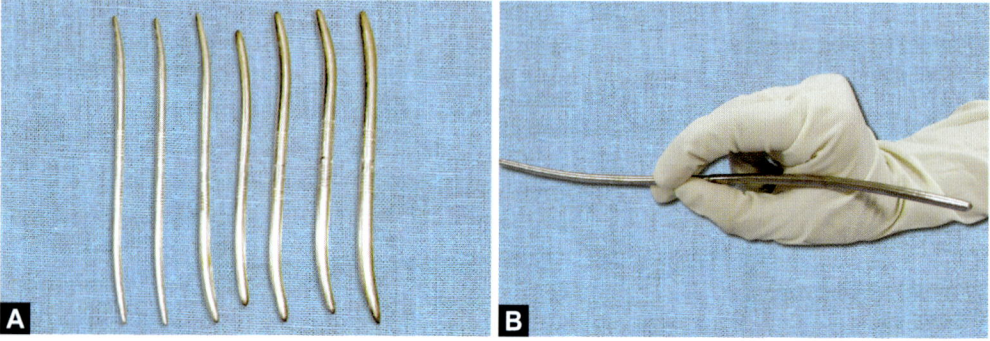

Figs. 15A and B: (A) Graduated set of Hegar dilators; (B) Cervical dilator.

closing the potential layers. Hemostasis must be confirmed after releasing the clamp. With the practice of infiltration of capsule by vasopressin, the use of these instruments has decreased.

CERVICAL DILATORS

Hegar Dilators

Hegar dilator is a smooth solid rod of stainless steel, gently curved either on one side or both sides; accordingly, it is a single-ended or a double-ended dilator. The size of the dilator is decided by its diameter, which usually ranges from 3 to 12 mm. The double-ended dilators are numbered from 3/4 to 17/18 mm indicating that diameter of one end is 3 mm and the other end is 4 mm. These are available in graduated sets with serially increasing sizes with a difference of 0.5 mm or 1 mm (Figs. 15 and 16A).

Technique of Use

Cervical dilatation is a painful procedure; paracervical block is required for cervical dilatation except in women requiring dilatation up to Hegar No. 4 dilator.

The patient is asked to empty the bladder and lie in dorsal or lithotomy position and a

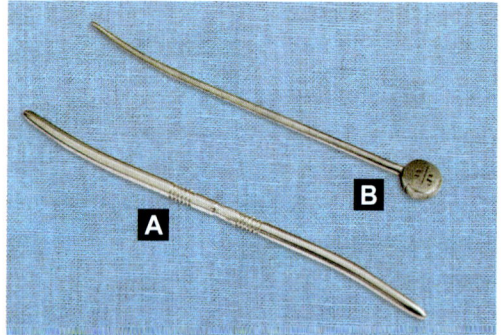

Figs. 16A and B: Cervical dilators. (A) Hegar dilator; (B) Hawkin dilator.

bimanual examination is carried out to know the position and size of uterus. The cervix is exposed with the help of a Sims speculum and anterior vaginal wall retractor and stabilized with a vulsellum. Uterocervical length is measured using a uterine sound except in pregnant women and women with suspected pyometra or carcinoma of the uterus due to increased risk of perforation. Cervical dilatation is done using graduated dilators in serial order beginning with 3/4 mm in size. It is important to apply traction to the cervix to decrease the angle between the cervical canal and uterine cavity facilitating the smooth entry of dilator in the uterus. Dilator should be held like a pen in the dominant hand with thumb and index, and middle fingers, ring,

Table 3: Indications for cervical dilatation in obstetrics and gynecology.	
Obstetrics	Gynecology
• Prior to suction evacuation of molar pregnancy • Prior to suction evacuation in first trimester termination of pregnancy • Retrograde dilatation of cervix when found closed at the time of hysterotomy or an elective cesarean section • For drainage of postpartum lochia	• Prior to endometrial curettage for abnormal uterine bleeding • In Manchester repair for aiding insertion of Sturmdorf suture and to prevent cervical stenosis • To drain uterine fluid contents as in conditions such as pyometra, hematometra, and hydrometra when secondary to cervical stenosis • Removal of intrauterine impacted intrauterine contraceptive device by curettage when other measures have failed • Prior to application of intrauterine source of irradiation, e.g., radium • Prior to operative hysteroscopy for removal of endometrial, placental or leiomyomatous polyp, septal resection • For diagnosis of incompetent cervix

and little fingers resting on the buttock. The dilator should be negotiated just beyond the internal os. The tip of the dilator can be lubricated to facilitate its passage through the internal os.

Extent of dilatation depends upon the procedure and diameter of the instrument to be passed in the uterus. For dilatation and curettage, cervix is dilated to not more than 8 mm. For termination of pregnancy, dilatation depends upon the period of gestation and the rule of thumb is that dilatation in millimeter is equal to the period of gestation in weeks. If the cervix is to be dilated more than 10 mm, a slow dilatation with a laminaria tent or misoprostol is indicated to prevent cervical insufficiency later on.

Indications

The indications of use of cervical dilators are listed in Table 3.

The two tests that are used for the diagnosis of incompetent cervix are:
1. *Inverse Palmer's test*: Passage of No. 8 Hegar dilator through internal os in nonpregnant state without resistance is suggestive of incompetent os.
2. *Shirodkar test*: When a size 8 Hegar dilator that has passed through internal os in a nonpregnant woman is withdrawn, there is a distinct snap as it passes out of internal os. Absence of this snap is suggestive of cervical incompetence.

Complications

- Perforation
- Cervical injury
- Postprocedure infection.

Other Dilators

Hank Dilator

Hank dilator is like Hegar dilator, except that it is less curved and the difference in diameter of successive dilators is 0.5 mm. Hence, dilatation of internal os is more gradual and less traumatic.

Pratt Dilator

Pratt dilators are shaped like Hegar, but they are half graduated, i.e., the difference between successive dilators is 0.5 mm, hence achieving smoother and lesser traumatic dilatation than the latter. The numbering of Pratt dilators corresponds to the circumference rather than the diameter as in Hegar dilators.

Hawkin Ambler Dilator

Hawkin Ambler dilators are single-ended cervical dilators, which come in sets of 16 starting from 3/6 and ending with 18/21. They are less curved than Hegar and have a disk-shaped finger grip at the nondilating end (Fig. 16B). The dilating portion is within the terminal 1.5 cm of the dilator with a difference of 3 mm in the diameter near the tip and the maximum dilating portion of the dilator.

CURETTES

Uterine Curette

Uterine curette is also known as Blake uterine curette. This instrument has a central shaft and one small oval loop at each end (Fig. 17). The loops are set at an angle to the shaft in order to facilitate curettage of the endometrium. The edge of the loop is either sharp or blunt.

Technique of Use

With patient in lithotomy position, the cervix is exposed with Sims speculum and anterior vaginal wall retractor and the anterior lip of the cervix is held with vulsellum or sponge-holding forceps. For curetting the anterior uterine wall, curette is held with three fingers below the curette and the thumb above the index finger is extended along the shaft of the instrument to prevent unguarded entry of the curette into the uterine cavity.

For curetting the posterior and sidewalls, the curette is held like a pen. All the uterine walls are systematically curetted until a grating sensation is felt, which occurs due to scraping of the curette against the fibrous tissue in basalis layer of endometrium. During endometrial curettage, approximately 60% of endometrium is sampled.

Indications

The sharp curette is used for curetting the endometrium in the nonpregnant state for the indications listed in Table 4. The blunt curette is used in obstetrics to decrease the risk of uterine perforation. However, some gynecologists prefer to use sharp curette for both obstetrical and gynecological indications due to better feel of walls with the sharp end.

The usual cervical dilatation required to pass the curette in uterine cavity is up to Hegar dilator No. 8.

Complications

- Uterine perforation
- Intrauterine infection

Table 4: Indications of using curette.

Obstetrical indications	Gynecological indications
• Check curettage for incomplete or inevitable abortion • After evacuation of hydatidiform mole	• Evaluation of endometrium in cases of abnormal uterine bleeding to rule out endometrial hyperplasia, carcinoma, and/or tuberculosis • *Infertility*: For documentation of ovulation and ruling out tuberculosis • To remove misplaced intrauterine contraceptive device

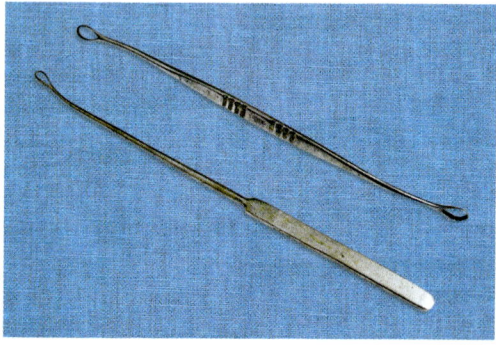

Fig. 17: Uterine curettes.

Chapter 52: Obstetrical and Gynecological Instruments

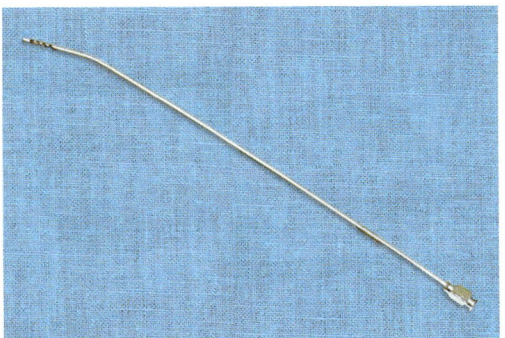

Fig. 18: Novak endometrial biopsy curette.

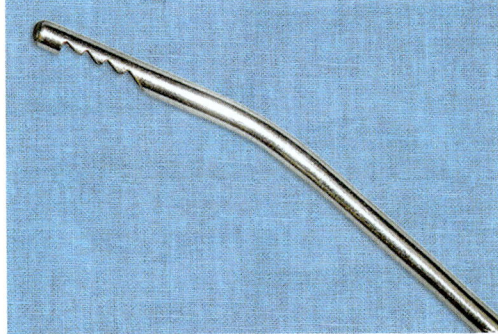

Fig. 19: Tip of Novak endometrial biopsy curette.

- Intrauterine synechiae
- Bleeding

Other Available Curettes

Randall Endometrial Biopsy Curette

Randall endometrial biopsy curette is a long, thin, tubular instrument curved near its tip to facilitate its entry into uterine cavity. Near its end, it has a notch with a sharp edge in its distal part so that during withdrawal of the instrument from the uterine cavity, it presses against the uterine wall and removes a strip of the endometrium, which enters the lumen of the instrument and is removed later on. As it is a thin instrument with an external diameter of 2 mm, it can be passed into the uterine cavity without dilating the cervix, hence the procedure can be done as an outpatient procedure. As it removes only a strip of tissue, it is not suitable in cases where focal lesions or carcinoma is suspected.

Novak Endometrial Biopsy Curette

Novak endometrial biopsy (EB) curette (Fig. 18) is like Randall curette, except that instead of a single notch with a cutting edge (Fig. 19), it has four notches in succession. This increases the efficiency in curetting the endometrium.

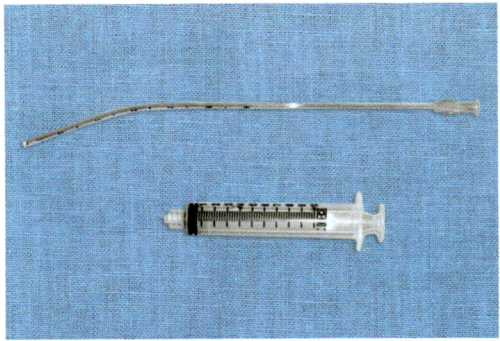

Fig. 20: Pipelle's endosampler.

Pipelle Endometrial Sampler

Pipelle endometrial sampler is a long hollow instrument with a piston at its distal end, which when withdrawn after entering the uterine cavity creates a negative suction pressure. The procedure can be done as an outpatient department (OPD) procedure without any anesthesia (Fig. 20).

EPISIOTOMY SCISSORS

Episiotomy scissors is a stainless steel scissors sterilized by dipping into Lysol or glutaraldehyde. The blades are angled on side and tip of one of the blades is blunt. This angulation makes it convenient to give an episiotomy as

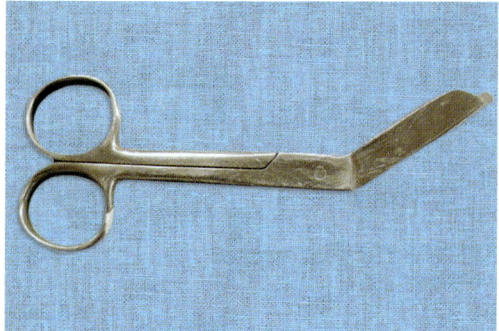

Fig. 21: Episiotomy scissors.

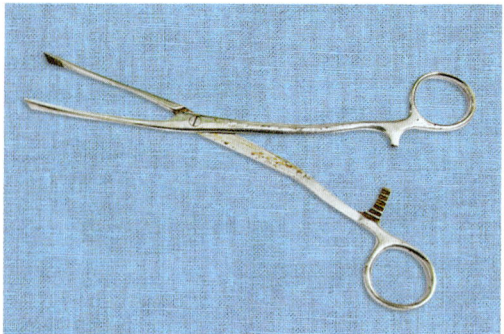

Fig. 22: Green Armytage forceps.

it prevents butting of the instrument against the patient's vulva, if straight scissors were used. The blade with blunt tip is introduced between the perineum and fetal head to prevent injury to the fetal head (Fig. 21).

Complications

- Injury to the fetal scalp
- Injury to the rectum and anal canal.

GREEN ARMYTAGE FORCEPS

Green Armytage forceps instrument has triangular solid tips with transverse serrations, a solid ratchet lock that makes its grip secure (Fig. 22).

Advantages

Green Armytage forceps is atraumatic and achieves hemostasis by compressing the bleeding edges.

Indications

To hold the cut edges of the lower uterine segment after extraction of fetus in CS to achieve hemostasis and lift the edges to define them better for facilitating suturing. Ideally six Green Armytage forceps are required during CS, one each for the angles, which bleed the most and two for each flap of uterine incision. However, one can manage with four also two for angles and two for lower edge. These cannot be used for upper segment CS as the edges are thick and cannot be held with Green Armytage forceps or sponge-holding forceps, instead Allis forceps must be used. It may be used in place of sponge-holding forceps to explore the cervix for cervical tears and repair them.

KARMAN CANNULA

Karman cannula is a flexible, transparent polythene cannula with a rounded tip. It is available in different sizes depending on its external diameter 4–12 mm. The smallest 4 mm cannula can be inserted into the uterine cavity without dilatation of the cervix. It has a rounded tip and two subterminal sharp triangular openings with overhanging convex hoods. Its tip bends without blocking its opening (Fig. 23).

Indications

- Medical termination of pregnancy during first trimester by suction evacuation. The size of the cannula selected is equal to the number of weeks of gestation or one less. The internal os is dilated by a dilator one

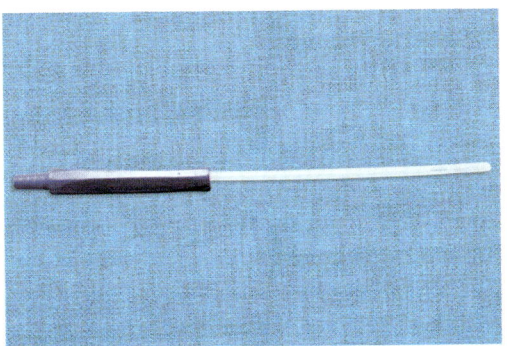

Fig. 23: Karman cannula.

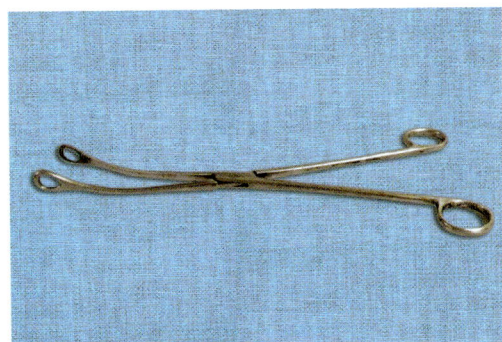

Fig. 24: Kelly Forceps.

size bigger than the Karman cannula to be used. The movement of the cannula in the uterine cavity is to and fro and rotatory.
- Completion of inevitable abortion during first trimester.
- For menstrual regulation.
- Evacuation of molar pregnancy.
- Endometrial aspiration biopsy.

Kelly's Forceps (Fig. 24)

It is long and curved forceps without lock with serrated ring jaws, slightly curved at the tip. Its length is 33–35 cm, major diameter of inner ring is 11–15 mm, and minor diameter of inner ring is 8–8.8 mm. The angle of the forceps tip on a horizontal plane is 5°.

Indication

For postplacental insertion of intrauterine device after vaginal delivery that is within 10 minutes of removal of placenta.

Technique of Use

Check woman's record to ensure that she is an appropriate client for IUCD and she has given her consent. Rule out contraindications of IUCD such as rupture of membranes for more than 18 hours, chorioamnionitis, and unresolved PPH.

Inspect perineum, labia and vaginal walls for lacerations. If lacerations are not bleeding heavily, insert the IUCD and repair if needed.

Gently visualize and clean cervix with antiseptic solution two times using two separate cotton swabs with povidone iodine or chlorhexidine. Wait for 2 minutes to allow the antiseptic to work. Gently grasp the anterior lip of the cervix with the ring forceps up to the first lock.

Grasp IUCD with long placental forceps in the sterile package using a no-touch technique. It should be held just on the edge of the placental forceps so that it can be easily released from the instrument when opened. Apply gentle traction on the anterior lip of the cervix using the ring forceps and insert IUCD into lower uterine cavity. Avoid touching the walls of vagina. Introduce the placental forceps with the IUCD carefully into the lower uterine cavity. Once the placental forceps is in the lower uterine cavity, lower the ring forceps holding the anterior lip of the cervix. Move the left hand to the woman's abdomen and push the entire uterus superiorly (upward). This is to straighten out the angle between the vagina and the uterus, so that the instrument can easily move upward toward the uterine fundus. Gently move placental forceps upward toward the fundus following the curve of the uterine cavity taking care not to apply excessive force. Always keep the instrument closed so that the IUCD is not dropped accidentally in the mid-portion of the uterine cavity. Confirm that the end of placental forceps has reached the fundus and tilt the forceps slightly inward. When it reaches the uterine fundus, one will feel resistance and will also feel the thrust of the instrument at the fundus of the uterus with her left hand which is placed on the abdomen. Open placental forceps and release the IUCD at the fundus. Sweep placental forceps to side wall of the uterus. Stabilize the uterus until the placental forceps is completely out of the uterus. Then the instrument is slowly withdrawn, keeping it slightly open always. If the instrument closes and catches the strings of the IUCD, it can accidentally pull the IUCD down from its fundal position, increasing the risk of expulsion.

LANE'S TISSUE FORCEPS

Lane's tissue forceps is a heavy 15 cm long fenestrated forceps with a single tooth and a lock made of stainless steel (Fig. 25).

Indications

- To hold the rectus sheath for retraction during abdominal operations with transverse incisions.
- To hold the polyp or fibroid in polypectomy or myomectomy operation.
- To hold the towels during draping.

LEECH WILKINSON CANNULA

Leech Wilkinson cannula is a 28 cm long tubular instrument with a spiral cone at one end and a Luer lock mount at the other end. Usually it has a stylet long with it to ensure patency (Fig. 26).

Indications

Leech Wilkinson cannula is used for doing tubal patency tests such as:
- Hysterosalpingogram (HSG)
- Chromopertubation
- Hydrotubation
- Sonosalpingography.

Technique of Use

The use of the instrument does not require any anesthesia. With the patient in lithotomy or dorsal position, the cervix is exposed with a vaginal speculum and anterior lip held with vulsellum. The tip of the cannula is placed at the external os and it is rotated clockwise, so that its tip advances in the cervical canal and the cannula gets fixed to the cervix. The spiral cone achieves

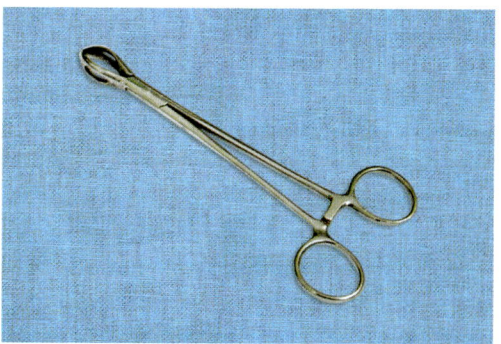

Fig. 25: Lane's forceps.

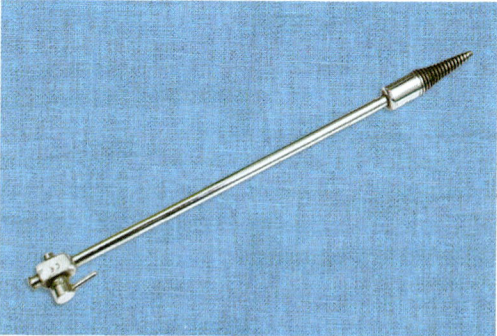

Fig. 26: Leech Wilkinson cannula.

a watertight fit and prevents leak of any dye back into vagina. It is important not to screw in the cannula more than what is required, as sometimes in an acutely anteverted or retroverted uterus, the cannula may be screwed against the uterine wall and result in resistance to the dye, when it pushed in uterine cavity and intravasation of dye due to trauma to the myometrium.

MYOMA SCREW

Myoma screw is an instrument that has a screw with a pointed tip at one end and a handle at the other end (Fig. 27).

Indications

- To fix the myoma after the capsule is cut open and to give traction to facilitate the enucleation of myoma from its bed.
- To give traction to the uterus during hysterectomy to lift it out of pelvis and facilitate placement of clamps.

Technique of Use

The myoma or uterus is stabilized, the tip of the screw is fixed on the surface and with constant screwing movements, the instrument is screwed carefully into the tissue ensuring that the screw remains inside the myoma or uterus and does not injure the surrounding structures.

NEEDLE HOLDER

The needle holders have ring finger grips and a ratchet lock at the distal ends. There is a groove on the inner side to stabilize the needle. They can be straight or curved (Heaney) and long or short (Figs. 28A and B). The curved needle holders are especially useful for vaginal surgeries, where the angled head allows the placement of curved needles and sutures at various angles with relative ease.

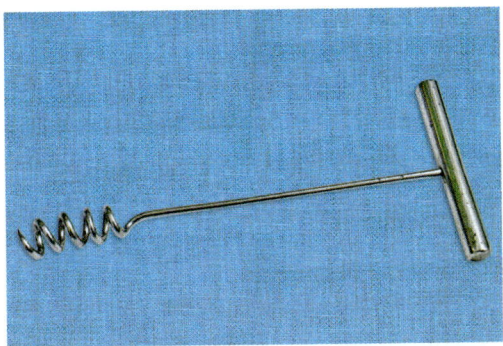

Fig. 27: Myoma screw.

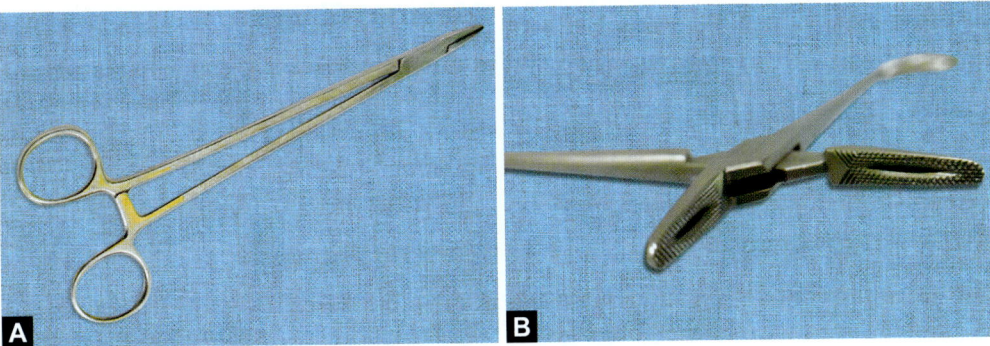

Figs. 28A and B: (A) Needle holder; (B) Needle holder with groove.

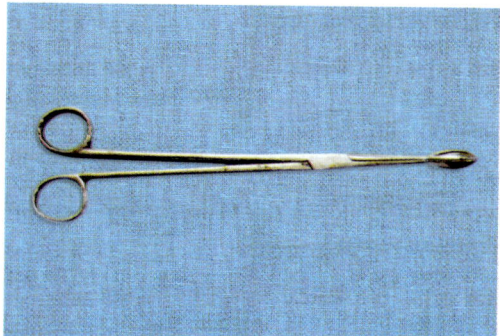

Fig. 29: Spoon-shaped blunt fenestrated end of ovum forceps.

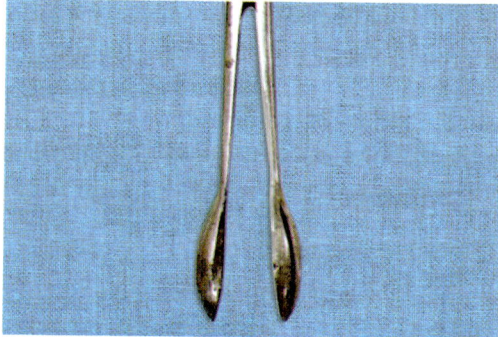

Fig. 30: Ovum forceps.

These are useful for placing sutures deep within the pelvis. The needle should be caught at the junction of anterior two third and posterior one third.

OVUM FORCEPS

Ovum forceps has spoon-shaped, blunt fenestrated ends that come in contact with each other when the forceps is closed (Figs. 29 and 30). There is no catch on the handles so that any structure held inadvertently is not crushed and traumatized but gets released when the instrument is drawn out.

Technique of Use

With patient in lithotomy or dorsal position, the cervix is exposed with Sims speculum and anterior vaginal wall retractor and held with vulsellum. The ovum forceps is held with thumb and middle or ring finger of the right hand and one or two fingers in between along the length of the instrument to steady it, and the closed instrument is passed into the uterine cavity through a dilated cervix with the palm facing either up or down. The jaws are opened inside the uterine cavity, the products of conception are grasped, and the forceps is withdrawn along with the products.

Indications

- First and second trimester inevitable and incomplete abortion to remove products of conception from uterus
- Removal of pedunculated uterine polyp or endometrial polyp
- Removal of foreign body from the uterus or vagina.

Complications

- Uterine perforation and injury to intra-abdominal structures
- Incomplete removal of products of conception.

PEDICLE CLAMPS

Maingot Clamp

Maingot clamp is a 20.5 cm long instrument with its blades that are curved. One blade has a longitudinal ridge, which fits into the longitudinal groove on the other blade (Fig. 31). The tips of the blades have one in two teeth, which prevent the clamped structures from slipping off. The blades can be tightened with a ratchet lock on the handles. The longitudinal groove in the clamp ensures complete occlusion of the vessels in the pedicle clamped.

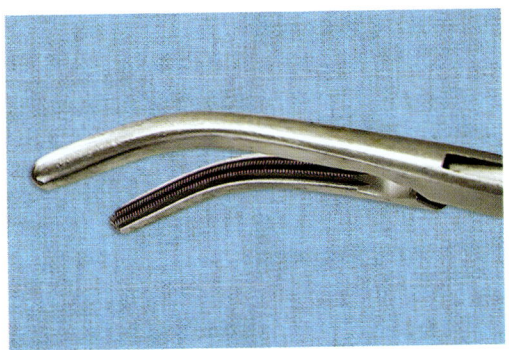

Fig. 31: Maingot clamp with curved blade and longitudinal groove.

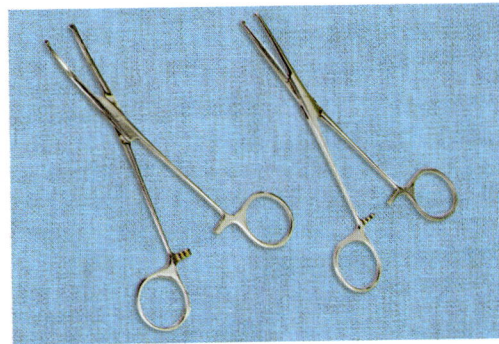

Fig. 32: Kocher's clamps.

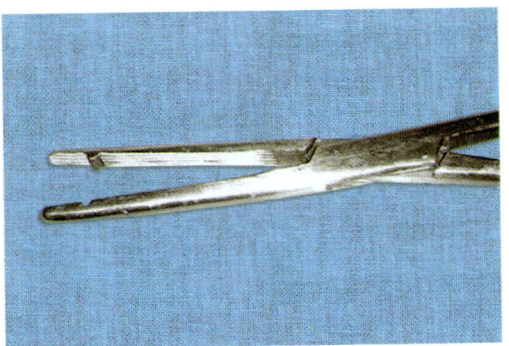

Fig. 33: Heaney clamp with subterminal notch and no tooth.

Kocher's Clamp

Kocher's clamp was invented by a surgeon Emil Theodor Kocher in 1882. This has transverse serrations on the blades and a tooth. It can be straight or curved (Fig. 32).

Indications

- It is used for clamping the pedicles during hysterectomy.
- To hold tough structures like sheath to retract the upper flap in a transverse incision.
- Clamping the umbilical cord of the newborns.
- To do artificial low rupture of membranes.

Heaney Clamp

Heaney clamp is like Kocher's clamp except that its blades have oblique serrations thus reducing the risk of structures slipping from the clamp. There is no tooth at the tip hence the risk of accidental trauma to tissues during application of clamp is less (Fig. 33). The subterminal transverse ridge and notch pa tern on the blades add to the security of the clamp.

Indications

- In hysterectomy, to clamp the pedicles like uterosacral ligaments, uterine blood vessels, and cornual structures or infundibulopelvic ligaments
- In oophorectomy for ovarian cyst or tumor
- For removal of pedunculated leiomyoma for clamping the pedicle
- In salpingectomy for tubal ectopic gestation
- In cesarean hysterectomy
- To hold the uterus during abdominal hysterectomy by applying clamps on either side of the uterus
- Clamping the umbilical cord of the newborns
- Artificial low rupture of membranes.

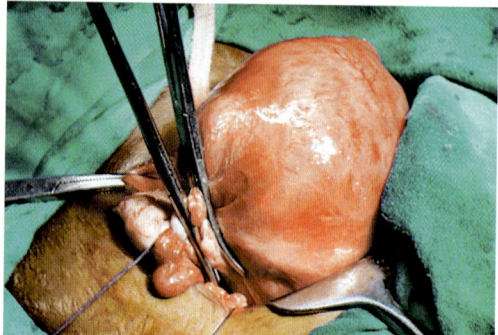

Fig. 34: Application of pedicle clamp.

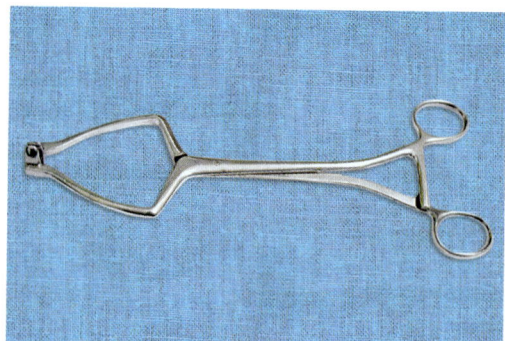

Fig. 35: Shirodkar cervical clamp.

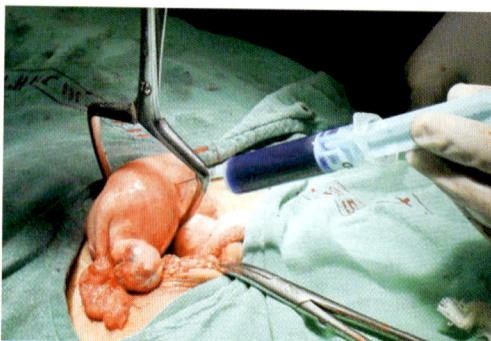

Fig. 36: Use of Shirodkar cervical clamp during tuboplasty.

Technique of Application of Clamp

Pedicle clamp is applied with the curve facing the structures to be removed, so that the ligature can be placed around the clamped pedicle easily (Fig. 34).

Shirodkar Cervical Clamp

Shirodkar cervical clamp is a uterus holding clamp. This instrument has convex curved blades so that the uterus may be accommodated in between without compression. The ends have suitably curved transverse bars. A ratchet lock is present on the handles (Figs. 35 and 36). It is applied with its blades placed in front and behind the uterine isthmus. The lock is tightened sufficiently to occlude the cervical canal.

Indications

- In uterine sling surgery for uterine prolapse, e.g., Shirodkar sling, Purandare's sling, etc.
- In tuboplasty, to occlude the isthmus of uterus for testing tubal patency by transfundal injection of methylene blue solution.
- It also holds and steadies the uterus to steady the Fallopian tubes in tubal recanalization.
- In salpingectomy, for tubal ectopic gestation.
- To lift the uterus during repair of vesicovaginal fistula (VVF) by the abdominal route and in Moschcowitz culdoplasty.

Disadvantage

As the blades run on the anterior and posterior surface of the uterus, any intervention on either surface of the uterus is not possible.

Shirodkar Hook

Shirodkar hook is shaped like a sound but has a hook at its tip. It is used for removal of a misplaced IUCD or stents left in the uterine

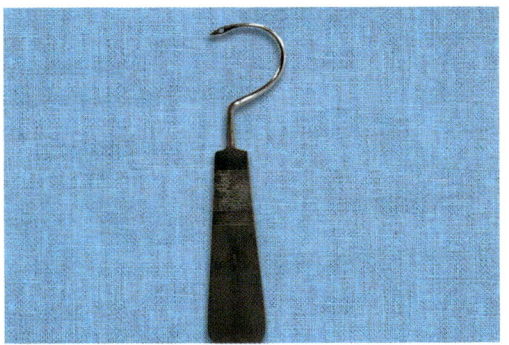

Fig. 37: Shirodkar needle.

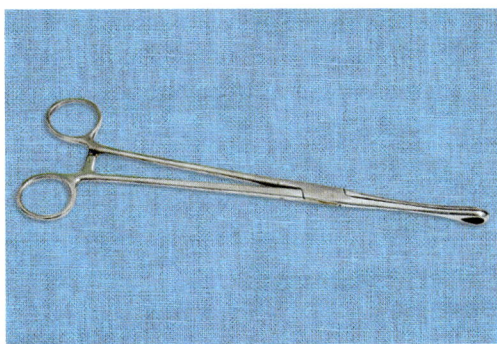

Fig. 38: Sponge-holding forceps.

cavity after interstitioisthmic anastomosis for blocked tubes at cornual ends.

Shirodkar Needle

Shirodkar needle is a 5 cm, half circle and blunt-tipped needle with a subterminal eye. The needle is attached to stout long handles at right angles (Fig. 37). These are available in pairs, right and left. It is used for placement of Shirodkar cervical cerclage for the management of incompetent cervix.

Sponge-holding Forceps

Sponge-holding forceps is a long instrument usually 22.5 cm in length with ring-shaped ends, which have transverse serrations on its inner surface for better grip. A ratchet catch on the handle locks the blades on closure and prevents the sponge from slipping (Fig. 38).

Indications

- Used for preparation of vagina, vulva, and abdominal wall before any surgery.
- To hold the cervix during pregnancy for indications as listed in Box 1.
- For cervical exploration in women with postpartum hemorrhage (PPH), the cervical rim is traced with the help of three sponge-holding forceps, one at 12 o'clock position and the other two tracing the entire cervical rim clockwise. For repair of cervical tear, the cervix is drawn downward with two sponge-holding forceps applied to the lower ends of the torn edges of cervix; thus, apex of the tear is visualized and the tear sutured by passing the first stitch beyond the apex to secure the bleeding vessel.
- During CS, sponge holder is used for blunt dissection by a folded gauge piece for pushing the bladder down so as to

Box 1: Indications for holding anterior lip of cervix.

- Second trimester incomplete abortion
- Insertion of Foley catheter for second trimester extra-amniotic ethacridine lactate infusion for medical termination of pregnancy
- For cervical cerclage
- For diagnosis and repair of cervical tear
- To remove placental bits and membranes from the uterus
- To pack uterine cavity in uncontrolled primary postpartum hemorrhage (PPH)
- For balloon tamponade in intractable PPH
- Postplacental intrauterine contraceptive device insertion

separate it from lower uterine segment and to hold the cut edges of the lower uterine segment for hemostasis and to facilitate suturing.
- To remove the products of conception in incomplete abortion and inevitable abortion, if ovum forceps is not available.
- To hold a sponge to swab blood from a distance during any operation.
- To press on an oozing area with a swab for hemostasis during an operation.
- It is used as a temporary atraumatic clamp over the ovarian vessels in the infundibulopelvic ligaments during myomectomy, metroplasty, and salpingostomy.
- To hold the bowel and omentum away from the field of operation by a swab during vaginal hysterectomy.

TENACULUM

Tenaculum is similar in design to vulsellum, except that there is a single tooth at the end of each blade and is straight. It provides more secure grip and is especially suitable for a small cervix as in a nulliparous woman. However, the risk of cervical tissue getting torn is greater, if excessive force is used (Fig. 39).

UTERINE SOUND

Uterine sound is an olive-pointed malleable instrument 25–27.5 cm long with distal 5 cm as the handle. It is graduated in inches or centimeters and is bent at an angle of 150° at 2.5 inches from its tip. The tip is around 2 mm in diameter, so that it passes into the cervical canal without any dilatation (Figs. 40A to C).

Indications

The indications of use of uterine sound are listed in Box 2.

Technique of Use

After doing a per vaginal examination, position and size of the uterus is noted. Posterior

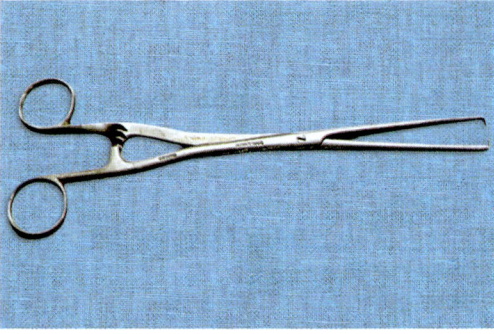

Fig. 39: Tenaculum and showing the tooth.

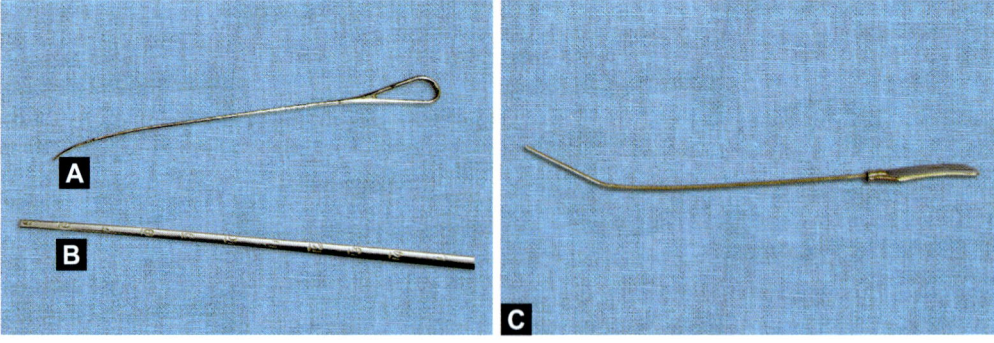

Figs. 40A to C: (A) Uterine sound; (B) Markings on uterine sound; (C) Curved proximal end.

vaginal wall is retracted with Sims speculum and the cervix is held with a vulsellum. Sound is held gently in a pen holding position and is passed into the cervical canal. At the level of internal os, resistance is felt, this gives the total cervical length that is combined supravaginal and intravaginal lengths; the sound is then passed further till the resistance by the uterine fundus is felt. This gives the total uterocervical length. Thus, the length of supravaginal portion of cervix can be calculated by subtracting the length of portio vaginalis from the total length of cervix.

For passage into an anteverted (AV) uterus, the sound is held almost vertically with angle directed toward the patient, while for passage into a retroverted (RV) uterus, it is held in such a way that its handle lies below the level of the tip of sound, the angle facing the floor.

Contraindications

- Pregnancy
- Malignancy
- Pyometra.

> **Box 2:** Indications of using uterine sound.
>
> - To confirm position of uterus as assessed on per vaginal examination
> - To measure the uterocervical length (UCL) (normal 7–9 cm)
> - For assessment of supravaginal elongation of cervix
> - Before intrauterine contraceptive device (IUCD) insertion for measuring UCL
> - Before doing dilatation and curettage (D and C) and other minor gynecological procedures
> - To diagnose and differentiate a uterine polyp from chronic uterine inversion—the sound can pass by the side of polyp unlike in inversion
> - To sound presence of foreign body, e.g., misplaced IUCD in the uterus
> - *To diagnose a missing IUCD*: By taking X-ray of the pelvis anteroposterior/lateral views with sound or another IUCD in uterine cavity
> - *For diagnosis of cervical stenosis*: Failure to pass the sound through the cervix

Complications

Perforation

As the diameter of the instrument is very small and it is blunt tipped, in case of perforation, the likelihood of complications such as injury to adjacent structures and bleeding is minimal. The perforation usually heals spontaneously. The procedure is abandoned till the next cycle and the patient is managed conservatively with vital monitoring and abdominal girth charting for early detection of any intraperitoneal bleed for 24 hours. In case the perforation occurs with patient in OT with facilities for laparoscopy, the procedure can be completed under laparoscopic guidance.

VAGINAL SPECULUMS

Sims Speculum

Sims speculum was designed by Marion Sims. Because of its peculiar shape, it is also called Duckbill speculum. It has a handle in center and the blades at right angles to the handle (Fig. 41). The blades are rounded at the end to be atraumatic and a trough runs along the entire length of the instrument. The blood or secretions collect in the concave blade and, if excessive, drain along the trough. It is either double-ended or single-ended. The double-ended speculum has two blades of different

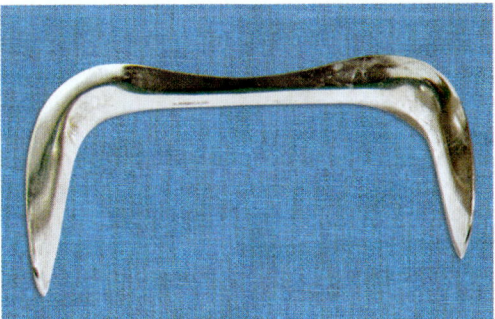

Fig. 41: Double-bladed Sims speculum.

Table 5: Cervical and vaginal lesions diagnosed by speculum examination.

Vaginal lesions	Cervical lesions
• Vaginitis and vaginal discharge • *Prolapse*: Cystocele, urethrocele, rectocele, enterocele • Anterior vaginal wall cyst • Gartner's cyst • Vesicovaginal fistula • *Foreign body*: Ring pessary • *Congenital malformations*: Vaginal septum • Vaginal carcinoma • Vaginal warts • Vaginal extension of carcinoma cervix • Secondaries of choriocarcinoma in suburethral region	• Hypertrophy of the cervix • Inflammation of the cervix nabothian follicles • Cervical erosion • *Cervical polyp*: Endometrial, mucus, and fibroid polyp • *Cervical tumors*: Fibroid • *Cervical ulcers*: Tuberculosis, syphilis • *Old cervical tears*: Ectropion • *Cervical growth*: Cancer, tuberculosis, and warts

Table 6: Minor and major procedures in which Sims speculum is used.

Minor procedures	Major procedures
• Pap smear for cervical cancer screening • Vaginal or cervical discharge for culture sensitivity • Cervical biopsy • Insertion/removal of IUCD • Polypectomy • Hysterosalpingography • Hysteroscopy • Culdocentesis/Colpotomy • Insertion of radium in uterine cavity	• Vaginal hysterectomy • Manchester repair • Sacrospinous hysteropexy • Sacrospinous colpopexy • Vesicovaginal fistula repair • Rectovaginal fistula repair

Table 7: Obstetrical indications for using Sims speculum.

Obstetrical condition	Purpose of use
Premature rupture of membranes	• To confirm diagnosis by visualizing leaking per vaginam • To collect liquor for culture and sensitivity • To observe cervix for its length and dilatation of os
Antepartum hemorrhage	To rule out local cause
Postpartum hemorrhage (PPH)	• To rule out trauma of cervix and vagina • To repair cervical and vaginal tears • To pack the uterine cavity and/or vagina for uncontrolled PPH
Dilatation and curettage or suction evacuation	For incomplete abortion or hydatidiform mole

sizes at each end. There are three sizes of blades available depending upon the width of the blades small, medium, and large. It is used to retract the vaginal walls, usually the posterior vaginal wall, but sometimes may be used for retracting anterior vaginal wall. The broader end is used for multiparous women and the narrower end for nulliparous women.

Indications

- Sims speculum is used for routine per speculum examination in gynecology OPD to visualize the cervix and the vagina to diagnose any lesion or condition (Table 5)
- Carrying out minor and major procedures (Table 6)
- Obstetrical indications (Table 7).

Technique of Use

Sims speculum can be used with the woman in dorsal, lithotomy or Sims position. The dorsal position is when the patient is lying on her back with legs flexed at hip and knee joints and her buttocks at the edge of the table. Sims position is left lateral position with right knee flexed against the abdomen.

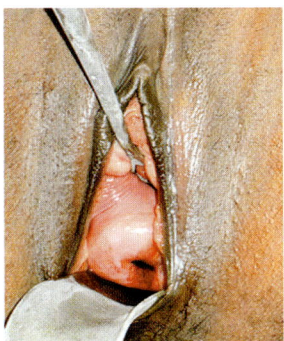

Fig. 42: Use of Sims speculum and anterior vaginal wall retractor to visualize cervix.

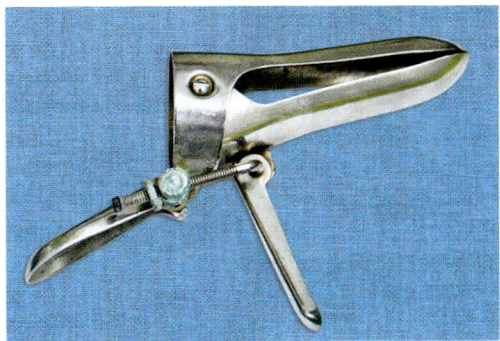

Fig. 43: Cusco's speculum.

It is helpful in visualizing lesions on the anterior vaginal wall such as vesicovaginal fistula as there is no need for using an anterior vaginal wall retractor in this position.

The blade of the speculum is lubricated with jelly or moistened with saline to facilitate insertion. The labia minora are held apart by thumb and index finger of the nondominant hand usually the left hand and the blade is inserted in between the thumb and index finger. The transverse blade is introduced in the introitus in oblique and once in the vagina, it is rotated to transverse position so that it retracts the posterior wall of vagina. This is done to prevent its contact with urethra, which is sensitive and may cause pain (Fig. 42). Often Sims anterior vaginal wall retractor is used along with it for adequate exposure of cervix. The posterior vaginal wall is examined as the speculum is withdrawn.

Disadvantages

Sims speculum is not self-retaining; if any procedure needs to be carried out by the examining physician, an assistant is needed to hold the speculum. The patient needs to be at the edge of the table for using this instrument.

Advantages

Sims speculum does not require any maintenance and is atraumatic.

Cusco's Speculum

Cusco's speculum is a bivalve self-retaining vaginal speculum. It retracts both anterior and posterior vaginal walls for better visualization of cervix and can be fixed after opening the blades by tightening the screw (Fig. 43).

Advantages

Cusco's speculum is self-retaining and can be used for carrying out minor procedures such as colposcopy, endometrial biopsy, Copper T insertion, cervical cauterization, polypectomy, and collection of the cervical or high vaginal swab for culture without any assistance.

Disadvantages

The visualization of vagina is limited compared to Sims speculum as Cusco's speculum covers two walls at a time and cannot be used for major surgical procedures (Fig. 44). It has a screw, so unlike Sims speculum it needs maintenance, and can get out of order. It is

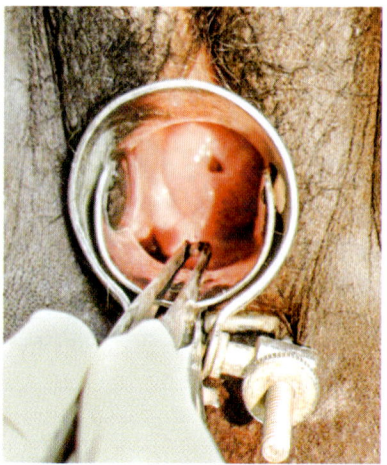

Fig. 44: Normal cervix visualized with Cusco's speculum.

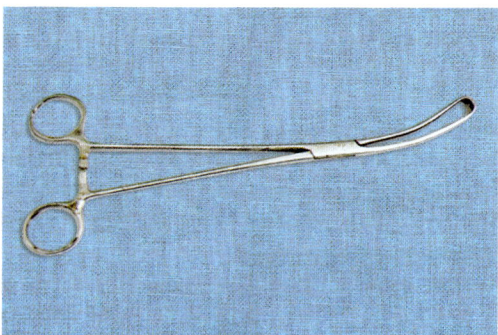

Fig. 45: Vulsellum with teeth.

more traumatic than Sims speculum hence its use is avoided, while examining a woman suffering from antepartum hemorrhage.

Vulsellum

Vulsellum is a 28 cm long instrument with blades gently curved on one side. The tips of the blade have two in three teeth, i.e., two teeth on one blade fit in between three teeth on the other blade ensuring good grip on the structures held (Fig. 45). The curve on the blade ensures that the fingers do not obstruct the field of vision when cervix is held during vaginal surgery. It is usually used to hold the anterior lip of the nonpregnant cervix, but sometimes for holding the posterior lip.

Indications

- To hold and steady the cervix during:
  - Sounding of uterus and measuring the uterocervical length
  - To assess cervical descent in women with a large cystocele or in a woman planned for nondescent vaginal hysterectomy
  - To diagnose stress urinary incontinence (SUI) in the presence of a massive prolapse of uterus with a large cystocele.
- To carry out procedures on cervix such as cervical biopsy, trachelorrhaphy, electrocauterization, endocervical curettage, and rapid/slow cervical dilatation
- To carry out procedures on uterus such as endometrial aspiration or curettage, polypectomy, insertion of IUCD, first trimester medical termination of pregnancy (MTP), HSG, drainage of hematometra or pyometra
- To hold the cervix to give traction, while clamps are being placed during vaginal hysterectomy.

Conditions where vulsellum is used for holding posterior lip of cervix:

- To carry out procedures in pouch of Douglas or cul-de-sac—culdocentesis, colpotomy, and culdoscopy
- Examination of enterocele and rectocele
- In nondescent vaginal hysterectomy
- In cases where anterior lip of cervix is absent or eaten up due to a growth or trauma.

Wertheim's Vaginal Clamp

Wertheim's vaginal clamp has long L-shaped blades with transverse serrations in the

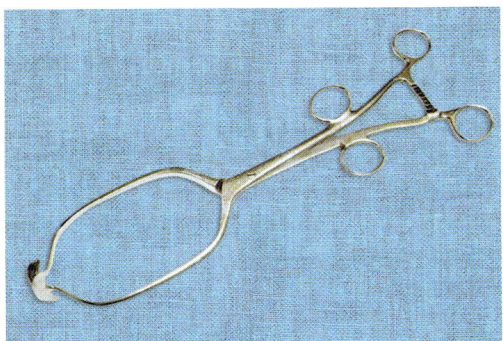

Fig. 46: Wertheim's vaginal clamp and its application.

Technique of Application of Clamp

Wertheim's vaginal clamp is used during Wertheim's hysterectomy. It is applied so that the angle of the L lies at the lateral angle of the vagina. After dividing the paracolpium and parametrium, the clamp is applied over the vagina on either side and then vagina is cut below the clamp. This prevents the spread of malignant cells from the surface of the tumor into the peritoneal cavity during hysterectomy for carcinoma cervix.

vertical portion of the L and longitudinal serrations in the horizontal portion of the L (Fig. 46). This makes the serrations to lie at right angles to the muscles and fibrous strands of vagina, hence minimizing the chance of slippage.

Although most of the instruments have been described, the list is not all inclusive. It is important that during their regular postings in the outpatient and inpatient department, operation theater, labor room, and casualty, students should carefully observe the procedures carried out, the instruments used and their correct technique of use.

53: Endoscopic Equipment and Instruments

Aruna Nigam, Arpita De

INTRODUCTION

There has been a great revolution in the surgical approaches in the last two decades. The surgical methods have traveled from the era of open surgeries to laparoscopic and robotic surgeries. In contrast to conventional open surgeries, laparoscopic surgery depends not only on the skill of the surgeon but also on the technology used to design specialized instruments as well. Over the last two decades, there has been a quantum leap in the technology used in the cameras and instrument designing. The instruments are computer designed; there are microprocessors in place to modify energy delivery and there are several safety features, which increase the scope and safety of laparoscopic surgeries.

There are two broad categories of equipment and devices used in laparoscopic surgeries:
1. Laparoscopic trolley.
2. Handheld instruments.

LAPAROSCOPY TROLLEY (FIG. 1)

Laparoscopy trolley consists of the monitor, insufflator, light source, hysteromat, cautery generator, and a shelf for the gas cylinder.

Monitor

The monitor can be a simple two-dimensional (2D) monitor or a better and clearer three-dimensional (3D) monitor connected to the camera system. The 3D monitor is compatible with a 3D camera system.

Camera System (Fig. 2)

To start with, people use to operate through a single-chip camera but with the advancement in technology, most of the setups are now using a three-chip camera or high definition (HD) camera system. The 3D camera system gives advantage of sharper image and better depth perception. This enables tricky dissection and difficult suturing in complex situations such as endometriosis and oncosurgeries. Most of the latest camera monitor units can be attached to a recorder for the videos to be recorded. Every company has different panels in the front to adjust the

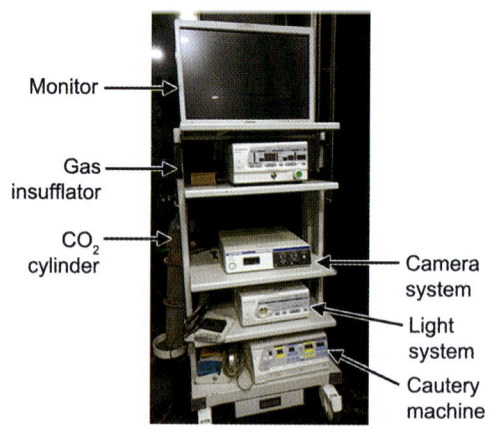

Fig. 1: Comprehensive laparoscopic trolley.

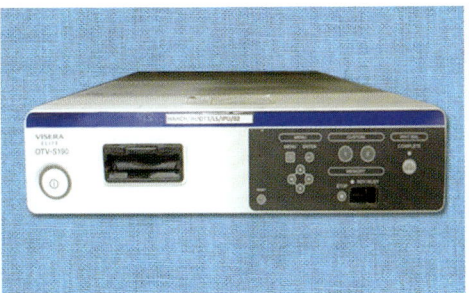 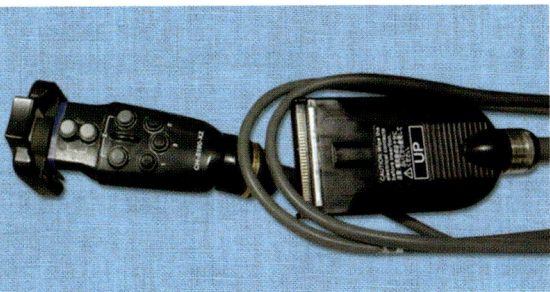

Fig. 2: Camera system.

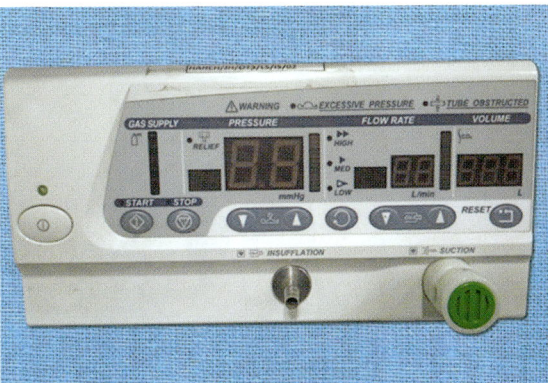 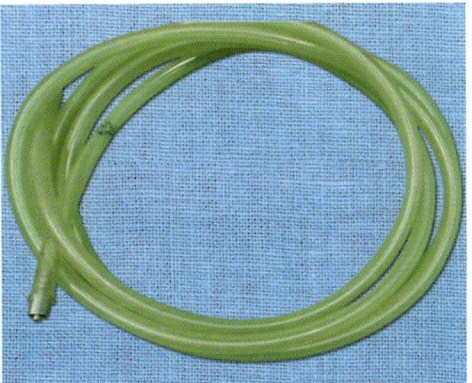

Fig. 3: Pneumoinsufflator and gas cable.

picture quality according to requirement. The camera system has a connection with the monitor as well as the camera cord. Once the camera is attached to the laparoscope, the first step is to do the white balance to adjust the natural colors. The camera itself has few buttons for adjusting the focus, zooming, saving images, and white balancing while doing surgery. During surgery, the camera should be covered by a sterilized camera cover.

Gas Insufflator (Fig. 3)

The insufflator regulates the rate of inflow of gas to create or maintain the pneumoperitoneum. It shows the intra-abdominal pressure and the total volume of gas used in real time. These three readings, i.e., intra-abdominal pressure, rate of gas flow, and the volume of gas used along with the status of gas inside the CO_2 cylinder, are shown on the panel. There is a gas cable (Fig. 3) which connects the insufflator to the Veress needle or any of the ports for inflow of gas.

Light Source (Fig. 4)

The light source is attached to the laparoscope by a cable which allows light to reach inside the abdomen without any reduction in its intensity. The intensity of light can be adjusted from the light source. Light cable has fiberoptic fibers, which can get damaged if they are not handled with care, affecting the quality of light. The source of light in light system can be a halogen bulb or a xenon bulb.

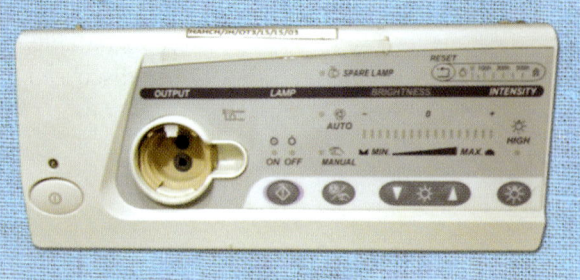
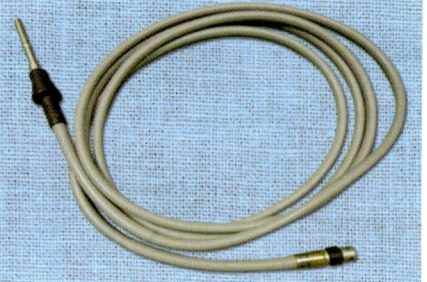

Fig. 4: Light source and fiberoptic cable.

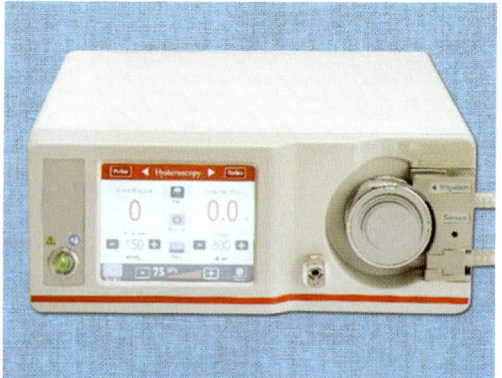

Fig. 5: Fluid management system: Hysteromat.

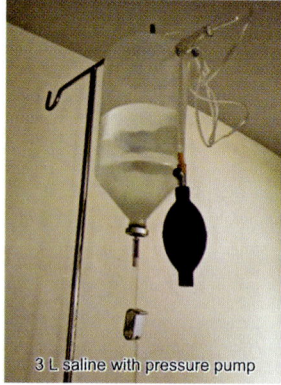

Fig. 6: Indigenous fluid management system.

The halogen bulb emits yellow light whereas the xenon bulb emits white light which is brighter with lesser heat generation.

Cautery Generator

The cautery generator has the option of unipolar, bipolar, and blend current. It has the provision for setting the intensity of current flow for each of these current types (see Fig. 1). Most of the generators are compatible with laparoscopic, hysteroscopic, and open surgery cauterization instruments.

Fluid Management System (Fig. 5)

This system provides an accurate and easy measurement of fluid balance and intrauterine pressure in a closed system during hysteroscopy. It regulates the amount of fluid that goes into the uterus, reflects and maintains the desired pressure within the uterus, and measures the volume of fluid coming out of uterus. It is essential to use the hysteromat in all the operative hysteroscopic procedures to avoid any fluid overload and subsequent complications.

The intrauterine pressure is usually adjusted at 70–80 mm Hg. Higher pressures (up to 125–150 mm Hg) may sometimes be required for visualization in patients with intrauterine bleeding, a large uterus, or in the presence of fibroids or adenomyosis with decreased myometrial distensibility. A higher intrauterine pressure can lead to increased absorption of the distending medium.

For diagnostic hysteroscopic procedures, a handmade pressure device (Fig. 6) can also be used to push fluid under pressure into the uterine cavity. The pressure is created with the help of a rubber bulb attached to one end of an intravenous (IV) set, the other end of which is fixed at the top of an inverted plastic 1 or 3 L saline bottle. Another IV infusion set is connected to the mouth of the bottle with its free end connected to the inflow channel of the diagnostic sheath. It is a low-cost option for pushing distension medium in uterus under pressure but can neither regulate the pressure nor increase the pressure to high levels, as in a hysteromat.

LAPAROSCOPIC INSTRUMENTS AND EQUIPMENT

The choice of laparoscopic instruments varies from surgeon to surgeon. Many factors such as cost, durability, whether for single use or multiple uses, curved or straight, traumatic, or atraumatic decide the choice of instruments. Unlike conventional open surgeries, the success and safety of a laparoscopic procedure are largely dependent on the instruments used.

The reusable instruments have a higher initial cost but are more cost effective to the patients. The staff needs to be trained in proper cleaning and sterilization of these instruments. Single-use instruments, on the other hand, do not need repeated sterilization and maintenance checks and are safe as regards transmission of infection and insulation is concerned but are expensive to the patients. There is a serious concern when single-use instruments are reused. Repeated handling and sterilization may damage the instrument and its insulation, thus compromising safety. Single-use instruments also raise concerns on disposal as they are usually made of plastic and are nonbiodegradable.

The instruments that will be discussed in this chapter are as follows:
- Laparoscope (telescope)
- Insufflation needles
- Trocars and cannulas
- Hand instruments
- Electrodes and electrosurgical cables
- Harmonic scalpel and vessel sealing devices
- Suction and irrigation cannula
- Uterine manipulators
- Tissue retrieval devices
- Port closure needles.

Laparoscope (Figs. 7A and B)

Laparoscope is a rigid endoscope used to illuminate the abdominal cavity and capture images during laparoscopic surgery. It is available in various sizes—5 and 10 mm outer diameter. It has two channels—one has glass fibers to transmit light from an external source into the abdomen. These run throughout the length of the scope and encircle the outer part of the telescope. The second channel is a central part that has multiple rod lenses throughout the length of the scope to capture images. It has two ends—ocular end that is connected to the camera and distal end that has the objective which can have angles of view ranging from 0° to 120°. The commonly used objectives are 0° which give a panoramic view and 30° to see the anterior abdominal wall or lateral pelvic wall, posterior surface of uterus, in depth or work around large masses. Telescopes with smaller caliber have poorer image quality due to lesser transmission of light. Flexible telescopes and 3D telescopes are also available. In hysteroscopy telescopes with smaller caliber, usually 4 mm and with a 30° angle

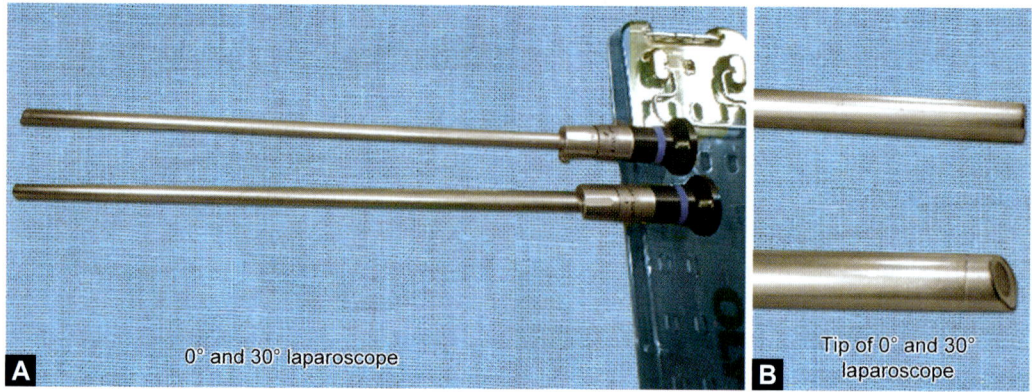

Figs. 7A and B: Laparoscope.

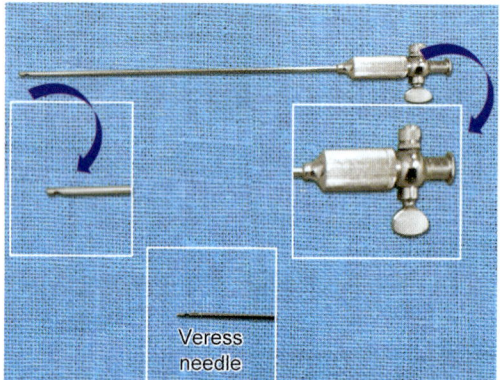

Fig. 8: Veress needle.

of view are used to facilitate visibility of all uterine walls, especially the cornual ends due to limited maneuverability of the telescope through the cervix.

Insufflation Needles

Veress needle (Fig. 8) is used to create pneumoperitoneum before the introduction of primary trocar and cannula. It has an outer cannula with a sharp beveled pointed tip guarded by an inner blunt stylet (zoom-in image of Fig. 8). During introduction of the Veress needle in the abdomen, the blunt stylet gets pushed into the cannula due to the resistance offered by the abdominal wall and the sharp beveled end of the outer cannula facilitates abdominal entry. Once the Veress needle enters the abdomen, the inner blunt stylet pops out by a spring action due to a sudden reduction in the resistance guarding the sharp tip of the outer cannula to prevent injury to abdominal organs. The needle can then be attached to the gas tube and the gas enters the peritoneal cavity through a lateral hole in the stylet.

It is available in different lengths—80, 100, and 120 mm. The required length is decided according to the thickness of the abdominal wall.

Technique of Insertion

The preferred site of insertion is the umbilicus as there is no fat or muscle between the skin and the fascia at this site. In case adhesions are expected at this site due to previous scar, entry through Palmer's point is preferred. It is a point 3 cm below the left costal margin in the the midclavicular line. Care is taken to rule out splenomegaly before inserting the needle through Palmer's point.

With the patient in lithotomy position, a small incision is given in the umbilicus. The patency and spring action of the needle is checked, and the needle is held like a dart and introduced through the skin at an angle of 45°. Two clicks are felt and heard, one at the time of piercing the rectus sheath and another the parietal peritoneum and the needle can be felt free in the peritoneal cavity. The entry should be controlled.

The intraperitoneal placement of the needle can be checked by various methods which are as follows:
- Place a drop of saline on the hub of the needle and lift the abdominal wall; the drop is sucked in.
- Push 5 mL of saline in the peritoneal cavity and then attempt to aspirate it. No fluid can be aspirated if the needle is in the peritoneal cavity.
- The pressure at which CO_2 flows in is single digit, i.e., ≤10 mm Hg, when the needle is in the peritoneal cavity.
- Liver dullness gets obliterated if gas is flowing intraperitoneally.

Complications

Extraperitoneal insufflation: One can attempt laparoscopy by Hasson technique or direct trocar entry if there is no risk of adhesions.

Injury to bowel, bladder, or major vessel: In this case, the needle is kept in place and abdomen is entered by laparoscopy or laparotomy by an alternate site to fix the injury.

Trocars and Cannulas (Fig. 9)

The trocar is a sharp stylet that is introduced through the cannula. They are available for both 5 and 10 mm ports. The conical or pyramidal tip trocars are more commonly used. A blunt tip trocar is also available to renegotiate the layers in case the cannula is accidentally pulled out or in open technique.

Cannulas are the outer sheaths of the sharp trocars used for entering the abdomen.

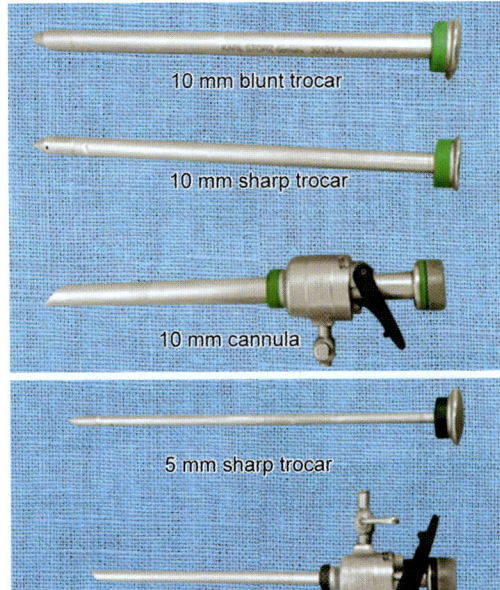

Fig. 9: Trocars and cannulas.

After entry, the trocar is withdrawn and the cannula is left behind through which the laparoscope or the hand instruments are inserted. Cannulas may be made of metal or plastic. They are designed to prevent reflection inside. On the top, all cannulas have a valve system which allows movement of the instruments without letting the pneumoperitoneum to leak.

Optical trocars are available to visualize the structures which are negotiated during intraperitoneal entry. Hasson trocar cannula and blunt obturator can be used in cases of open entry in the abdominal wall.

Hand Instruments

Most of the hand instruments can pass through the 5 or 10 mm ports. The lengths should be such that half of the instrument should be inside the abdomen and half should be outside. Accordingly, there

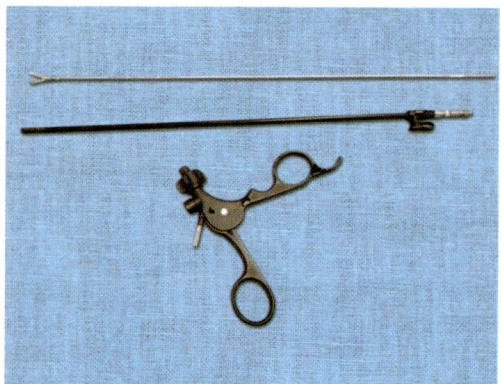

Fig. 10: Hand instrument insert, outer tube, handle.

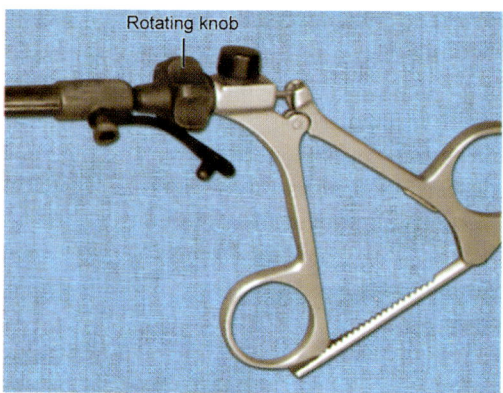

Fig. 11: Handle with lock.

are smaller instruments of 18–25 cm for the pediatric cases and longer instruments of 36–45 cm for the adults.

Each hand instrument is comprised of an insert which has a specialized tip, an insulated outer tube within which the insert slides in, and a handle for manipulation (Fig. 10). All these parts are detachable and need to be cleaned separately. Some inserts have just an opening and closing function while others have more range of functions such as angulation. It may be a grasper or scissors. The outer insulated sheath prevents electrical injury to the internal viscera.

The handles may be with or without a lock. The lock may have a ratchet (Fig. 11) to adjust the pressure on the jaws. The lock avoids fatigue on the fingers, especially when structure must be held with traction for a long time. A rotating knob may be present on the handle to rotate the tip inside the abdomen instead of rotating the arm, thus easing the manipulation of the tissues.

Common hand instruments used in gynecological surgeries are mentioned below.

Grasper

Grasper is the one of the most used instruments. It can be atraumatic with or without fenestrations, or toothed for a firmer hold on the tissues. Bowel graspers are usually fenestrated, while Babcock can be used for grasping tubes. Claw grasping forceps are available even for 10 mm port, which are used for tissue retrieval through the central port. The tips may be single-action jaws, where only one jaw moves, or double-action jaws, in which both jaws move. In single-action jaws, more force can be applied, while double-action jaws have a wider opening. This enables more maneuverability during dissection (Figs. 12A to D).

Scissors (Fig. 13)

Scissors can be straight, curved, hooked, or serrated. In laparoscopy, scissors not only help in cutting but with closed jaws can aid in dissecting planes as well. They have a very important role in lysis or removal of adhesions near vital structures such as bowel or ureter where it is not safe to use energy source for adhesiolysis. Unlike energy devices, the surgeon has a complete control over the targeted tissues. There are insulated scissors available to which cautery lead may be attached to the handles and monopolar cautery can be used.

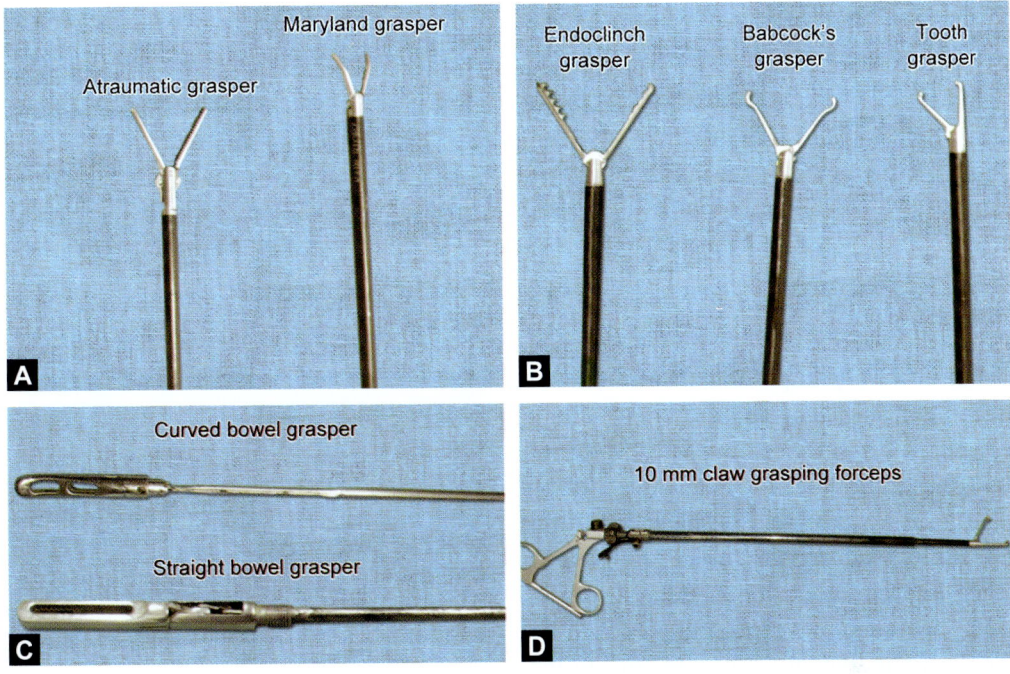

Figs. 12A to D: Different types of graspers.

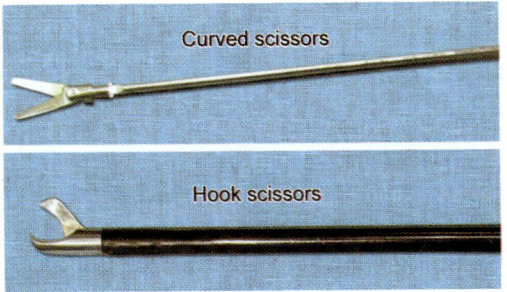

Fig. 13: Scissors.

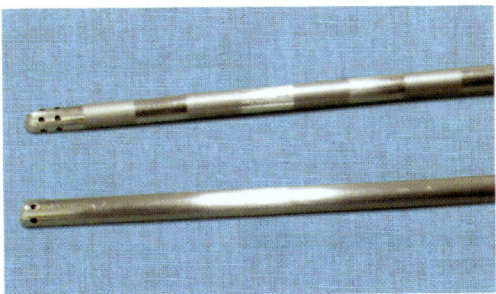

Fig. 14: Suction irrigation cannula.

Different scissors have different advantages. Straight scissors enable one to control the depth till which cutting is required. The fixed jaw is kept downward, and the mobile jaw is placed upward. Curved scissors are more commonly used as both the limbs are better seen under laparoscopy and they can be easily manipulated during dissection. There is a special hook scissors which has C-shaped blades. These enable the jaws to hold and stabilize the tissues before cutting them.

Suction Irrigation Cannula (Fig. 14)

Laparoscopic suction irrigation cannula enables both suction of the intra-abdominal contents and irrigation for peritoneal lav-

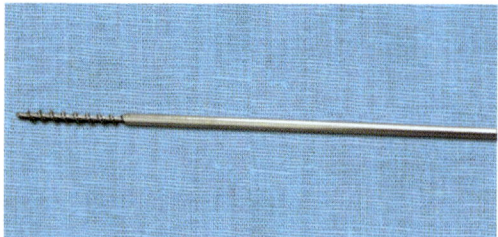

Fig. 15: Myoma screw.

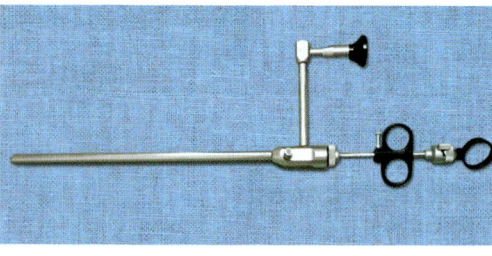

Fig. 16: Laparocator.

age. It is a very important instrument for hydrodissection that is atraumatic blunt dissection. It has two channels near the handle—one is the inlet for irrigation and the other for the attachment of the suction tubing. The tips are of two types—one is open ended and the other one is smooth tipped, which has a smooth closed end. The latter one does not allow the bowel to stick to the suction tip. Suction cannulas are available in 5 and 10 mm sizes. The 10 mm suction cannula is essential when there is massive intraperitoneal bleeding with big clots as in ruptured ectopic.

Myoma Screw (Fig. 15)

Myoma screw is used both in myomectomies and in hysterectomies. It is fixed to the myoma or myometrium by screwing it into the tissue for giving proper traction. The tips can be long or short depending on the size of the myoma or uterus which needs traction.

Laparocator (Fig. 16)

All laparoscopic sterilizations can be done through this single instrument by a single incision for the central 10 mm port. It has prongs to pick up a loop of fallopian tube and an applicator for pushing the falope rings over the loop.

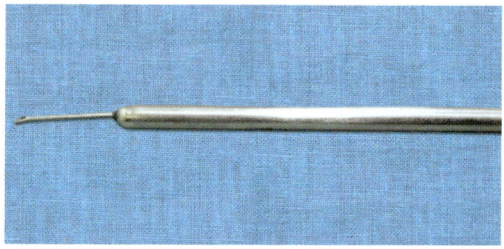

Fig. 17: Laparoscopic aspiration needle.

Laparoscopic Aspiration Needle (Fig. 17)

This long needle can be used to aspirate tuboovarian abscesses or ovarian cysts. It is also used for pushing in the saline with adrenalin or only saline for hydrodissection. During hydrodissection, the bevel of the needle is introduced into the capsule of the ovary or myoma. Fluid pushed through it demarcates a plane of dissection. Such infiltration is required in myomectomies or complex surgeries such as endometriosis to reduce blood loss.

Needle Holders (Fig. 18)

Endosuturing is possible with good sturdy needle holders. The tips may be curved or flat and tooth or nontooth. Firm pressure is needed on the needle, so needle holders always have single action jaws. The handles have a locking and unlocking mechanism for firmly holding the needle during manipulation. Usually, endosuturing can be done with two needle holders or one needle holder and one grasper.

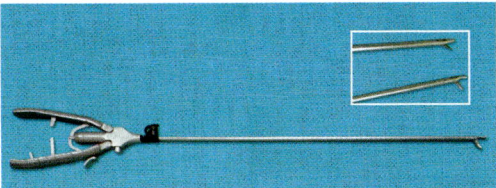

Fig. 18: Needle holders with curved and straight tips in inset.

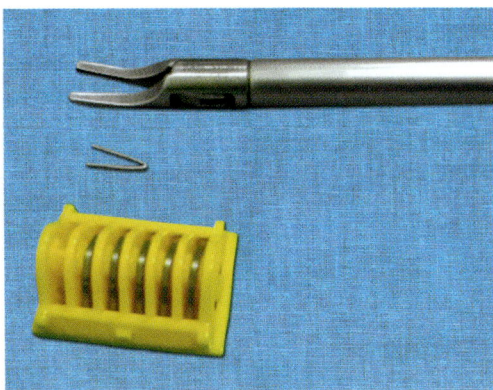

Fig. 19: Laparoscopic clip applicators.

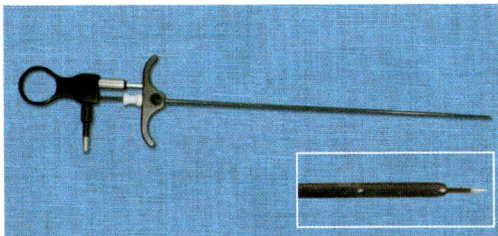

Fig. 20: Ovarian drilling needle.

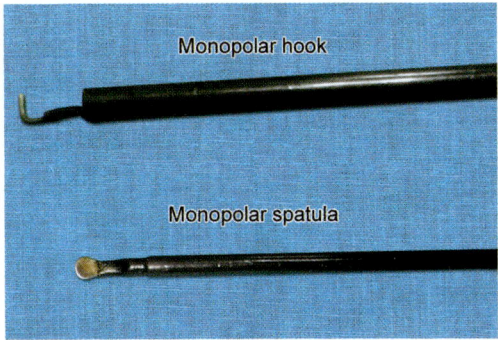

Fig. 21: Electrodes.

Laparoscopic Clip Applicators (Fig. 19)

Clips are required in gynecological surgeries for clipping the uterine arteries at their origin. This may be required in radical hysterectomies or when massive hemorrhage is anticipated. Clip applicators may be factory preloaded or loaded prior to application during surgery. While applying the clip, the jaws should be perpendicular to the artery and both the jaws should be visible to avoid inadvertent inclusion of any other tissue.

Ovarian Drilling Needle (Fig. 20)

This is specially used for drilling ovaries in women with polycystic ovarian syndrome (PCOS) resistant to medical treatment. The instrument is connected to monopolar cautery lead. This destroys the ovarian cortex containing follicles for a depth of 4 mm only so that no extracortical tissue is destroyed. It is recommended that only 4 holes (3–6), 4 mm deep, are made in each ovary with a coagulating current of 40 W. This is a second-line treatment for women with PCOS which are either resistant to oral ovulogens or fail to conceive with oral ovulogens. This procedure is associated with complications such as increased risk of adhesions around the ovaries and decrease in ovarian reserve; hence, it requires an informed decision by the patient.

Coagulating and Dissecting Electrodes

Both monopolar and bipolar electrodes are available. Monopolar electrodes (Fig. 21) can be in the form of different shaped hooks or

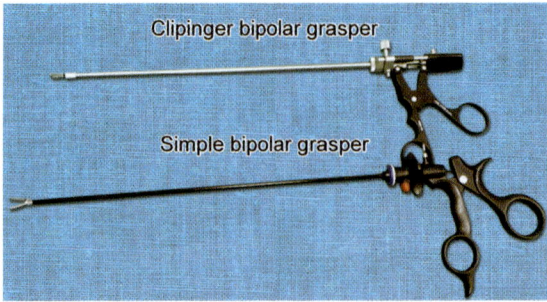
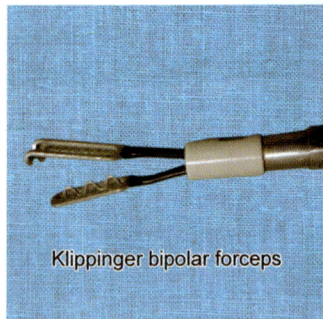
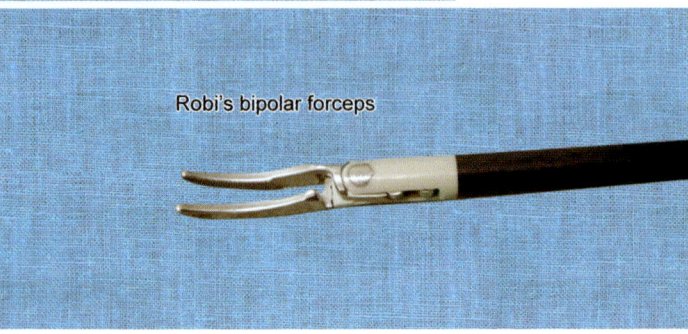

Fig. 22: Bipolar forceps.

they may be attached to other hand instruments such as scissors. Monopolar spatula, balls, or needles are also used in different clinical scenarios. In gynecological surgeries, monopolar hook is commonly used for procedures such as vault incision in hysterectomy or for giving incision over myoma. It can be used for resection, dissection, and coagulation. Monopolar current travels through the body to reach its return plate, thus increasing the chances of damage to other organs or to the skin. There are higher chances of injury due to insulation failure or inadvertent direct or capacitive coupling. The chances of injuries increase where multiple instruments are in close vicinity to each other like single-port laparoscopy or in robotic surgery.

In bipolar forceps (Fig. 22), the current flow is from one jaw to the other, reducing the chances of thermal damage. Whenever possible, bipolar forceps should be used instead of monopolar electrodes. Vessels are cauterized with maximum efficiency and safely with bipolar forceps. Bipolar instrument is essential in gynecological surgeries.

Ultrasonic Scalpel (Fig. 23)

Surgery in the last two decades has been revolutionized with the use of ultrasonic vibrations in laparoscopy. It was first introduced by "Ethicon division of Johnson and Johnson" and was named as the harmonic scalpel. It is one of the most popular energy devices. These ultrasonic vibrations cut and coagulate at the same time, thus mitigating the need for frequent change of instruments.

Mechanism of Action

The ultrasonic generator converts the ultrasonic energy to mechanical energy. A piezoelectric crystal located at the tip of the hand piece vibrates at the rate of 55,000 Hz and

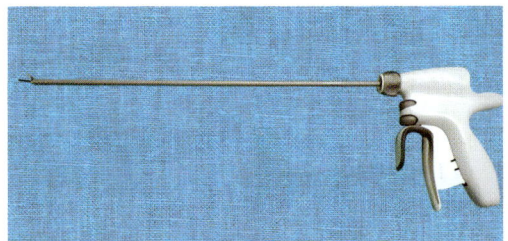 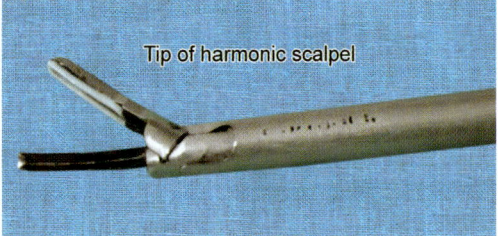

Fig. 23: Harmonic scalpel.

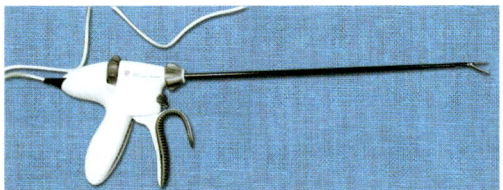

Fig. 24: Enseal, an advance bipolar device.

generates a mechanical force. The range of peak tissue temperatures is much lower (60–100°C) compared with those produced by electrocautery (200–300°C). The inactive white blade holds the tissue while the active blade delivers high-grade frictional force. This coagulates the tissue proteins which form a coagulum for vessel sealing and enables coaptation of the tissues as well. With the use of harmonic scalpel, there is precise dissection, good hemostasis, minimum thermal spread, and minimum smoke production, and hence an increased safety profile of this instrument. Vessels up to 5 mm diameter can be coagulated safely by the harmonic shears.

Advanced Bipolar Tissue Sealers (LigaSure and Enseal)

They are advanced bipolar devices (Fig. 24) which provide a combination of high pressure and energy to seal and then transect vessels. They provide better hemostasis, less thermal spread, and improved ergonomics. They can coagulate vessels up to 7 mm in diameter. These devices also have a feedback-controlled response system which automatically stops further energy delivery when the seal cycle is complete.

Hybrid Energy Devices (Thunderbeat by Olympus)

The hybrid energy devices deliver advanced bipolar and ultrasonic energy simultaneously contributing to high performance and efficiency in vessel sealing as well as accurate and faster tissue dissection. Like advanced bipolar tissue sealers, this too has a tissue impedance feedback system which stops further delivery of energy when sealing is complete and autostop of ultrasonic cutting when tissue transection is complete. It can dissect like ultrasonic shears and coagulate vessels up to 7 mm diameter like advanced bipolar devices. This dual action increases maneuverability and reduces operating time.

Uterine Manipulators

Different uterine manipulators are available to aid laparoscopic hysterectomies. There is Rumi manipulator, Mangeshkar manipulator, and some others. Mangeshkar manipulator (Figs. 25A and B) is an assemble of many components. It can antevert or retrovert the uterus and can push a cup around the cervix

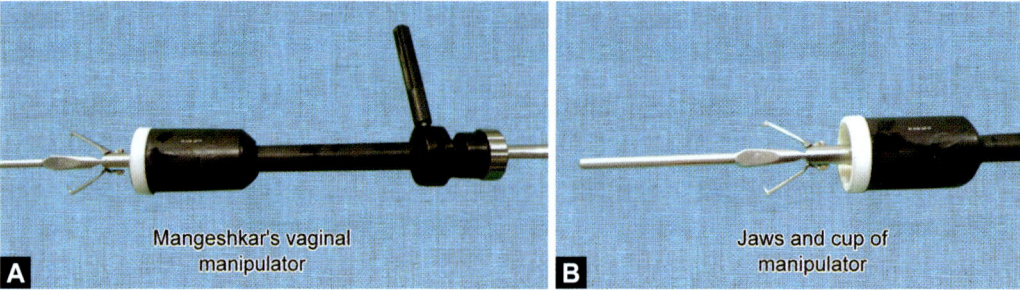

Figs. 25A and B: Uterine manipulators.

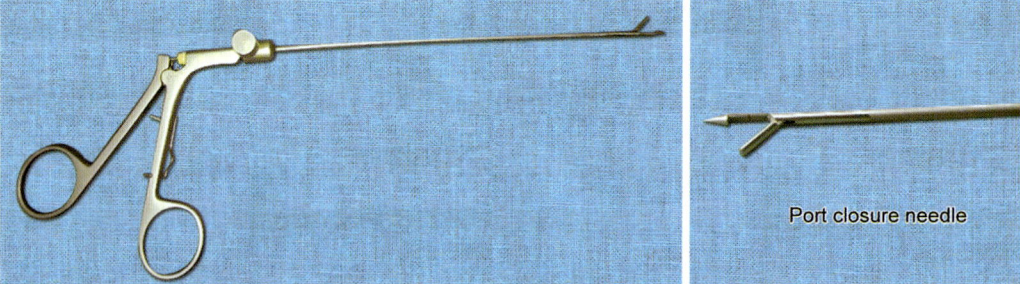

Fig. 26: Port closure needle.

for delineation of the fornices and provides a firm plastic surface for cutting of vault without thermal damage to other structures.

Morcellators

Morcollator is an instrument which minces bulky tissues inside the abdomen, like myoma after myomectomy or uterus after hysterectomy, for ease of tissue retrieval. It consists of a grasper which pulls the tissue inside a cylinder and the cutting jaws inside the cylinder to mince the tissues. However, during morcellation, many small tissue pieces are spilled into the peritoneal cavity which is a serious concern. It has led to cases of disseminated leiomyomatosis and dissemination of leiomyosarcoma or other abnormal cells. These complications are more difficult to treat compared to the primary disease. The Food and Drug Administration (FDA) has issued a warning against the use of power morcellators. In present day, minimal access surgery and morcellation are advisable only inside an endobag.

Port Closure Needle (Fig. 26)

They are special needles which are used to stitch the fascial defects with ports >10 mm size. They are like the cobbler's needle. A 5 mm telescope is used to visualize the closure of the port site. The tip holds the suture and pierces the rectus in the central port and leaves one end of the suture in the abdomen. The needle is then pierced again through the other side of the port. The suture is feed in its jaw and the needle is pulled out, thus leaving a loop which closes the fascial defect.

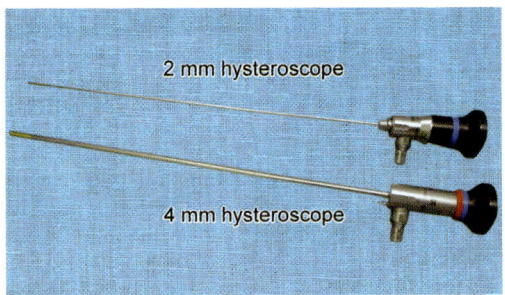

Fig. 27: Hysteroscope.

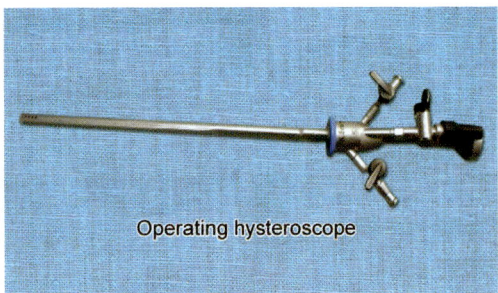

Fig. 28: Operating hysteroscope.

HYSTEROSCOPY INSTRUMENTS

An assembled diagnostic hysteroscope comprises a telescope, an inner sheath through which saline flows inside and an outer sheath through which saline flows out of the uterine cavity. There has been a constant effort to reduce the diameter of the hysteroscope. At present, narrow lumen scopes are available for performing outpatient diagnostic hysteroscopy without anesthesia. These hysteroscopes can be rigid or flexible. Surgeries inside the uterus can be done either with operating hysteroscope or with a resectoscope.

Telescope (Fig. 27): Hysteroscopic telescope come in various diameters (2 and 4 mm) and angulation of the lenses, i.e., 0°, 12°, 30°, and 70°. In gynecology, we use 30° hysteroscope for better end-on view of endometrial cavity.

The operating hysteroscopic sheath (Fig. 28) has a fine channel through which ancillary instruments (5 French diameter) can be inserted inside the uterine cavity. The operating hysteroscope has a total of 4.9 mm diameter and the operating channel has a 2 mm diameter.

The commonly used ancillary instruments are scissors, graspers, and biopsy forceps (Fig. 29). These are commonly used for polypectomy, excision of endometrial

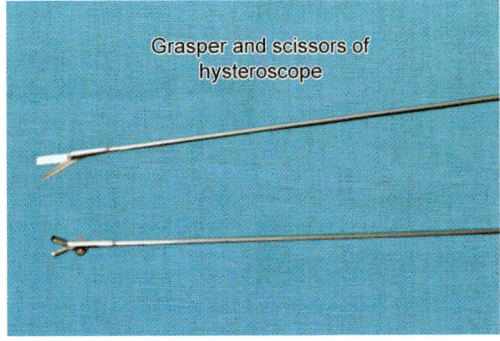

Fig. 29: Grasper and scissors of hysteroscope.

adhesions, removal of misplaced intrauterine contraceptive device (IUCD) and for taking directed endometrial biopsies. Though the ancillary instruments can be flexible, rigid, or semirigid, most surgeons prefer the semirigid ones. The semirigid instruments are easier to manipulate and are more durable. The flexible instruments are fragile, less durable, and have less stability. They are appropriate for reaching the cornual or uterotubal junctions.

The resectoscope used for myoma resection is assembled from three parts (Fig. 30). It has a working element on which electrodes are attached. This working element has a spring system which enables the surgeon to push the electrode into full view when using it. The working element with the loaded electrode is then introduced in the inner sheath

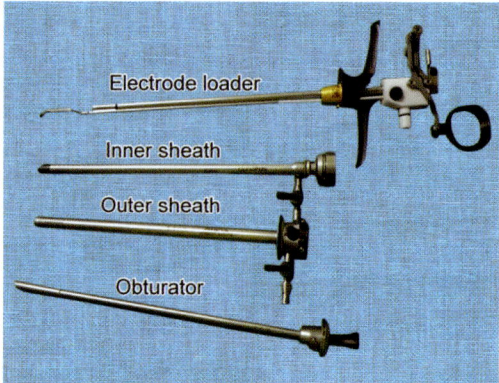

Fig. 30: Resectoscope.

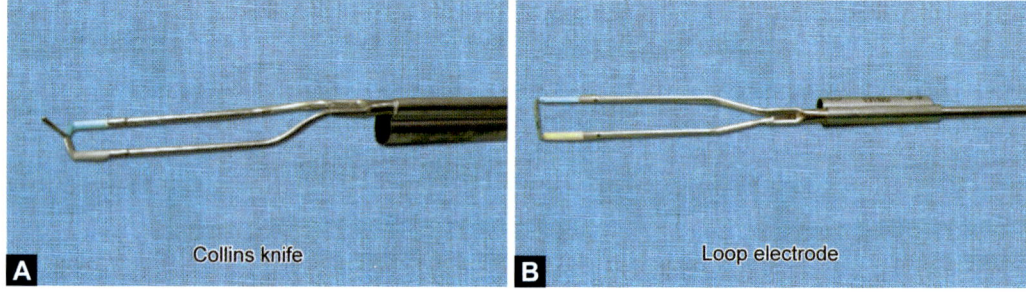

Figs. 31A and B: A Collins knife and a loop electrode.

and then in the outer sheath. The inner sheath is for fluid entry. The outer sheath has multiple holes for the fluid to come out and has a ceramic tip to avoid thermal injury by the active electrode. Initially, after cervical dilatation, outer and inner sheath with an obturator is introduced in the uterine cavity. After negotiating the internal os, the obturator is withdrawn and the working element with the telescope is inserted. This safeguards the telescope and the electrode. The diameter of telescope is 4 mm and that of outer sheath is 8–9 mm. Many surgeons prefer to prime the cervix with misoprostol tablets and then dilate the cervix.

Electrodes Used in Resectoscope

Electrodes can be monopolar or bipolar. The monopolar electrodes need an electrolyte poor media such as glycine to distend the uterine cavity. Glycine gets absorbed into the bloodstream and can cause fluid overload and electrolyte imbalance with a fluid deficit of 500–1,000 mL. Inflow and outflow need to be measured and the fluid not accounted for is the amount that has entered the blood. With the use of bipolar electrodes, normal saline can be used as a distention medium instead of glycine and a fluid deficit of up to 2.5 L can be tolerated. However, bipolar electrodes are more expensive (Fig. 31B).

Most of the procedures such as myomectomy and polypectomy use the loop electrode. A ball electrode is available for hemostasis and thermoablation of endometrium. A knife (Collins knife) is used for septum resection (Fig. 31A).

STERILIZATION OF LAPAROSCOPIC INSTRUMENTS

Sterilization of instruments should be as per the manufacturer's specifications. All laparoscopic instruments should be disassembled and thoroughly cleaned with distilled water. The instruments are then air dried. The sterilization methods depend on the time available and the material of the instrument.

Autoclaving by means of steam sterilization is the safest and most cost-effective method of sterilization. However, the complex laparoscopic systems cannot be autoclaved and need chemical sterilization.

Chemical sterilization of instruments is most done by ethylene oxide (EtO) gas. It is suitable for endoscopes, plastics, rubbers, and complex laparoscopic systems as well. Sterilization takes 3–6 hours. An adequate aeration period of 8–20 hours should be given as any remaining fume is highly toxic. EtO therefore is usually done 1 day prior to the surgery.

Glutaraldehyde 2% solution (Cidex) is a good sterilizing solution, especially for instruments with lenses but not for the laparoscopic camera and cables. After disassembly and cleaning of the instruments, they should be completely immersed in the glutaraldehyde solution for 10–12 hours. The instruments should be properly washed before use, preferably three times with sterile water. Cidex should not be used >15 times or >21 days, whichever comes earlier.

For faster sterilization, Cidex OPA is available. It is 0.55% orthophthalaldehyde. It is a gentle chemical disinfectant which can be used for all delicate instruments as well. For manual sterilization, 12-minute soaking is adequate. It has a 2-year shelf period and an open bottle can be used for 75 days.

Formalin chambers were very popular for small setups and for carrying sterilized instruments to other places. Airtight formalin chambers are available in which the unassembled parts are kept for sterilization. About 8–10 tablets of formalin are put inside, and the fumes should be in contact with the instruments for >12–24 hours. However, lately, its use is wrapped up in controversy due to its carcinogenic potential.

Other sterilizing options include gas plasma sterilizers and systems using peracetic acid.

To summarize, minimal access surgery is mostly about the knowledge of the correct anatomy and the biophysics of the instruments. The surgeon should know the limitations of all devices and which one is to be used where. There is a continuous advancement in equipment and instrumentation based on different technologies. The surgeon should be abreast with recent advancements.

SUGGESTED READING

1. Dutta DK, Dutta I. The harmonic scalpel. J Obstet Gynaecol India. 2016;66(3):209-10.
2. Frascà C, Degli Espodti E, Arena A, Tuzzato G, Moro E, Martelli V, et al. Can in-bag manual morcellation represent an alternative to uncontained power morcellation in laparoscopic myomectomy? A randomized controlled trial. Gynecol Obstet Invest. 2018;83(1):52-6.
3. Hegde CV. Mangeshikar uterine manipulator. J Obstet Gynaecol India. 2016;66(2):134-6.
4. Law KS, Abbott JA, Lyons SD. Energy sources for gynecologic laparoscopic surgery: a review of the literature. Obstet Gynecol Surv. 2014;69(12):763-76.
5. Mishra RK. Textbook of Practical Laparoscopic Surgery, 3rd edition. New Delhi: Jaypee Brothers Medical Publishers; 2013.
6. Sabnis RB, Bhattu A, Vijaykumar M. Sterilization of endoscopic instruments. Curr Opin Urol. 2014;24(2):195-202.
7. Vilos GA, Rajkumar C. Electrosurgical generators and monopolar and bipolar electrosurgery. J Minim Invasive Gynecol. 2013;20(3):279-87.

54 Cardiotocography

Vidhi Chaudhary, Shalini Malhotra

INTRODUCTION

Cardiotocography (CTG) is a technical method for recording of the pattern of fetal heartbeat using principles of ultrasound. The machine used for monitoring is called a cardiotocograph. CTG is used both antenatally (before birth) and during labor to monitor the fetus for any signs of distress.

EXTERNAL VERSUS INTERNAL FETAL HEART RATE MONITORING

External fetal heart rate (FHR) monitoring involves the placement of two transducers on abdomen of a pregnant woman. One transducer records the FHR using ultrasound. The other transducer monitors the intrauterine pressure during labor. It is prone to signal loss, causing inadvertent monitoring of the maternal heart rate or artefacts leading to double counting. The signal loss is common in women with high body mass index (BMI) and or uncooperative patients. External monitoring may not detect fetal arrhythmias accurately.

Internal measurement involves inserting a pressure catheter into the uterine cavity, as well as attaching a electrode to fetal scalp (can be applied in breech) to measure the fetal heart electrical activity (R-R interval in QRS complexes). Cervical dilatation and ruptured amniotic membranes are the prerequisites. It should not be used in patients with active infection, genital herpes, active hepatitis B, human immunodeficiency virus infection, in suspected fetal blood disorders, uncertain presenting part, an unengaged presentation, extreme preterm fetus, antepartum hemorrhage, and placenta previa.

Monitoring of Twins

Continuous external FHR monitoring of twin gestations during labor should preferably be performed with dual channel monitors that allow simultaneous monitoring of both FHRs with a difference of 20 beats in calibration of both probe recordings to have separate tracings using the same machine.

INDICATIONS OF CARDIOTOCOGRAPHY MONITORING

The evidence for continuous CTG monitoring, as compared with intermittent auscultation, in both low and high-risk labors is scientifically inconclusive. The only benefit of CTG has been the decrease of the occurrence of neonatal seizures with no effect on the overall incidence of perinatal mortality or cerebral palsy.[1,2] The routine uses of admission CTG for low-risk women presenting in labor result in increase in cesarean section

rates with no improvement in perinatal outcomes.[3] However, experts agree that continuous CTG monitoring should be considered in the following cases:
- High risk of fetal hypoxia/acidosis, e.g., hemorrhage and maternal pyrexia, fetal growth restriction, and meconium-stained liquor
- Epidural analgesia
- Abnormalities detected during intermittent fetal auscultation
- Induced or augmented labor
- Previous cesarean section.

MATERNAL POSITION FOR CARDIOTOCOGRAPHY ACQUISITION

Position preferred for CTG monitoring is lateral recumbent or half-sitting position. Maternal supine position may cause aortocaval compression by gravid uterus, thereby affecting placental perfusion and fetal oxygenation thereby causing misinterpretation of results.

PAPER SCALES AND SPEED FOR CARDIOTOCOGRAPHY INTERPRETATION

The horizontal scale for CTG measures the "paper speed" and available options are usually 1, 2, or 3 cm/min. Speed of 1 cm/min provides sufficient details for clinical analysis and has an advantage of reducing tracing length. The vertical scale records the fetal heart rate and are usually at 20 or 30 bpm/cm. The paper scales used in each center should be the one with which healthcare professionals are most familiar. Change in the paper scales to which the staff is unaccustomed may lead to erroneous interpretations of CTG features. For example, at 3 cm/min variability may appear reduced to a clinician familiar with the 1 cm/min scale, while it may appear exaggerated in the opposite situation.

EVALUATION OF BASIC CARDIOTOCOGRAPHY FEATURES

Normal baseline:
- Normal FHR is considered as 110–160 bpm. Preterm fetuses tend to have values toward the upper end of this range and postterm fetuses toward the lower end. The mean FHR rounded to increments of 5 bpm during a 10-minute segment, excluding accelerations, decelerations, and periods of marked FHR variability.

  The baseline must be for a minimum of 2 minutes (not necessarily contiguous) in any 10-minute segment, or the baseline for that segment is defined as "indeterminate."
  - *Bradycardia*: A baseline FHR <110 bpm for >10 minutes—possible causes are maternal hypothermia, administration of beta-blockers, and fetal arrhythmias such as atrioventricular block.
  - *Tachycardia*: A baseline FHR >160 bpm for >10 minutes—possible causes are initial hypoxia due to compensatory catecholamine release, maternal pyrexia, chorioamnionitis, beta agonist drugs, and fetal arrhythmias.
  - *Periodic pattern*: FHR pattern associated with uterine contraction.
  - *Episodic pattern*: FHR pattern not associated with uterine contraction.
- *Baseline variability*: It is the fluctuation in baseline fetal heart rate. These fluctuations are irregular in amplitude and frequency. Variability is measured

from the peak to the trough of the FHR fluctuations and is quantitated in bpm. Variability is classified as follows:
- *Absent*: Amplitude range undetectable
- *Minimal*: Amplitude range detectable but ≤ 5 bpm
- *Moderate*: Amplitude range 6–25 bpm
- *Marked*: Amplitude range >25 bpm.
- *Reduced variability*: It occurs due to central nervous system hypoxia or acidosis causing decreased sympathetic and parasympathetic activity. Important causes include previous cerebral injury, infection, and administration of central nervous system depressants or parasympathetic blockers.
- *Increased variability (saltatory pattern)*: Beat-to-beat variability of 25 bpm or more. It is caused by fetal autonomic instability or hyperactive autonomic system.

Patterns

- *Acceleration*: Abrupt increase in FHR above the baseline of 15 bpm lasting for at least 15 seconds but <2 minutes at 32 weeks or more period of gestation and 10 bpm for at least 10 seconds if the period of gestation is <32 weeks. It is a sign of a neurologically responsive fetus that does not have hypoxia or acidosis. The absence of accelerations in an otherwise normal intrapartum CTG does not indicate hypoxia or acidosis. Accelerations lasting for ≥2 minutes but <10 minutes is a prolonged acceleration but if it lasts for ≥10 minutes, it is a baseline change.
- *Early deceleration*: Gradual decrease in FHR and return to baseline corresponding with uterine contraction. It is ≥30 seconds from onset to nadir of deceleration and is visually apparent. The onset, nadir, and recovery of the deceleration are coincident with the beginning, peak, and ending of the uterine contraction, respectively. They are caused by fetal head compression and do not indicate fetal hypoxia or acidosis.
- *Late deceleration*: Gradual decrease in FHR and return to baseline corresponding with uterine contraction starting after the onset of contraction, with the nadir of the deceleration occurring after the peak of uterine contraction and recovery after the end of contraction. It is ≥30 seconds from onset to nadir of deceleration and is visually apparent. These are due to chemoreceptor-mediated response to fetal hypoxemia.
- *Variable deceleration*: Abrupt decrease in FHR below the baseline by 15 bpm lasting for at least 15 seconds but <2 minutes and not related to uterus contractions They are the most common type of decelerations during labor and are caused by baroreceptor-mediated response to increase in arterial pressure, which occurs with umbilical cord compression. They are concerning if they last for >60 seconds, reduced baseline variability within the deceleration, failure to return to baseline, biphasic (W) shape and no shouldering.[4]
- *Acute prolonged deceleration*: This is decrease of FHR by >15 bpm below the baseline lasting for at least 2 minutes but <10 minutes from onset to return to baseline. They indicate acute hypoxemia. It is caused by abruptio, uterine rupture, cord prolapse, and maternal seizure.
- *Sinusoidal pattern*: It is a smooth, sine wave-like pattern of amplitude of 5–15 bpm, and a regular frequency of 3–5 cycles per minute. It occurs in association with severe fetal anemia, such as anti-D alloimmunization, fetal–maternal hemorrhage, twin-to-twin transfusion syndrome, and ruptured vasa previa. It is also seen in cases of

acute fetal hypoxia, infection, cardiac malformations, hydrocephalus, and gastroschisis.
- *Pseudosinusoidal pattern*: This is a pattern resembling the sinusoidal pattern but with a more jagged "saw-tooth" appearance rather than the smooth sine-wave form. Its duration seldom exceeds 30 minutes and it is characterized by normal patterns before and after. Events causing these patterns are maternal analgesia and during periods of fetal sucking.

INTERPRETATION

Cardiotocography Trace Interpretation: Guiding Principles

Pneumonic DR C BRAVADO is used for interpretation of FHR tracings or CTGs. This includes the following steps:
- DR *Define Risk*: Whether low or high risk
- C   *Comment on contractions*: Frequency and intensity
- Bra *Baseline fetal heart rate*: Normal, bradycardia, or tachycardia
- V   *Variability beat to beat*: Absent, minimal, moderate, or marked
- A   *Accelerations*: Present or absent >15 bpm for ≥15 seconds
- D   *Decelerations*: Early, late, or variable
- O   *Overall*: Assessment category I, II, or III (Box 1).

MANAGEMENT: CLINICAL DECISION

Several factors, such as gestational age and medication administered to the mother, can affect FHR features, so CTG analysis must be integrated with other

Box 1: NICHD three-tier FHR classification system.[5]
- Category I:
  FHR tracings include all of the following:
  - *Baseline rate*: 110–160 bpm
  - *Baseline FHR variability*: Moderate
  - *Accelerations*: Present or absent
  - Late or variable decelerations absent
  - Early decelerations present or absent
- Category II:
  Includes all FHR tracings not categorized as Category I or Category III
- Category III:
  FHR tracings include either:
  - Fetal heart rate tracing includes sinusoidal pattern or absent baseline variability with recurrent late decelerations, recurrent variable decelerations, or bradycardia

Note: The presence of fetal heart rate accelerations, even with reduced baseline variability, is a sign of the baby being healthy.

(FHR: fetal heart rate; NICHD: National Institute of Child Health and Human Development)

clinical information for adequate management. Generally, if the fetus continues to maintain a stable baseline and a reassuring variability, the risk of hypoxia to the central organs is very unlikely. Clinical decisions must be interpreted according to the management principles given in Table 1.

Clinical Example 1

Cardiotocography trace of primigravidae at 38 weeks of gestation with mild preeclampsia in early labor. When the trace began, rate is 130 bpm. Initially, there is no acceleration with reduced variability. This is sleep pattern. As trace continues, beat-to-beat variability improves to 10–15 bpm, with 4–5 accelerations of >15 bpm lasting for >15 seconds. Trace is reassuring and set at 1 cm/min (Fig. 1).

Table 1: Clinical management according to categorization of CTG.

Category	Management
Category I or normal	Normal labor monitoring. Discontinue CTG, unless clinically indicated

Category II or suspicious	• Correct any underlying causes such as hypotension or uterine hyperstimulation
	• Perform a full set of maternal observations
	• *Start one or more conservative measures:*
	  – Encourage the woman to mobilize or adopt an alternative position (and to avoid being supine)
	  – Offer intravenous fluids if the woman is hypotensive
	  – Reduce contraction frequency by reducing or stopping oxytocin if it is being used and/or offering a tocolytic drug (subcutaneous terbutaline 0.25 mg)
	• Inform an obstetrician or senior midwife
	• Document a plan for reviewing the whole clinical picture and the CTG findings
	• Brief woman and her birth companion(s) about what is happening and take her preferences into account

Pathological or Category III	• Obtain a review by an obstetrician and a senior midwife
	• Exclude acute events (e.g., cord prolapse, suspected placental abruption, or suspected uterine rupture)
	• Correct any underlying causes such as hypotension or uterine hyperstimulation
	• Start 1 or more conservative measures
	• *If the cardiotocograph trace is still pathological after implementing conservative measures:*
	  – Obtain a further review by an obstetrician
	  – Offer digital fetal scalp stimulation and document the outcome.
	  – If the cardiotocograph trace is still pathological after fetal scalp stimulation: Consider fetal blood sampling and expediting the birth

• Need for urgent intervention Acute bradycardia, or a single prolonged deceleration for 3 minutes or more	• Urgently seek obstetric help • If there has been an acute event (e.g., cord prolapse, suspected placental abruption or suspected uterine rupture)—expedite the birth • Correct any underlying causes such as hypotension or uterine hyperstimulation • Start conservative measures • Expedite the birth if the acute bradycardia persists for 9 minutes • If the fetal heart rate recovers within 9 minutes, reassess the decision to expedite the birth and involve laboring women in decision-making.

Case 1: Cardiotocography Interpretation (Fig. 1)

DR: Define Risk—High Risk (primigravida, preeclampsia)
C: Contractions—nil
BR: Baseline rate—normal
V: Variability—reduced, <5 bpm for first 10 minutes, then improves to >5 bpm
A: Accelerations—nil in first 15 minutes (sleep pattern), followed by more than two accelerations in last 15 minutes suggestive of fetal wakeful state after sleep)
D: Decelerations—absent
O: Overall—category I trace

Plan to watch for spontaneous progress as early labor.

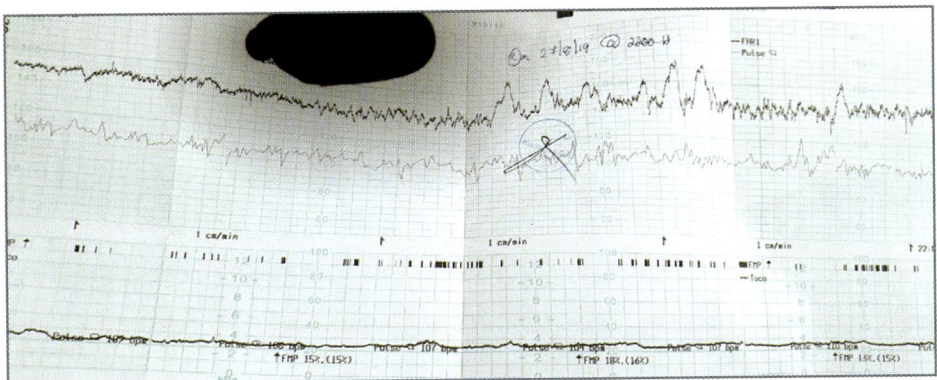

Fig. 1: Uppermost trace—fetal heart rate, middle light trace—maternal pulse, and lowermost trace—uterine activity.

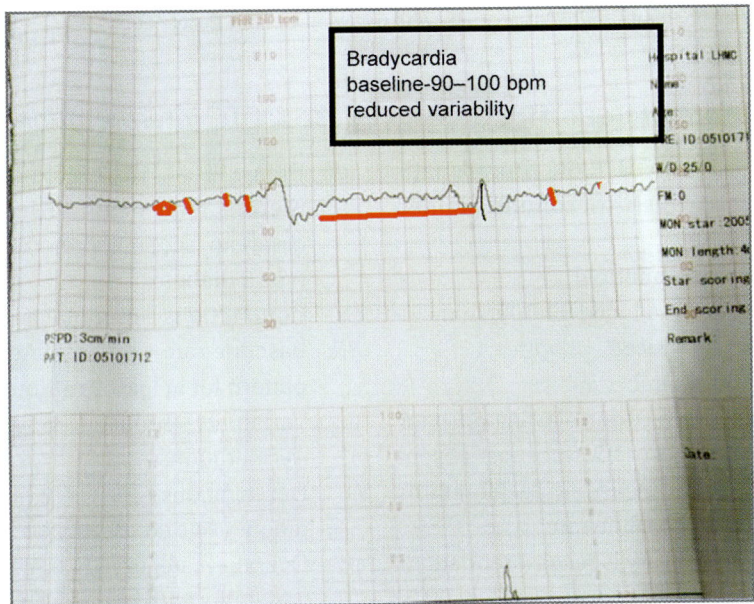

Fig. 2: Bradycardia (baseline 90–100 bpm) with reduced variability.

Clinical Example 2

Multigravida G2P1L1 at 37 + 4 weeks of gestation with intrahepatic cholestasis of pregnancy in active labor had the following CTG. Prolonged bradycardia 80–85 bpm with reduced variability (2–3 bpm). Immediate vaginal examination revealed 5 cm cervical dilatation 75% effacement, with vertex at -1 station and thick meconium with no improvement on scalp stimulation. Immediate emergency cesarean was done. Baby was resuscitated and was healthy (Fig. 2).

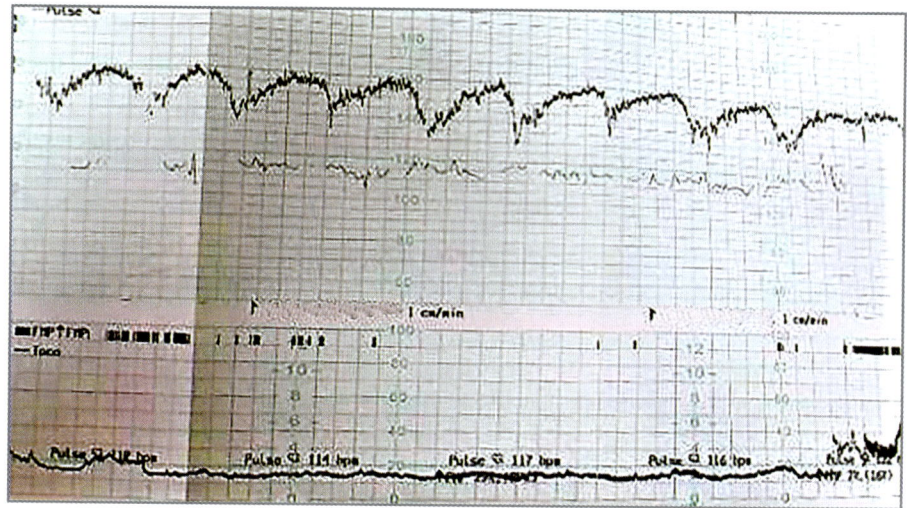

Fig. 3: No baseline heart rate, reduced variability with recurrent variable decelerations.

Case 2: CTG Interpretation

- *DR*: Define Risk—HIGH RISK (Intrahepatic cholestasis, thick meconium-stained liquor)
- *C*: Contractions—minimal
- *BR*: Baseline rate—reduced 90–100/min
- *V*: Variability—reduced, <2 bpm
- *A*: Accelerations—nil
- *D*: Decelerations—recurrent, lasting <15 bpm
- *O*: Overall—category III trace as absent variability with recurrent decelerations with reduced baseline rate

Immediate delivery is recommended.

Clinical Example 3

A 35-year-old G2P1L1 with previous intrauterine death and previous cesarean section at 36 weeks with type 2 diabetes mellitus showing variable decelerations. Patient was taken for emergency cesarean after stabilization. Baby had acidemia and needed admission in neonatal intensive care unit (Fig. 3).

Case 3: CTG Interpretation

- *DR*: Define Risk—HIGH RISK; previous intrauterine fetal death (IUFD), previous cesarean section, preterm (36 weeks), type 2 diabetes
- *C*: Contractions—minimal
- *BR*: Baseline rate—no baseline as no stable pattern for at least 2 minutes
- *V*: Variability—reduced, <5 bpm
- *A*: Accelerations—nil
- *D*: Decelerations—recurrent variable decelerations as no contractions recorded
- *O*: Overall—category III trace no baseline variability with recurrent decelerations

Immediate delivery is recommended.

Clinical Example 4

A gravida 6 para 4 with one miscarriage, previous all normal vaginal deliveries at 38 weeks in spontaneous labor arrives in labor room. After detailed review, maternal condition is stable and CTG in done to establish fetal condition (Fig. 4).

Chapter 54: Cardiotocography

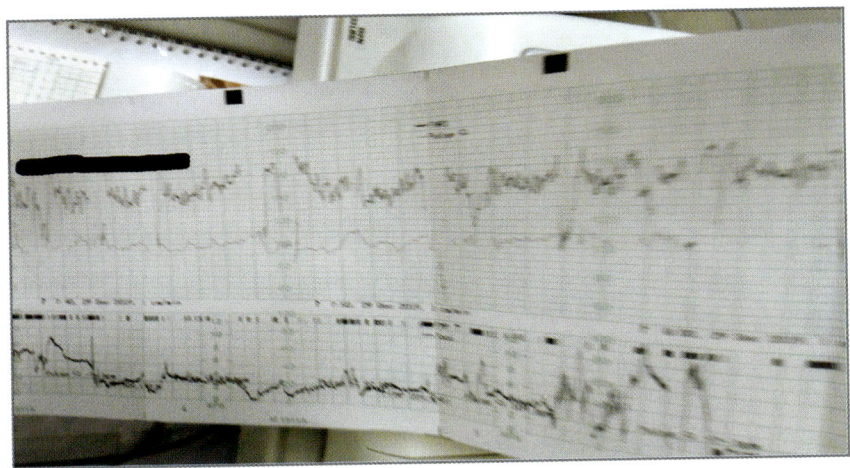

Fig. 4: Normal baseline rate, with recurrent early decelerations.

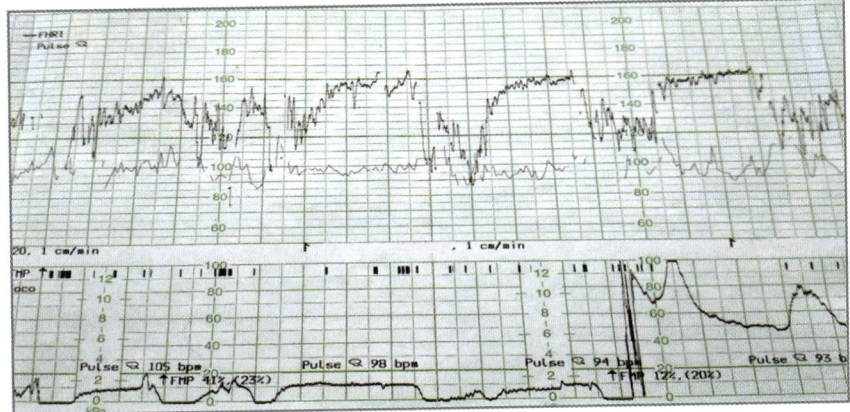

Fig. 5: Shift of baseline with persistent variable decelerations.

Case 4: CTG Interpretation

DR: Define Risk –LOW RISK (para 4, previous all normal vaginal deliveries)
C: Contractions—irregular, low amplitude
BR: Baseline rate—normal, 144 bpm
V: Variability; normal, >5 bpm
A: Accelerations—present
D: Decelerations—four, sharp possibly early decelerations
O: Overall—category I trace; observe for spontaneous progress

Clinical Example 4 Continues

After 4 hours, CTG is reconnected as patient complains of more pain abdomen with blood-stained discharge (Fig. 5).

Interpretation:
DR: Define Risk—LOW RISK (para 4, previous all normal vaginal deliveries)
C: Contractions—irregular, low amplitude initially but high amplitude later—possibly loss of contact of probe and thus not recording initially—need to palpate

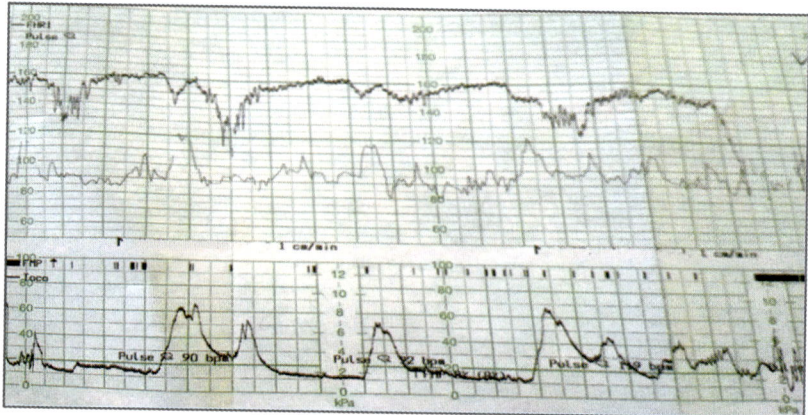
Fig. 6: Absent variability with recurrent late decelerations.

strength of contractions manually till probe is reconnected
- BR: Baseline rate—normal, 160 bpm (shift of baseline)
- V: Variability—normal, >5 bpm
- A: Accelerations—absent
- D: Decelerations—variable decelerations present with both last recorded contractions
- O: Overall—category II trace—baseline shift, decelerations variable but persistent with each recorded contraction

Thus, vigilant monitoring is continued with CTG.

Next trace after 30 minutes (Fig. 6):
Interpretation:
- DR: Define Risk—High RISK (para 4, previous all normal vaginal deliveries with previous category II CTG)
- C: Contractions—regular, increasing amplitude
- BR: Baseline rate; normal, 160 bpm
- V: Variability—absent <2 bpm
- A: Accelerations—absent
- D: Decelerations—late decelerations
- O: Overall—category III as shift of baseline to 160 bpm with reduced variability with late decelerations

Immediate delivery is mandatory.

Management: Since the patient was only 6 cm dilated, with fully effaced cervix, membranes were ruptured and blood-stained liquor was noted; urgent cesarean section, category I, was done and placental abruption was found. The baby did well after resuscitation.

LIMITATIONS OF CARDIOTOCOGRAPHY

- CTG analysis has considerable intra- and interobserver disagreement.
- Suspicious and pathological tracings have a limited capacity to predict metabolic acidosis and low Apgar scores, i.e., a large percentage of cases with suspicious and pathological tracings do not have adverse neonatal outcomes.
- However, there remains a strong association between certain FHR patterns and hypoxia/acidosis. Hence, they are sensitive indicators, but have a low specificity and low positive predictive value.

As per current evidence, limited benefit of continuous CTG in labor for all women is 50% reduction in neonatal seizures with no differences in the incidences of overall perinatal mortality and cerebral palsy. However, it was recognized as per the International Federation of Gynecology and Obstetrics (FIGO) consensus guidelines that the trials were underpowered to detect differences in these outcomes.[6] It is worthwhile to note that continuous CTG was associated with a 63% increase in cesarean delivery and a 15% increase in instrumental vaginal deliveries.[7]

KEY POINTS

- Intrapartum fetal monitoring is to identify situations that precede hypoxia/acidemia to avoid fetal injury and institution of appropriate management.
- Always use DR C BRAVADO pneumonic to interpret a CTG.
- Put all risk factors from the case details.
- Note maternal temperature, pulse, drugs administered, etc., as they affect fetal heart rate.
- Before reporting any CTG as category II or III, please review previous CTG as a previous pattern might suggest changes that are progressing.
- When in doubt, ask for FRESH EYES (SECOND OPINION) as a single observer following a case might get biased. This helps in those traces which are unclear though not category I.
- A shift of baseline always suggests a progressive change and thus, should be noted.
- When baseline variability is reduced, even shallow decelerations <10 bpm are considered significant. These two features, when present together, predict poor outcome unless immediate action is taken.
- Cesarean sections are not done for fetal distress noted on CTG. Urgent delivery is indicated when category III CTG is noted and delivery not imminent vaginally. This clearly explains that CTG interpretation decides timing of delivery depending on stage of labor-not mode of delivery.
- Using common terminology to report CTG helps all to speak same language, reducing communication misunderstandings.

REFERENCES

1. National Institute for Health and Care Excellence. (2014). Clinical guideline: Intrapartum care for healthy women and babies. [online] Available from: https://www.nice.org.uk/guidance/cg190/resources/intrapartum-care-for-healthy-women-and-babies-pdf-35109866447557. [Last accessed March, 2020].
2. Ayres-de-Campos D, Spong CY, Chandraharan E. FIGO consensus guidelines on intrapartum fetal monitoring: Cardiotocography. Int J Gynaecol Obstet. 2015;131(1):13-24.
3. Devane D, Lalor JG, Daly S, McGuire W, Cuthbert A, Smith V. Cardiotocography versus intermittent auscultation of fetal heart on admission to labour ward for assessment of fetal wellbeing. Cochrane Database Syst Rev. 2012;2:CD005122.
4. Holzmann M, Wretler S, Cnattingius S, Nordstrom L. Cardiotocography patterns and risk of intrapartum fetal acidemia. J Perinat Med. 2015;43(4):473-9.
5. Robinson B. A review of NICHD standardized nomenclature for cardiotocography: The importance of speaking a common language when describing electronic foetal monitoring. Rev Obstet Gynecol. 2008;1(2):56-60.
6. Royal College of Obstetricians and Gynaecologists. The use of electronic fetal monitoring. Evidence-based clinical guideline, number 8. London: RCOG Press; 2001
7. Alfirevic Z, Devane D, Gyte GM. Continuous cardiotocography (CTG) as a form of electronic fetal monitoring (EFM) for fetal assessment during labour. Cochrane Database of Syst Rev. 2013;5:CD006066.

SUGGESTED READING

1. American College of Obstetricians and Gynecologists (2019). ACOG Committee Opinion: Limit Intervention during labour and birth. [online] Available from https://www.acog.org/Clinical-Guidance-and-Publications/Committee-Opinions/Committee-on-Obstetric-Practice/Approaches-to-Limit-Intervention-During-Labor-and-Birth?IsMobileSet=false. [Last accessed March, 2020].
2. American College of Obstetricians and Gynecologists. ACOG Practice Bulletin No. 106: Intrapartum fetal heart rate monitoring: nomenclature, interpretation, and general management principles. Obstet Gynecol. 2009;114(1):192-202.
3. Macones G. Management of intrapartum category I, II, and III fetal heart rate tracings. [online] Available from https://www.uptodate.com/contents/intrapartum-category-i-ii-and-iii-fetal-heart-rate-tracings-management. [Last accessed March, 2020].
4. National Institute for Health and Care Excellence. (2014). Intrapartum care (NICE guideline CG190). [online] Available from https://www.rcog.org.uk/en/guidelines-research-services/guidelines/intrapartum-care-care-of-healthy-women-and-their-babies-during-childbirth-nice-clinical-guideline-190/. [Last accessed March, 2020].

55 Forceps and Ventouse

Anuradha Singh

INTRODUCTION

Operative vaginal delivery refers to emergency assisted delivery using either ventouse cup or forceps for extraction of the baby. The choice of instrument depends upon skill of the operator, availability of instrument, and clinical circumstances. There is a wide variation in the rates of operative vaginal deliveries all over the world ranging from 1.5 to 15% with an average of 10%. There is a general decline in the rate of operative vaginal deliveries with ventouse becoming more popular.[1] Operative vaginal delivery has the potential for increased morbidity for both the mother and the baby. It is therefore important to perform operative vaginal delivery only when indicated by a skilled operator and after ensuring that all prerequisites are fulfilled.

INDICATIONS

The indications for performing operative vaginal delivery are listed in Box 1.

CONTRAINDICATIONS

There are a few contraindications for operative vaginal delivery and these are classified as relative or absolute (Table 1).

For a successful and safe operative vaginal delivery, all the prerequisites should be fulfilled irrespective of the urgency to deliver the baby (Box 2). A detailed abdominal and pelvic examination is required. For labor room procedures verbal consent should be obtained prior to assisted vaginal birth and discussion documented in the notes later on.

Box 1: Indications for operative vaginal delivery.

Maternal
- Maternal exhaustion, distress, and ineffective pushing
- Prolonged second stage (>2 hours in a primigravida and >1 hour in multigravida and 1 hour extra with epidural in both)
- *Compromised maternal condition*:
  - Cardiac disease—class III or IV
  - Pulmonary disease
  - Severe hypertension or eclampsia
  - Neurological disease with weakness

Fetal
- Suspected fetal compromise in the second stage of labor
- Fetal malposition [occiput transverse (OT) and occiput posterior (OP)]
- *Fetal malpresentation*: After-coming head of breech and face presentation
- Cord prolapse

VENTOUSE VERSUS FORCEPS EXTRACTION

When compared with forceps, there is increased incidence cephalohematoma, subgaleal, and retinal hemorrhage with ventouse delivery. It is less likely than forceps to result in successful vaginal delivery. There is less use of regional and general anesthesia, lesser serious maternal injuries and less pain after delivery.

Table 1: Contraindications for operative vaginal delivery.

Absolute contraindications	Relative contraindications
For both forceps and ventouse delivery: • Any contraindication to vaginal delivery • Inexperienced operator • Incompletely dilated cervix • Unknown fetal position • Unengaged head • Malpresentation, e.g., brow or face (mentoposterior) • Suspected CPD *Ventouse delivery:* • Preterm < 32 weeks gestation (risk of intracranial hemorrhage and cephalhematoma) • Face presentation, after-coming head of breech	• Baby has predisposition to fracture (e.g., osteogenesis imperfecta) • Baby diagnosed with or has a suspected bleeding disorder like hemophilia or alloimmune thrombocytopenia • Women on oral anticoagulants • Hepatitis B, hepatitis C and HIV due to increased risk of vertical transmission

(CPD: cephalopelvic disproportion; HIV: human immunodeficiency virus)

Box 2: Prerequisites for operative vaginal delivery.

- Head is engaged < one-fifth palpable (one pole) per abdomen
- Cervix should be fully dilated and effaced
- Membranes should be ruptured
- Favorable presentation
- Exact position of fetal head and asynclitism should be known
- Pelvis should be adequate
- Bladder should be empty
- Verbal and written informed consent documented in case notes
- Adequate analgesia and anesthesia: Pudendal block and/or perineal infiltration
- Facilities for emergency lower segment cesarean section (LSCS) in case of failed procedure

Whereas when compared with ventouse delivery, forceps delivery is less likely to result in neonatal morbidity, more likely to result in maternal soft-tissue injury, more likely to result in successful vaginal delivery over a shorter time frame, and suitable for assisted vaginal delivery of less than 32 weeks gestation. Unlike ventouse forceps can be applied for face presentation and after-coming head of breech.

FORCEPS DELIVERY

Classification of Forceps Delivery

Forceps delivery classification is based on two most important factors, which influence the risk of operative vaginal delivery to the mother and newborn; the station and rotation of the head (Box 3).

Rotational delivery carries an additional risk and requires specific expertise, and training. In this situation, manual rotation followed by forceps extraction or ventouse extraction is preferred.

About the Instrument

The forceps have two branches each comprising of a blade, shank, lock, and handle (Fig. 1). There are two curves, a pelvic curve which conforms to the curve of pelvic canal and a cephalic curve that conforms to the shape of fetal head. The blades are fenestrated and joined to the handle by a shank. The lock between the two blades can be an English lock or a sliding lock. Usually, it is an English lock. The functions of the instrument are traction and rotation. The correct application can be ascertained by certain points listed in Box 4.

Box 3: Classification of forceps deliveries (American College of Obstetricians and Gynecologists, 2015).[2]

Outlet forceps
- Scalp visible at introitus without separating labia
- Head is at or on the perineum
- Sagittal suture in anteroposterior (AP) diameter or right or left occiput anterior or posterior position
- Rotation does not exceed 45°

Low forceps
- Leading point of fetal skull is at ≥ +2 cm and not on the pelvic floor (station ≥ +2/5 cm station

It has two subdivisions:
- Rotation is ≤45°
- Rotation >45°

Mid-forceps rotational (Kielland)
- Head is engaged (at least 0 station) but leading point is above +2 cm station (that is 0 to +1/5 cm)

Box 4: Checking the appropriateness of forceps application.
- Forceps are easily locked
- Sagittal suture should be perpendicular to the plane of shanks of the forceps
- The blades should be equidistant from the sagittal suture in occipitoanterior position and from midline of face and brow in occipitoposterior position
- The posterior fontanel should be midway between the blades and one fingerbreadth above the plane of the shanks
- A small, but equal amount of fenestration should be felt on each blade

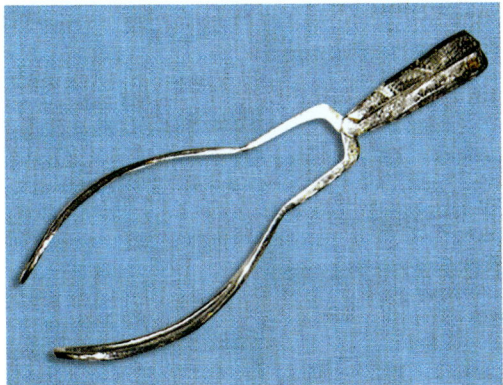

Fig. 1: Outlet forceps.

When correctly applied, the blades grasp the head at right angles to the submentovertical diameter. There is a greater likelihood of the forceps slipping if large amount of fenestration is palpable. If the application is not appropriate, the blades should be unlocked, removed, and reapplied.

Technique of Forceps Delivery

With the women in dorsal lithotomy position and after fulfilling the prerequisites, the two blades of the forceps are identified and locked (ghost application). The left blade is applied first by holding it in the left hand of the obstetrician parallel to the opposite inguinal ligament. It is applied on left side of maternal pelvis, while the operator's right hand displaces the posterior and lateral vaginal wall and guides the placement of the blade. Similarly, the right blade is inserted on the right side of maternal pelvis, while the left hand displaces the lateral and posterior vaginal wall and guides the placement of the blade. The blades are articulated. The appropriateness of application is checked and gentle traction is applied along the pelvic axis during uterine contractions intermittently.

There are two components of traction, i.e., direction and force. The direction of traction must be along the pelvic axis that is perpendicular to the various pelvic planes. It will depend on the station and position of head. The force of pull should be applied with a finger placed between the two shanks and keeping the forearms flexed. It is gradually increased with the uterine contraction and slowly released as the contraction passes off. The delivery should be accomplished with two to three pulls with application of moderate force or else procedure is abandoned.

As the head nears delivery episiotomy is given, if required. The forceps' blades are removed in the opposite order to application once head is nearly delivered. The perineum, vagina, and cervix are explored for any tears after the delivery of the baby. A single dose of intravenous amoxicillin and clavulanic acid is recommended to reduce maternal infection.

Complications

Forceps delivery may be associated with traumatic injuries to the mother and the baby. The frequency of occurrence can be minimized by properly selecting the cases and fulfilling all the prerequisites. The complications are listed in Table 2.

VENTOUSE DELIVERY

About the Instrument

Ventouse delivery essentially consists of a ventouse cup, which is applied to the fetal head and connected to a suction machine with connecting tubes. There are many types of cups available. They are broadly divided into rigid metal cups and soft silastic cups. These are available in various sizes ranging from 40 to 60 mm (Fig. 2). The soft cups are mostly wider 60 mm in diameter. The edge of the metal cup is curved so that the rim has a smaller diameter than the cavity. When the negative pressure is created after the cup is placed against the fetal scalp, the air is sucked out and the scalp is sucked into the cup to form a chignon. The silastic cup is wider malleable and trumpet shaped. Another hand held ventouse Kiwi OmniCup Vacuum is available (Fig. 3). It has the advantage of being small in size, single use, and obstetrician operated, but has higher failure rates compared to conventional cups.

A negative pressure of 0.8 kg/cm^2 is applied after the cup has been correctly placed and checked for any inclusion of maternal tissues. With metal cup, the pressure is raised gradually at the rate of 0.2 kg/cm^2 every 2 minutes to a maximum of 0.8 kg/cm^2.

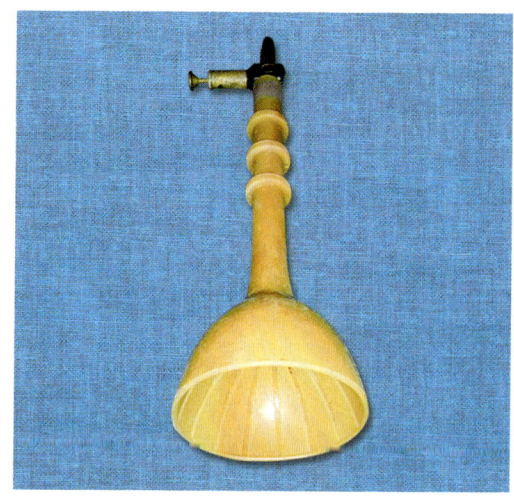

Fig. 2: Ventouse silastic cup.

Table 2: Complications of forceps delivery.

Maternal complications	Fetal complications
• Extension of episiotomy and anal sphincter laceration • Perineal tears, cervical tears, vaginal lacerations, and rarely uterine rupture • Postpartum hemorrhage • Retention of urine and urinary tract infection • Postpartum endometritis • Vesicovaginal and/or rectovaginal fistula • Urinary and/or rectal incontinence • Dyspareunia	• Intracranial hemorrhage • Tentorial tears with supratentorial, subdural or subarachnoid hemorrhage • Skull fractures • Facial nerve palsy • Facial laceration or abrasions • Injury to soft tissues, eyes, etc. • Retinal hemorrhage

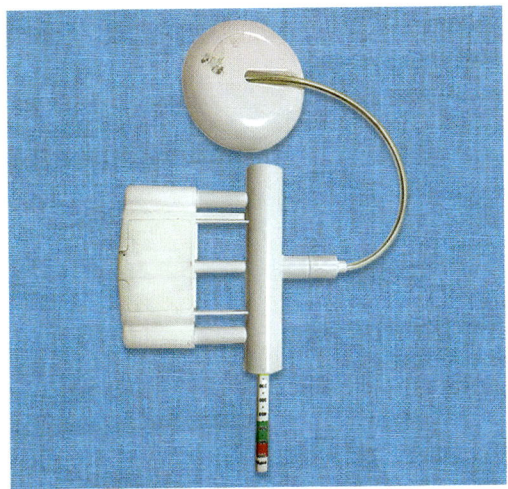

Fig. 3: Ventouse Kiwi OmniCup.

However, with soft cups the pressure can be increased to 0.8 kg/cm² within 1 minute. Soft cups have higher failure rates, but fewer scalp injuries compared to rigid cups.

Indications

They are essentially the same as that of forceps delivery. However, it is contraindicated in face or any other nonvertex presentations, fetal coagulopathy, recent scalp blood sampling, and in fetuses of <34 weeks gestation. It is used with caution in fetuses between 34 and 36 weeks gestation.

Technique

Vacuum extraction may be undertaken using rapid or gradual method of suction using either mechanical or electrical suction. Fetal injuries increase with increasing duration of procedure. It is essential to avoid shearing forces on the scalp to reduce the risk of subgaleal hematoma by proper application of cup and direction of pull.

The woman is positioned in dorsal lithotomy and after fulfilling prerequisites, and under all aseptic precautions, the cup is inserted in the vagina. The cup should be placed over the sagittal suture as near the occiput as possible to aid in flexion of head during traction. If applied anteriorly towards the anterior fontanel it will result in deflexion of the head.

If the fetal head is in posterior position, place the center of the cup over the flexion point, which is 3 cm in front of posterior fontanel over the sagittal suture. Aim to apply the cup as far back as possible. After the placement a check is made by sweeping a finger all around the cup to exclude entrapment of any maternal tissue beneath the cup. Negative pressure of 0.8 kg/m² is then created as mentioned above.

Traction in applied gently along the pelvic axis in coordination with maternal expulsive efforts and uterine contractions. Traction should be applied perpendicular to the fetal head with the right hand of the operator, while the left hand stabilizes the cup and detects the slipping of the cup early. No attempt is made to rotate the cup. By aiding in flexion of head, traction results in autorotation by bringing the occiput in contact with pelvic floor. The pressure is maintained in between the contractions. Adequate descent should be verified during each pull. If the cup dislodges it is reapplied. The negative pressure is released and cup removed once the head crowns or distends the perineum. The genital tract is explored for any injuries after the delivery.

If there is minimal or no descent after two consecutive pulls or the cup dislodges once senior support should be sought. The procedure is abandoned if there are two POP offs or fetal head does not come on to perineum after 3 pulls. If the head is on the perineum three additional gentle pulls can be used to ease the head. Sequential use of ventouse and forceps may result in increased maternal and neonatal morbidity and is discouraged except in the hands of an experienced and skilled obstetrician.

Table 3: Complications of ventouse delivery.

Maternal complications	Fetal injuries
• Suction injury to the vaginal mucosa or cervix by getting included under the cup • Perineal trauma • Postpartum hemorrhage	• Superficial scalp injuries • Cephalohematoma • Subgaleal hematoma • Intracranial hemorrhage • Jaundice • Retinal hemorrhage • Neonatal mortality especially with subgaleal hematoma

The reasons for a failed ventouse delivery include improper placement of cup, incorrect application of traction; either oblique to fetal head or not along the axis of pelvic canal, presence of a large caput following prolonged second stage, inadequate suction due to faulty equipment or inclusion of vaginal, or cervical tissue under the cup and an inexperienced operator.

Complications

There are more fetal injuries than maternal injuries with ventouse delivery as compared to forceps delivery. The maternal and fetal complications associated with ventouse delivery are given in Table 3.

The superficial scalp injuries and cephalohematoma have a good prognosis, but subgaleal or subaponeurotic hematoma is associated with a high neonatal mortality.

For safe ventouse delivery it is recommended that same classification, indications, and contraindications should be observed as are applicable for forceps. Ventouse should not be applied to unengaged head that is leading bony point above zero station. It should be applied by an experienced operator and the operator should abandon the procedure if there is no descent with three pulls or the cup dislodges two times with traction.

KEY POINTS

- Operative vaginal delivery has a definite place in modern obstetrics.
- Thorough knowledge of the indications, contraindications, and prerequisites is essential for the obstetricians to decide regarding the most suitable mode of delivery for each woman.
- Both forceps and ventouse are potentially hazardous in inexperienced hands.
- Choosing the right instrument and applying it skillfully can result in optimum outcome.
- Informed consent and documentation is important for avoiding medicolegal litigations in the unfortunate event of adverse outcome.
- Single dose IV prophylactic antibiotic is indicated.

REFERENCES

1. Bofll JA, Rust OA, Perry KG, Roberts WE, Martin RW, Morrison JC. Operative vaginal delivery: a survey of fellows of ACOG. Obstet Gynecol. 1996;88(6):1007-10.
2. Committee on Practice Bulletins—Obstetrics. Practice Bulletin No. 154 Summary: Operative Vaginal Delivery. Obstet Gynecol. 2015;126: 1118-9.

SUGGESTED READING

1. Hobson S, Cassell K, Windrim R, Cargill Y. No. 381-Assisted Vaginal Birth. J Obstet Gyanecol Can. 2019;41:870-82.
2. RCOG (2020). Operative Vaginal Delivery (Green-top Guideline No. 26). [online] Available from https://www.rcog.org.uk/en/guidelines-research-services/guidelines/gtg26/.

56 Contraception

Harkiran Kaur Narang, Anju Yadav

INTRODUCTION

Regulation of fertility is one of the many traits that make us human. From 1921, when Marie Stopes set up the first birth control clinic in UK, we have come a long way in acceptability and practice of contraception. The question in the minds of many people today is not whether to use contraception or not but rather which method to use. In a couple not using any contraceptive method, the fertility rate is 80–90% in 1 year.

An ideal contraceptive is one that can offer total protection against pregnancy, is convenient to use, and is free from side effects. We do not have one yet, but we have come quite close to it. The availability of many methods to choose from has led to the "cafeteria approach" to contraception, which involves couples making an informed choice regarding the method they wish to use. The use of contraceptive not only helps couples in controlling their family size but also protects the women from morbid after effects of an unintended pregnancy.

The methods of contraception can be classified as given in Table 1.

Contraceptive methods are of two types: (1) User dependent and (2) method depend-

Table 1: Methods of contraception.

Temporary methods	Permanent methods	Emergency contraceptives

• Natural methods
• *Barrier methods*:
  – *Male*: Condoms
  – *Female*:
    » Condoms
    » Cervical caps
    » Diaphragms
    » Sponge
• *Intrauterine devices*:
  – Hormonal
  – Nonhormonal (including postpartum intrauterine device)
• *Hormonal methods*:
  – Combined (E + P): Pills, patches, rings, and injectables
  – Progestogen-only pills, injectables, and implants
• *Nonhormonal pills*: Centchroman
	• *Male*: Vasectomy
	• *Female*: Tubectomy
	  – Laparoscopic
	  – MiniLap
	  – Vaginal
	  – With laparotomy or cesarean section
		• Hormones:
		  – Levonorgestrel
		  – Combined oral contraceptive pills
		  – Ulipristal acetate
		• Copper intrauterine contraceptive device

ent. User-dependent methods include oral contraception, patches, barrier methods, and fertility awareness-based methods, all of which need compliance of the user to be effective. Method-dependent contraceptives once accepted, are effective till the method expires. Long-acting reversible contraceptives (LARCs), such as intrauterine contraceptive devices (IUCDs) and implants, are method dependent. The failure rates with "user-dependent contraceptive" methods are more than those with "method-dependent contraceptive" methods.

Table 2: World Health Organization (WHO) eligibility criteria for contraception.[1]

WHO eligibility criteria for contraception	Category
A condition for which there is no restriction for use of the contraceptive method	1
A condition, where the advantages of using the method generally outweigh the theoretical or proven risks	2
A condition, where the theoretical or proven risks usually outweigh the advantages of using the method	3
A condition, which represents an unacceptable health risk if the contraceptive method is used	4

Counseling

Counseling is the process of helping a woman make an informed and voluntary decision about the method she wants to accept for contraception. It should follow the GATHER (Greet, Ask, Tell, Help, Explain, and Return) approach (refer to Chapter 57 on Medical Termination of Pregnancy and Sterilization).

PRESCRIBING A CONTRACEPTIVE: WHAT TO BEAR IN MIND?

Not all contraceptives are suitable for everyone and everyone has different requirements. It is mandatory to take a detailed history and do a thorough examination before prescribing any contraceptive. Reference to the World Health Organization (WHO) medical eligibility criteria (MEC)[1] is useful in assessing the suitability and safety of any contraceptive method in each clinical scenario. The WHO MEC classify the contraceptive use into four categories, according to the safety of the method in any clinical condition (Table 2).

Natural or Conventional Methods

These include breastfeeding, abstinence, sex without penile–vaginal intercourse, coitus interruptus (withdrawal method), and fertility awareness methods.

Breastfeeding

Breastfeeding can be used as an effective method of contraception for 6 months provided the woman practices exclusive breastfeeding, i.e., no substitute breastmilk and interval between feeds not >6 hours and menstrual period has not returned. This is also known as lactational amenorrhea method (LAM). Frequent sucking causes a high level of prolactin secretion in the mother with suppression of ovulation. It is 98% effective during first 6 months postpartum, if menses have not resumed and if the woman is exclusively breastfeeding.

It is economical, effective, promotes bonding between mother and baby, decreases the postpartum blood loss, and helps in involution of uterus. It is also helpful in postpartum weight loss.

Coitus Interruptus (Withdrawal Method)

During sexual intercourse, erect penis is withdrawn just before ejaculation by the partner.

Semen is discharged outside the vagina. It is a widely practiced method all over the world, in all cultures and by people of all religions. It has a high failure rate due to deposition of sperm through pre-ejaculate secretions or occasionally deposition of small quantity of semen in vagina before withdrawal. It is 70–85% effective.

It is acceptable to many religious groups and societies, cost effective, and used widely all over the world. Responsibility for contraception is shared by the male partner. There are no side effects. However, it is not suitable for those with premature ejaculation, who cannot control their buildup to ejaculate, and adolescents. It does not offer protection against sexually transmitted disease (STD) and acquired immunodeficiency syndrome (AIDS).

Fertility Awareness Methods

Women learn to recognize the fertile days of the menstrual cycle over several months and avoid intercourse or use the barrier methods on those days. Fertility awareness methods include the following: calendar method, basal body temperature (BBT), cervical mucus method, and sympto-thermal method.

Fertilization is avoided by abstinence or by use of barrier method preventing the sperm from entering the cervix and uterus during the fertile phase of the cycle. These are 80–90% effective.

These methods have no physical side effects. These are free and inexpensive, responsibility is shared by both partners, and are acceptable to all religions and cultures; their effectiveness and use can be increased by concomitant use of the barrier method during the preovulatory phase (first half of the cycle) and fertile period. Training the couples in these methods also increases awareness and knowledge about reproduction. However, they do not offer protection against STD and AIDS.

The disadvantages are that training in the method is required by a counselor. It requires abstinence or use of barrier method to be practiced for 10-15 days in each cycle. It demands commitment from both partners. It is not effective with irregular cycles and infection. Spermicidal use interferes with the mucous method. Febrile conditions interfere with the BBT method.

- *Calendar (rhythm) method*: The woman keeps a record of six menstrual cycles and then calculate the fertile days. From the record, the longest and shortest cycles are chosen. Subtract 20 from the shortest cycle and 10 from the longest cycle some use 18 and 11 days, respectively, e.g., shortest cycle is 26 days and longest cycle is 34 days (26−20 = 6 and 34−10 = 24). The abstinence or barrier method must be practiced from day 6 to day 24 of the cycle.
- *Basal body temperature*: This method identifies the day of ovulation but not the beginning of the fertile period. Hence, for the effectiveness of this method, intercourse is to be avoided during the first half of the cycle until 3 days after the temperature has risen or backup barrier method can be used. Record the temperature every morning before getting up from bed as soon as the woman is awake. The special BBT thermometer is useful. Record the temperature on BBT chart as a dot and connect the dots with a line. When BBT has risen 0.2–0.5°F and remains elevated for 3 days, the fertile phase is over.
- *Cervical mucus method*: Fertile period is indicated by a sensation of wetness at vulva or when vaginal discharge increases. To observe mucus, one can wipe vulva with a tissue paper when one

feels or sees mucus. The partner should use condom till 4 days after the peak symptom day. Peak symptom day is the day of maximum mucus. Spermicides, vaginal infection, drugs, and intercourse can affect normal pattern of a woman's cervical mucus. Mucus can be recorded on daily basis in a chart.

- *Sympto-thermal method*: This method combines cervical mucus method and BBT. Beginning of fertile period is indicated by cervical mucus or even by calendar method and the end of fertile period by BBT. Fertile period ends 4 days after peak mucus or 3 days after sustained rise of BBT, whichever is later.

Barrier Methods

Barrier methods consist of two components—mechanical and chemical, and are available for both male and female partners. The concept is to create a barrier between the cervicovaginal surface and the ejaculate.

Male and female condoms also protect against acquisition of sexually transmitted infections (STIs). Thus, they have the additional benefit of reducing the risk of ectopic pregnancy and tubal factor infertility.

The success of barrier methods is largely dependent on the user. Failure rates with typical usage are double or more than that with ideal usage.[2]

Condoms

Condoms can be used as a primary or as an additional method of contraception with other methods for double protection. Various types of condoms available are—latex, nonlatex (silicone), and deproteinized latex. They are about 15–20 cm in length, 3–3.5 cm in diameter, and 0.003–0.007 cm in thickness,

lubricated or nonlubricated. When using additional lubricants with latex condoms, water or silicone-based lubricants are recommended as oil-based lubricants can damage latex. The use of condoms lubricated with nonoxynol-9 is not recommended as there is no evidence that this improves the efficacy.

Male condoms (Fig. 1) are 98% effective in preventing pregnancy, but only when used consistently and correctly.[3] The failure rate ranges from 2 to 20%. Failure rate is 2% in a perfect user but about 20% in a typical user. Besides inconsistent or incorrect use, failure can also be due to condom breakage or slippage. Breakage rates range from 1 to 8 per 100 episodes of vaginal intercourse and slippage from 1 to 5 per 100 episodes.[4] Breakage rates are higher with anal intercourse.

Female condoms (Fig. 2) are also available and are made of polyurethane and prelubricated with silicone. They serve the same functions as male condoms but have higher failure rates, are costlier, and are more

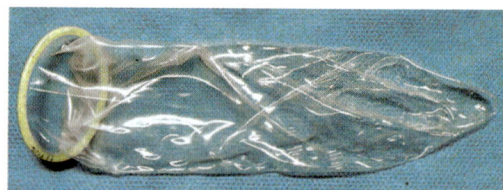

Fig. 1: Male condom.

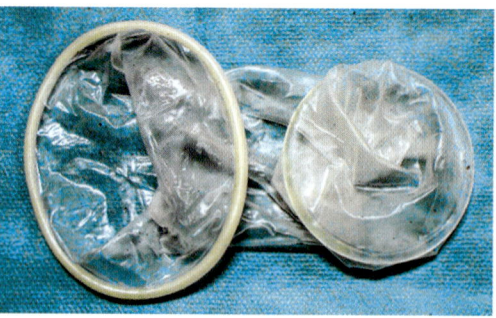

Fig. 2: Female condom.

cumbersome to use. High slippage rates are associated with its use. Additional spermicide need not be used.

Technique of use of male condom: The couple should be counseled that for condom to be effective as a contraceptive method, it should be used for every act of intercourse, irrespective of whether the woman is in the safe or unsafe period of menstrual cycle. The male partner is counseled to roll it over an erect penis after pinching the tip of the condom just before inserting penis in the vagina. This will provide some space at the tip of condom to accommodate the ejaculated semen and prevent overflow of the semen and resultant failure. After the sexual intercourse, it should be removed along with the penis from the vagina before erection is lost, holding the edge of the condom at the base of the penis to prevent any spillage of semen. It should then be discarded carefully after tying a knot at the top to prevent spillage and wrapping it in a paper.

Spermicides

Spermicides comprise a chemical or a surface-active agent capable of destroying sperms and are available in various forms or vehicles such as tablets, pessaries, creams, jellies, foam tablets, and contraceptive films. The failure rate with a typical user is 29% compared to 18% in a perfect user.[2]

They may be used in addition to any method but are required to be used with vaginal caps and diaphragms. They need to be reapplied for every act of intercourse and can prove messy to use. The disadvantage beside the high failure rate is possible allergy, vaginal dryness, or soreness.[4]

Contraceptive Sponge

Contraceptive sponge is a system for sustained release of spermicide and absorption of semen. It is inserted vaginally after moistening. Its efficacy is higher than spermicidal jellies and tablets, but since it does not come in different sizes, parous women are likely to have higher failure rates.

Vaginal Diaphragm

Vaginal diaphragm is a safe method of contraception with minimal side effects. It is a circular membrane of latex or silicone attached peripherally to a rim. It comes in sizes ranging from 50 to 105 mm in diameter with increments of 2.5–5 mm. The correct size is the largest that be comfortably fitted behind the pubic symphysis to the posterior fornix.

Successful use of the diaphragm depends on the fit, which in turn is dependent on the vaginal and perineal musculature. The size should be assessed by the healthcare provider. Weight gain or loss and vaginal delivery can alter the vaginal caliber thus necessitating an annual check for the size. The failure rate is 16% in a typical user compared to 6% in a perfect user.[2]

Risks: Urinary tract infections are two- to three-fold more common among diaphragm users than among women using oral contraception.[4] Possible explanations could be incomplete voiding due to urethral compression, perineal handling at the time of insertion, and removal or alteration of the vaginal flora by spermicide leading to bacteriuria with *Escherichia coli*. Improper fitting or prolonged retention can cause vaginal erosions.

Storage: Natural latex rubber will degrade over time. Depending on usage and storage conditions, latex diaphragm should be replaced every 1–3 years. Silicone diaphragms may last much longer up to 10 years. Upon removal, a diaphragm should be cleansed with warm water and a mild unperfumed soap before storage in a cool, dry place. It should not be cleaned with detergent. The diaphragm must be removed for cleaning at least once every 24 hours and can be reinserted immediately.[5]

It is advisable to check the diaphragm for any holes or tears prior to use. Any discoloration, however, does not decrease the efficacy.

Vault Cap

In women with vaginal laxity or prolapse, a diaphragm will not stay in position anteriorly and a vault cap is indicated. This fits in the vaginal vault covering the cervix and suction is maintained by contact between the entire rim of the cap and the vaginal fornices. The bowl of the cap is shallow and will therefore accommodate a short cervix.

Cervical Cap

Cervical caps are used with a spermicidal cream or jelly and are fitted on the mouth of the cervix. For a better fit and effectiveness, it is important that the cervix is parallel sided. If it is conical or points backward, there is a risk that the cap will dislodge during intercourse. It is available in various types, latex or silicone, and in various sizes. The reported failure rates with a nulliparous typical user is 16% compared to 9% in a perfect user and the failure rates are double in multiparous women.[2]

There is no evidence that the use of cervical caps causes dysplastic changes in the cervix. Use of spermicides and or diaphragms with spermicide can disrupt the cervical mucosa, which may lead to increased viral shedding and human immunodeficiency virus (HIV) transmission to uninfected sexual partners. There is little evidence that these methods reduce the rate of HIV transmission.[3]

Diaphragms and caps should be inserted no longer than 3 hours prior to intercourse with spermicidal cream or jelly. Spermicide should be reapplied if sex is to take place and the diaphragm or cap has been in situ for 3 or more hours, or if sex is repeated with the method in place. A diaphragm or cap should not be removed until at least 6 hours after the last episode of intercourse.

In women with history of toxic shock syndrome, diaphragms and caps are in category 3 of the WHO eligibility criteria.

Intrauterine Contraceptive Devices

Mechanism of Action

All intrauterine devices (IUDs) including inert devices exert a foreign body reaction including infiltration of endometrium with leukocytes and macrophages. Copper can enhance this reaction as well as cause alteration in local fluids that impair the viability of gametes and impede fertilization.

Levonorgestrel intrauterine system (LNG-IUS) works by its effect on cervical mucus and endometrium by preventing sperm penetration and fertilization, respectively. Condoms or abstinence need to be advised for 7 days after inserting LNG-IUS unless the current contraceptive method is still effective to allow for the time it becomes effective.

Types of Intrauterine Devices

Intrauterine devices can be nonhormonal or hormonal. The various types of IUDs have special characteristics and duration of action. The details of each are as described in Table 3.

The differences between hormonal and nonhormonal devices are listed in Table 4.

Table 3: Details of various types of intrauterine devices.

Copper (Cu) devices	Lifespan	Remarks
CuT 380A (Figs. 3 and 4)	8–10 years	Barium-impregnated polyethylene frame with a copper wire and two copper sleeves on horizontal arms providing a surface area of 380 mm^2
CuT 380Ag	4 years	Barium-impregnated polyethylene frame with a copper wire and with a silver core to prevent fragmentation and increase the life of copper
Multiload 375	5 years	Flexible arms with plastic fins on the horizontal arms to decrease expulsion
Cu SAFE	5 years	Bent horizontal arms to accommodate inside the uterine cavity
LNG-IUS (Figs. 5A and B)	5 years	T-shaped device with a collar attached to the vertical arm containing 52 mg levonorgestrel, released initially at a rate of 20 µg/day
Progestasert	1 year	Vertical arm contains a capsule with 38 mg progesterone releasing at a rate of 65 µg/day

(LNG-IUS: levonorgestrel intrauterine system)

Table 4: Comparison of hormonal and nonhormonal intrauterine devices.

	Copper T 380A	LNG-IUS
Blood loss	More	Less
Dysmenorrhea	More	Less, used for treatment of dysmenorrhea
Expulsion	Less	More
Failure rate	0.8% in first year of use	0.2% in first year of use
Effect	8–10 years	5 years

(LNG-IUS: levonorgestrel intrauterine system)

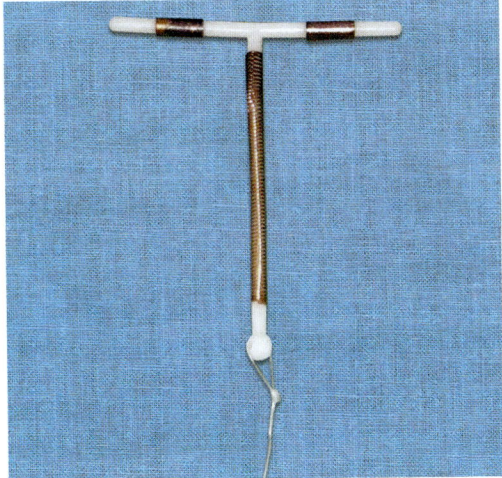

Fig. 3: Copper T 380A.

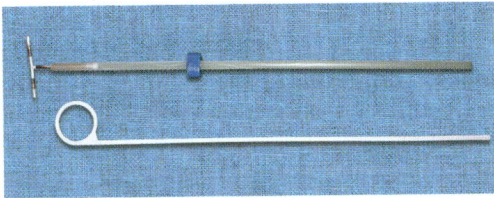

Fig. 4: Copper T with applicator.

Technique for insertion

Pre-insertion: Provided it is reasonably certain that the woman is not pregnant, an IUD or IUS may be inserted at any time during the menstrual cycle, but for the LNG-IUS, if the woman is amenorrheic or it is >5 days

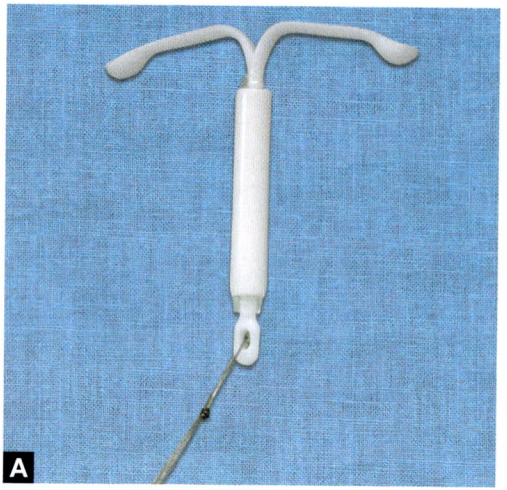
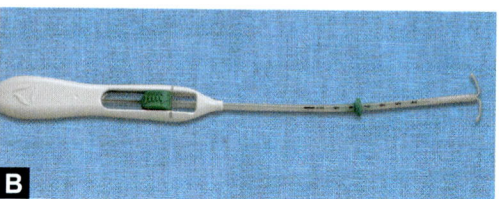

Figs. 5A and B: Hormonal intrauterine contraceptive device. (A) Levonorgestrel intrauterine system; (B) Levonorgestrel intrauterine system with applicator.

since her period started, she should use barrier contraception for the first 7 days after insertion.[6]

Intrauterine devices can be inserted immediately after first or second trimester abortion or postplacental, i.e., within 10 minutes of the delivery of placenta, or postpartum within 48 hours of delivery and at any time after the abortion or 4 weeks postpartum, irrespective of the mode of delivery.

The clinical history should be taken as a part of the routine assessment for intrauterine contraception to assess suitability of the woman for use of the method and to identify those at increased risk of STIs. This includes women, who are under 25 years of age, have more than one partner, or if woman's regular partner has other partners. Bimanual examination should be done to rule out pelvic inflammatory disease. Prophylactic antibiotics may be offered to those at high risk of STIs.[4]

Vasovagal syncope may occur at the time of insertion due to cervical dilatation. This may in turn increase the risk of seizures in patients with epilepsy. Local application of lignocaine jelly, paracervical block, or non-steroidal anti-inflammatory drugs (NSAIDs) given 2 hours prior to insertion can ease the pain associated with insertion. Transient bacteremia following replacement of IUCD has been identified but does not warrant antibiotic prophylaxis for endocarditis. In women with previous endocarditis or a prosthetic heart valve replacement, intravenous antibiotic prophylaxis is required to protect the woman against bacterial endocarditis during IUD insertion or removal.

Insertion: After ensuring that the eligibility criteria are fulfilled, i.e., the woman has regular menstrual cycles with normal flow is in a stable monogamous relationship, has low risk for STIs, and is not pregnant, an informed consent is taken. The woman is asked to evacuate her bladder. She is asked to lie in dorsal position with legs drawn up and buttocks at the edge of the table. A per speculum and per vaginal examination is done to rule out any cervical or vaginal pathology and pelvic inflammatory disease and to note the size and position of the uterus.

The posterior vaginal wall is retracted with Sims' speculum and anterior lip of cervix is held with vulsellum. The cervix is cleaned with a betadine swab. Uterine sound is introduced and uterocervical length is measured. The guard on the inserter is adjusted according to the measured uterocervical length and the horizontal limbs of the copper (Cu) T (see Fig. 4) are inserted in the inserter by a no-touch technique. The tip of the plunger is placed in contact with the end of the vertical limb of CuT. The whole assembly is introduced in the uterine cavity keeping the plunger in same position till the guard is in contact with the external os. The plunger is stabilized and the inserter is withdrawn to release the Cu device in the uterine cavity and then both the plunger and inserter are removed together. The threads attached to the device are trimmed to about 1 inch from the external os. The instruments are removed, and the client is handed over the cut threads and made to feel them to apprise her of what to feel when she puts her finger in the vagina for checking the threads postmenstrual.

Postinsertion: The woman should be offered advice to check the IUD threads after menses and seek medical assistance at the earliest if she cannot feel the threads. A routine follow-up visit is suggested after the first menses following the insertion. The woman is counseled regarding the likelihood of heavy periods for first 3–6 months for which she is prescribed some hemostatic agent such as tranexamic acid 1 g every 6–8 hours and a hematinic preparation to prevent anemia. She is informed of the danger signals such as lower abdomen pain, foul-smelling vaginal discharge, fever, missed periods, and missing threads, and asked to report immediately to the hospital.

Any copper IUD fitted after the age of 40 years can be left in situ until the menopause. The IUS lasts for 5 years but, if fitted after the age of 45 years and the woman remains amenorrheic, it can stay in place until the menopause.[7]

Contraindications

The contraindications to the use of copper and progesterone-containing IUDs are tabulated in Box 1.

Side Effects and Complications

The risk of developing pelvic inflammatory disease following IUD insertion is very low, <1 in 100 in women at low risk of STIs. It is

Box 1: Contraindications for use of intrauterine device.

Medical eligibility criteria (MEC) category 3 or 4:
- Distortion of uterine cavity
- Evidence of STD/PID/genital TB/puerperal sepsis/postabortion sepsis
- HIV WHO stage 3 or 4 (can be continued if condition develops while using the method)
- Unexplained vaginal bleeding
- Cervical cancer
- Persistently elevated or declining hCG levels in GTN
- Insertion > 48 hours or < 4 weeks postpartum
- *For Cu devices*: Severe thrombocytopenia
- *For LNG-IUS*:
  – Acute DVT/PE
  – Ischemic stroke
  – History of breast cancer
  – Liver tumor

Note: LNG-IUS may be useful in the treatment of menorrhagia associated with thrombocytopenia.[8]
(DVT: deep vein thrombosis; GTN: gestational trophoblastic neoplasia; hCG: human chronic gonadotropin; HIV: human immunodeficiency virus; LUG-IUS: levonorgestrel intrauterine system; STD: sexually transmitted disease; PE: pulmonary embolism; PID: pelvic inflammatory disease; TB: tuberculosis; WHO: World Health Organization)

maximum within the first 21 days of insertion and is usually due to preexisting infection with chlamydia or gonorrhea.

Intrauterine devices may be expelled, but the incidence is 2–8%; maximum expulsion is in the first 3 months of insertion.

The overall risk of ectopic pregnancy with IUD is very low, at about 0.1% in 5 years. The EURAS–IUD study reported an ectopic pregnancy rate for the 52 mg LNG-IUS of 0.02 per 100 woman-years and for the Cu-IUD, a rate of 0.08 per 100 woman-years.

If a woman becomes pregnant with IUD in situ, the risk of ectopic pregnancy is about 1 in 20 and she should seek advice to exclude ectopic pregnancy.[6] The overall risk of ectopic pregnancy is reduced with the use of IUDs, as compared to the women not using any contraception. No device is associated with a lower rate of ectopic pregnancy. There is no delay in return to fertility.

Follow-up and Management of Problems

The first follow-up visit is recommended after the first menses or 3–6 weeks after insertion to exclude infection, perforation, or expulsion. For heavier and/or prolonged bleeding associated with use of an IUD, NSAIDs and/or tranexamic acid are useful. Irregular bleeding is common with LNG-IUS for the first 6 months followed by amenorrhea. Dysmenorrhea increases with copper devices and decreases with LNG-IUS.

If a woman becomes pregnant with an intrauterine pregnancy, advise removal of the IUD or IUS before 12 weeks' gestation, whether she intends to continue the pregnancy or not. Limited evidence suggests that removal of IUD where possible by 12 weeks can help reduce but not eliminate the risks of infection, miscarriage, and preterm labor.

In women presenting with history of missing threads, after eliciting the history whether the device has been expelled or not, a per speculum and per vaginal examination is done. Per speculum examination to see if the threads are lying coiled in the vagina and per vaginal examination to rule out pregnancy as sometimes the threads are pulled up due to the enlarging uterus. If the threads are not visualized on per speculum examination and pregnancy is ruled out, then an ultrasound examination of the uterus is indicated to see if the device is in the uterine cavity. If the uterine cavity is empty, a plain X-ray of lower abdomen and pelvis, both anteroposterior and lateral views, with a uterine sound or a fresh IUD inserted in uterine cavity is offered to visualize the lost IUD and appreciate its relative position to the uterus and pelvis.

Postpartum IUCD

Immediate postpartum period is an ideal time to educate and counsel a woman for contraception to promote spacing or limiting family. Postpartum IUCD (PPIUCD) is an ideal method to fulfil any of the above objectives. Both CuT 380A and CuT 375 are approved for this purpose. PPIUCD can be postplacental inserted within 10 minutes of placental expulsion following vaginal delivery, intracesarean, i.e., during cesarean, after placental delivery, before closing the uterine incision, or within 48 hours of vaginal delivery. IUCD should not be inserted from 48 hours to 6 weeks following delivery due to the risk of infection and expulsion.

Counseling: The ideal time for counseling for PPIUCD is antenatal period and it is documented on the antenatal card. But it can be done during admission to labor room in early labor or before elective CS or on first postpartum day. The woman should not be

Box 2: Contraindications of PPIUCD.
MEC 3 and MEC 4 Criteria for PPIUCD: • Between 48 hours and 6 weeks after delivery • Chorioamnionitis • Prolonged rupture of membrane >18 hours • Puerperal sepsis • Unresolved PPH

(MEC: medical eligibility criteria; PPIUCD: Postpartum IUCD; PPH: postpartum hemorrhage)

Box 3: Advantages and disadvantages of PPIUCD.
Advantages: • Convenient, saves time and additional visit • Safe, as it is certain that woman is not pregnant • High motivation of client and family members for an effective spacing method • No risk of uterine perforation as the wall of the contracted uterus is thick • Reduced perception of initial side effects such as bleeding and cramps due to normal puerperal changes • Reduced chances of heavy bleeding due to lactational amenorrhea • No effect on quality of milk • Woman has an effective method of contraception before discharge from the hospital • Convenient for the service provider as it is certain that woman is not pregnant, convenient as it does not require additional evaluation, minimal requirements of instruments, equipment, and helps reduce the overcrowding of outpatient facilities *Disadvantage*: The limitations are same as that with interval insertion, except that the risk of expulsion is higher

counseled for the first time in active phase of labor as she may not be able to exercise free choice due to stress.

The key messages for PPIUCD include the importance of initiating family planning method soon after delivery as fertility may return within 4–6 weeks if not breastfeeding.

Contraindications: The contraindications MEC category 3 and 4 for PPIUD are listed in Box 2.

Advantages and disadvantages: The advantages and disadvantages of PPIUCD are listed in Box 3.

Hormonal Contraception

Hormonal contraceptives can be either combined estrogen and progesterone or progesterone-only contraceptives. The combined estrogen and progesterone contraceptives are available as oral pills, patches, vaginal rings, or injectable preparations. The progesterone-only contraceptives are available as pills, implants, and injectable preparations. The failure rates of all combined preparations are 8% in a typical user and 0.3% in a perfect user.[2]

Combined Oral Contraceptive Pills

Mechanism of action: The combined oral contraceptive (COC) pills work primarily by inhibiting ovulation through their action on the hypothalamic–pituitary–ovarian axis by lowering the levels of luteinizing hormone (LH) and follicle-stimulating hormones. The progesterone component mediates through changes in cervical mucus preventing sperm penetration and changes in endometrium that interfere with implantation.

Classification of combined oral contraceptive pills: Combined oral contraceptive pills are classified into various generations based on the estrogen content and progesterone component. All modern pills are low-dose pills containing <50 μg of ethinyl estradiol (EE). The third-generation pills contain newer progesterones, which have lesser metabolic and androgenic effects but higher risk of venous thromboembolism. The classification of COCs is given in Table 5.

The pills can be monophasic or multiphasic. In monophasic pills, same dose of estrogen and progesterone is administered throughout the cycle; however, in multiphasic

Table 5: Classification of combined oral contraceptive pills.	
Generation	Composition
First generation (Figs. 6A and B)	EE 50 µg + LNG or norethindrone
Second generation	EE 20, 30, 35 µg + LNG or norethindrone (see Fig. 4)
Third generation	EE 20, 30, 35 µg + Desogestrel, gestodene, or norgestimate

(EE: ethinyl estradiol; LNG: levonorgestrel)

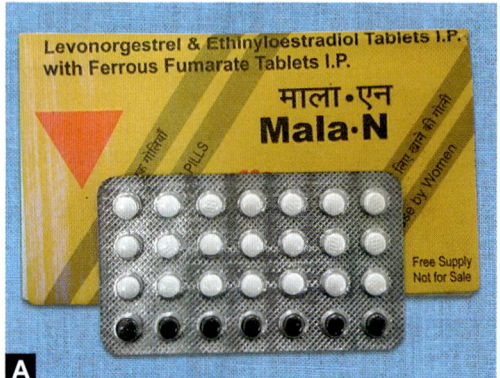 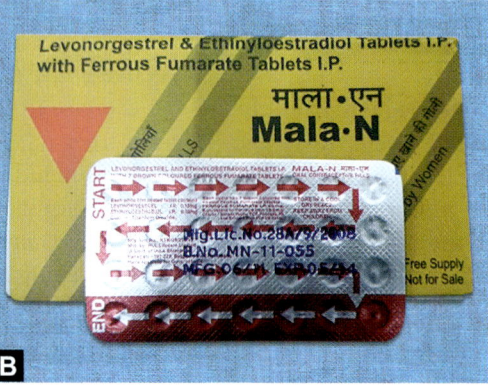

Figs. 6A and B: Mala N combined oral contraceptive pills. (A) Front view; (B) Back view.

pills, the estrogen and progesterone content of the pills varies with the phase of cycle and simulates the hormonal changes of a normal cycle. The advantage of the multiphasic pills is lesser amount of hormone administration per cycle.

The combined or oral contraceptive pills, such as Mala N tablets containing 30 µg of EE and 150 µg LNG, are supplied free of cost by the Government of India (GOI). Each packet has 28 tablets, 21 active tablets, and 7 iron-containing tablets. The back side of the pack gives the directions on where to start the packet from (Figs. 6A and B).

Regimes: Tailored regimes for monophasic preparations can be prescribed. The conventional regime is a 21 days' cycle. However, lately extended duration regime has been introduced, which include continuous intake of pills for 3–4 months and pill-free intervals of either 4 days or the conventional 7 days. Extended duration of pill intake lowers the frequency of bleeding episodes and is preferred by many women. Shortened pill-free intervals also decrease the amount of bleeding in the cycle and reduce the contraceptive failure rate by reducing the risk of breakthrough ovulation.

Contraindications: The contraindications to oral contraceptive pills are listed in Table 6.

When to start:

Conventional start: It is started from day 1 up to and including day 5 of normal menses or abortion. It can be started after 6 months of delivery in lactating mothers after confirming that the woman is not pregnant and from day 21 if not lactating.

Quick start: Combined pills can be started at any time, provided it is certain that the woman is not pregnant.

Table 6: Contraindications to oral contraceptive pills.[1]

WHO category 3	WHO category 4
Age >35 years, smoker or stopped smoking for <1 year	Age >35 years, smoker, smoking >15 cigarettes per day
Body mass index ≥35	Current ischemic heart disease/stroke
Moderate hypertension (systolic blood pressure 140–159 or diastolic 90–99 mm Hg)	Severe hypertension (systolic >160 mm Hg or diastolic >100 mm Hg) multiple risk factors for arterial cardiovascular disease such as older age, smoking, diabetes mellitus, and hypertension
History of breast cancer of >5 years back	Current breast cancer
Family history of venous thromboembolism in first-degree relative <45 years of age	Past or current history of venous thromboembolism in the woman or positive for antiphospholipid antibodies or thrombogenic mutations
Immobility unrelated to surgery	Major surgery with prolonged immobilization

Side effects: Some patients experience nausea with the pill. If the patient vomits within 3 hours of ingestion of the pill, it is advisable to take it again. Antiemetics may be prescribed initially to prevent pill-associated nausea. Cyclical weight gain, bloatedness, water retention, headaches, and breast tenderness are also seen. It is less with low-dose estrogen-containing pills. Headaches are one of the most common side effects and reduce with duration of use.

One of the most important side effects is breakthrough bleeding. It mostly occurs during the first three cycles of pill use as the endometrium adapts itself to lesser thickness and decidualization. It is important to rule out local causes, pregnancy, and errors in pill taking prior to assigning the cause of bleeding as breakthrough bleeding. Taking the pill with enzyme-inducing drugs such as rifampicin, and antiepileptics can also cause bleeding and reduce the efficacy of the pills.

Risks: The absolute risk of venous thromboembolism (VTE) with combined pill use is 5–12/100,000 woman-years; an increase up to 3–5.5 fold compared with nonusers 2/100,000 woman-years, but the absolute risk is still low, and considerably lower than the risk in pregnancy 60/100,000 woman-years. It is more with third-generation pills compared to second-generation pills 25/100,000 woman-years versus 15/100,000 woman-years.[9]

The risk of VTE is highest in the first 4 months following initiation of combined hormonal contraception. The risk reduces after 1 year and remains stable thereafter. It remains higher than that of nonusers until the contraceptive is stopped. The risk also increases with age, restarting the pill after a break of at least 1 month and in the presence of other risk factors. Risk increases with doses of EE >50 µg.

Newer combined pills with drospirenone have the same risk profile as the second-generation pills. Diane (cyproterone with EE) is not licensed for contraceptive use alone as it has a higher risk of VTE than conventional low or standard-dose pills.

Levonorgestrel, norethisterone and its prodrugs (such as ethynodiol diacetate) cause slight decrease in high-density lipoprotein (HDL) cholesterol levels. This increases the risk for atherosclerosis and ischemic heart disease. Desogestrel and gestodene do not have these effects. The risk of MI does not vary clearly with the type of progestogen but some studies suggest that the risk is lower with third-generation progestogen compared to second generation.

There may be a very small increase in the absolute risk of ischemic stroke associated with COC use, but with the presence of additional risk factors, the use becomes unacceptable. For OC pill users, who are heavy smokers the relative risk of myocardial infarction (MI) may be 10 times that of smokers who do not use the pill. Pill users with hypertension have a three-fold increased risk of MI compared with pill users without hypertension. While the use of the COC pill is an independent risk factor for ischemic stroke, the risk is doubled in patients, who are hypertensive and trebled in those who smoke.[10]

The prevalence of breast cancer is low in the young reproductive age group women. A large meta-analysis of case-control studies from 25 countries showed an increased risk of breast cancer whilst using COC (relative risk 1.24, 95% CI 1.15–1.33), which is approximately an increase of 24% above the background risk. This study suggested that any excess risk of breast cancer associated with COC use increases quickly after starting, does not increase with duration of use, and disappears within 10 years of stopping COC use.[10]

For women with a family history of breast cancer, there is an increased risk of breast cancer compared to women with no family history. Although the background risk is increased, current evidence shows that risk of breast cancer among women with a family history is not increased further by using COCs.

The use of oral contraceptives for >5 years increases the risk of cervical cancer. Women, who use the pill for 10 years from the age of 20, have an increased cumulative incidence of cervical cancer at the age of 50 years from 38 cases per 10,000 (in never users) to 45 cases per 10,000. The risk returns to the level of never users after 10 years.[11]

Noncontraceptive benefits: Other than a reliable method of contraception, the use of combined pills is associated with several noncontraceptive benefits (Table 7). COCs are recommended as chemoprophylaxis in women at risk of endometrial or ovarian cancer.

Table 7: Noncontraceptive benefits of combined oral contraceptives.

Cyclic	Noncyclic
Decrease in dysmenorrhea	Use produces fewer symptomatic fibroids and functional ovarian cysts
Decrease in menorrhagia	Less benign breast disease
Decrease in premenstrual syndrome	Reduced risk of pelvic inflammatory disease and ectopic pregnancy
Improve anemia	Reduced risk of ovarian, endometrial, and colon cancer

Missed pills: If one or two pills are missed or the woman has started the new pack 1 or 2 days later, she is advised to take the hormonal pill as soon as possible or two tablets at the scheduled time. There is no or little risk of pregnancy.

If she misses three or more pills in 1st or 2nd week or started the pack 3 or more days late, she is advised to take the hormonal pill as soon as possible and continue with the remaining scheduled pills. In addition, she needs to use a backup method for next 7 days and consider taking emergency contraceptive if she has had sex in last 72 hours.

If she has missed three or more pills in the 3rd week, she is advised to take the hormonal pill as soon as possible and continue with remaining hormonal pills but discard nonhormonal pills and start with a new pack the next day. In addition, she needs to use a backup method for next 7 days and consider taking emergency contraceptive if she has had sex in last 72 hours.

If she has missed any nonhormonal pill, she should discard that pill and continue with the scheduled pills and start the new pack once as usual.

If she vomits within 2 hours of ingestion of pill, she should take another pill from the pack and continue taking scheduled pills.

Drug interactions: Combined hormonal contraceptives (CHC) pills interact with drugs such as antibiotics, which are enzyme inducers. Therefore, in patients on long-term enzyme-inducing drugs such as rifampicin, a contraceptive method such as progestogen-only injectables, copper-bearing or progesterone IUD should be preferred. In women who are on short-term treatment with an enzyme-inducing drug and who do not wish to change from a combined oral pills, oral preparations containing at least 30 μg EE, a patch or a vaginal ring along with some additional contraception should be advised as the contraceptive efficacy of the pills is reduced. An extended regimen can be used with a hormone-free interval of 4 days. Additional contraception should be continued for 28 days after stopping the enzyme-inducing drug. Additional contraceptive precautions are not required during or after courses of antibiotics that do not induce enzymes.

In women on antiepileptic drugs, the metabolism of which is affected by combined oral contraceptive pills, close monitoring of serum levels of antiepileptic drugs should be done when they are prescribed CHC pills.

Combined Injectable Contraceptives

Combined injectable contraceptives (CICs) provide for the release of a natural estrogen plus a progestogen. The mode of action is same as that of oral contraceptive pills, i.e., inhibition of ovulation, except that the first-pass metabolism by the liver is avoided with injectable contraceptives, thereby minimizing the effect of estrogen on the liver.

Two CIC formulations available are Cyclofem and Mesigyna, which are administered at an interval of 4 weeks; Cyclofem contains medroxyprogesterone acetate 25 mg plus estradiol cypionate 5 mg and Mesigyna contains norethisterone enanthate 50 mg plus estradiol valerate 5 mg. Estradiol is a naturally occurring estrogen, which is less potent, has a shorter duration of effect, and is more rapidly metabolized than the synthetic estrogens used in other contraceptive formulations such as COCs, combined contraceptive patch (P), and combined contraceptive ring (R). The estrogen-related side effects such as effect on blood pressure, hemostasis and coagulation, lipid metabolism and liver function are less with CIC than with other formulations. The effect of CICs continues for some time after the last injection. These are not available in India.

Combined Contraceptive Ring

Contraceptive ring (NuvaRing) is a flexible transparent ring of a nonbiodegradable material which releases 15 μg EE and 120 μg etonogestrel, which is a metabolite of desogestrel over 24 hours (Fig. 7). It is available in only one size 54 mm in diameter and 4 mm thickness. It acts by inhibiting

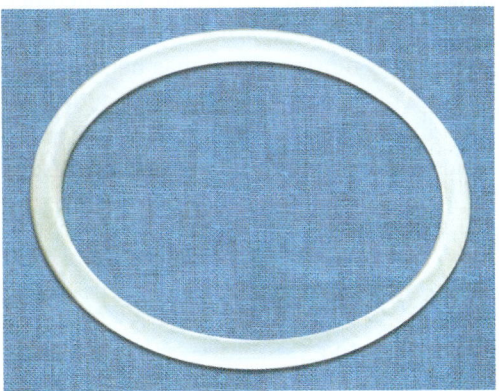

Fig. 7: Combined hormonal contraceptive ring.

ovulation. It is inserted vaginally by the patient once a month. In 1-month period, it is removed 3 weeks after insertion for withdrawal bleeding and a new ring is inserted 7 days later.

Since, unlike diaphragm, it has no role as a barrier, it can be placed in the vagina without the need for it to surround the cervix. If the ring is removed and not replaced in 3 hours, then additional method of contraception is recommended till the ring has been in place for 7 days. Although removal of the ring for intercourse is not recommended, if it is removed then it needs to be replaced within 3 hours. Vaginal flora or cervical cytology is not affected by the presence of the ring. Contraceptive ring is available in India.

Combined Contraceptive Patch

A transdermal patch (Evra) is 5 × 5 cm in size, containing 600 µg EE and 6 mg norelgestromin, is to be applied weekly for 3 weeks. It can be applied to the same or different site every week. If there is a delay of 24 hours or more in application of new patch after accidental detachment, a new patch cycle should be started along with backup contraception for 1 week. Emergency contraception is not required, if there has been regular patch use for a week before and after the hormone-free interval. If there has been an unscheduled patch detachment (partial or complete) for 48 hours or more, or there has been continued use of the same patch for an additional 48 hours or more on week 1, consider emergency contraception if unprotected sexual intercourse (UPSI) has taken place during the hormone-free interval, or week 1.

Progestogen-only Hormonal Contraceptives

Progestogen-only hormonal contraceptives are available as pills, injectables, subdermal implants, and intrauterine systems. Pills and injectables are available in India, whereas implants are not available. They mainly act through alteration in cervical mucus to prevent the ascent of sperms to the upper genital tract.

Progestogen-only Pills

Mode of action: In addition to making the cervical mucus hostile to sperm penetration, there is variable rate of inhibition of ovulation. With conventional progestogen-only pills (POPs) containing LNG, norethisterone, or ethynodiol diacetate, about 60% of cycles are anovulatory whereas with desogestrel-containing pills, up to 97% of the cycles are anovulatory.

For maintaining contraceptive efficacy of POPs, regular daily intake of pills is important. Ideally, a pill should be taken at or around the same time every day and there should be no pill-free interval. If taken consistently and correctly, POPs are >99% effective in preventing pregnancy.[2]

Contraindications: The use of POPs is safe in some women where COCs are contraindicated such as lactating women in first 6 months, women with history of thromboembolism. The contraindications to the use of POPs are listed in Table 8.

When to start: The POPs can be started at any time within the first 21 days postdelivery, immediately after a miscarriage, or day 1–5 of menses. Starting any time, after this provided pregnancy is ruled out, requires the use of additional contraception for 48 hours.

Additional contraception is also required if liver enzyme-inducing drugs are co-prescribed with POPs.

Missed pills: Traditional pills if taken >3 hours late or desogestrel pill taken >12 hours late, require additional contraception to be used for 48 hours after taking the missed pill.

Table 8: Contraindications to the use of progestogen-only pills.

MEC category 3	MEC category 4
History of breast cancer	Unexplained vaginal bleeding
Acute DVT/PE	Current breast cancer
	Liver cirrhosis
	Hepatic adenoma

(DVT/PE: deep thrombosis/pulmonary embolism; MEC: medical eligibility criteria)

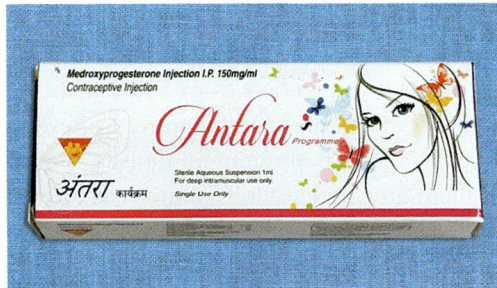

Fig. 8: Injectable medroxyprogesterone acetate.

Progestogen-only Injectable Preparations

Mode of action: Progestogen-only injectable preparation acts primarily by inhibition of ovulation and by making the cervical mucus unfavorable to sperm penetration.

Available preparations: The two preparations available for intramuscular use are depot medroxyprogesterone acetate (DMPA) 150 mg every 3 months or 300 mg every 6 months and norethisterone enanthate (NET-EN) 200 mg every 2 months. Both injections can be given 2 weeks earlier or later without any additional need for contraception. The failure rate is 3% with a typical user compared to 0.3% with a perfect user.[2]

Intramuscular MPA is provided free of cost by the GOI by the name of "Antara" (Fig. 8).

An aqueous suspension of DMPA is also available usually in a prefilled syringe that should be stored at room temperature and in a horizontal position. Syringes should be shaken vigorously before use to ensure complete suspension of the contents. The solution should be administered using the prepacked needle and can be self-administered.

Norethisterone enanthate is a thick, oily fluid that is drawn up into a syringe; the ampule should be immersed in warm water before use to reduce the viscosity. Both NET-EN and DMPA should ideally be administered as a deep intramuscular injection in the upper arm in deltoid muscle or buttocks in gluteal muscle or anterior outer thigh.

When to start: Ideally, first injection should be given between days 1 and 5, both inclusive of a normal menstrual cycle or an abortion. No additional contraception is required in such circumstances. Injections may also be initiated at any other time in the menstrual cycle if the clinician is reasonably certain that the woman is not pregnant. Additional contraception barrier method or abstinence should be advised for 7 days after initiation to allow for onset of action.

These can be safely administered to breastfeeding women and may be initiated up to postpartum day 21 with immediate contraceptive cover, but if initiated after day 21, then condoms or abstinence is advised for first 7 days. The GOI recommends administration of injection MPA after 6 weeks in breastfeeding mothers.

Side effects and risks: Side effects include irregular bleeding, weight gain, and breast tenderness. Irregular bleeding is common in the first few months of use. The amount and frequency of bleeding reduce with each reinjection progressing to amenorrhea in majority of the women by the end of 1 year. EE given as a COC pill and mefenamic acid may be effective in the management of unacceptable breakthrough bleeding due to thin endometrium associated with its use. There is no protection from STDs with the use of injectable contraceptives. Reversible decline in bone mineral density is seen without any increase in fracture risk. Hence, DMPA is not recommended as the first choice in women <18 years of age or >45 years.

There is a delay in return to fertility. Effect of Depo-Provera on menstrual cycles and fertility remains for 6–8 months after the last injection.

Noncontraceptive benefits: It is cost-effective and improves dysmenorrhea and the symptoms of endometriosis. The associated amenorrhea helps to build iron stores in anemic women.

Progesterone Implants

Progesterone implants are inserted into the medial aspect of the upper arm. They provide highly effective contraception that is independent of intercourse. Training is required to learn the method of insertion and removal. The failure rates are 0.05%.

Mechanism of action: Sustained levels of hormone are maintained in the circulation. Contraceptive effect is due to progestogenic effects on the endometrium and cervix and in the case of Implanon, the primary mode of action in addition to the above is inhibition of ovulation.

Available types: Two types of implants available are Nexplanon and the Implanon. Nexplanon has barium sulfate impregnated within it making it possible to detect its position using X-ray. Both have etonogestrel as the progestogen component. Norplant was previously available as a contraceptive implant.

Implanon is a 4 cm long flexible rod containing 68 mg etonogestrel, formerly known as 3 keto-desogestrel. The hormone is released at an initial rate of 67 µg/day decreasing to 30 µg/day after 2 years. It is to be replaced every 3 years.

How to start: Insertion can be done anytime from day 1 to 5 of menses. Insertion at any other time provided the clinician is sure that patient is not pregnant requires additional contraception for 7 days from the day of insertion.

Nonhormonal Oral Contraception

Centchroman

Centchroman or ormeloxifene is a nonsteroidal, nonhormonal, once-a-week contraceptive developed by the Central Drug Research Institute, Lucknow. It acts as selective estrogen receptor modulator (SERM). In some tissues/organs of the body, it has weak estrogenic action (e.g., bones) while in others, it has strong antiestrogenic action (e.g., uterus and breasts). It is available free of cost in the GOI contraceptive basket under the name Chayya. It is a tablet containing 30 mg of ormeloxifene Figure 9.

Mode of action: Centchroman acts by causing asynchrony between the embryo and preparedness of the uterine cavity critical for nidation or embedding of the blastocyst.

Centchroman suppresses endometrial proliferation and decidualization and alters biochemical parameters of implantation.

It accelerates in tubal transport of embryo and blastocyst development, and delays shedding of zona pellucida (the covering of the ovum) causing the embryo to move into the uterine cavity before it is ready to receive it.

How to start: Show the packet of Centchroman to the client as instructions are being given and explain the timing of starting the pill and the schedule to be

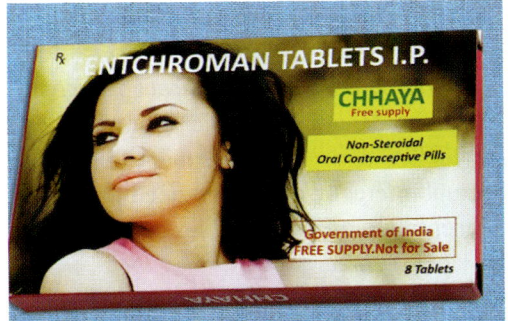 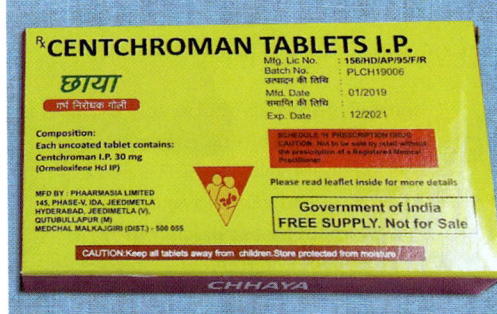

Fig. 9: Chayya (Centchroman or ormeloxifene).

followed. Take the first tablet on the first day of the menstrual period, second tablet on the fourth day, and subsequent tablets twice a week on the same days of the week (e.g., Wednesday and Sunday) for the first 3 months. After the first 3 months, take the tablet once a week on the same day of the week.

Explain that the periods may be delayed. If one pill is forgotten, take it the next day as soon as you remember it. If you forget it for 2 or more days, but <7 days, continue normal schedule, but use condoms to be sure of preventing pregnancy for rest of the cycle. If forgotten for >7 days, discontinue and start all over again like a new user beginning with the next menstrual period and taking it twice a day. Meanwhile, use condoms as a backup method.

Contraindications: The contraindications are listed in Box 4.

However, it is appropriate for any woman in the reproductive age group, who desires a highly effective contraceptive with minimal side effects and immediately after abortion or delivery.

Emergency Contraception

Unprotected sexual intercourse (UPSI) or intercourse when the method of contraception is not yet effective or use of hormonal contraception with liver enzyme-inducing drugs

> **Box 4:** Contraindications to use of Centchroman.
>
> *Absolute contraindications*:
> Centchroman should not be given in the following conditions:
> - History of jaundice or diseases of liver current or in the last 6 months
> - History of polycystic ovarian disease
> - Cervical dysplasia
>
> *Relative contraindications*:
> Centchroman should be considered carefully in the following conditions:
> - History of tuberculosis
> - History of kidney disease
> - Lactating mothers in the first 6 months postpartum

or a ruptured condom can necessitate use of emergency contraception.

Available Methods

Various methods can be used for emergency contraception. These are copper-bearing intrauterine device (Cu-IUD) that can be inserted up to 120 hours after the first episode of UPSI. It has a low documented failure rate. Antiprogesterone ulipristal acetate (UPA) 30 mg can be given up to 120 hours of UPSI. It is the only oral emergency contraceptive licensed for use between 72 and 120 hours. LNG 1.5 mg stat has been demonstrated to be effective up to 96 hours of UPSI. It has a high failure if used between 96 and 120 hours. Emergency

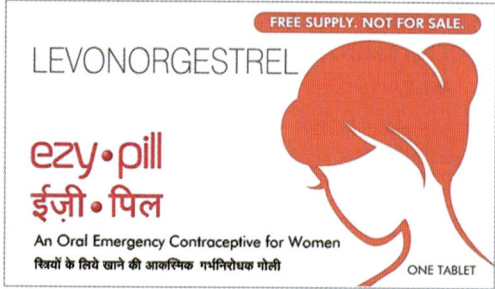

Fig. 10: Ezy pill containing 1.5 mg of levonorgestrel.

contraceptive pill is provided free of cost by GOI as Ezy pill containing 1.5 mg of LNG (Fig. 10) in public sector and is available in the market as I pill.

Mechanism of action: Copper is toxic to the ovum and sperm, thus Cu-IUD is effective for emergency contraception. If fertilization has already occurred, there is an anti-implantation effect immediately after insertion. The precise mode of action of LNG is incompletely understood, but it is thought to work primarily by inhibition of ovulation. Administration of LNG appears to prevent follicular rupture or cause luteal phase dysfunction. LNG taken prior to the LH surge has been shown to result in ovulatory dysfunction in the subsequent 5 days. LNG can thus inhibit ovulation for 5–7 days, by which time any sperm in the reproductive tract will have become nonviable. The closer to ovulation the treatment is given; the less likely it is to interfere with this process.

The primary mechanism of action of UPA is thought to be inhibition or delay of ovulation. If administered immediately before ovulation, UPA has been shown to suppress growth of lead follicles. There is evidence to suggest that UPA can prevent ovulation after the LH surge has started, delaying follicular rupture up to 5 days. Administration of UPA at the time of the LH peak or after it has been shown to be ineffective in delaying follicular rupture.

Oral emergency contraception (EC) methods do not provide a continuing contraceptive cover for subsequent unprotected sexual intercourse. Women need to use contraception or refrain from sex to avoid further risk of pregnancy.

Side effects: Women should be advised to seek medical advice if they vomit within 3 hours of taking LNG pill or within 3 hours of administration of UPA. A repeat dose of the same method with an antiemetic or Cu-IUD may be offered if appropriate. UPA should not be used in women taking liver enzyme-inducing drugs and for 28 days after these drugs are stopped. Also, UPA should not be used concomitantly with drugs that increase gastric pH.

Menstrual disturbances can occur after oral EC use. If there is any doubt about whether menstruation has occurred, a pregnancy test should be performed 3 weeks after unprotected sexual intercourse has occurred.

Headache, nausea, and altered bleeding patterns are side effects common to oral EC.

There are no known teratogenic effects on the fetus if the pregnancy cannot be prevented. This could be possible since the ECPs are taken long before organogenesis starts.

KEY POINTS

- A cafeteria approach should be followed while counseling a couple for contraception.
- The couple should be asked about their knowledge of various methods and their experience of using any method.
- Then they are explained about various options, their advantages and disadvantages and helped in taking an informed

decision about the method they want to opt for.
- A method-specific counseling is done to provide detailed information of the method chosen.
- Government of India has added injection MPA (Antara), Centchroman (Chhaya), and Emergency contraceptive pill (Ezy pill) to its armamentarium.

REFERENCES

1. A WHO family planning cornerstone. Medical eligibility criteria for contraceptive use, 4th edition. Geneva: Reproductive Health and Research, World Health Organization; 2009.
2. Trussell J. The essentials of contraception: efficacy, safety, and personal considerations. In: Hatcher RA, Trussell J, Nelson AL, Cates W, Stewart FH, Kowal D (Eds). Contraceptive Technology, 18th revised edition. New York: Ardent Media Inc; 2004.
3. Faculty of Sexual and Reproductive Healthcare RCOG Clinical Guidance. Barrier Methods for contraception and STI prevention. Clinical Effectiveness Unit Guidance Document. England: Faculty of Sexual and Reproductive Healthcare; 2011.
4. Speroff L, Fritz MA. Clinical Gynecologic Endocrinology and Infertility. Part 3 contraception, 7th edition. Philadelphia: Lippincott Williams and Wilkins; 2005. pp. 827-1010.
5. Richard A. Diaphragm Fitting. Am Fam Physician. 2004;69(1):97-100.
6. National Institute for Health and Clinical Excellence (2005). Long-acting Reversible Contraception. Clinical Guideline 30. [online]. Available from https://www.nice.org.uk/guidance/cg30. [Last accessed March, 2020].
7. Wu JP, Pickle S. Extended use of the intrauterine device: A literature review and recommendations for clinical practice. Contraception. 2014;89(6):495-503.
8. Schaedel ZE, Dolan G, Powell MC. The use of the levonorgestrel-releasing intrauterine system in the management of menorrhagia in women with hemostatic disorders. Am J Obstet Gynecol. 2005;193(4):1361-3.
9. Royal College of Obstetricians and Gynaecologists (2010). Venous thromboembolism and hormonal contraception. Green-top Guideline 40. [online] Available from https://www.rcog.org.uk/en/guidelines-research-services/guidelines/gtg40/. [Last accessed March, 2020].
10. Collaborative Group on Hormonal Factors in Breast Cancer. Breast cancer and hormonal contraceptives: collaborative reanalysis of individual data on 53,297 women with breast cancer and 100,239 women without breast cancer from 54 epidemiological studies. Lancet. 1996;347(9017):1713-27.
11. International Collaboration of Epidemiological Studies of Cervical Cancer, Appleby P, Beral V, Berrington de González A, Colin D, Franceschi S, et al. Cervical cancer and hormonal contraceptives: collaborative reanalysis of individual data for 16,573 women with cervical cancer and 35,509 women without cervical cancer from 24 epidemiological studies. Lancet. 2007;370(9599):1609.

SUGGESTED READING

1. Family Planning Division, Ministry of Health and Family Welfare, Government of India (2013). IUCD reference Manual for Medical Officers and Nursing Personnel. [online] Available from: https://nhm.gov.in/images/pdf/programmes/family-planing/guidelines/IUCD_Reference_Manual_for_MOs_and_Nursing_Personne_-Final-Sept_2013.pdf. [Last accessed March, 2020].
2. Family Planning Division, Ministry of Health and Family Welfare, Government of India (2013). Reference Manual for Male Sterilization. [online] Available from https://nhm.gov.in/images/pdf/programmes/family-planing/guidelines/Reference_Manual_for_Male_Sterilization-NSV-Oct_2013.pdf. [Last accessed March, 2020].
3. Family Planning Division, Ministry of Health and Family Welfare, Government of India (2014). Reference Manual for Female Sterilization. [online] Available from

https://www.ukhfws.org/uploads/documents/doc_3768_ref-manual-for-female-sterilization.pdf. [Last accessed March, 2020].

4. Family Planning Division, Ministry of Health and Family Welfare, Government of India (2014). Standards and Quality Assurance in Sterilization Services [online] Available from https://www.ukhfws.org/uploads/documents/doc_3768_ref-manual-for-female-sterilization.pdf. [Last accessed March, 2020].

5. Family Planning Division, Ministry of Health and Family Welfare, Government of India (2016). Reference Manual for Injectable Contraceptive (DMPA). [online] Available from https://www.nhmmp.gov.in/WebContent/FW/Guideline2017/Injectable_Manual.pdf. [Last accessed March, 2020].

6. Family Planning Division, Ministry of Health and Family Welfare, Government of India (2016). Reference Manual for Oral Contraceptive Pills. [online] Available from https://nhm.gov.in/images/pdf/programmes/family-planing/guidelines/Reference_Manual_Oral_Pills.pdf. [Last accessed March, 2020].

7. World Health Organization (2015). Improving Access to Quality of Care in Family Planning: Medical Eligibility Criteria for Contraceptive Use. [online] Available from https://apps.who.int/iris/bitstreamhandle/10665/61086/WHO_RHR_00.02.pdf?sequence=1&isAllowed=y. [Last accessed March, 2020].

57

Medical Termination of Pregnancy and Sterilization

Raina Chawla

INTRODUCTION

Medical termination of pregnancy (MTP) refers to induced abortion or willful termination of pregnancy before the period of viability. Every year about 80 million unintended pregnancies occur worldwide and more than half of these, nearly 46 million, are terminated each year, many of which are illegal.[1] In order to curb the large numbers of illegal abortions, the Medical Termination of Pregnancy (MTP) Act was introduced in India in 1971 and later amended in 2002.[2]

Liberalization of induced abortions was approved by the Indian Parliament in 1971 and was implemented from April 1972. The main objective of the act was to reduce maternal mortality by decreasing unsafe abortions. The Act permits termination of pregnancy till 20 weeks in the circumstances listed in Box 1.

The Act specifies that abortion procedures can only be performed by doctors who have received adequate training. For the termination of pregnancies till 12 weeks, certification of one qualified doctor is enough; however for pregnancies between 12 and 20 weeks, two doctors must give their approval. MTP can only be performed at a clinic or hospital established or maintained by the government or an institute approved by the government for this purpose.

In 2002, certain amendments were made in the Act, which included substituting the word "lunatic" by "mentally ill," formulation of district level committees, and making termination by unregistered practitioners and those performed in unregistered places a punishable offence.[2]

In January 2020, the Union Cabinet approved a bill that proposes amendments to the current Act. As per the Ministry of Health and Family Welfare, these amendments include: Enhancing the upper gestational limit from 20 to 24 weeks for special categories which will be defined, upper gestational limit not to apply in cases of substantial fetal abnormalities diagnosed at the Medical Board, and name and other particulars of a woman whose pregnancy has been terminated shall not be revealed, except to a person authorized in any law.[3]

Box 1: Indications for medical termination of pregnancy (MTP) under MTP Act.

- Where the continuation of pregnancy would involve a risk to the life of the pregnant woman or grave injury to her physical or mental health
- Where substantial risks exist to the child being born with serious physical or mental abnormality
- Pregnancy due to rape
- Pregnancy due to failure of contraception

MEDICAL TERMINATION OF PREGNANCY

Prerequisites for Medical Termination of Pregnancy

Prerequisites for MTP include a detailed history, thorough examination, preprocedure counseling, relevant investigations, and informed consent.

History and Examination

History and examination are useful in confirming pregnancy, assessing the exact period of gestation and determining any associated gynecological or medical condition.

History essentially includes the date of woman's last menstrual period (LMP), pattern of menstrual cycle, parity, live births, abortions, any previous cesarean, contraceptive use, reasons for MTP, any significant medical illness, pelvic or abdominal surgery, and any known drug allergies.

Examination entails reviewing her general health and any coexisting medical conditions. It also includes confirming intrauterine pregnancy and determining the size of the uterus on pelvic and/or abdominal examination and whether it corresponds to the gestational age. For example, a large for date uterus suggests a possibility of mistaken dates, fibroid uterus, multiple pregnancies, or molar pregnancy. A pelvic examination also detects any signs of reproductive tract infection, which need to be treated prior to any procedure.

Preprocedure Counseling

Counseling is essential and it should be confidential. It should include a discussion on the reason for seeking MTP, various options available for termination of pregnancy, technical details of the method chosen, duration of the procedure, management of pain, type of anesthesia if a surgical procedure is involved, safety, complications, and follow-up care. It is also a good opportunity to review the contraceptive method being used by the couple and do method-specific counseling.

Investigations

The investigations required prior to MTP include hemoglobin (Hb), blood group, and Rh typing. However, in some women with clinical suspicion of ectopic pregnancy, an ultrasound of pelvis is indicated to confirm intrauterine pregnancy.

Consent

A written and informed consent needs to be taken in a language clearly understood by the patient explaining the type of procedure (medical/surgical), alternatives available, likely complications, and failure rates. Consent of the patient undergoing the procedure is enough and consent of spouse or partner is not mandatory.

Methods of Medical Termination of Pregnancy

Methods of MTP are medical or surgical and depend upon the period of gestation of the woman seeking MTP.

First-trimester Medical Termination of Pregnancy

Termination of pregnancy in the first trimester can be carried out by either medical or surgical method. The preferred method up to 7 weeks of gestation is medical method and from 6 to 12 weeks is surgical method.

Medical Method

Procedure: The Ministry of Health and Family Welfare released guidelines on Comprehensive Abortion Care in 2018. For medical abortion, a combination of two drugs is used; Mifepristone and misoprostol which are approved for medical methods for abortion. Mifepristone is a derivative of norethindrone and is an antiprogestin. It binds to progesterone receptors in the endometrium and decidua resulting in necrosis and detachment of the conceptus. It also softens the uterus and causes mild uterine activity. Mifepristone also sensitizes the uterus to the effect of prostaglandins. Misoprostol is a prostaglandin E1 analog which binds to myometrial cells causing strong uterine contractions, cervical softening, and dilatation.[4]

- *First visit (day 1)*:
  - After a careful history, the woman is examined to confirm the pregnancy and assess the uterine size.
  - She is counseled and an informed written consent is obtained.
  - Mifepristone 200 mg is administered orally.
  - Anti-D (50 µg) is given to women who are Rh-negative.
  - Patient is instructed to maintain a menstrual diary and explained about the possibility of spotting, which should not be considered as a sign of menstruation.
  - Backup facility address, and phone numbers should be given where she can contact in emergency.
  - She is instructed to return to the clinic after 48 hours.

A small percentage (3%) may expel products of conception with mifepristone alone, but the total drug dosing with misoprostol must be completed. Home administration of misoprostol may be allowed at the discretion of the provider. It can improve privacy, convenience, and acceptability of the services, and safety is not being compromised. The woman should have access to 24-hour emergency services. She should also be instructed on how and when to use an additional dose of misoprostol.

- *Second visit (day 3)*:
  - History of any bleeding or side effects should be noted.
  - *Administer misoprostol*:
    - 400 µg by sublingual, buccal, vaginal, or oral route for gestational age up to 7 weeks *or*
    - 800 µg by sublingual, buccal, or vaginal route for gestational age up to 9 weeks.

Additional dose of misoprostol should be repeated in the below-mentioned circumstances:

- The woman vomits within half-an-hour of the intake of oral misoprostol.
- There is no vaginal bleeding even after 24 hours of misoprostol administration (a woman reporting no bleeding or very light bleeding suggests that either there is a continuing pregnancy or that the treatment is not working).
- If there is excessive bleeding.

If the bleeding does not get controlled even after the repeat dose of misoprostol, surgical evacuation may be considered:

- For vaginal use, misoprostol tablet should be moistened with a few drops of water and introduced vaginally. The woman is instructed to rest in bed for half-an-hour.
- She is observed for 4 hours in the clinic/hospital.
- Pulse and blood pressure are monitored, and any side effects noted.
- The time of start of bleeding and expulsion of products is noted.
- A pelvic examination is done before the woman leaves the clinic, and if internal

- os is open and products are partially expelled, a digital evacuation is done.
- Drugs for pain relief are prescribed.
- Patient should be advised to abstain from intercourse or to use condoms, till the next visit.
- She is instructed to take adequate rest and avoid going out of station.
- She should report in case of excessive pain or bleeding.
- *Third visit (day 15)*:
  - A clinical history and pelvic examination should be done to ensure that there are no complications.
  - Ultrasonography (USG) is advised if history and examination do not confirm expulsion of products of conception.
  - If she is still having irregular bleeding it suggests retained products which may require evacuation and curettage.
  - The woman should be informed that her next periods may be delayed, but she should come for a check-up if she does not get period in 6 weeks.
  - Contraceptive advice is given and appropriate contraception is provided.

Adjunct medications such as prophylactic antibiotics are usually not required following a medical method of MTP unless there is evidence of vaginal infection. Analgesics are prescribed for pain relief.

Side effects and complications of medical methods: Common side effects with medical abortion include abdomen pain, bleeding per vaginum, fever, nausea and vomiting, diarrhea, headache, chills, dizziness, and fatigue. A detailed description of complications is as given below.

- *Failure*: The term failure with medical abortion is used when a surgical curettage is performed for any reason including clinician's decision, patient's choice or a true drug failure. True drug failure is defined as the presence of cardiac activity 2 weeks following mifepristone and misoprostol administration. It occurs in <1% of women and pregnancy should be terminated by surgical evacuation in these women.
- *Missed ectopic*: Ectopic pregnancy should be excluded, if the woman does not expel products following therapy and/or is having persistent pain.
- *Heavy bleeding*: Preabortion counseling should emphasize that bleeding is likely to be heavier than menses, comparable to that of a miscarriage. She should be told that soaking two pads per hour for 2 hours in a row is expected at the time of peak cramping, which is often the case when the expulsion of products of conception occurs. However, if this persists and or the woman feels dizzy, she should report in emergency and consult doctor. Severe bleeding necessitating a surgical curettage is reported in <1% of patients.[5]
- *Abdominal cramps*: Crampy abdominal pain is experienced by most women for a short time, coinciding with expulsion of products of gestation. Pain relief is an important part of the therapy. The perception of pain is modified by fear, anxiety, and emotions. It often responds to acetaminophen (paracetamol). Pain usually subsides once the products are expelled.

Persistent pain, with failure to respond to these drugs for several hours, warrants evaluation for other causes, such as ectopic pregnancy, infection, or incomplete abortion:

- *Fever or a feeling of warmth*: It is thought to be related with the use of prostaglandin analogs. It is usually short lived and resolves spontaneously. Acetaminophen

given for pain relief also takes care of fever, but if temperature exceeds 100.4°F (38°C) or persists for several hours, despite antipyretics, infection should be ruled out.
- *Incomplete abortion*: Women having a persistent gestational sac without cardiac activity 2 weeks after mifepristone and misoprostol administration are diagnosed to have incomplete abortion. Such women usually do not have pregnancy-related symptoms and often expel the products spontaneously. The clinician must understand that during medical abortion, once the gestational sac is expelled, the uterus will normally contain blood, blood clots and decidua, which appear as hyperechoic tissue on USG. In the absence of excessive bleeding, these patients should be followed conservatively.

Risk of teratogenesis: Mifepristone has no known teratogenic effects. Misoprostol exposure is associated with multiple congenital defects. Möbius sequence is known to occur after misoprostol administration and includes congenital facial paralysis with or without limb defects. It is, therefore, advisable to terminate pregnancy surgically in case of failure with medical methods:
- *Delay in onset of next menses*: Next menstruation occurs 3–6 weeks after the abortion and is usually normal. Contraception should thus be initiated within 15 days of abortion to avoid an unwanted pregnancy.

Surgical Methods

Surgical methods include vacuum aspiration and dilatation and evacuation. Of these, vacuum aspiration is preferred, as it is faster and associated with less blood loss. Vacuum aspiration can be electrical or manual.

Preprocedure assessment and preparation: Cervical priming ahead of surgical procedure is preferred by some if the period of gestation is >8 weeks. It facilitates cervical dilatation and reduces the risk of complications such as cervical injury, uterine perforation, hemorrhage, and incomplete abortion. The most used cervical priming agent is 400 µg misoprostol 3 hours prior to the procedure given sublingual or 4 hours prior if given vaginally.

Surgical abortion is performed either in a hospital or in a dedicated facility. The procedure can be performed under paracervical block and intravenous analgesia; general anesthesia may be preferred if the size of the uterus is large or if the patient so desires.

The steps of the surgical procedure are described in Box 2.
- *Manual vacuum aspiration*: The manual vacuum aspiration (MVA) syringe is a 60-mL syringe with a double valve. It is

Box 2: Steps of dilatation and evacuation.
- The patient is asked to empty her bladder
- Under all aseptic precautions, vulva and vagina are painted with antiseptic solution and draped with clean drapes
- A bimanual examination is done to determine the position and size of uterus
- Sims speculum is inserted
- 1 mL of 1% lignocaine is injected into the cervix at 12 o'clock position and the anterior lip of the cervix is then held with a vulsellum or long Allis forceps; traction on the vulsellum straightens the angle between the cervical canal and uterine cavity
- 4–5 mL lignocaine (1%) is injected at 4 and 8 o'clock positions each at the cervicovaginal junction about 1 cm deep, after ensuring that needle is not in a vessel
- Cervix is then dilated serially with Hegar dilators
- A plastic cannula is inserted in the uterus, connected with a tubing to suction machine (600 mm Hg) or a MVA syringe and the products of conception are aspirated till the uterine cavity is empty

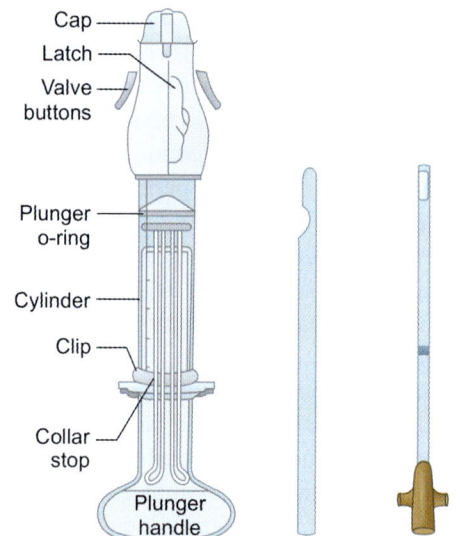

Fig. 1: Manual vacuum aspiration (MVA) syringe and cannulae.

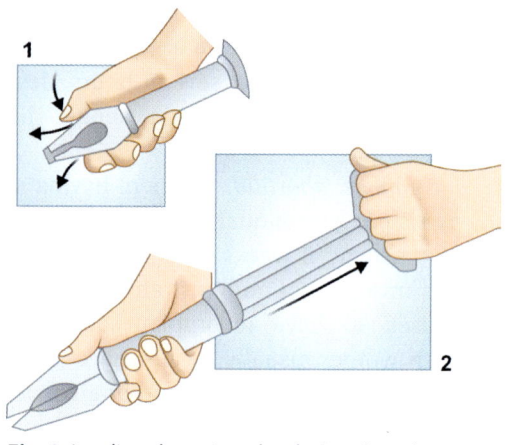

Fig. 2: Loading the syringe by closing the valves.

Table 1: Color coding of suction cannulae.	
Diameter of cannulae (mm)	Color
4	Yellow
5	Green
6	Blue
7	Tan
8	Ivory
9	Dark brown
10	Dark green
12	Dark blue

connected to a flexible plastic cannula (Fig. 1). These cannulas are available in different sizes (4–12 mm) and are color-coded according to their size (Table 1). It is easy to handle, dismantle, and clean these cannulas.

The syringe is first loaded by locking both the valves (Fig. 2) and the syringe is charged by creating vacuum by pulling out the plunger with the valves locked (Fig. 2). The cannula of the right size is selected. The rule of thumb is to select the number corresponding to the weeks of gestation, e.g., 8 mm cannula will be chosen for MTP of 8 weeks' pregnancy. The cervical dilatation is done up to a dilator size one number more than the number of weeks of gestation, to avoid use of force to introduce the cannula. The cannula is inserted through the cervix towards fundus keeping it below the fundus and then the charged syringe is attached to it. The pinch valve is released, and vacuum is transmitted to the uterus. Rotatory and back forth movements of the cannula are done and the products of conception are aspirated into the syringe till the uterine cavity is empty (Fig. 3). The signs of complete evacuation are given in Box 3.

Postprocedure curettage is usually not recommended, except in cases where there is a doubt of retained products.

The material aspirated is placed in a glass container containing water or sieved. Fresh placental tissue floats in water and chorionic villi appear as soft, fluffy, feathery and discernible finger-like projections. The tissue is sent for histopathological confirmation if in doubt. This is helpful in detecting molar pregnancy if vesicles are seen, and suspecting

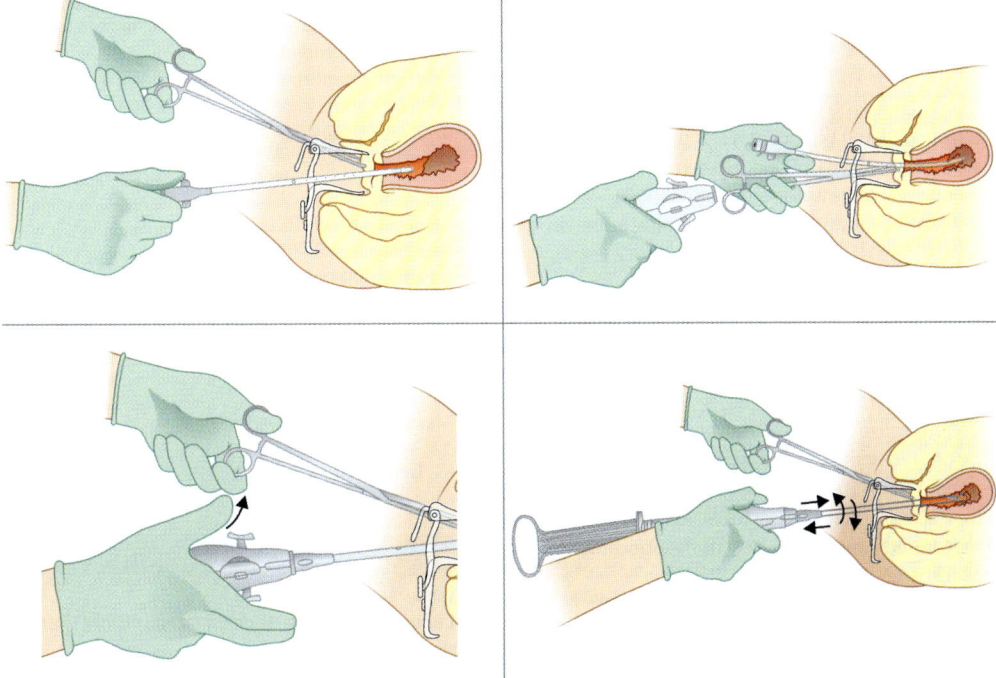

Fig. 3: Evacuating the uterine cavity.

Box 3: Signs of complete evacuation.
• No tissue only foamy bubbles are seen through the cannula
• Gritty feeling of cannula against uterine walls
• Internal os grips around cannula

ectopic pregnancy or incomplete abortion, if adequate tissue is not obtained:

- *Electrical vacuum aspiration*: The procedure is like an MVA, except that the suction pressure is electrically produced using an electric suction machine. The differences in the MVA and electrical vacuum aspiration (EVA) are depicted in Table 2. However, for first trimester MTP by vacuum aspiration, the Royal College of Obstetricians and Gynecologists (2004)[6] recommends the use of either electric or manual aspiration devices, as both are effective and acceptable to women and clinicians.

Table 2: Differences between MVA and EVA.

MVA	EVA
Portable	Not portable
Not dependent on electricity	Dependent on electricity
Suitable even for rural/primary care setup	Not suitable
Cannula can be used as a dilator	Metal dilator needed
360° rotation possible	180° either side due to kinking of tubing
Precreated vacuum suction en mass	Takes time to create required vacuum (600–650 mm Hg) suction in pieces
Chances of damage due to uterine perforation are less (vacuum decreases or breaks with uterine perforation preventing suction of mesentery and or intestines)	Chances of damage are more (continuous vacuum endangers suction of mesentery and or intestines)

(MVA: manual vacuum aspiration; EVA: electrical vacuum aspiration)

Box 4: Surgical abortion—postprocedure care and follow-up.

- Prophylactic antibiotics are given postprocedure doxycycline (100 mg bd for 7 days) with metronidazole (400 mg tid for 7 days) is preferred
- All nonsensitized RhD-negative women should be given anti-D immunoglobulin G (IgG) immunoprophylaxis following surgical abortion; 50 μg anti-D if the gestational age is <12 weeks
- Initial follow-up visits after 2 weeks or earlier if she develops any of the following danger signals; severe lower abdominal pain, fever, heavy and persistent vaginal bleeding, foul-smelling discharge per vaginum
- *Contraceptive advice*: An intrauterine device can be offered at the time of aspiration/evacuation if there is no infection; oral contraceptives can be started within a week; tubal ligation can be performed concomitantly with the abortion procedure

Box 5: Complications of surgical procedures.

- *Immediate complications*:
  - Complications of local anesthesia
  - Vasovagal syncope
  - Cervical laceration
  - Perforation
  - Hemorrhage
- *Early complications*:
  - Persistent bleeding
  - Retained products
  - Pelvic infection
  - Continuing pregnancy
- *Delayed complications*:
  - Asherman's syndrome
  - Rh sensitization
  - Subfertility
  - Cervical insufficiency

Box 6: Signs of uterine perforation.

- Loss of resistance
- Length of instrument negotiated is more than the assessed uterine size
- Excessive bleeding
- Visualization of bowel or omentum through cannula
- Severe abdominal pain or shock

- *Dilatation and evacuation*: The initial steps in this procedure are the same as those for an MVA or EVA. Following dilatation of the internal cervical os, an ovum forceps is introduced into the uterine cavity in a closed position. Once inside the uterine cavity, it is opened and rotated for 90° in a clockwise and anticlockwise manner, closed as to hold fetal tissue tightly and is then taken out. This is repeated till the fetal tissue is entirely evacuated. Check curettage is then done to ensure all the contents have been evacuated.

Postprocedure care and follow-up: Majority of patients undergoing surgical abortion require a short postoperative stay unless general anesthesia has been given. The important aspects of postprocedure care and follow-up are listed in Box 4.

Complications of surgical methods: Complications can be immediate, early, or delayed with long-term adverse consequences (Box 5).

Uterine perforation: Uterine perforation is a rare, but potentially serious complication. It occurs in 0.1–0.28% of all surgical abortions. Nulliparity and increasing gestational age are risk factors for perforation. An increase of 2 weeks in the gestational age increases the risk of perforation by 1.4-fold.[7]

The signs of perforation are listed in Box 6. Depending on the site and instrument causing perforation it can lead to vascular injury or injury to the bowel or bladder. The damage is likely to be more if perforation occurs with a sharp curette or suction cannula due to negative pressure compared to that with a dilator, which is blunt.

Perforation can be prevented by prior ripening of the cervix. Proper assessment of the size and direction of the uterus is done so that the dilator is directed accordingly. While introducing instruments, traction is applied on the Allis forceps or vulsellum holding the cervix, to straighten the uterocervical axis. Gradual and careful dilatation of cervix is done, Karman's cannula is introduced in the uterine cavity with its tip below the fundus in the center of the uterine cavity.

When perforation occurs or is suspected, the procedure should be stopped and completed under direct observation, i.e., laparoscopy or laparotomy. The patient should be kept under observation. If there is a strong suspicion or actual diagnosis of injury to the intestines and/or omentum or uncontrolled hemorrhage, laparotomy should be performed. Laparoscopy is useful in a stable patient to assess the extent of perforation and damage to adjacent organs.

Second-trimester Medical Termination of Pregnancy

Second-trimester abortions accounts for 10–15% of all induced abortions.[8] In the last two decades, improvements in medical methods for second-trimester abortions have made this procedure much safer and more easily accessible. MTP Act permits termination up to 20 weeks' gestation; anything beyond this is unprotected by the MTP Act and is considered illegal.

Because of the potential for heavy vaginal bleeding and serious complications, it is advisable that second-trimester terminations take place in a healthcare facility where blood transfusion and emergency surgery including laparotomy are available. The combination of mifepristone and misoprostol is now an established and highly effective method for second-trimester abortion. Where mifepristone is not available or affordable, misoprostol alone can be used and is effective, although a higher total dose is needed and efficacy is lower than for the combined regimen. Efforts should be made to reduce unnecessary surgical evacuation of the uterus after expulsion of the fetus. Methods such as intrauterine instillation of hypertonic saline and extra-amniotic ethacridine instillation are now outdated and have no place in modern obstetrics.

Surgical procedures like dilatation and evacuation are usually carried out in the rare event of a failed trial with medical methods and should be carried out by well-trained personnel. Hysterotomy is rarely indicated.

Medical Methods

Medical methods include misoprostol alone or a combination of mifepristone and misoprostol. Misoprostol initiates cervical dilatation and uterine contractions. It is the most used method for second trimester terminations. Various protocols have been stated, most of which recommend repeated doses of 200–600 µg at 3–12 hourly intervals. Overall, when misoprostol is used alone, 400 µg appears to be the minimum effective dose. Repeating the dose approximately every 3–4 hours for five doses is effective and shortens the induction to abortion time.[9]

The vaginal route is the more effective route with respect to induction to abortion interval. Side effects include retention of placenta and uterine rupture, which is more common in a previously scarred uterus. The use of mifepristone prior to misoprostol reduces the induction abortion interval.

Prostaglandin F2α can also be used for medical abortion in second trimester. It is indicated in a dose of 250 µg (2.5 mg) intramuscularly every 3 hours to a total of 10 doses. The drug is associated with diarrhea and vomiting so antiemetics and antidiarrheal agents should be administered prophylactically. Prostaglandin F2α is contraindicated in women with asthma as it causes bronchospasm.

Surgical Methods

Surgical methods include dilatation and evacuation and hysterotomy. Dilatation and evacuation is not a popular method for second-trimester abortion in most countries. It requires considerable cervical dilatation and involves prior preparation of the cervix with osmotic dilators or prostaglandins to safely achieve dilatation for smooth passage of instruments into the uterine cavity to remove the products of conception. It can be done under ultrasound guidance to minimize the risk of perforation, which is the most significant complication associated with this procedure. Other complications are as with first-trimester dilatation and evacuation, i.e., infection, hemorrhage, and retained products though these occur more frequently with second-trimester MTP.

Hysterotomy is a procedure-like cesarean section in which an incision is made on the uterus in lower uterine segment if possible and the endometrial cavity is evacuated through abdominal route for second-trimester abortion. Hysterotomy is seldom required as an elective procedure. However, it may be indicated in certain situations like hemorrhage in second-trimester MTP and failed MTP, especially in patients with previous caesarean sections in which misoprostol is relatively unsafe.

Follow-up and postabortion contraception counseling: Follow-up and postabortion contraception counseling is an important component of patient management as it can effectively reduce the incidence of MTPs. The key messages for counseling include:
- She should wait at least 6 months before trying to conceive again as it reduces the chances of low birth weight, premature birth, and maternal anemia.
- Fertility returns quickly, within 10–11 days after first-trimester abortion or miscarriage and within 4 weeks after a second-trimester abortion or miscarriage.
- She can choose from available family planning methods that can be started at once.
- If a woman decides not to use contraceptives at this time, providers can offer information on all available methods and from where to obtain them. Providers can also offer condoms, oral contraceptives, or emergency contraceptive pills for women to take home and use later.
- To avoid infection, she should not have intercourse until bleeding stops. If being treated for infection or vaginal/cervical injury, she should wait until she is fully healed.

Method-specific counseling should follow if she chooses any family planning method (Table 3).

STERILIZATION

Both male and female sterilization are permanent methods of contraception. Female sterilization is the most widely used contraceptive method in the world. It is a procedure safe, highly efficacious, cost-effective requiring a single act of compliance, that separates contraception from sexual activity and do not rely on partner behavior. Sterilization's ability to achieve long-term contraception with a single event is unique and is an important reason for its popularity. This feature makes sterilization an ideal method of permanent contraception in developing countries where access to healthcare providers is limited. Although vasectomy is faster, safer, less complex and less costly, equally effective compared to female sterilization, more women than men undergo sterilization procedures.

Table 3: Time of initiation of contraceptive methods after abortion.

After medical abortion with mifepristone and misoprostol	• Combined oral contraceptive pills • Progestin only pills	• Can be started on 3rd day or 15th day of medical abortion protocol, if there are no medical contraindications
	• Centchroman pills	• Can be started on the 3rd day of medical abortion protocol
	• Injection DMPA	• Can be started on the 3rd day of medical abortion protocol
	• Condoms	• Can be used as soon as sexual activity is resumed
	• IUCD	• Can be inserted once the abortion is complete (around day 15) and the presence of infection is ruled out
	• Female sterilization	• Can be performed after the first menstrual cycle
After surgical abortion	• Combined oral contraceptive pills	• Can be started immediately
	• Progestin only pills	• Can be started immediately
	• Centchroman pills	• Can be started immediately
	• Injection DMPA	• Can be started immediately
	• Condoms	• Can be started immediately
	• IUCD	• Can be inserted immediately when infection and injury to the genital tract are ruled out or resolved
	• Female sterilization	• Can be performed concurrently or within 7 days postabortion provided woman is eligible by the minilaparotomy as well as laparoscopic methods

Female Sterilization

The various methods of female sterilization are as listed in Box 7.

Counseling

Counseling is the process of helping women make informed and voluntary decision about the method she wants to accept for contraception. It should follow the GATHER approach. (Table 4)

Before the woman signs the consent form, it is important that she is informed of all available methods of family planning and should be made aware that for all practical purpose sterilization is a permanent method. She should be counseled in the language she understands. She should be made to understand what will happen before, during, and after the surgery, and potential complications. She should be told that it will not affect her strength or her ability to perform normal day-to-day functions and that it does not protect against reproductive tract infections (RTIs), sexually transmitted infections (STIs), or human immunodeficiency virus (HIV)/acquired immune deficiency

Box 7: Methods of female sterilization.

- *Associated with pregnancy*:
  - *Postpartum*: With cesarean section or minilaparotomy
  - *Postabortion*: Laparoscopic or minilaparotomy
- *Interval*:
  - *Abdominal*: Minilaparotomy or with laparotomy (Pomeroy or modified Pomeroy, Uchida, Irving, fimbriectomy, partial salpingectomy)
  - Laparoscopic (fulguration, clips, and rings)
- Vaginal
- Hysteroscopic
- Hysterectomy

Table 4:	GATHER approach for contraceptive counseling.
G	Greet the woman
A	Ask if she is aware of or using any contraceptive method
T	Tell her about all available methods
H	Help her choose a suitable method
E	Explain her about the chosen method in details
R	Return (ask her to return for follow-up)

Box 8: Eligibility criteria for female sterilization.[10]
- Clients should be married (including ever married)
- Female clients should be below the age of 49 years and above the age of 22 years
- The couple should have at least one child whose age is above 1 year unless the sterilization is medically indicated
- Clients or their spouses/partners must not have undergone sterilization in the past (not applicable in cases of failure of previous sterilization)
- Clients must be in a sound state of mind to understand the full implications of sterilization
- Mentally ill clients must be certified by a psychiatrist and a statement should be given by the legal guardian/spouse regarding the soundness of the client's state of mind

syndrome (AIDS). It is important for her to know that a reversal of this surgery is possible, but that it is a major surgical procedure and its success cannot be guaranteed. She must be encouraged to ask questions to clarify her doubts, if any. Her decision should be voluntary.

Preprocedure Assessment

Preprocedure assessment is important to evaluate the woman for her eligibility for undergoing sterilization prior to surgery. This includes her medical history, physical examination, and laboratory investigations as specified below.

Demographic information: The required information includes age, marital status, occupation, religion, educational status, number of living children, and age of the youngest child.

Medical history: History of illness to screen for any prolonged medical illness or chronic disorder. Her immunization status for tetanus is assessed. Any current medications such as last contraceptive used or any other medications is noted.

Menstrual history: This includes the date of last menstrual period and current pregnancy status.

Obstetric history: This includes the number of living children the woman has and the age of the youngest child.

Physical examination: This includes general condition, pulse, blood pressure, respiratory rate, temperature, body weight, and pallor. Auscultation of heart and lungs, examination of abdomen, pelvic examination, and other examinations as indicated by the client's medical history or general physical examination are carried out.

Laboratory examination: Blood test for Hb, urine analysis for sugar and albumin, and other laboratory examinations as indicated.

There are no absolute medical contraindications for performing female sterilization. However, there are certain conditions that require doctors to be cautious, to delay the surgery, to refer the client to an especially equipped center or to counsel the client to go in for alternative method of contraception. If the Hb is <7 g/dL, the procedure should be delayed until the anemia is corrected. If Hb is between ≥7 and <10 g/dL, the procedure can be conducted in a routine setting, but with extra preparation and precautions.[8] The eligibility criteria for female surgical sterilization procedures outlined by Government of India serve as guidelines for case selection based on the clinical findings of the client (Box 8).[10]

Table 5: Timing of the female sterilization.

Situation	When to perform
Having menstrual cycles	• Any time within 7 days of start of her menstrual cycle • Any time of menstrual cycle, provided it is reasonably certain that she is not pregnant
Switching from another method	• *OCP*: To be done any time but she is advised to continue the pill until the pack is finished to maintain regularity of her cycle • *IUCD*: To be done anytime concurrently with removal of IUCD
No monthly menstrual bleeding, e.g., lactational amenorrhea	Any time provided it is reasonably certain that she is not pregnant
After childbirth	• Within 7 days after giving birth (only postpartum minilaparotomy tubectomy can be performed) • Any time 6 weeks or more after childbirth if it is reasonably certain she is not pregnant (interval sterilization)
After MTP	• Concurrently with surgical MTP or within 7 days post MTP • Laparoscopic tubal occlusion procedure can be performed only in MTPs up to 12 weeks of gestation • In case of medical abortion, the tubectomy should be done after next menstrual cycle
After miscarriage or abortion	Within 7 days if no complication
After using emergency contraceptive pills	Within 7 days after the start of her next monthly bleeding or any other time if it is reasonably certain she is not pregnant

Timing of the Procedure

Female sterilization can be performed at various times as described in Table 5.[9]

Laparoscopic tubal ligation should not be done concurrently with second-trimester abortion and in the postpartum period as the tubes are thick and edematous.

Minilaparotomy

The operation is performed under local anesthesia or general anesthesia. After aseptic cleaning of the abdomen and placing sterile drapes, the abdomen is opened in layers through a small incision. The site of the incision depends on the size of the uterus. For puerperal sterilization subumbilical incision is placed 2 finger breadth or 3–4 cm below the level of the fundus, whereas in interval sterilization, the incision is suprapubic 2.5 cm above the pubic symphysis.

After opening the parietal peritoneum, the pelvic structures are identified. The fallopian tubes are identified. This is done by tracing the tubes till the fimbrial ends. It is important not to confuse the round ligament with the fallopian tubes. The tubes are held with atraumatic Babcock's forceps.

Tubal ligation is then performed using one of the techniques as described below.

Pomeroy technique: In this method, a loop of 2–3 cm of the isthmic portion of the tube is made approximately 2–3 cm from the cornual end of the tube. It is elevated to expose the vascular supply of the mesosalpinx. A strand of absorbable suture material chromic catgut no. 1-0 is passed through an avascular portion of mesosalpinx to ligate the base of the loop till it blanches. The stump ligature is held with an artery forceps and the mesosalpinx is pierced with an open blade of the Metzenbaum scissors above the ligature and

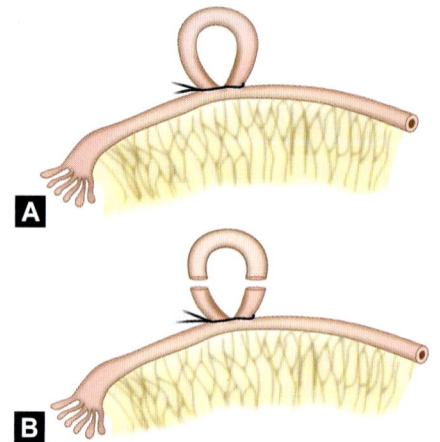

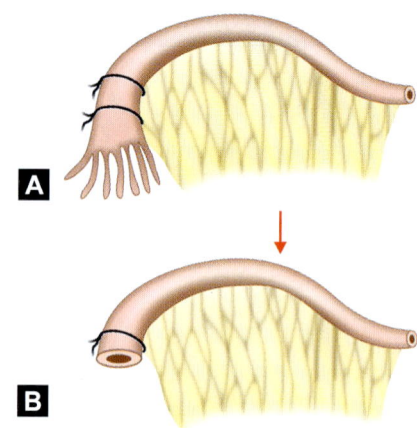

Figs. 4A and B: Pomeroy's technique of tubal ligation. (A) Loop of fallopian tube in isthmic portion; (B) Excision of a segment of fallopian tube.

Figs. 5A and B: Kroener technique of tubal ligation. (A) Fallopian tube tied near fimbrial end; (B) Fimbrial end excised.

approximately 1 cm of the tube is excised, leaving a 0.5 cm stump on either side (Figs. 4A and B).

The stump is checked for hemostasis. The same is repeated on other side. The two ends fall apart once the suture gets absorbed subsequently.

Irving technique: In Irving technique, the tube is doubly ligated with chromic catgut about 2.5 cm from the uterine cornu and then severed in between the sutures. The sutures on the medial ends of the tube are kept long for traction. This medial tubal end is mobilized by dissecting it from the mesosalpinx.

A small tunnel is made on the posterior surface of the uterus near the cornu and the medial stump is buried into this. The lateral stump is peritonized by burying it into the mesosalpinx. This technique has a very low failure rate.

Uchida technique: Saline with epinephrine is injected into the mesosalpinx, which is then cut open and the tube is pulled out to form a loop. A portion of the tube is removed after ligating it at two sites and the medial stump is buried into the mesosalpinx.

Fimbriectomy (Kroener Technique): The fimbrial end of the tube is doubly ligated with silk sutures and then removed (Figs. 5A and B). It is a simple procedure, but has very poor chances of successful recanalization subsequently.

Madlener technique: In Madlener technique, a loop of tube is made as in Pomeroy technique in the isthmic portion of the tube and the base is crushed and ligated with silk, a nonabsorbable suture. It is a simple procedure, but has high failure rates. It is not advocated for postpartum women as the ligature may slip or become loose when the fallopian tube involutes in the postpartum period.

Parkland technique: An avascular area in the mesosalpinx adjacent to the tube is identified and perforated with a small artery forceps and the jaws opened to separate the tube from the adjacent mesosalpinx for about 2.5 cm. The freed tube is ligated proximally and distally with chromic catgut suture and the intervening segment is excised with

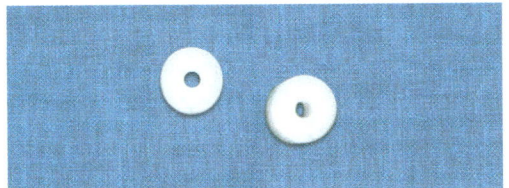

Fig. 6: Falope rings.

scissors. It is preferred when the tube is adherent and thick and it is difficult to make a loop.

Laparoscopic Sterilization

Laparoscopic sterilization is a safe, simple, and effective minimally invasive procedure. It can be performed under local anesthesia as an outpatient procedure and is commonly performed in sterilization camps.

Methods of tubal occlusion in laparoscopic sterilization:

Falope ring: Falope ring was introduced by Yoon in 1974.[11] It is the most used device for laparoscopic tubectomy. The rings are made of silicone rubber with 5% barium sulfate to make them radiopaque. The outer diameter is 3.6 mm, inner diameter is 1 mm, and thickness is 2.2 mm (Fig. 6). A specially designed laparoscope is loaded with two Falope rings and introduced inside the abdominal cavity. After identifying one of the fallopian tubes, the prongs of the applicator are pushed out, the tube grasped about 3 cm from the cornual end of the uterus, and the prongs are closed. The tube is then pulled into the applicator with simultaneously slowly pushing the laparoscope inside the abdomen. The ring is then pushed over the tube. This is repeated on the other tube (Fig. 7).

Clips: Two types of clips are available, the spring-loaded clip (Hulka-Clemens clip) and silicone titanium clip (Filshie clip). The

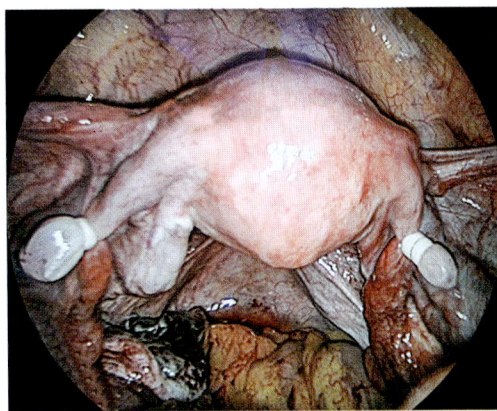

Fig. 7: Bilateral laparoscopic ligation.

Hulka-Clemens clip consists of two plastic jaws with interlocking teeth. The jaws are held together by a stainless-steel spring, which is pushed forward to lock the clip in place over the tube. A clip is placed on the isthmus on each tube 2–3 cm from the uterus with a special straight type laparoscope. The Filshie clip is made of titanium with the inner surface of silicone. The latest clips have hinged jaws that open and close easily, allowing easy removal and repositioning when needed.

Bipolar electrocoagulation: The current from an electrocautery machine enters and leaves the body tissues from the same grasping forceps. The forceps grasps the mobile midportion of the tube and current is passed for about 10 seconds from a bipolar generator. The fulguration involves only a small portion of the tube and its adjacent mesosalpinx. However, due to lateral spread of thermal damage to adjacent tissues, electrocoagulation is not recommended and rarely used.

Contraindications: The contraindications to laparoscopy are listed in Box 9. In all these cases, minilaparotomy is preferred.

Box 9: Contraindications to laparoscopic sterilization.
- Heart disease
- Severe respiratory dysfunction
- Hiatus hernia
- History of previous intestinal surgery
- Puerperium/post second-trimester abortion

In India, the Ministry of Health and Family Welfare has issued Standards for Female Sterilization (2006)[10] which were revised in 2014.[9] These are to be followed while performing sterilization. These are listed in Box 10. In addition to this, certain precautions should be observed while applying Falope rings (Box 11).

Complications: Complications, though rare, are possible and should be kept in mind while performing this procedure. Minor complications include abdominal wall hematoma, surgical emphysema, and uterine injury. Serious and more dangerous complications include anesthetic hazards, injury of larger vessels, intestinal injury, thermal injury if electrocoagulation is used, mediastinal emphysema and cardiorespiratory embarrassment.

Failure rates: The typical failure rate following female sterilization by tubal ligation is 0.4% [World Health Organization (WHO)].[12] In India, large studies report a failure rate of 0.2–1.3% with laparoscopic sterilization.[13]

Vaginal Tubal Ligation

Tubal ligation by the vaginal route is not very popular. The procedure is performed as an interval procedure, but due to its high failure rate and increased rate of complications such as bleeding and infection, it is now rarely performed in favor of the easier options as mentioned before.

Box 10: Standards for laparoscopic sterilization.[10]
- To avoid hypoventilation, the patient must not be placed in the Trendelenburg position in excess of 15°
- A uterine elevator should be used to facilitate visualization of the fallopian tube
- Pneumoperitoneum should be created with Veress needle
- Insufflation of the abdomen with carbon dioxide is the preferred method
- Intra-abdominal pressure must not exceed 15 mm of mercury. Slow insufflation with a graded insufflator and gradual desufflation must be done
- The skin incision should not exceed the diameter of the trocar
- The trocar is to be angled toward the hollow of the sacrum; the operator must lift the anterior abdominal wall before introducing the trocar
- Tubal occlusion must always be done with Falope rings; cautery should not be used
- Surgeon should remove all the gas from abdominal cavity before removing the trocar

Box 11: Practical tips while applying Falope rings on fallopian tubes.
- Fallopian tube should be drawn slowly and smoothly into the sleeve of the laparoscope after proper identification
- Length of the tube included should be just necessary to provide adequate occlusion. Too short or too long loop should be avoided to prevent failures or excessive damage to the tube, respectively
- Avoid pulling up the tube and once the tube is caught between the prongs, the laparoscope is pushed close to the tube before the ring is applied. This is to prevent injury to the mesosalpinx and or tube
- Applying rings on thick, edematous or fixed tubes should be avoided
- After ligating both tubes, the operator should systematically inspect the pelvis to verify that both tubes are now occluded and that there is no unusual bleeding or visceral injury

Hysteroscopic Sterilization (Essure)

The microcoil "Essure" is a spring-like device. This is introduced using a hysteroscopic inserter into the uterus and then into the cornual end of each fallopian tube. In 3 months' time, scar tissue grows into the device and plugs the fallopian tube. This can be performed as an outpatient procedure. The microcoil insertion is successful in 90–95% of women.[14] The placement of Essure must always be confirmed by X-ray or USG after 3 months, until then the woman must not have unprotected intercourse. It has not yet been introduced in India. Since 2013, the product has been controversial, with thousands of women reporting severe side effects leading to surgical extraction of the coil. In February 2016, the Food and Drug Administration (FDA) issued a "black box" label to warn the public about the harmful complications associated with the use of this device and requested the manufacturers to follow 2,000 women for at least 3 years, comparing the effectiveness and safety of the device with other surgical contraceptive methods. In April 2018, the FDA restricted sale and use of Essure.

Male Sterilization

Despite male sterilization (vasectomy) being an easier, safer, and less costly procedure, it remains far less commonly performed procedure as compared to female sterilization as a permanent method of contraception. Newer improvements in the technique, especially the "no scalpel" technique developed in China have further popularized this procedure. The eligibility criteria as outlined by Government of India are listed in Box 12.[9]

Counseling

Counseling is the process of helping the patient make informed and voluntary decisions about fertility. Counseling should be in the language that they understand.

Box 12: Eligibility criteria for male sterilization.

- Client should be married
- Client should ideally be below the age of 60 years
- The couple should have at least one child whose age is above 1 year unless the sterilization is medically indicated
- Client or their spouse or partner must not have undergone sterilization in the past (not applicable in the cases of failure of previous sterilization)
- Client must be in a sound state of mind to understand the full implications of sterilization
- Mentally ill person must be certified by a psychiatrist and a statement should be given by the legal guardian/spouse regarding the soundness of the client's state of mind

The following steps must be taken before the client signs the consent form:

- Patients must be informed of all the available methods of family planning and made aware that for all practical purposes this operation is a permanent one. An informed decision for sterilization must be made voluntarily.
- Patients should be made to understand what will happen before, during, and after the surgery, and potential complications.
- It should be explained that it is a permanent procedure for preventing future pregnancies.
- It is a surgical procedure that has a possibility of complications, including failure, requiring further management.
- It does not affect sexual pleasure, ability, or performance.
- It does not affect the client's strength or his ability to perform normal day-to-day functions.
- After vasectomy, it is necessary to use a backup contraceptive method until azoospermia is achieved (usually this takes 3 months).

- Sterilization does not protect against RTIs, STIs, and HIV/AIDS.
- A reversal of this surgery is possible, but the reversal involves major surgery and its success cannot be guaranteed.

Preprocedure Assessment

Preprocedure assessment includes case selection, preoperative assessment, review of the surgical procedure, and postoperative care. It is essential to ensure that the consent for surgery is voluntary and well-informed and that the client is physically fit for the surgery. Preoperative assessment can also provide an opportunity for overall health screening and treatment of reproductive tract infections.

Demographic information: This includes age, marital status, occupation, religion, educational status, number of living children, and age of youngest child. Some of this information is required for assessing if the client is eligible for undergoing the procedure.

Medical history: It is important to screen the client for severe anemia, acute febrile illness, jaundice, chronic systemic disease, bronchial asthma, heart disease, uncontrolled diabetes, hypertension, thyrotoxicosis, severe nutritional deficiencies, and sexual impairments or sexual problems. The immunization status for tetanus; current medications, if any; current contraceptive method being used by the couple; and the last menstrual period (LMP) of the wife should also be enquired.

Physical examination: The pulse, blood pressure, temperature, general condition, and nutritional status of the client are assessed. The penis, testicles, and scrotum are examined. Further examination is done as indicated by the client's medical history. Laboratory evaluation includes Hb level, urine analysis for sugar, and any other investigation as indicated.

Contraindications

There are no absolute contraindications for performing male sterilization. There are certain conditions that require caution, delay, or referral to a specially equipped center. The eligibility criteria for male surgical sterilization procedures outlined by Government of India family planning serve as guidelines for case selection based on the clinical findings of the client.[10]

Timing of Surgical Procedure

Male sterilization can be done at any convenient time on healthy clients.

Surgical Technique

The procedure is usually performed under local anesthesia (1% lignocaine) and can be either a conventional vasectomy or a non-scalpel vasectomy (NSV).

Conventional vasectomy: The conventional vasectomy operation is performed either with two incisions located at the root of the scrotum on either side or with one incision in the midline. The length of each incision should not be >2 cm. Smaller incisions will minimize the chances of complications. The midscrotal part of the vas should be removed. It must not be cut close to the epididymis, over the convoluted part of the vas deferens. The vas must be separated from the tissues and excised in all cases. The portion excised should not be >1 cm in length. Removal of the excess length of the vas may make a recanalization operation difficult, if it is required in the future. The cut ends of the vas must be tied with 2-0 silk and the sheath of the vas that is the spermatic fascia should be interposed between the two cut ends. The skin incision should be closed with nonabsorbable sutures and covered with a piece of sterile gauze. Before closing the wound, all bleeding points must be tied so as to ensure complete hemostasis and to prevent bleeding or hematoma formation. Use of tincture of benzoin causes excoriation of the scrotal skin and should therefore be avoided for dressing. The patient should wear a suspensory bandage for 1 week to support the scrotum, until the stitches are removed.

Nonscalpel vasectomy: The basic difference between the NSV procedure and the conventional technique is in the surgical approach to the vas, which is through a small puncture in the scrotum rather than by a cut with a scalpel. The surgical procedure of vas ligation is the same as in the conventional method. Long-term clinical reports have shown that NSV is less invasive than the conventional technique, causes fewer complications and takes much less time.

The procedure involves fixation, puncture, and delivery of vas followed by ligation. The site of fixation and puncture of the vas will be at the junction of the upper and the middle third of the scrotum on the midline.

The vas is fixed in the midline at the junction of its upper one third and lower two third by a vas fixation forceps. This is done by the three-finger technique. The skin is then punctured with a vas dissection forceps, the vas is dissected out, and the bare vas is delivered out of the puncture hole, ligated and excised. About 1 cm length of the bare vas should be ligated and excised. The removal of the excessive length of vas may make the recanalization operation difficult, if it is required by the client in the future.

The cut ends of the vas should be tied with nonabsorbable suture material (2-0 silk) and the sheath of the vas should preferably be interposed between the two cut ends.

The opposite vas must be fixed exactly in the same manner using the three-finger technique at the lower end of the previously made puncture hole. It should be punctured and delivered in the same way through the earlier hole without increasing its size.

After the excision and ligature of both the vas, the puncture site is inspected for any bleeding. If there is none, the puncture site should be dressed with a small piece of gauze. This should be retained for 48 hours. No stitch is applied since the puncture contracts and is nearly invisible after the removal of the instruments.

The patient should wear his normal snugly fitting underwear or use scrotal support with suspensory bandage.

Postoperative Care

The patient should be discharged when the following conditions are met: 30 minutes have passed after the surgery, patient is alert, and the ambulatory and vital signs are stable and normal.

Analgesic and other medicines if needed must be provided or prescribed prior to sending the patient home. Following vasectomy, he should wear tight undergarments to keep the scrotum well-supported and preventing the subsequent possibility of bleeding and hematoma formation.

Clear postoperative instructions should be given to the patient. He can resume normal work after 48 hours and return to full activity, including cycling, after 1 week following surgery. He resumes a normal diet as soon as possible and is advised to take analgesics as per need. He is asked to keep the operated area clean and dry, and not disturb or open the dressing. The patient may bathe after 24 hours, while keeping the operated part of the body protected. If the dressing becomes wet, it should be changed. After 48 hours, the dressing may be taken off. He may have intercourse whenever it is comfortable after the surgery, but must be told that he does not become sterile immediately after the operation and that he, or his wife or partner will have to use another method of contraception for 3 months following vasectomy or until the semen analysis shows no sperms. The client must use condoms if his wife or partner is not using contraception.

He is instructed to report to the doctor or the clinic, if there is excessive pain, fainting, fever, bleeding, increase in scrotal size or pus discharge from the operated site. He should return to the clinic in case of conventional vasectomy for removal of stitches and postoperative checkup in 7 days and report for semen analysis after 3 months.

Complications of Male Sterilization

Intraoperative complications:

- *Transient drop in blood pressure or dizziness due to vasovagal attack*: In such cases, the procedure should be delayed, and the patient allowed to rest. The head end of the bed should be lowered, and the leg end raised. An intravenous injection of atropine (0.6 mg) may be given if there is bradycardia. It can be repeated if the baseline pulse rate is not achieved within 1–2 minutes. Oxygen should also be administered simultaneously.
- *Convulsions and reactions to local anesthesia*: In such cases, first and foremost, maintain the patency of airway and give 100% oxygen inhalation. If convulsions persist, injection diazepam 5–10 mg intravenous may be given. Administration of intravenous fluids is generally not needed but may be done depending on the case. In such an event, surgery should be stopped, and the patient is allowed to recover. Further surgery should be performed only at a center with a full range of services.
- *Injury to testicular artery*: This complication is very rare, but if it does occur, first pressure should be used to tamponade both ends of the vessel. Subsequently, both ends of the artery must be ligated.

Immediate complications:
- *Swelling of the scrotal tissue, bruising and pain*: These minor complications often disappear without treatment within 24–48 hours. Ice packs, scrotal support, and simple analgesics may provide relief.
- *Hematoma*: If small, it can be treated by scrotal support, analgesics, and antibiotics. A large hematoma may need evacuation, antibiotics, and further treatment. If a hematoma is detected early, it is desirable to cut the stitches, remove the clots, and look for the bleeding or oozing points, which should be tied.

Infection:
- *Stitch abscess*: To be treated with removal of stitch, drainage, dressings and antibiotics.
- *Wound sepsis*: In case of severe sepsis, the wound should be opened, and the pus drained. Further treatment should include application of dressings and administration of antibiotics and analgesics.
- *Orchitis*: Cases must be treated with antibiotics, analgesics, scrotal support, and bedrest. Severe orchitis may need hospitalization.

Delayed complications:
- *Sperm granuloma*: This can occur either at the site of the vas occlusion or over the epididymis. Majority of these are symptomless and respond to analgesics and anti-inflammatory drugs. Very occasionally, a persistent and painful granuloma may necessitate surgical intervention.
- *Psychological problem*: It is uncommon; however, discussion of the problem,

Table 6: Financial incentives under the National Family Welfare Program.

Contraceptive methods	Incentives		
	Acceptors	Motivators	Service provider
PPIUCD	₹ 300	₹ 150	₹ 150
Female sterilization (tubectomy)	₹ 600 for (BPL + SC + ST)/ ₹ 250 for (above poverty line)	₹ 150	₹ 75
Male sterilization (vasectomy)	₹ 1,100	₹ 200	₹ 100

(PPIUCD: postpartum intrauterine contraceptive device)
NB: No incentive is paid in case of medical method of abortion (MMA).

Table 7: Available benefits under the Family Planning Indemnity Scheme.

Section		Coverage
Section I (A-D): For beneficiaries		Limits
I A	Death following sterilization (inclusive of death during process of sterilization operation) in hospital or within 7 days from the date of discharge from the hospital	₹ 2 lakh
I B	Death following sterilization within 8–30 days from the date of discharge from the hospital	₹ 50,000/-
I C	Sterilization failure	₹ 30,000/-
I D	Cost of treatment in hospital and up to 60 days arising out of complication following sterilization operation (inclusive of complication during process of sterilization operation) from the date of discharge	Actual not exceeding ₹ 25,000/-
Section II: Empanelled doctors under Public and Accredited Private/NGO Sector and Health Facilities under Public and Accredited Private/NGO sector		
II	Indemnity coverage up to 4 cases of litigations per doctor and per health facility in a year	Up to ₹ 2 lakh per case of litigation

clarification of the role of sterilization, and answering questions are important steps. Appropriate referral should be given to the patient.

- *Failure of vasectomy*: Incidences of failure are quite low but may occur because of technical deficiencies in the surgical procedure or as a result of spontaneous recanalization. The patient's wife should be offered MTP or should be medically supported throughout pregnancy. The patient should be offered a repeat surgery, as indicated.

Financial Incentives under the National Family Welfare Program

Under the National Family Welfare Program, the Government of India gives incentives for acceptors of various family planning methods. Incentives are also offered to the motivators and service providers for their services. The incentive money is transferred to the account of the beneficiary by DBT (Direct Bank Transfer) to ensure transparency. The various incentives offered under the Family Welfare Program are given in Table 6.

Family Planning Indemnity Scheme[15]

As per the directives of Hon'ble Supreme Court, the Union of India brought into effect an Insurance Policy for all States/UTs with effect from November 29, 2005 to provide compensation for postoperative complications, failure of sterilization or death attributable to the procedure of sterilization. The scheme thereafter has been modified as "Family Planning Indemnity Scheme" and is operational from April 1, 2013.

The available benefits under the Family Planning Indemnity Scheme are given in Table 7.

KEY POINTS

- Medical termination of pregnancy and sterilization are both important components of the Family Welfare Program.
- It is important to select the right procedure for the right patient for optimum outcome and minimum complications.
- Preprocedure counseling, informed consent, and postprocedure advice are as important as the procedure itself.

REFERENCES

1. World Health Organization (2012). Safe and unsafe induced abortion: global and regional levels in 2008, and trends during 1995-2008. [online] Available from https://www.who.int/reproductivehealth/publications/unsafe_abortion/rhr_12_02/en/. [Last accessed March, 2020].
2. The Medical Termination of Pregnancy Act, 191 no. 34 of 1971. [online] Available from http://www.mp.gov.in/health/acts/mtp%20Act.pdf [Accessed September, 2014].
3. Press Information Bureau, Government of India. (2020). [online] Available from https://pib.gov.in/PressReleasePage.aspx?PRID=1600916 [online]. [Last accessed on March, 2020].
4. Ministry of Health and Family Welfare, Government of India. (2018) Comprehensive Abortion Care. Training and Service Delivery Guidelines, 2nd edition. [online] Available from: https://nhm.gov.in/New_Updates_2018/NHM_Components/RMNCHA/MH/Guidelines/CAC_Training_and_Service_Delivery_Guideline.pdf. [Last accessed March, 2020.
5. Kruse B, Poppema S, Creinin MD, Paul M. Management of side effects and complications inmedical abortion. Am J Obstet Gynecol. 2000;183:S65-75.
6. Royal College of Obstetricians and Gynaecologists. The Care of Women Requesting Induced Abortion (Evidence-based Clinical Guideline No. 7). London: RCOG Press; 2004.
7. Goldberg, Dean G Kanf MS, Youssof S, Darney PD. Manual versus electric vacuum aspiration for early first-trimester abortion: a controlled study of complication rates. Obstet Gynecol. 2004;103(1):101-7.
8. Statham H, Solomou W, Green J. Late termination of pregnancy: law, policy and decision making in four English fetal medicine units. BJOG. 2006;113(12):1402-11.
9. Ministry of Health and Family Welfare, Government of India. (2014). Reference Manual for Female Male Sterilization.[online] Available from. http://www.tnhealth.org/dfw/notification/manuals/Ref%20Manual%20for%20Female%20Sterilization.pdf. {Last accessed on March, 2020].
10. Division of Research Studies and Standards, Ministry of Health and Family Welfare, Government of India. (2006). Standards for Female and Male Sterilization Services. [online] Available from http:// nrhm.gov.in/images/pdf/guidelines/ nrhm-guidelines/family-planning/std-for-sterilization-services.pdf [Last accessed March, 2020].
11. Brenner WE, Edelman DA, Black JF, Goldsmith A. Laparoscopic sterilization with electrocautery, spring-loaded clips, and Silastic bands: technical problems and early complications. Fertil Steril. 1976;27(3): 256-66.
12. World Health Organization. (2015). Medical Eligibility Criteria for Contraceptive Use, 5th edition. [online] Available from https://www.who.int/reproductivehealth/publications/

family_planning/MEC-5/en/. [Last accessed March, 2020].
13. Shilpa Vishwas, Rokade J, Mule V, Dandapannavar S. Female sterilization failure: Review over a decade and its clinico-pathological correlation. Int J Appl Basic Med Res. 2014;4(2):81-5.
14. Povedano B, Arjona JE, Velasco E, Monserrat JA, Lorente J, Castelo-Branco C. Complications of hysteroscopic Essure® sterilisation: report on 4306 procedures performed in a single centre. BJOG. 2012;119(7):795-9.
15. Family Planning Division, Ministry of Health & Family Welfare, Government of India. (2016). Manual for Family Planning Indemnity Scheme. [online] Available from http://upnrhm.gov.in/assets/site-files/family_planning/4.Manuals_of_FP-2015-16/FPIS_Manual.pdf. [Last accessed March, 2020].

SUGGESTED READING

1. Family Planning Division, Ministry of Health & Family Welfare, Government of India (2016). Manual for Family Planning Indemnity Scheme [online] Available from: http://upnrhm.gov.in/assets/site-files/family_planning/4.Manuals_of_FP-2015-16/FPIS_Manual.pdf. [Last accessed March, 2020].
2. Ministry of Health and Family Welfare, Government of India (2014). Reference Manual for Female Male Sterilization [online] Available from: http://www.tnhealth.org/dfw/notification/manuals/Ref%20Manual%20for%20Female%20Steri l ization.pdf. {Last accessed on March, 2020].
3. Ministry of Health and Family Welfare, Government of India (2018). Comprehensive Abortion Care. Training and Service Delivery Guidelines, 2nd edition [online] Available from: https://nhm.gov.in/New_Updates_2018/ NHM_Components/RMNCHA/MH/ Guidelines/CAC_Training_and_Service_ Delivery_Guideline.pdf. [Last accessed March, 2020.
4. World Health Organization (2015). Medical Eligibility Criteria for Contraceptive Use, 5th edition [online] Available from: https://www.who.int/reproductivehealth/publications/family_planning/MEC-5/en/. [Last accessed March, 2020].

58 Government Initiatives to Improve Maternal and Neonatal Health

Monika Datta

INTRODUCTION

An obstetrician puts his/her knowledge and skills to achieve a healthy mother and newborn as an outcome of a pregnancy in his/her care. In addition to their knowledge and skills, there are other factors which can influence the outcomes which include timely access to obstetric care, sociocultural and economic barriers, lack of awareness about the required care and its availability, literacy levels, nutritional status, and other environmental factors, many of which are not directly in the purview of the health departments. A holistic approach toward address of these issues is required for optimizing maternal and neonatal outcomes.

Sustainable Development Goals (SDGs), articulated by the global community, show that governments are now working in that direction. Seventeen SDGs have been identified and SDG 3 is "Good health and well-being." Targets for achievement under this goal include reduction in maternal mortality ratio (MMR) to <70 and reduction in neonatal mortality rate (NMR) to <12 by 2030.

India, with world's 17% population, contributes significantly to the global maternal and newborn deaths and thus, has a vital role to play in global SDG achievement. Government is fully committed to achievement of these targets and has undertaken many initiatives.

Some of the initiatives are listed here.

Provision of Accredited Social Health Activist

Provision of an Accredited Social Health Activist (ASHA) in rural areas (1 for every 1,000 population) and vulnerable urban areas (1 for every 2,000 population) to make the women aware of the early and complete antenatal care (ANC) and to mobilize her to the nearest public healthcare facility for accessing the care. ASHA is incentivized for the early registration, complete antenatal checkup, and institutional delivery and three postnatal visits. There is emphasis on early identification of the high-risk cases and ensuring her safe delivery. ASHA is a valuable resource for reaching out and holding on to the high-risk women throughout pregnancy and attainment of safe delivery. Obstetricians in first referral units (FRUs) and district hospitals must therefore understand and use this enablement judiciously.

Provision of Auxiliary Nurse Midwife

Under this, one Auxiliary Nurse Midwife (ANM) is provided for every 10,000 population. Each primary healthcare facility has ANMs who are responsible for line listing of all pregnant women in their area and ensure complete ANC and safe delivery with the help of the ASHAs of her area. The aim is to ensure 100% institutional deliveries. Following delivery, each newborn and especially those at a higher risk are followed up for appropriate care. Early diagnosis and effective management of anemia is one of the vital activities. Complete and timely immunization and nutritional and growth surveillance of infants and children are also the mandates of the ANM. Counseling on reproductive health, family planning methods, and safe abortion services are parts of the package of services the ANM provides. Obstetricians and pediatricians in public healthcare facilities must utilize this human resource through their capacity building and effective liaison with them.

Home-based Newborn Care (HBNC)

Under this initiative, all ASHAs are trained in making home visits for checking postpartum progress and well-being of mothers and newborns using a simple checklist and counseling for breastfeeding, diet, etc. ASHA makes six home visits in case of an institutional delivery and seven visits in case of a home delivery upon fixed intervals. At every visit, she enquires about certain signs and symptoms and weighs and examines the baby. Upon coming across a mother or a newborn showing any danger signs or symptoms which requires higher level care, the woman is referred to the nearest primary or secondary healthcare facility. If required, ASHA accompanies the patient to the referral facility. Growth monitoring with special emphasis on tracking of low birth weight babies and mobilizing the women for timely and complete immunization of newborns and infants are also key activities of ASHA.

Capacity Building of the Staff at Various Levels of Healthcare Facilities

For provision of optimum antenatal, intranatal, and postnatal care, modules/manuals laying detailed guidelines have been prepared and are used for training staff at various levels. The various guidelines, namely Anemia Mukt Bharat, Diagnosis and Management of Gestational Diabetes Mellitus, Prevention and Management of Postpartum Hemorrhage, Lactation Management, National Immunization Schedule, etc., have been brought out by the Ministry of Health and Family Welfare, Government of India (MOHFW, GOI). Skill laboratories/stations are being set up at medical colleges and district hospitals for skill enhancement and training on newer strategies for Care Around Birth (CAB) through "Dakshata" trainings.

Strengthening of the Health Infrastructure at the Primary Level and the Delivery Points

District hospitals and FRUs are being strengthened in terms of the required equipment and manpower. All FRUs are to have a blood bank or a blood storage facility. Government is providing funds for setting up of High Dependency Units (HDUs) and Obstetric Intensive Care Units (ICUs) in district hospitals and medical college hospitals for optimum management of obstetric emergencies and complications. In order to ensure quality-assured care, government is building new maternity and child health (MCH) blocks and augmenting the bed capacity in already existing ones.

Ensuring Quality in Care—"LaQshya" (Labor Room Quality Improvement Initiative)

Compliance with Standard Operating Protocols for intranatal and postnatal care is being reinforced through a quality assessment and improvement process under National Quality Assurance Program. A subset dealing with the labor room and maternity care has been labeled as LaQshya. As a part of the Quality Certification, the assessment of labor room/maternity operating theater (OT) is done using exhaustive checklists designed to gage the status of service availability, quality in clinical care, inputs, infection control mechanisms, support services, patient satisfaction scores, outcomes, and existing quality management systems. In LaQshya assessments, there is a special emphasis on respectful maternity care and the new concept of allowing birth companion in labor room. Apart from the enhanced outcomes, recognition and quality branding of the institution also gets certain monetary incentive with LaQshya certification.

Operationalization of Newborn Stabilization Units and Special Newborn Care Units

Facility-based newborn care (FBNC) is another key initiative being implemented under the National Health Mission (NHM) to reduce the neonatal mortality. This includes setting up of Newborn Care Corners (NBCCs) at all delivery points to provide essential newborn care, Newborn Stabilization Units (NBSUs) at the Community Health Centers and FRUs for management of selected newborn conditions and to stabilize serious and sick newborns before referral to higher centers.

District hospitals and subdistrict hospitals with annual delivery load of >3,000 deliveries are being provided with Special Newborn Care Units (SNCUs) to provide care for sick newborns:

Operationalizing referral linkages

Defining and optimizing referral linkages for delivery, especially high-risk deliveries, is also an important activity without which the service delivery loop is not completed.

Ambulances for MCH Services

In many states, transporting pregnant women for delivery and back home after discharge is a part of the ambulance services.

Reproductive and Child Health (RCH) Portal

Tracking of eligible couples, pregnant women, and newborns through IT-based enablement. RCH portal is a web-based IT platform in which the ANM captures the information about the eligible couples and their protection status, pregnant woman, and the details of the ANC parameters, delivery, newborn details, status of weight and immunization. Reports of details of high-risk women, services overdue and newborns at risk, etc., are generated from the portal and used for effective tracking and follow-up.

Kilkari

This is a mobile service that delivers time-sensitive 72 audio messages (voice call) about pregnancy and child healthcare directly to the mobile phones of pregnant women/

mother/parents. For this, beneficiary must be registered on RCH portal with correct phone number and correct last menstrual period (LMP).

Maternal Death Audit

Audit of every maternal death is done at the facility level, designated officials at the district/state level to find gaps, filling of which can prevent maternal deaths.

In addition to these institutional mechanisms, certain specific schemes are also being implemented by the Government which are described in the following text.

GOVERNMENT SCHEMES FOR BENEFICIARIES

Janani Suraksha Yojana

Janani Suraksha Yojana (JSY) is an intervention aimed at reducing maternal and neonatal mortality by promoting institutional delivery among the poor pregnant women. Scheme is funded by Central Government through NHM across the nation with special focus on low performing states. It provides cash incentive to women availing complete ANC and institutional delivery.

ASHA, who works as a link between the community and the healthcare providers, is also incentivized for facilitating access to the complete ANC package and institutional delivery. Scheme focuses on the poor pregnant women. States having high home delivery rates, namely Uttar Pradesh, Uttaranchal, Bihar, Jharkhand, Madhya Pradesh, Chhattisgarh, Assam, Rajasthan, Orissa, and Jammu and Kashmir, have been named as low performing states (LPS) while the remaining states are categorized as high performing states (HPS).

Eligibility for the Scheme

- *Below poverty line (BPL) certification*: This is required in all HPS states. However, where BPL cards have not yet been issued or have not been updated, states/UTs have formulated a criterion for certification of poor and needy status of the expectant mother's family by empowering the Gram Pradhan or ward members to issue such certificates.
- *Beneficiary registered under the scheme must have a JSY card along with the MCP (Mother and Child Protection) card*: The woman must be registered with a primary healthcare facility and with the help of the area ASHA must avail the antenatal services. The ANM and Medical Officer prepare a microplan to ensure the safe delivery and appropriate postpartum care. Services provided at each ANC visit are recorded on the MCP card. This and the JSY card are seen before paying the assistance money.
- The woman must provide the bank details and Aadhaar for payment.

Cash Assistance Amount (in INR)

The cash assistance amount (in INR) is given in Table 1. Direct Benefit Transfer (DBT) mode is used for the payment to beneficiaries. Payment is made into the Aadhaar-linked bank account of beneficiary via Public Finance Management System (PFMS) portal. This is an IT-enabled payment gateway.

Janani Shishu Suraksha Karyakaram

With Janani Shishu Suraksha Karyakaram (JSSK), though the institutional deliveries increased in number, there was still a

Table 1: Cash assistance amount (in INR) in Janani Suraksha Yojana.

Category	Rural			Urban		
	Mother's package	ASHA's package	Total	Mother's package	ASHA's package	Total
LPS	1,400/-	600/-	2,000/-	1,000/-	200/-	1,200/-
HPS	700/-		700/-	600/-		600/-

(ASHA: accredited social health activist; HPS: high performing states; LPS: low performing states)

significant number of women not accessing the health facilities for delivery. Many who agree to institutional delivery refuse to stay in the hospital for 48 hours which is the period for most of the postpartum complications. Out-of-pocket spending (OOPs) on transport, medicines, investigations, and food during hospital stay were factors preventing access to safe delivery services.

Janani Shishu Suraksha Karyakaram was launched with the objective of minimizing OOPs on pregnancy, delivery, spending on sickness of neonate to zero, and is unmistakably a giant leap toward achievement of "Health for all". Initiative entitles all pregnant women delivering in public health institutions, irrespective of socioeconomic status, to free and no-expense delivery, including caesarean section.

As per the scheme, no user charges would be levied and all expenses related to delivery in a public health facility would be borne by the government. The entitlements include:

- *For the mother*:
    - Free drugs and consumables
    - Free essential diagnostics (blood, urine, ultrasonography, etc.)
    - Free antenatal and delivery services including cesarean section
    - Free blood, if so required
    - Free diet during hospital stay
    - Free transport from one facility to another in case of referral
    - Free transport from home to hospital and back to home
    - No user charges to be levied.
- *For the sick newborn*:
    - Free drugs and consumables
    - Free essential diagnostics (blood, urine, ultrasonography, etc.)
    - Free blood, if so required
    - Totally free treatment and no user charges of any kind
    - Free transport from one facility to another in case of referral
    - Free transport from home to hospital and drop back to home.

The scheme is funded by central government through NHM. Under the scheme, no cash benefit is provided to the beneficiary. All public health facilities providing antenatal, delivery, and neonatal healthcare are provided additional funds to enable them to fill up their gaps in supply chain mechanisms, diagnostic services, blood transfusion facility, and ensure that beneficiaries do not spend any money from their pocket on these items. Funds also support provision of food during the hospital stay and transport services.

Though JSY and JSSK have increased the access to institutional deliveries to a significant extent, operational bottlenecks at the level of hospital administrators in local procuring and tedious record keeping are preventing optimum utilization of this scheme in some states. Also, under JSY, the DBT mode through PFMS and Aadhaar-linked bank account of a onetime cash assistance is resulting in lesser number of beneficiaries getting the assistance.

Pradhan Mantri Surakshit Matritva Abhiyan

Both JSY and JSSK have managed to draw pregnant women to the public health institutions for delivery, but this has not resulted in the expected quantum fall in maternal mortality. Around 61.8% women receive first ANC in first trimester (RSOC) and the full ANC coverage which includes a minimum of four ANC visits and two Tetanus Toxoid injections; provision of 100 iron and folic acid (IFA) tablets is as low as 20%. This indicates that quality of ANC, despite availability of treatment guidelines, provisions for regular trainings, and supportive supervision and outreach platforms such as Village Health and Nutrition Day (VHND), is a matter of great concern.

In order to augment the range of existing services for completeness and quality, Pradhan Mantri Surakshit Matritva Abhiyan (PMSMA) has been launched to cover over 3 crore pregnant women in the country. Under the campaign, a minimum assured package of ANC services is provided to the beneficiaries on the 9th day of every month to ensure that every pregnant woman receives at least one checkup in the second and third trimesters of pregnancy. Level-appropriate components of the ANC are delivered at identified public health facilities and accredited private healthcare facilities volunteering for the PMSMA.

The services are provided by the Medical Officer and/OB-GY (Obstetrics-Gynecology) specialist and if required OB-GY volunteers from private sector. PMSMA focuses on detection, referral, treatment, and follow-up of high-risk pregnancies and efforts are made through the ASHAs and ANMs to track the women left out or dropped out and bring them back into the loop of services. PMSMA platform is also used to generate demand through Information Education and Communication (IEC), Interpersonal Communication (IPC), and Behavior Change Communication (BCC) activities.

Pradhan Mantri Matritva Vandana Yojana

Pradhan Mantri Matritva Vandana Yojana (PMMVY) is a centrally sponsored scheme being implemented by the Ministry of Women and Child Development. It is implemented with the objective of providing nutritional support to the pregnant woman, making her aware and facilitate access to complete antenatal, natal, and postnatal services and newborn care. It also provides a partial wage compensation to women for wage-loss during childbirth and childcare.

It is a conditional cash transfer scheme for pregnant and lactating women of 19 years of age or above for the first live birth. INR 5,000/- are disbursed directly into the woman's account through PFMS portal in three installments upon fulfillment of certain conditions, given in Table 2.

Table 2: Conditions for cash transfer scheme for pregnant and lactating women.

Instalments	Conditions	Amount
First	Requires the mother to register her pregnancy in the MCP card along with required documents within 150 days from LMP	1,000/-
Second	At least one antenatal checkup can be claimed post 180 days of pregnancy	2,000/-
Third	• Childbirth is registered • Child has received first cycle of immunizations of BCG, OPV, DPT, and hepatitis B	2,000/-

(BCG: bacillus Calmette-Guérin; DPT: diphtheria-tetanus-pertussis; LMP: last menstrual period; MCP: mother and child protection; OPV: oral polio vaccine)

Rashtriya Bal Swasthya Karyakram

Rashtriya Bal Swasthya Karyakram (RBSK) is an important initiative aiming at early identification and intervention for children from birth to 18 years to cover four "Ds," namely Defects at birth, Deficiencies, Diseases, and Development delays including disability. RBSK includes comprehensive newborn screening at birth for neural tube defects, Down syndrome, cleft lip and palate/cleft palate, talipes (clubfoot), developmental dysplasia of the hip, congenital cataract, congenital deafness, congenital heart diseases, and retinopathy of prematurity.

Mother Absolute Affection Programme

Breastfeeding within an hour of birth could prevent 20% of newborn deaths. Infants who are not breastfed are 15 times more likely to die from pneumonia and 11 times more likely to die from diarrhea than children who are exclusively breastfed. Breastfeeding is a critical child survival intervention. Mother Absolute Affection (MAA) Programme focuses on awareness campaigns through health systems to improve the breastfeeding indicators. It targets pregnant and lactating mothers, family members, and society in order to promote optimal breastfeeding practices.

It includes strengthening of lactation support services at public health facilities through trained healthcare providers and through skilled community health workers. Under the program, there are provisions for recognition and incentivization of health facilities achieving high rates of breastfeeding through robust lactation management processes.

Surakshit Matritva Aashwasan

Surakshit Matritva Aashwasan (SUMAN) is an overarching initiative for *"Zero Preventable Maternal and New-born Deaths"* launched by the Ministry of Health, Government of India, in October 2019. Taking into consideration various ongoing schemes for maternal and new-born healthcare, the initiative seeks to ensure and enforce guaranteed access to free and quality-assured services delivered with respect for women's autonomy and dignity with zero tolerance for denial of services.

The initiative emphasizes on:
- Zero tolerance for any negligence
- Integration of existing initiatives (JSSK, PMSMA, LaQshya, FRUs, etc.)
- Respect for women's autonomy, dignity, feelings, and choices
- 100% maternal death reporting and reviews
- Grievance redressal mechanism
- Client feedback mechanism
- Awards to champions
- Community level maternal death reporting
- Community engagement and mega IEC/BCC
- Intersectoral convergence.

Delivery of promised healthcare services, entitlement schemes, reporting and review of every maternal death, robust feedback mechanisms, and time-bound grievance redressal form the core intent of the initiative.

There are many initiatives and programs in place to facilitate quality care to the pregnant women and their newborn. All healthcare providers should aim at providing quality obstetric care that is safe, timely, effective, equitable, efficient respectful, and patient centric. Quality of obstetric care is the predictor of quality of life of our future generations.

Index

Page numbers followed by b refer to box, f refer to figure, fc refer to flowchart, and t refer to table

A

Abdomen 34
    computed tomography of 49, 348
    ultrasonography 35, 89, 348
        examination of 82
Abdominal circumference 189-191
Abdominal examination 12, 96, 124, 257, 283, 330, 353, 418, 450
Abdominal pain 49, 51fc, 52, 60, 248, 353, 437
    causes of 49, 253
    differential diagnosis of 50t
Abdominal wall
    edema of 162
    hematoma 343
Aberrant right subclavian artery 132, 133
Abnormal behaviour 269, 272fc
    causes of 270
    differential diagnosis of 270, 270b
Abnormal uterine bleeding 301, 302, 330, 332, 353
    differential diagnosis of 301, 301b
Abnormal visual score 430
Abortion 6, 32, 36, 158, 343, 347
    complete 32, 158
    incomplete 32, 35, 158, 607
        septic 50
    inevitable 32, 158, 343
    mid-trimester 50
    missed 32
    post second-trimester 618
    recurrent 25
    second-trimester 611, 612
    septic 34, 86, 148
    surgical 610b, 613
    threatened 32, 35, 343
Abruption 25, 219
Abscess 354, 449, 461
    diverticular 354
    formation 498
    injection site 252, 253f
    pyogenic 92
    stitch 622
    tubo-ovarian 86
Acanthosis nigricans 28, 430
Accredited Social Health Activist 626, 630
    provision of 626
Acetic acid 506, 508, 509t, 511, 512f
    acetowhite negative 507f
    acetowhite positive 507f
    visual inspection with 308, 506, 506t

Achalasia 73
Achilles tendon 95
Acid-fast bacilli 106, 252, 309
    sputum for 106
Acne 415
    depict adrenal maturation 442
Acorn cannula 479
Acquired anal incontinence, differential diagnosis of 390t
Acrochordons 430
Acute respiratory distress syndrome 101, 102, 105
Addison's disease 73
Adductor deformity, bilateral 336
Adenoma, hepatic 146
Adenomyoma 353
Adenomyosis 302, 309f, 310, 329, 331, 336, 343, 358
    ultrasound appearance of 309f
Adnexa 329
Adnexal torsion 50
Adrenal hyperplasia, nonclassic congenital 428
Adrenal insufficiency, autoimmune primary 418
Adrenal pathology, screening for 174
Adrenarche 415, 442
Adrenocorticotropic hormone 440
    stimulation test 438
Advanced bipolar
    devices 559
    tissue sealers 559
Advanced cardiovascular life support 228, 231, 235-237
Advanced trauma life support system 228
Airway 92, 236, 237
    disease 108
    obstruction, upper 101
Alanine
    aminotransferase 75
    transaminase 151, 152
Albumin 151
    serum 152
Alcohol 192, 377
    withdrawal 92
Alkaline phosphatase 150-152
Alkalosis, hypochloremic 77
Allergic dermatitis 111, 399
Allergies 103
Allis forceps 523, 524f, 524t, 534
Alopecia 415

Alpha-2 globulins 117
Alpha-adrenergic
    agonists 377
    blockers 377
Alpha-fetoprotein 213, 357
Alpha-methyldopa 428
Ambiguous genitalia 437
Amebiasis 344
Amenorrhea 32, 414, 415, 417
    causes of 415
    differential diagnosis of 416t
    management of 425t
    primary 414, 420fc, 424
    secondary 414, 415, 417, 421fc, 424
American Academy of Pediatrics 40
American College of Obstetricians and Gynecologists 40, 342
Amniocentesis 129, 219
Amniotic fluid 69f, 122
    biochemical analysis of 142
    testing of 141f
    embolism 92, 100, 101, 108
    index 70, 97
    qualitative assessment of 491
Amniotomy 491
    complications of 492
    contraindications 492
    indications 491
    preprocedure assessment 492
    surgical technique 492
Amsel's criteria 68b, 296
Amylase, serum 56, 230, 257
Anal canal 390
    length 395
Anal contraction, voluntary 370
Anal incontinence 265, 266, 389, 396fc, 498
    postpartum 264
Anal intercourse 390
Anal intraepithelial neoplasia 510
Anal manometry 395
Anal sphincter
    anatomy of 496f
    resting tone 370
Anal wink reflex 370, 370f, 382
    interpretation of 393fc
Anaphylaxis 100, 101
Androgen 430
    insensitivity syndrome 416, 418, 424, 425t
    secreting tumors 427

Anemia 9f, 10f, 21, 54, 77, 111, 122,
    148, 209, 217, 257, 270
  absence of 117
  aplastic 302
  autoimmune hemolytic 220
  causes of 163, 165, 165t
  chronic 157, 158
  combined 158
  megaloblastic 117, 151
  severe 101
  sideroblastic 151
  type of 163, 163t
Anesthesia
  general 252
  local 610, 622
Aneuploidy 192
  screening for 212
Aneurysm
  aortic 343
  needle 524, 525f
  splenic 50
Angina, abdominal 343
Angiogram, pulmonary 107
Angiotensin-converting enzyme 181
  inhibitors 377
Ankle
  jerk 95
  reflex 95f
  swelling 182
Anomaly scan 194, 215
Anorectal anatomy 496
Anorexia 182
  nervosa 418
Anosmia 443
  history of 415
Antacids 80
Antenatal care 3b, 23, 234
  aim of 3
  complete 626
Antenatal management 185
Antenatal steroids, administration
    of 122
Antenatal visits, schedule of 4t
Anterior vaginal wall
  retractor 285f, 286f, 525, 525f, 545f
  visualization of 367f
Antiandrogens 433
Antibiotics 80, 92
  prophylaxis, intravenous 588
Antibody testing 326
Anticardiolipin antibody 174
Anticholinergics 377
Anticoagulants 302, 310
Anticonvulsant 192
Anti-D antibody
  levels 221
  titer of 29
Antidepressants 377
Anti-double-stranded DNA
    antibodies 29

Antiepileptics 417
Antifungal agents 412
Antigen-antibody complexes 410
Antihypertensive agents 176
Anti-inflammatory agents 413
Antimalarials 92
Anti-Müllerian hormone 321
Antineoplastic agents 192
Antinuclear antibody 175
  identification of 175
Antiphospholipid antibody 29, 30, 174
  immunoglobulin G 29
  syndrome 25, 28, 29, 31, 170, 175,
    192
Antipruritic agents 412
Antipsychotics 302, 377, 417
Antithrombin 29
Antitubercular drugs 417
Antral follicles 320f
Anus 284
Anxiety 101
Aorta, coarctation of 170
Aortic dissection 100
Appendicitis 50, 73, 86, 343, 346
Arcuate uterus 480
Arnaux sign 212
Arrhythmias 100, 101, 182
Arterial blood
  gas 105, 232, 252
    analysis 89, 106, 230
    partial pressure of oxygen in 108
Arterial carbon dioxide tension 100
Arteriovenous malformation 92
Artery forceps 525, 525f
Arthritis 28
Artificial insemination 326
Ascites 182
Asherman's syndrome 416, 417, 419,
    610
  diagnosis of 424
Aspartate
  aminotransferase 75, 172
  transaminase 151, 152
Aspiration pneumonitis 101
Aspirin 101
Assisted reproductive techniques 209,
    313, 326
Asthma 101-103, 108
Atrophic external genitalia 363f
Atrophy, vaginal 335
Attention deficit hyperactivity
    disorder 85
Attitude 54
Auscultation 17, 56, 104, 183, 212,
    245, 283
Autoimmune disease 124
Autoimmune disorders 33, 422
Autosomal dominant 143
  trait 137

Auxiliary nurse midwife 626
  provision of 626
Axillary freckling 436
Axillary hair 442
Axonal swelling 174
Ayre's spatula 286, 287f, 503f, 505, 525,
    526, 526f
  indications 526
  technique 526
Azithromycin, oral 83
Azoospermia, obstructive 326

B

Babinski's response 96
Bacillus Calmette-Guérin 631
Backache 210
Bacterial vaginosis 62, 64f, 65, 67, 69,
    69t, 290, 294
  diagnosis of 68b, 296
Bad obstetric history 25, 29t, 30, 30fc
  causes of 25b
Baden-Walker halfway system 366
Barbiturates 122
Barrier methods 584
Bartholin's cyst 407f
Bartholin's gland 290, 338
  infections of 335
  palpation of 285f
Basal body temperature 583
Basal pneumonia 50
Basic life support 235-237
Behçet's disease 409
Below poverty line certification 629
Benzodiazepines 122
Berry aneurysm, ruptured 92
Beta globulins 117
Beta-adrenergic agonists 377
Beta-human chorionic
    gonadotropin 36, 38, 347
Beta-thalassemia 192
Biceps
  jerk 96
  reflex 96f
Bicornuate 323f
  uterus 481f
Bile acids 150, 151
  chelating agent 120
  elevated serum 153
  total serum 118
Biliary tract disease 73
Bilirubin 150
Biometry 194
Biophysical profile 119, 125, 199
  modified 125
  score 70
Biopsy 385, 519
  cannula 477
  specimens, methods of 411
Biparietal diameter 191

Index

Bipolar electrocoagulation 617
Bipolar forceps 558*f*
Birth
  preterm 31, 85
  vaginal 202
Bishop's score 19
  modified 19*t*
Bladder 216, 242
  carcinoma 354
  catheters 526
  diary 378
  distended 212, 354
  function 242, 377*t*
  sound 529, 529*f*
    indications 529
Bleeding 160, 241, 241*f*
  causes of 32*b*, 40*b*
  disorders 302, 307*b*
  in early pregnancy 32
  in late pregnancy 40
  intermenstrual 301
  per vaginum 32, 35, 36*t*, 38*fc*, 41, 46*fc*, 47*fc*
    causes of 40
  persistent 610
  severity of 303
  vaginal 32
Blighted ovum, ultrasound image of 36*f*
Blindness, cortical 174, 176
Blood
  brain barrier 174
  cells 82*f*
  chronic loss of 160
  count, complete 56, 72, 75, 88, 96, 104, 150, 163, 166, 172, 230, 232, 257, 258, 272, 331, 332, 347, 401, 412, 422
  culture 89
  glucose 75, 257
  grouping 29, 230
  investigations, basic 422
  loss 270, 587
    vaginal 34
  pressure 3, 11, 34, 46, 62, 94, 103, 170, 171, 182, 203, 282
    diastolic 171
    high 102
    measurement 12*f*
    recording 282*f*
    systolic 171
  stained vaginal discharge 291
  sugar
    levels 117
    random 97
  toxicology studies 230
  transfusion, massive 101
  urea 29
    nitrogen 56, 75
Blumer's shelf 450

Blurred vision 248
Body mass index 8, 28, 31, 192, 193, 203, 279, 279*t*, 305, 316, 326, 363, 378, 429, 564
Bone 598
  age 439
  marrow aspiration 165
  mineral density 422
Bonney's myomectomy clamp 529
Bonney's test 285*f*, 365*f*, 379, 379*f*
Bormal umbilical artery 196*f*
Bowel
  complaints 250, 264
  disease, inflammatory 50, 329, 335, 336, 343, 390, 408, 445
  echogenic 131-133
  function 242
  injury 485
  obstruction 343
  problems, differential diagnosis of 265*t*
Bradycardia 28, 418, 565, 569*f*
Bradykinins 119
Brain
  abscess 270
  imaging 271
  natriuretic peptide 107
  tumor 111
Braxton Hicks contractions 50
Breast 598
  abscess 453
    lactational 244*f*
  benign lumps of 452*t*
  bilateral 458*f*
  cancer 278, 459
    early stages of 449
  carcinoma of 450
  clinical examination of 452
  complaints 250
  complications 251, 258
  conditions 259*f*
  development, stages of 434, 435*f*
  discharge 449
  disorders, benign 459
  engorged 244*f*, 251, 252*f*
  examination 12, 34, 81, 243, 260, 280, 305, 378, 392, 418, 450
  fibrocystic disease of 456
  lump 449, 454*fc*
    diagnosis of 452
    differential diagnosis of 449, 449*b*
    management of 453*t*
  malignant lumps of 452*t*
  pain in 449
  pathology, treatment of 449
  self-examination 451*f*
  self-palpation, position for 451*f*
  swollen 248
  tender 248

  tissue
    palpation of 458*f*
    proliferation of 457
    ultrasonography 460
Breastfeeding 242, 582, 627, 632
  practice 259
Breathing 92, 236, 237
  difficult 248
  shortness of 248
Breathlessness 100, 109, 449
  acute onset 109
  differential diagnosis of 101*t*
  presence of 102
British Association for Sexual Health and HIV 296
British Society for Colposcopy and Cervical Pathology 308
Broad ligament 354
  hematoma 158
Budd-Chiari syndrome 146, 147
Bulbocavernosus reflex 382
Bullous pemphigoid 111
Burning micturition 5
Burns 335
Burr cells 172

C

Cachexia 182
Cafe-au-lait spots 436
Caffeine 377
Calcineurin inhibitors, topical 413
Calcitriol 402
Calcium
  channel blockers 260, 377
  serum 75
Calendar method 583
Calymmatobacterium granulomatis 411
Camera system 549*f*
Campylobacter 80
Cancer
  cervix 302
  screening technique 502
  vulval 399
Candida
  albicans 64
  infection 62, 63
  vaginitis 290
  vulvovaginitis 403*f*, 406*f*
  wet smear 295*f*
Candidal discharge 293*f*
Candidiasis 62, 67, 69, 335, 399, 412
  thick curdy white clumpy discharge in 64*f*
Cannulas 553
Carbon
  dioxide 484
  monoxide poisoning 101
Carcinoembryonic antigen 357

Carcinoid syndrome 80, 119
Carcinoma 343, 450
  body uterus 309f
  cervix 288
  colon 278, 354
  endometrial 310
  epithelial 353
  hepatocellular 146
  invasive 514
Cardiac arrest 237
Cardiac defect 139
Cardiac failure
  clinical features of 182t
  congestive 171
Cardiff count to ten method 122
Cardiomyopathy 101, 180
  peripartum 101
Cardiorespiratory embarrassment 210
Cardiotocography 70, 89, 123, 124, 177, 564
  acquisition, maternal position for 565
  interpretation 565, 568
  limitations of 572
  monitoring, indications of 564
  trace interpretation 567
Cardiovascular examination 162, 182, 186, 255
Cardiovascular system 12, 88, 95, 161, 171, 226, 282, 378
  evaluation of 229
  examination of 104, 203
Carpal tunnel syndrome 28
Cash transfer scheme 631t
Cauda equina 390
Celiac disease 445
Cells, abnormal 65
Cellulitis 260
Centchroman 311, 417, 598, 599f, 601
  Acts 598
  use of 599b
Central nervous system 53, 86, 95, 227, 390, 436, 437, 439, 450
  infections 270
  tumors of 73
Cephalopelvic disproportion 576
Cerebral
  malaria 92, 270
  palsy 564
  redistribution 195
Cerebroplacental ratio 189-191, 195, 199
Cerebrospinal fluid 271, 272
Cerebrovascular accident 92
Cervical
  amputation 329
  atresia 329
  biopsy 515
  cancer 291, 307f, 501
    advanced 353

  diagnosis of 501, 502, 509
  screening 501, 501b
cap 586
carcinoma 304, 501
conization 516
consistency 19
descent 329
dilatation 19, 530, 562, 564
  indications for 531t
ectropion 32, 40, 290
erosion 32, 35, 40, 62, 63, 290, 302, 306f
excitation pain 293
incompetence 25, 29, 31
infections 32
insufficiency 610
laceration 610
  repair of 499f
length 19
lesions 510t, 514t, 544, 544t
mucus 69f
  method 583
pathology 588
polyp 35, 62, 63, 290, 302, 544
position 19
punch biopsy forceps 515f
stenosis 329, 416
tear 491, 499
  cervix for 534
trauma 485
tumors 32
Cervicitis 293
Cervix 63, 390, 477
  anterior lip of 308f
  colposcopic examination of 513t
  erythema of 64f
  holding anterior lip of 541b
  laceration 498
  normal 512f, 546f
    well-stained 508f
  posterior lip of 308f
  single 481f
  surface of 502
  surgery on 290
  tumors of 40
  visual inspection of 508b
  visualization of 286f, 308f
Cesarean delivery 186, 201
Cesarean section 201
  lower segment 47, 253
  previous 201, 202b, 205fc
  wound 244f
    inspection of 245f
Chadwick's sign 18
Chancroid 339, 408, 410
Chayya 599f
Cheilosis 162
Chemotherapy 335
Chest 95
  auscultation of 104

  evaluation of 229
  examination 255
  pain 102, 248, 449
    history of 180
  trauma 101
  X-ray 29, 30, 105, 106, 180, 185, 186
Chikungunya 86
Chlamydia 294, 302
  antibody test 326
  cultures 348
  trachomatis 62, 86, 291, 294, 326, 411
Chlorides 117
Cholecystitis 50, 73, 86
Cholelithiasis 57f, 146, 147, 150
Cholestyramine 120
Chorioamnionitis 50, 158, 492
Chorioangioma, placental 220
Chorionic villus sampling 129, 138, 143, 219
Chorionicity, determination of 214
Chromopertubation 323f, 324
Chromosomal abnormality 25, 127, 418
  parental 25
Chromosomal anomaly, risk of 139t
Chromosomal microarray 139, 140, 142
Chronic disease 158, 450
Chronic medical disorders 192
Chronic obstructive pulmonary disease 102, 192
Ciprofloxacin 83
Circulation 92, 236
Circumvallate placenta 192
Cirrhosis 146
  primary biliary 146
Clindamycin 69
Clitoral index 430
Clitoral prepuce 338
Clitoris 284
  enlargement of 419
Clobetasol propionate 402
Clostridioides difficile infection 84
Clotrimazole 402
  vaginal pessary, topical 69
Clubbing 28, 103
Clue cells, presence of 68
Coagulation disorder 160
Coagulation profile 35, 44, 153
Coagulogram 184
Cocaine 101
Coccydynia 343
Coitus interruptus 582
Cold extremities 87
Cold knife conisation 517
  advantages of 517t
  disadvantages of 517t
Collin's cannula 479
Collin's knife 562, 562f
Color Doppler 45
  ultrasound 385

Colposcope 510*f*
Colposcopic grading systems 514
Colposcopy 509, 511, 511*f*
  facilitates visualization 509
  guided cervical biopsy 515
  indications of 511*b*
  unsatisfactory 514, 516
Colpotomy 475, 486, 487
Coma 91
Community Health Centers 628
Complex laparoscopic systems 563
Compression ultrasonography 107
Computed tomography 51, 57, 75, 174, 230-232, 252, 256, 272, 357, 358, 385, 386
  pulmonary angiography 107
  scan 118, 231
Condom 62, 63, 584
  female 584, 584*f*
  male 584, 584*f*, 585
Condyloma 507
Condylomata 512
Cone biopsy 516
  indications of 516*b*
Congenital anomaly 122
  absence of 190*t*
  recurrence of 136*t*
Congenital disorder 335
Congenital malformations 544
  type of 139*t*
Conization 517
Conjunctiva
  inspection of 9*f*
  normal 280*f*
  pale 160*f*
Conscious pain mapping 350
Consciousness 235
  level of 74
Constipation 50, 210, 242, 267, 343, 377, 415
  chronic 362
  postpartum 265
Constrictive pericarditis 10
Contact dermatitis 111, 406*f*
  irritant 111
Continuous electronic fetal monitoring 231, 232
Contraception 187, 581, 582*t*, 584
  emergency 304, 599
  methods of 581, 581*t*
  nonhormonal oral 598
  oral emergency 600
Contraceptive 335
  advice 610
  combined hormonal 311, 595, 595*f*
  counseling 614*t*
  history 159, 160, 243, 304, 314, 346
  hormonal 302, 417, 591
  implant 598
  long-acting reversible 582

  patch, combined 596
  pills
    combined oral 433, 591, 594*t*
    emergency 601
    oral 304, 330, 332, 336, 346, 461, 592*t*, 593*t*
    prescribing 582
    progestogen-only hormonal 596
    ring, combined 595
    sponge 585
Conventional pap smear 501, 503*b*
  requirements for 502
Convulsions 6, 91, 92*b*, 248, 622
  control of 98
  differential diagnosis of 92*b*
  history of 148
Coombs test
  direct 222
  indirect 29, 221, 222
Copious grayish white discharge 64*f*
Copper T 587*f*
Cord prolapse 492
Cordocentesis 219
Core needle biopsy 453
Corpus luteum 321*f*
  cyst 353
  hematoma 343
  ruptured 50
Costovertebral angle 347
Cough 102, 377
  acute 102
  chronic 362
  impulse 368
  nocturnal 182
COVID 19 86, 101
Cracked nipple 244*f*, 259*f*
Cramps, abdominal 606
C-reactive protein 56, 88
Creatine kinase muscle brain 184, 186
Crichton's method 17*f*
Crigler-Najjar syndrome 152
Criminal Law Amendment Act 462
Crohn's disease 73, 80, 343, 354, 390
Crown rump length 213
  measurement 213*f*
Culdocentesis 348, 475, 486, 487*t*
  complications 487
  contraindications of 486, 486*t*
  indications of 486, 486*t*
  procedure 486
Cullen's sign 34
Curved artery forceps 525*f*
Cusco's bivalve self-retaining vaginal speculum 285*f*
Cusco's speculum 285, 285*f*, 487, 503, 508, 545, 545*f*, 546*f*
  advantages 545
  disadvantages 545
Cushing's syndrome 170, 418, 427, 430
Cyanosis 28, 54, 91, 103

Cyclical abdominal pain, history of 415
Cyclical progestins 311
Cyclosporine 428
Cyproterone acetate 433
Cyst 354, 453
  endometriotic 353
  hemorrhagic 348*f*
  sebaceous 407*f*
Cysticercosis 92
Cystitis 86, 336, 344, 346
  acute 50
  interstitial 336, 343
Cystocele 528
Cystometry 383
Cystoscopy 384
Cystourethritis 343
Cystourethroscopy 383
Cytology 501
Cytomegalovirus 21, 25, 86, 131, 137, 154
Czerny's retractor 523*f*

D

Daily oral iron supplementation 23
Danazol 428
Dandy-Walker malformation 139
Danger signals 248*b*
D-dimer 107
Death
  intrauterine 81, 119, 219
  perinatal 206
Deaver retractor 523, 523*f*
  indications 523
Deep tendon reflexes 95
  delayed relaxation of 28
Deep vein thrombosis 102, 260, 589
  features of 260
Defecography 396
Dehydrated dry tongue 81*f*
Dehydration 77, 79, 270
Dehydroepiandrosterone sulfate 423, 430, 431, 439, 440
Delayed puberty 442, 446*fc*
  causes of 442
  differential diagnosis of 442*b*
Delirium 375
Delivery
  cesarean section 219
  history of 240
  vaginal 219
Dementia 390
Dengue 86
  serology 89
Deoxyribonucleic acid 220, 221, 410, 467, 501
  double-stranded 30, 175
  test 505
Depot medroxyprogesterone acetate 4, 304, 314, 330, 417
Depression
  postnatal 279

postpartum 269, 270, 272
severe 248
somatic manifestation of 343
Dermatitis
    atopic 413
    herpetiformis 409
    irritant 399
    vulvar 402
Dermatosis
    course of 115
    preexisting 111
Desogestrel, metabolite of 595
Dexamethasone suppression
    test, interpretation of 432t
Diabetes 25, 28, 111, 117, 124, 192, 399, 415
    in Pregnancy Study Group India 21
    mellitus 25, 29-31, 122, 142, 257, 278, 292, 362, 390, 400, 422
    gestational 6, 209, 217, 627
    history of 93, 304
    type 2 428
    uncontrolled 31
Diagonal conjugate 19, 20, 20f
Diaphragms 586
Diarrhea 79, 80, 83fc, 84, 266, 390, 415
    acute 79, 80, 82
    causes of 79, 80t
    chronic 79
    classification of 79t
    infectious 80
    persistent 79, 80
    postpartum 265
    types of 79
Dichorionic diamniotic pregnancy, diagnosis of 214
Dietary deficiency 160
Diethylstilbestrol 502
Differential leukocyte count 70, 257
Diffuse chronic villitis 192
Digital rectal examination 288
Digoxin 73
Diphtheria-tetanus-pertussis 631
Dipstick test 173
Direct immunofluorescence test 118f
Discharge
    from nipple 459f
    per vaginum 61, 65, 66fc, 241, 241f, 298b, 298fc
Discoid rash 28
Discordant growth, monitoring of 215
Disseminated intravascular coagulation 94, 151
Diuretics 377
Diverticulitis 50, 336, 343
Doppler
    fetal monitor 229
    flow studies, abnormal 216
    pulsatility index 194

Double-dye test 384
Double-ended dilators 530
Dovetail appearance 393f
Down syndrome 21
Doxycycline, oral 83
Doyen retractor 522, 523f
    disadvantage 522
    indications 522
Drugs 92, 111, 270, 310
    abuse 92, 192
    enzyme-inducing 599
    history 242, 392, 417
    intake, history of 115, 181
    intolerance 73
    toxicity 73
Dry vaginal mucosa 368f
Dubin-Johnson syndrome 146, 152
Duckbill speculum 543
Duct papilloma 461
Ductal carcinoma in situ 461
Ductus venosus 191, 195, 198f, 199
    flow 195
    normal waveform of 198f
Duodenal atresia 139
Dye test 384
Dyselectrolytemia 117, 485
Dysentery 79, 80
Dysfunctional uterine bleeding 301
Dyskinesia 443
Dysmenorrhea 303, 314, 328, 332fc, 587
    causes of 329b, 329f
    differential diagnosis of 328
    impact of 333
    primary 328-330, 333, 343
    refractory 333
    secondary 278, 329, 343
Dyspareunia 334, 340, 340fc, 400, 495
    causes of 335f
    deep 314, 334
    differential diagnosis of 335, 335b
    primary 334
    secondary 334
Dyspnea 91, 100, 105fc, 180, 182
    acute 108t
    causes of 100
    physiological 100, 101, 108
Dysuria 263, 400

E

Ears, examination of 418
Ecchymosis 162
Echocardiogram 105
Echocardiography 29, 185, 186
Echogenic intracardiac focus 132, 133
Eclampsia 91, 146, 149, 150, 170, 235, 270
    principles of management of 97, 98b

Ectopic pregnancy 6, 32, 36, 50, 219, 336, 343, 347, 606
    acute ruptured 50, 158
    chronic 354, 358
    unruptured 349f
Edema 111, 162, 280, 281f
    macular 174
    pedal 10, 11f, 171
    pitting 161f
    pulmonary 98, 101, 108
Elective repeat cesarean
    delivery 201
    section 201
Electrical vacuum aspiration 38, 609
Electrocardiogram 29, 75, 97, 180, 271, 272, 371
Electrocardiography 30, 105, 106, 175, 184, 186, 261
Electrodes 557f
Electroencephalogram 97, 272
Electroencephalography 271
Electrolyte
    abnormalities 235
    disturbances 270
    imbalance 77, 79
    replacement of 84
    serum 56, 89, 117, 184, 230, 257
Electrophoresis 165
Eliciting scar tenderness 204f
Elliptocytosis, hereditary 158
Elschnig spots 174
Embden-Meyerhof pathway
    defects 158
Embolism 92, 481, 485
Embryo transfer 326
Emesis
    gravidarum 73
    pregnancy-unique
        quantification of 74
Encephalitis 86, 270
Encephalopathy
    hypoxic ischemic 206
    postinfectious 92
End-diastolic blood flow, absent 190, 199
Endocarditis 588
Endocervical brush 286, 287f, 306, 307f, 526f
Endocervical canal 478
Endocervical curettage 516
    indications for 516
Endocervical polyp 306f
Endocervical smear 503f
Endocervix 466
Endocrinal diseases 170
Endocrine disorders 158, 427
Endocrinopathies 302
Endometrial biopsy 319, 325, 475, 477f
    complications of 478, 478b
    contraindications of 476, 476t

indications of 476, 476t
preprocedure
considerations 476
procedure 477
Endometrial cancer 278, 302, 353
risk of 425
Endometrioma 331, 348f
bilateral 349f
Endometriosis 326, 329, 333, 343, 344, 358
Endometritis 251, 329
atrophic 302
Endometrium
biopsy of 424
histopathology of 319f
proliferative 320f
secretory 321f
Endoscopy 59, 82
lower gastrointestinal 75, 82
End-to-end repair 497f
Enema 394
Engorgement 258
Entamoeba histolytica 80, 82
Enterocele 368t
Enzyme
deficiencies, inherited 158
linked immunosorbent assay 81, 401, 412
Eosinophilia 117
Epididymis 620
Epilepsy 415
history of 93
principle of management of 98b
Episiotomy 335, 491, 493, 496
complications 495
diagnosis 496
incision 494f
indications 493
mediolateral 494t
midline 494, 494t
palpating 246f
procedure 494
scissors 533, 534f
complications 534
suture materials for repair 494
technique of repair 495
timing of procedure 494
type of 494
Epithelial cell abnormality 504
Epstein-Barr virus 154
Erosive lichen planus 406f
Erythema multiforme 409
Erythrocyte sedimentation rate 117, 412, 422
Escherichia coli 585
Esophagitis, ulcerative 77
Estradiol, serum 423
Estrogen
effect of 595
producing ovarian tumors 302, 310

progesterone challenge test 422
receptor modulator 598
Ethinyl estradiol 447, 591, 592
Ethylene oxide 563
Ethynodiol diacetate 596
Excoriation 621
Expected date of delivery 3, 4, 86, 232
External anal sphincter 395, 496
muscle 389
External cephalic version 219
External fetal heart rate 564
monitoring 564
External genitalia 363, 393
examination of 63, 363, 380, 419, 437
Extraperitoneal insufflation 553
Extra-urethral incontinence 375
Eyes 162
examination of 418
Ezy pill 600f

F

Facial puffiness 171
Failed ventouse delivery 580
Fallopian tube 616f, 618b
carcinoma 354
excision of segment of 616f
loop of 616f
Falope ring 617, 617f, 618b
Family Planning Indemnity
Scheme 623t, 624
Fat necrosis 449, 453
Fatigue 180, 182
Fatty liver, acute 52
Febrile conditions 583
Fecal impaction 390
Fecal incontinence 370
management of 397fc
Feces 399
Federation of Gynecology and Obstetrics 573
Feet, edema of 182
Female metal catheter 526, 528, 528f
Female sterilization 612, 613
eligibility criteria for 614b
methods of 613b
timing of 615t
Femur
length 190, 191
short 132, 133
Fern test 65, 66, 69f
Ferriman-Gallwey scoring 429f, 436
Fertility
awareness methods 583
regulation of 581
Fetal
anomaly 124, 215
management of 143fc
autopsy 142

blood disorders 564
condition 199
demise, intrauterine 123, 192
growth
charts 190
monitoring of 215
restriction 7, 14, 77, 122, 124, 189-191, 195, 199, 220
head, descent of 17f
heart rate 63, 96, 161, 199, 567, 569f
abnormalities 81
monitoring, internal 564
heart sound 43, 46, 47, 123, 161, 162, 231
auscultation of 17f
hydrops, nonimmune 220
infections 192
testing for 194
injury 492, 580
karyotyping 138, 194
loss 77
macrosomia 212, 496
movements 122, 122b
absent 123fc
node 36f
physiology 227
position 122
sleep 122
status, direct assessment of 491
surveillance 185
transplacental hemorrhage 219
weight, estimated 189-191, 199
Fetoscopy 219
Fetus
hemolytic disease of 219, 221
multiple 212
number of 162
presentation of 162
Fever 85, 86fc, 88fc, 146, 242, 248, 250, 405, 606
causes of 85, 86t
consequences of 87f
differential diagnosis of 251t
history of 113
low-grade 146, 250
Fiberoptic ductoscopy 461
Fibrinogen degradation products 97, 153
Fibroadenoma 452, 453
Fibroadenosis 449
Fibroblast growth factor 443
Fibrocystic disease 453, 456, 461
Fibroids 14, 59f, 302, 310, 329, 331, 336, 358
degenerating 343
polyp 302, 306f, 329
red degeneration of 50
uterus 347
Fibromyalgia 336, 343
Fibrosis, cystic 101, 316, 317

Filariasis 260
Filshie clip 617
Fimbriectomy 616
Fimbrioplasty 33
Financial Incentives Under National Family Welfare Program 623
Finasteride inhibits 433
Fine needle aspiration 453
  biopsy 357, 460
  cytology 358
First information report 464
First-trimester 5, 17, 50, 146
  combined test, report of 127f
  medical termination of pregnancy 604
  screening 128, 129
  serum screening 212
  uterine artery 194
Fissure in Ano 336
Fistula 62
Flat nipple 243f
Fluconazole 402, 412
  oral 69
  antifungal 402
Fluid
  management system 550f
  overload 101, 485
  replacement 82, 84
Fluorescence in situ hybridization 131, 139
Fluorescent treponemal antibody absorption test 26, 29
Focal neurological deficit 436
Folate deficiency 77f
Foley catheter 526, 527t, 529
  adult 527f
  indications 526
  pediatric 527f
Folic acid 117, 163
  antagonists 192
  deficiency 163
  anemia 158
Follicle-stimulating hormone 318, 414, 420-422, 430, 438, 440, 442, 444, 446, 591
Follicular cyst 353
Folliculitis 111
Food and Drug Administration 69
Food poisoning 73
Forceps delivery 576
  classification of 576, 577b
  complications of 578, 578t
  instrument 576
  technique of 577
Forensic science laboratory 467
  sample collection for 468
Foul-smelling
  lochia 248
  vaginal discharge 257
    causes of 257b
    history of 304

Fox Fordyce disease 399
Free beta-human chorionic gonadotropin 127
Functional gonadotropin deficiency 442
Fundal grip 15
Fundal height 13, 14, 123, 212
  assessment of 13f, 124
  estimation of 13t
  measurement 193
Fundus examination 173
Fungi 399

G

Gait 103
Galactocele 453
Galactography 460
Galactorrhea 305, 418, 436, 457
  history of 415
Galactosemia 422
Gallstones 50, 57f
Gamma-glutamyltransferase 151
Gartner's cyst 361, 528
Gas flow, rate of 549
Gastric malignancy 73
Gastroenteritis 73, 86, 343, 344, 346
  acute 50, 54
Gastrointestinal malignancy 343
Gastrointestinal system 227
Gastrointestinal tract 79, 302
Gastroparesis 73
Gastroschisis 139, 192
Genital examination 63
Genital herpes 335, 399, 406f, 408, 564
  simplex 412
Genital hiatus 366
Genital injuries 462
Genital lesion 404
Genital pain, persistent 334
Genital tract
  evaluation of 229
  malignancy 62
Genital ulcers 404, 408
  differential diagnosis of 404, 404t
  examination of 410t
Genitalia
  examination of 88, 162, 284f, 292, 316, 317, 338
  normal external 363f
Germ cell
  carcinoma 353
  tumor 353
Gestation
  multiple 192
  period of 4, 14, 33, 38, 47, 93, 123, 212b
Gestational age 189, 190, 195, 227, 231
  correct estimation of 194
  large for 189
  small for 189, 195, 199

Gestational sac, intrauterine 36f
Gestational trophoblastic
  disease 32, 101
  neoplasia 302, 589
Giemsa stains 410, 411
Gilbert's syndrome 152
Girth, abdominal 14, 14f
Glandular cells 504
  atypical 512
Glandular enlargement 405
Glandular lesion 516
Glasgow coma scale 94
Glossitis 162, 281f
Glucose
  6-phosphate dehydrogenase deficiency 158, 163
  tolerance test 29, 137
Glutaraldehyde 563
Glutathione precursor 120
Glycine 486
Glycosylated hemoglobin levels 137
Goiter 28
Gonadotropin-dependent precocious puberty 436, 439
Gonadotropin-releasing hormone 415, 439, 440, 443, 446, 484
  agonist 337, 350
  deficiency 443
Gonorrhea 348
Goodell's sign 18
Gram stain 64, 65, 67, 410
  bacterial vaginosis 67f
  candidiasis 67f
  smear 66f, 295f, 296f
  trichomoniasis 67f
Grand mal seizures 170
Granuloma 477f
  formation 481
  inguinale 339, 408, 410
Graspers, types of 555f
Graves' disease 171
Gray scale ultrasound 45
Green Armytage forceps 534, 534f
  advantages 534
  indications 534
Grey Turner's sign 34
Growth
  abnormalities 215
  chart
    in small for gestational age 195f
    role of 190
  factor-1, insulin like 431
  restriction
    asymmetrical 190
    symmetrical 190
Guilt 336
Gynecological history 315
Gynecological pain 344
Gynecological surgeries 376

Gynecology 275
    minor procedures in 475, 475b
Gynecomastia, absence of 317

H

Haemophilus ducreyi 411
Hair 10
    distribution 317
    growth, assessment of 429f
Hand instruments 553, 556, 556f
Hank dilator 531
Harmonic scalpel 559f
Hawkin ambler dilator 530f, 532
Hay criteria 296
Head circumference 191, 247
Headache 169, 248, 443, 600
    history of 415
    severe 176
Health infrastructure, strengthening of 627
Heaney clamp 539, 539f
    indications 539
Hearing loss, history of 415
Heart
    defect, congenital 192
    disease 25, 28, 29, 158, 179, 186fc, 618
        acquired 180
        congenital 180, 215
        cyanotic 192
        diagnosis of 104, 179
        differential diagnosis of 180b
        functional classification of 181t
        ischemic 100, 101, 180, 184
        mimicking 180t
        rheumatic 92
        valvular 101
    failure, congestive 10
    murmurs, grading of 184t
    rate 247
    sound, third 182
Heartburn 50
Heavy menstrual bleeding 301, 606
Heavy periods 304
Hegar dilators 530, 530f
    complications 531
    graduated set of 530f
    indications 531
    technique of 530
Hegar sign 18
Helmet cells 164f
Hemangioma, placental 192
Hematocolpos 419, 424
Hematocrit 105, 223
Hematological diseases 101
Hematoma 158, 354, 449, 622
    subaponeurotic 580
    subcapsular hepatic 50
    subgaleal 580

Hematometra 329, 353, 419, 424
Hematuria, occult 165
Hemoglobin 21, 117, 150, 158, 172, 604
    electrophoresis 59
    glycated 29
Hemoglobinopathies 160, 165
Hemoglobinuria, paroxysmal nocturnal 158
Hemogram, complete 35, 44, 117, 184
Hemolysis
    acute 73
    elevated liver enzyme, and low platelet syndrome 73, 94, 97, 145-147, 150, 152, 154, 172, 254
Hemolytic uremic syndrome 172
Hemoperitoneum 58f
Hemorrhage 92, 270, 485, 610, 612
    antepartum 6, 25, 40, 160, 219, 564
    concealed accidental 14
    fetomaternal 25, 220
    gastrointestinal 50
    postpartum 154, 160, 209, 251, 279, 304, 527, 541, 591, 627
    retinal 575
Hemorrhoids 40, 201, 336
Hepatic disorder 445
Hepatic dysfunction 77
Hepatic encephalopathy 97, 148, 270
    grades of 149t
Hepatic failure 92
    fulminant 145-147, 150
Hepatic impairment 399
Hepatic rupture 50, 146, 147, 150, 158
    traumatic 158
Hepatic ultrasound 154
Hepatitis 50, 54, 73, 137, 148
    A 111
    autoimmune 146
    B 111
        active 564
        core antigen 153
        surface antigen 21, 212, 297, 412, 468
    C 111
        antibodies 297
        virus 153, 153f, 412
    delta virus 153
    drug-induced 146, 147, 150
    E virus 154
    serology 117
    virus 153
Hepatosplenomegaly 162
Hernia 343
    diaphragmatic 73, 139, 192
    hiatus 618
    inguinal 418
    strangulated 50
Herpes simplex 86, 131, 137
    virus 154, 291, 339
        infections 21

Heteroechoic adnexal mass 37f
Hidradenitis suppurativa 399, 402
High definition camera system 548
High-density lipoprotein 432
    cholesterol levels 593
High-grade squamous intraepithelial lesion 504f
High-performance liquid chromatography 21, 153, 165, 166, 220
High-vaginal swab 272, 332
High-viscosity distension media 486
Hirsutism 427, 428b, 431fc, 433, 433fc
    diagnostic of 429
    differential diagnosis of 427, 427b
    history of 415, 427
    idiopathic 427
    investigations 430
    management 432
    severity of 428
Holoprosencephaly 139
Holter monitoring 184
Homan's sign 94, 252f
Hookworm 158
Hormonal intrauterine contraceptive device 588f
Hormonal methods 581
Hormone 302
    metabolites 120
    profile 438
    replacement therapy 305, 425, 447t
    serum luteinizing 438, 444
Hulka-Clemens clip 617
Human chorionic gonadotropin 75, 356, 589
Human immunodeficiency virus 81, 86, 92, 137, 154, 212, 280, 292, 401, 409, 412, 467, 468, 576, 586, 589, 613
    infection 257, 564
    testing 21
Human papilloma virus 501, 505
Human parvovirus 25
Humerus
    length 191
    short 132, 133
Hybrid energy devices 559
Hydatidiform mole 14, 212
Hydralazine 98
Hydramnios 50, 101
Hydrocephalus 138f, 139
Hydrocortisone 412
Hydronephrosis, mild 132
Hydrosalpinx 354
    bilateral 481f
    right-sided 480f
Hydroxyprogesterone 440
Hygroma, cystic 139

Hymen 284
    imperforate 329, 335, 419f
    rigid 335
Hyperaldosteronism, primary 170
Hyperandrogenic states 423
Hyperandrogenism 429
Hypercalcemia 73, 117
Hyperechoic serosa-bladder interface 45
    disruption of 45
Hyperemesis gravidarum 72, 73, 117, 145-147, 150, 152
    complications of 77b
Hyperglycemia 270
    postprandial 49
Hyperinsulinemia 430
Hyperkalemia 173, 235
Hyperkeratosis 507, 512
Hypermagnesemia 117
Hyperparathyroidism 117
Hyperphosphatemia 117
Hyperplasia
    congenital adrenal 430
    endometrial 302
Hyperprolactinemia 302, 432, 445, 457, 459, 461
Hypertension 28, 124, 169, 175fc, 177, 177fc, 192, 362
    causes of 170t
    chronic 97, 170, 192
    control of 98
    essential 170
    gestational 170, 177
    history of 93, 114, 304
    idiopathic 170
    portal 146
    pregnancy induced 163, 170
    secondary 170, 174
    severe 92
    tests for ascertaining chronicity of 175
    uncontrolled 101
Hypertensive disorders 6, 25, 169, 209, 217
Hyperthermia 270
    maternal 88
Hyperthyroidism 28, 73
Hypertrichosis 428
Hypertrophic scar, hyperpigmented 203f
Hypertrophy, left ventricular 183
Hypnotics 377
Hypoalbuminemia 117
Hypocalcemia 92, 97, 117
Hypoglycemia 92, 270
    fasting 49
Hypoglycemic agents 31
Hypogonadism
    permanent 447
    primary 442, 444
    secondary 326, 442

Hypokalemia 77, 92, 97, 173, 235
Hypomagnesemia 97
Hypomenorrhea 314, 457
Hyponatremia 77, 92, 97
Hypoplasia, marrow 163
Hypoplastic nasal bone 132
Hypoproteinemia 158, 165, 171
Hypotension 34, 87, 418
Hypothalamic disease 445
Hypothalamic disorder 415
Hypothalamic-pituitary-gonadal axis 436
Hypothalamic-pituitary-ovarian axis 414fc, 415, 591
    syndrome 302, 310
Hypothermia 87, 235, 270, 418
Hypothyroidism 28, 31, 73, 122, 124, 163, 270, 302
    central 445
Hypovolemia 235
Hypoxia 235, 270
Hysterectomy 311, 376
    total abdominal 358
    vaginal 529
Hysterosalpingo-contrast sonography 323
Hysterosalpingogram 480f, 481f
    abnormal 323f
    normal 480f
Hysterosalpingography 29, 322, 324, 331, 332, 424, 475, 478, 479f
    complications of 481, 481b
    contraindications of 478, 478t
    indications of 478, 478t
    interpretation of 480
    normal 323f
    preprocedure considerations 478
    pretreatment with analgesics 470
    procedure 479
    treatment with antibiotics 478
Hysteroscope 561f
    Grasper and scissors of 561f
    operating 561f
Hysteroscopy 29, 324, 331, 424, 475, 481, 482, 483f
    complications 483
    contraindications of 482, 482b
    gaseous 484
    indications of 482, 482t
    instruments 561
    liquid 485
    method 483
    operative 482
    procedure 483
Hysterosonography 324
Hysterotomy 612
    emergency 231
    resuscitative 238

I

Ichthyosis 111
Icterus, presence of 281f
Ileitis, terminal 343
Ileus 73
Iliopectineal lines 19
Immune thrombocytopenia 301
Immunofluorescence tests 117
Immunoglobulin E 112
Impetigo herpetiformis 117
In vitro fertilization 326, 425, 484
Incontinence
    overflow 263, 374
    prevalence of 389
Indian Council of Medical Research 163, 164
Indigenous fluid management system 550f
Indigo carmine test 68
Infarction 50
Infections 92, 260, 375, 399, 485, 612
    active 564
    bacterial 117, 412
    chronic 117, 163
    congenital 220
    gastrointestinal 343
    intrauterine 122
    maternal 25
    nonimmune 25
    postoperative 291
    presence of 160
    primary 411
    risks of 590
    systemic 270
Infertility 33, 313, 327
    causes of 313t
    duration of 314
    treatment for 480
    types of 314
Infiltrative diseases 442
Infiltrative disorder 163
Infusion site thrombophlebitis 252
Injectable medroxyprogesterone acetate 597f
Injury, electrosurgical 485
Insect bite, history of 115
Insemination, intrauterine 326
Insufflation needles 552
    complications 553
    technique of insertion 552
Interischial diameter, assessment of 20f
Interlabial sulci 338
Internal anal sphincter 391, 395, 496
    muscle 389
International Continence Society 366, 374
International Federation of Obstetrics and Gynecology 301, 302

International League Against
    Epilepsy 91
International Normalized Ratio 150, 153
Intestinal obstruction, acute 50
Intra-abdominal pressure 549
Intracytoplasmic sperm
    injection 326
Intrauterine contraceptive devices
    160, 302, 303, 310, 329, 330,
    337, 346, 484, 529, 561, 581,
    582, 586, 588, 590
    complications 589
    contraindications 589
    postpartum 590, 591b
    postplacental 240
    side effects 589
    technique for insertion 587
    types of 586, 587t
    use of 589b
Intrauterine pregnancy, early 36f
Intrinsic sphincter deficiency 387
Introitus 284
Iron 73
    deficiency 117, 163
        anemia 151, 158, 399
        early 163
        preparations 80
        stores 165
        studies 117
        serum 445
Irritable bowel syndrome 80, 329, 343,
    344, 415
Irving technique 616
Ischemia 73
Ischial spines 19
Ison criteria 296
Itching 111, 400, 405

J

Janani Shishu Suraksha
    Karyakaram 629, 630
Janani Suraksha Yojana 629, 630t
Jaundice 8, 54, 145, 145fc, 146, 154f,
    154fc, 156, 450
    causes of 147t
    differential diagnosis of 146, 146t,
        150t
    history of 114, 148
    management of 155
    mild 149
    severe 155f, 155fc
Joint, sacrococcygeal 19
Journey retractor 523
Jugular venous pressure 10, 94, 160,
    162, 180, 182
    elevated 182

K

Kala-azar, chronic 158
Kallmann's syndrome 316, 424

Karman cannula 475, 477, 534, 535f
    indications 534
Kartagener syndrome 316
Karyotype 326, 424
    abnormality, parental 31
Kell alloimmunization 220
Kelly's forceps 535, 535f
    indication 535
    technique of use 535
Kernig's sign 94, 95f
Ketoacidosis, diabetic 50, 73, 101
Kidney
    diseases 158
    disorder, chronic 415
    function test 35, 44, 56, 72, 104,
        117, 163, 166, 175, 232,
        257, 271, 272, 422
Kilkari 628
Kleihauer-Betke test 230
Knee
    jerk 95
    reflex 95f
Kocher's clamp 492, 539, 539f
    indications 539
Koilonychia 162
Korotkoff sound 11, 12
Korsakoff psychosis 73
Kroener technique 616, 616f
Krukenberg's tumor 450

L

Labetolol 98
Labia majora 338, 409
Labia minora 284, 338, 409
Labor
    after cesarean, trial of 201, 201b
    augmentation of 491
    induction of 101, 206, 491
    pains 50
    room quality improvement
        initiative 628
Lactate, serum 89
Lactational amenorrhea method 582
Lactic dehydrogenase 153, 357
Lactobacilli, absence of 67f
Lambda sign 214f
Landon vaginal retractor 528, 528f
    indications 528
Lane's tissue forceps 536, 536f
    indications 536
Laparoscope 551, 552f
Laparoscopic aspiration needle 556,
    556f
Laparoscopic clip applicators 557, 557f
Laparoscopic instruments
    and equipment 551
    sterilization of 563
Laparoscopic ligation, bilateral 617f
Laparoscopic sterilization 617, 618b
    standards for 618b

Laparoscopy 324, 349
    trolley 548
Laqshya 628
Laser conisation 518
    advantages of 519t
    disadvantages of 519t
Last menstrual period 3, 4, 14, 211,
    303, 604, 631
    date of 33, 53, 86, 228
Late pregnancy 158
    placental abruption 44f
Lax introitus 364f
Leech Wilkinson cannula 479, 536, 536f
    indications 536
    technique of use 536
Leg
    edema of 111
    swelling of 250, 260
    ulcers 28
    veins 260
Leiomyoma 354
Leopold's grips 212
Leopold's maneuver 15, 15f, 16, 16f
Leptin 424
Leptospirosis 146
Lesions
    benign 453t
    malignant 453t
    spread of 113
    systematic examination of 409
Lethargy 182
Leukocytes 586
Leukopeptidase, serotonin in 119
Leukoplakia 507, 512
Levator ani, assessment of tone of 369f
Levator tone, assessment of 369
Levonorgestrel 592, 593, 600f
    intrauterine system 304, 417, 586,
        587, 588f, 589
Lichen
    planus 111, 335, 399, 402, 409
    sclerosus 111, 335, 399, 402, 403f,
        406f
    simplex chronicus 335, 399, 402
Lid lag 28
Lid retraction 28
Lignocaine 92
    jelly, local application of 588
Lipase, serum 257
Liquid-based cytology
    advantages of 505t
    disadvantages of 505t
Liquor, amount of 162
Lithotomy position 552
Livedo reticularis 28
Liver
    biopsy 154
    cirrhosis of 456
    disease 111, 163, 165
        chronic 153

disorder 117, 422
  chronic 415
  failure 155, 155f
  function test 35, 44, 56, 72, 75, 88, 89, 97, 117-119, 151, 151t, 163, 165, 166, 172, 230, 232, 257, 272, 422
kidney microsomal antibodies 153
spontaneous rupture of 50
subscapular hematoma of 57f
with Doppler flow, ultrasound of 154
Loop electrode 562f
Loop electrosurgical excision procedure 511, 517, 518, 518f
Low platelet count 96
Lower abdominal pain 5, 250, 253, 254t, 342, 350fc, 351
  differential diagnosis of 343t
Lower limbs, swelling of 180
Low-molecular-weight heparin 31
Lugol's iodine 308f, 506, 507, 508, 509t, 512f
  application of 511
  test 508f
Lugol's staining 514
Lumbar puncture 271
Lump 456
  abdomen 359
    differential diagnosis of 353, 353t
  appendicular 354
  fixity of 452
Lung consolidation 106
Lupus anticoagulant 29, 174, 175
Luteinizing hormone 318, 414, 420, 421, 440, 442, 446, 591
Lymph node 10, 453
  supraclavicular 281f
Lymphadenopathy 162
Lymphogranuloma venereum 339, 408, 410
Lymphoma 119, 354

M

Mackenrodt's ligaments 288
Macrophages 586
Madlener technique 616
Magnesium 80
  sulfate 92, 98
  toxicity 238
Magnetic resonance imaging 29, 310, 349f, 420, 421, 446
  noncontrast 174
Maingot clamp 538, 539f
Mala N combined oral contraceptive pills 592f
Malabsorption 111, 160
  syndrome 117, 158, 192

Malar rash sparing nasolabial folds 28
Malaria 25, 86, 146, 192
  chronic 158
Malarial parasite 164f, 165
Male sterilization 612, 619
  complications of 622
  contraindications 620
  counseling 619
  demographic information 620
  eligibility criteria for 619b
  medical history 620
  physical examination 620
  postoperative care 621
  preprocedure assessment 620
  surgical technique 620
  timing of surgical procedure 620
Malecot's catheter 487
Mallory-Weiss tears 77
Malodorous discharge per vaginum 250, 257
Mammary duct ectasia 456, 460, 461
Mangeshkar manipulator 559
Manual vacuum aspiration 38, 607, 609
  syringe and cannulae 608f
Masses
  adnexal 37f, 212
  benign 452
  focal exophytic 45
  malignant 452
  retroperitoneal 354
  tubo-ovarian 258, 331, 343, 350f, 354
Massive abdominal distension 141f
Mastalgia 449
Mastitis 251
Maternal blunt abdominal trauma 219
Maternal collapse 234, 236fc
  differential diagnosis of 235t
Maternal death 206
  audit 629
Maternal disease 122
Maximum resting pressure 395
Maximum squeeze pressure 395
Mayer-Rokitansky-Kuster-Hauser syndrome 424
McCall culdoplasty 336
McCune-Albright syndrome 436
Mean corpuscular
  hemoglobin 21
  volume 21
Medical disorders 260
  cardiac 260
  hepatic 260
  history of 181
  renal 260
Medical eligibility criteria 582, 591, 597
Medical methods, side effects of 606
Medical termination of pregnancy 143, 219, 278, 304, 355, 546, 603, 604

and sterilization 603
  methods of 604
  prerequisites for 604
  provision for 470
  under MTP Act, indications for 603b
Medroxyprogesterone acetate 422
Membranes
  artificial rupture of 47, 491
  prelabor rupture of 192
Meningitis 73, 86, 92, 270
Menopause 335, 428
  premature 278
Menorrhagia 158, 330, 347
Menstrual cycles
  irregular 476
  number of 313t
Menstrual disturbances 600
Menstrual history 5, 33, 42, 53, 86, 93, 159, 160, 193, 211, 278, 292, 337, 346, 362, 377, 400, 417, 428, 450
Menstrual irregularity 433
  history of 428
Menstruation 301
Mental
  illnesses 272t
  retardation 390, 443
  status examination 382
Mesenteric artery syndrome, superior 50
Metabolic disorder 25, 92, 210
Methaqualone 409
Metoclopramide 428
Metronidazole 69, 92, 402
  oral 84
Metzenbaum scissors 615
Microcytic hypochromic red blood cells 163f
Microdeletion 137
Micro-laparoscopy 350
Middle cerebral artery 192, 195, 197f
  peak systolic velocity 215, 223, 224
Mid-luteal serum progesterone testing 319
Mifepristone 605
Migraine 73
Military antishock trousers 228
Milk production 258
Minilaparotomy 615
Miscarriage 26, 50, 85, 219, 590, 606
  recurrent 31
  first-trimester 29
  risk of 209
Misoprostol 605, 611, 613
  dose of 605
Missed pills 594, 596
Mittelschmerz pain 343, 344
Moist tongue 81f

Molar pregnancy 6, 35, 36, 37f, 158
    partial 219
Monochorionic diamniotic
    pregnancy 214
Monopolar electrodes 485
Mons pubis 409
Morning sickness 77
Morris retractor 522, 523f
Mosquito forceps 525f
Mother Absolute Affection Programme 632
Müllerian agenesis 415, 416, 418, 425t
Müllerian anomaly, obstructed 343
Müllerian duct anomalies 478
Müllerian fusion
    abnormalities 25
    defects 29
Multiple submucous myomas, hysteroscopic view of 483f
Multivitamin supplementation, absence of 74
Murmurs 162
    grade of 184
Muscle wasting 182
Muscular dystrophy 390
Myasthenia gravis 390
Mycobacterium tuberculosis 297
Mycoplasma hominis 326
Myelodysplasia 163
Myocardial dysfunction 108
Myocardial infarction
    acute 50
    inferior 73
Myofascial pelvic pain syndrome 336
Myoma 353
    beds 529
    screw 537, 537f
        indications 537
        technique of use 537
    submucous 325f, 484
Myxedema 117

N

Naegele's formula 4, 5
Nails 162
    examination of 9f
    normal 9f
    pale 9f, 161f, 280f
Narcotics 377
Nasal bone 130, 133
    absent 132
National AIDS Control Organization 297
National Family Welfare Program 623t
National Immunization Schedule 627
National Institute of Child Health and Human Development 567
Nausea 53, 72, 345, 600
    differential diagnosis of 73b
history of 73, 114
pregnancy-unique quantification of 74
Neck 10, 162
    rigidity 94, 94f
Neisseria gonorrhoeae 62, 291, 294
Neodymium-doped yttrium aluminum garnet 485
Neuritis, peripheral 111
Neurological disease 362
Neurological examination 370, 437
Neurological system 171
    evaluation of 229
Neuromuscular disease 101
Neuropathy, peripheral 162
Neurosarcoidosis 418
New York Heart Association 180
Nifedipine 98
Nipple 451
    discharge 456, 457fc, 459t, 460, 461, 461t
        bloody 461
        cytology 460
        differential diagnosis of 456, 456b
        examination 458
        history 457
        hormonal assessment 460
        investigations 460
        mammography 460
        management 461
    pain 456
    problems 259
    retracted 259
    sore 248
Nitrazine test 65, 67
Nitrofurantoin 101
Noninvasive prenatal testing 128, 130, 131, 133, 213
Nonscalpel vasectomy 621
Nonsexual hair growth 427
Non-steroidal anti-inflammatory drugs 54, 73, 80, 330, 332, 400, 461, 478, 588
Nonstress test 97, 119, 125
Norethindrone enanthate 417
Norethisterone 593
    enanthate 597
Normal Doppler flow studies 216
Normal pregnancy
    signs in 180t
    symptoms in 180t
Novak endometrial biopsy 475
    curette 533, 533f
N-terminal pro-brain natriuretic peptide 107
Nuchal fold thickness 131-133
Nuchal translucency 127, 128, 130, 213, 214f
Nucleic acid amplification test 296, 298
Nugent's criteria 296
Nutritional anemia 158

O

Obesity 28
    central 418
    extreme 336
Obstetric
    anal sphincter injuries 491, 496
    examination 183
    grips 14
    history 5, 42, 53, 63, 87, 93, 116, 160, 170, 193, 202, 211, 278, 315, 362, 377, 392, 417, 428, 450
    indications 532
    injury 390
    minor procedures in 491
    trauma 390
    ultrasound 174
Obstruction, intestinal 73
Oligohydramnios 122, 192, 216
Oligomenorrhea 301, 314, 457
Oliguria 87
Omphalocele 139, 192
Operative vaginal delivery 575
    contraindications for 575, 576t
    indications for 575b
    prerequisites for 576b
Ophthalmic examination 438
Opiate 417
    overdose 238
Optic
    atrophy 174
    neuritis 174
    neuropathy, ischemic 174
Optical trocars 553
Optimal breastfeeding practices 632
Oral cavity 162
Oral glucose tolerance test 24, 142, 212, 432
Oral polio vaccine 631
Oral rehydration solutions 83
Orchitis 622
Organophosphorus 92
Ormeloxifene 311, 599f
Orthopnea 102, 182
    degree of 102
Osiander's sign 18
Osteitis pubis 343
Osteoporosis 425
Ovarian cancer 278
Ovarian cyst 329, 336
    ruptured 343
    torsion of 50
    twisted 343
Ovarian drilling needle 557, 557f

Ovarian failure 415
    autoimmune premature 418
    premature 417, 422
Ovarian insufficiency, primary 420
Ovarian lumps 355
Ovarian remnant syndrome 343
Ovarian reserve 321
Ovarian stimulation, controlled 326
Ovarian torsion 73, 158
Ovarian tumor 14, 358
Ovarian vein 252
Ovary
    biopsy of 424
    D12 scan of 320f
    D15 scan of 321f
Ovulation induction 33, 326
Ovulatory cycles 476
Ovulatory dysfunction 310, 314, 326
Ovulatory function 319
Ovum forceps 538, 538f
    complications 538
    indications 538
    spoon-shaped blunt fenestrated
        end of 538f
    technique of use 538
Oxygen saturation 235
    measurement 105

P

Paget's disease 399
Pain 52, 241, 254, 404, 405
    calf 248
    character of 52
    duration of 52
    fear of 336
    gastritis-induced 53
    history of 304
    idiopathic 343
    in perineum 248
    intensity of 52
    loin 5
    lower abdomen 351fc
    myofascial 343
    nature of 330
    radiation of 52
    severe abdominal 248
    site of 51
Pallor 8, 103, 157, 165, 166fc, 167fc,
        280, 280f
    assessment of 203
    causes of 157
    conjunctival 9f
    differential diagnosis of 158t
    management of 165
    mucosa for 162
    severe 157
Palm, examination of 10f
Palmar's erythema 28
Palmer's test, inverse 531

Palpation 13, 55, 183, 245, 283, 338
Palpitations 180, 415
    history of 102
Pancreatic disorders 148
Pancreatitis 50, 73, 86
Pap smear 297, 307f, 316, 401, 516
    abnormal 504f, 505t
    advantages of 503t
    Bethesda system, reporting of 504b
    collection 287f
    disadvantages of 503t
    normal 505f
    positive 516
    reporting of 504
Pap test 315
Papillophlebitis 174
Paracentesis 348
Paracervical block 588
Paradoxical embolism 92
Paraovarian cyst, torsion of 50
Parasitic infections 86
Parathyroid hormone levels 117
Paravaginal cyst excision 376
Parental genetic testing 137, 138
Parkland technique 616
Partial thromboplastin time 153
Parvovirus 86, 220
Paternal phenotype, zygosity of 224
Pawlik's grip 15
Peak expiratory flow rate 108, 109
Pedicle clamp 538, 540
    application of 540f
Pediculosis pubis 399
Pedunculated myoma 361
    torsion of 50
Pelvic
    abscess 80, 258
    adhesions 329, 343
    assessment 19t
    congestion syndrome 329, 336, 343
    endometriosis 336
    examination 28, 56, 96, 204, 256,
        284, 316, 331, 347, 353,
        355, 419
        bimanual 73, 369
    floor muscle
        assessment of 381
        strength 370
    floor reconstructive
        procedures 376
    grip
        deep 16
        superficial 15
    infection 291, 333, 481, 610
        chronic 291
        history of 63
    inflammatory disease 33, 278, 302,
        310, 314, 329, 334-336,
        344, 350f, 478, 588, 589
        chronic 343

kidney 354
    mass 336
    organ prolapse 360, 371, 371fc
        differential diagnosis of 361t
        management of 371, 372fc
        quantification system 366t
    pain 278, 328, 342
        chronic 342
        diagnosis of 342
        surgery, previous 336
        ultrasonography 383, 424, 446
    veins 252, 260
Pelvis 210
    assessment of 19
    ultrasound 348
    ultrasound examination of 82
Pemphigoid gestationis 111-113, 114f,
        118, 118f, 119
    bullous stage of 114f
    prebullous stage of 114f
Penetration, fear of 336
Penicillin 92
Penile-vaginal intercourse 582
Peptic ulcer 50
    disease 73
Per abdomen examination 34, 42, 55,
        81, 149, 203, 212, 229, 244,
        256, 263, 292, 305, 316, 338,
        346, 355, 363, 378
Per rectal examination 288f, 356, 368,
        370, 394, 419
    bimanual 289f
Per speculum examination 28, 35, 43,
        63, 88, 162, 204, 229, 264, 284,
        285, 285f, 286f, 293, 305, 306f,
        307f, 338, 356, 367, 368, 380, 394
Per vaginal examination 35, 44, 81, 205,
        258, 264, 288, 356, 369, 381, 394
Percutaneous epididymal sperm
        aspiration 326
Periductal mastitis 456
Perimortem cesarean
    delivery, role of 231
    section 238
Perineal body 284, 360, 363
Perineal injuries, previous 335, 496
Perineal muscle layer, repair of 495
Perineal sensation 370
    examination for 382
Perineal tears 279
    classification of 496
    complete 364f
    old healed complete 393f
Perineal trauma 390
Perineorrhaphy 335
Perineum 338, 364f
    evaluation of 229
    examination of 363
    local examination of 264
Peripheral blood smear 163f, 164f

Index

Peripheral nervous system 390
Peripheral smear 96, 150, 163, 165, 166, 172, 232, 272, 332, 412
Peritonitis 73
Periumbilical skin, bluish discoloration of 34
Petechiae 162
Phenazopyridine 382
Phenothiazines 428
Phenytoin 98, 193, 428
Pheochromocytoma 170
    signs of 175
    symptoms of 175
Phobic reaction 336
Photopsia 176
Piles 158
Pills 591, 596
    combined 417, 594
    nonhormonal 581
    progestogen-only 596, 597t
Pimecrolimus 413
Pipelle endometrial biopsy sampler 475f, 533, 533f
Pituitary disease 445
Placenta
    anterior location of 122
    low lying 211
    manual removal of 219, 251
    previa 40, 43, 43t, 44f, 45, 157, 158, 192, 564
        morbidly adherent 45f, 45t, 192
    removal of 535
Placental abruption 40, 43, 43t, 50, 58f, 157, 158, 492
Placental alkaline phosphatase 357
Placental disease
    mild 191
    severe 191
Placental growth factor 176
Placental lacunae, presence of abnormal 45
Placental mosaicism 192
Plain disposable catheter 528, 528f
    indications 528
Planter reflex 96f
Plasma
    brain natriuretic peptide 107
    protein
        low pregnancy-associated 193
        pregnancy associated 127, 128, 184, 186
Platelet 172
    count 150, 172, 176, 230
Platonychia 162
Pleuritis 50, 101
Pneumoinsufflator and gas cable 549f
Pneumonia 86, 101, 106, 270
Pneumonitis 89
Pneumothorax 100, 101
    spontaneous 101

Polycystic ovarian syndrome 30, 278, 302, 304, 415, 421, 428, 431, 432, 557
Polyglycolic acid 494
Polyhydramnios 14, 122, 141f, 216
Polymerase chain reaction 142, 194, 220, 506
Polyneuropathy 390
Polyp 484
    endometrial 302
Pomeroy technique 615, 616f
Poorly formed flat nipple 259f
Porphyria 50, 73
Port closure needle 560, 560f
Positive aneuploidy screening test 127
Postabortal infections 291
Postcoital test 325
Posterior reversible encephalopathy syndrome 174
Posterior vaginal wall 308f, 508f, 545, 589
    visualization of 368f
Postnatal affective disorders 269
Postnatal urinary complaints 262t
Post-surgery cervical stenosis 353
Postvoid residual urine, assessment of 379
Potassium 117
    hydroxide 294, 339, 488
    hydroxide mount 489f
    serum 173
    titanyl-phosphate 485
Pouch of Douglas 35, 80, 287, 317, 347, 356, 360, 450, 486
Pradhan Mantri Matritva Vandana Yojana 631
Pratt dilator 531
Precocious puberty 434, 436b, 439fc, 440b
    causes of 436
    central 440
    differential diagnosis of 436b
    peripheral 440
Precoital stimulation, inadequate 336
Preeclampsia 73, 92, 97, 117, 146, 150, 152, 170, 192, 235, 270
    retinopathy of 173
    severe 50, 52
    symptoms suggestive of 5
    syndrome 170
Pregnancy 32, 290
    acute fatty liver of 50, 57, 73, 145-147, 150, 152, 154, 155
    atopic eruption of 111-113, 115f, 119
    cholestasis of 25, 152
    complications 310
    dating of 4, 4b, 213
    early 158
    fear 336

    hypertensive disorder of 25, 193
    intrahepatic cholestasis of 111-113, 117, 119, 145-147, 150-154
    intrauterine 36
    multiple 14, 73, 209, 210
    nausea and vomiting of 72, 76, 77
    normal vaginal discharge of 61f
    polymorphic eruption of 111-113, 114f, 119
    second-trimester medical termination of 611
    test 347, 419
    with pelvic mass 14
Premature rupture of membrane 65, 67, 69, 86, 250
Prenatal invasive diagnostic procedures 219
Preterm labor 6, 116, 122, 209, 590
    pains 50
Previous intestinal surgery, history of 618
Pritchard regime 98
Procidentia 369f
Proctitis 336
Proctosigmoidoscopy 394
Progesterone
    challenge test 422
    implants 598
Progestins 428
Prolactin 420, 421, 423
Prolapse 335, 544
    examination of 366
    quantification system 366
    with decubitus ulcer 302
Prophylactic antibiotics 588, 610
Prostaglandin 611
Prosthetic heart valve replacement 588
Protein 68
    C 29
    electrophoresis 117
    energy malnutrition 77
    S 29
    serum 165
Proteinuria 173
Prothrombin time 96, 152
Proximal vein compression ultrasonography 107
Prurigo nodules 115f
Pruritus 111, 112fc, 117, 147, 291, 404
    differential diagnosis of 111t
    history of 148
    management of 119fc
    systemic causes of 117t
    treatment of 412
    urgent evaluation of 120
    vulvae 399, 401fc, 402
        causes of 399, 399b
        management of 401
Pseudoprecocious puberty 436

Pseudotumor cerebri 73
Psoriasis 111, 114, 399, 402, 407f
Psychiatric illness, history of 417
Psychosis 399
   postpartum 270, 272
Pubarche 415
Puberty 290
   nomograms 444
Pubic angle 20
Pubic hair 442
   collection of samples of 463f
   development 418
      tanner stages of 435f
   distribution of 284
Pubic symphysis 14f, 615
Puborectalis sling 389
Pudendal block 491, 492, 493f
   complications 493
   contraindication 492
   indication 492
   technique 493
Pudendal nerve 493f
   block 492
   terminal motor latency 395
Puerperal pelvic infections 291
Puerperium 92b, 240, 250, 254t, 269, 270b, 272fc, 618
Pulmonary disease, chronic 101
Pulmonary embolism 100, 101, 108, 154, 175, 589, 597
Pulmonary function testing 108
Pulsatility index 197f, 199
Pulse 11, 103
   oximetry 97
   rate 34, 46, 162, 171, 235
   recording 11f, 282f
Pulseless electrical activity 236
Pulsus alternans 182
Purandare's sling 540
Pus cells 82f
Pyelectasis
   bilateral 132f
   mild 133
Pyelogram, intravenous 49, 385, 386
Pyelonephritis 73, 86, 158, 343
   acute 50
Pyometra 353
Pyosalpinx 354
Pyrexia 87, 88
Pyridium 382
   test 382
Pyruvate kinase deficiency 163

Q

Q fever 86
Q-tip test 365f, 380f
Quadruple test 129, 131, 131fc
Quinolones 83
Quintero classification 216t

R

Radiation
   colitis 80
   enteritis 390
   proctitis 390
   therapy 453
Radiographs, abdominal 256
Radiotherapy 335
Raised jugular venous pressure 171
Randall endometrial biopsy curette 533
Rape survivors, treatment of 462
Rapid plasma reagin 411
Rash
   erythematous 115f
   maculopapular 28
Rashtriya Bal Swasthya Karyakram 632
Recanalization 33
   operation 621
Rectal
   compliance, abnormal 390
   examination 450
   mucosa 389
   neoplasm 390
   prolapse 390
Rectocele 368t
Rectovaginal examination 56, 288f, 368
Rectovaginal fistula 390
Rectum, neoplasm of 390
Rectus
   muscle hematoma 50
   sheath hematoma 58f
Red blood cell 21, 151, 158
Red cell enzyme defect 25
Reflects ovarian maturation 442
Reflux esophagitis 73
Reid colposcopic index 514
Renal artery stenosis 170
Renal calculi 50
Renal disease 25, 28, 29, 111, 117, 139, 165, 170
   chronic 192
Renal disorders 422
Renal dysfunction 77
Renal failure 270
   chronic 117, 456
Renal function test 75, 88, 97, 165, 173, 230
Renal impairment 399
Renal parenchymal disease 170
Renal stones 73
Renal system 227
Reproductive tract infection 315, 613
   signs of 604
Resectoscope 562, 562f
Reserpine 428
Respiration 103
Respiratory complications 252
Respiratory dysfunction, severe 618
Respiratory rate 94, 162, 203, 235, 247, 282
Respiratory system 12, 95, 171, 227, 282, 378
   examination of 103

Respiratory tract infection 86
Restrict fluid infusion rate 98
Resuscitation 98
   cardiopulmonary 234
Reticulocyte count 163
Retinal artery 174
Retinal detachment 174
Retinal pigment epithelial lesions 174
Retinal vasospasm 176
Retractors, abdominal 522, 523f
Retroplacental sonolucent zone, loss of 45
Reversed arterial perfusion 209
Rh blood group system 219
Rh isoimmunization 31
Rh negative
   isoimmunized pregnancy, management of 224
   nonimmunized pregnancy, management of 222
   pregnancy 219
      management of 223fc
Rh sensitized pregnancy 29
Rheumatic fever, history of 181
Rheumatic valvular disease 179
Rhodes index 74
Rhythm method 583
Rib fracture 101
Ringer's lactate 38
Rotor syndromes 152
Routine cervical cytology 502
Rubella 21, 86, 137
Rudimentary horn 349f, 353
   pregnancy, rupture of 50

S

Sacral reflexes, neurological examination of 381
Sacrosciatic notch 19
Sacrospinous ligament 493f
Sacrum 19
Saline sonohysterography 308, 308f
Salmonella 80
   infection 149
Salpingoneostomy 33
Salpingo-oophoritis 329
Sarcoidosis 101
Sarcoma 353, 354
Scabies 111, 399
Scar
   dehiscence 50
      risk of 203
   endometriosis 495
   keloid 204f
   rupture 206
   type of 203
Schiller's iodine, application of 511
Schiller's test 515
Schistocytes 172
Schistosomiasis 165

Scintigraphy, pulmonary 107
Sclerosis, multiple 92, 336, 390
Scotomata 176
Screening tests 128
    degree of sensitivity of 128*t*
Scrotal skin 621
Secnidazole 402
Second-trimester 5, 50
    aneuploidy screening 130
    serum screening 213
Sedatives 377
    drugs alcohol, intake of 122
Seizures 443
    control of 98
    psychogenic nonepileptic 92
Sensitizing events 219*b*
Sepsis 94, 101
    causes of 50
    puerperal 270
Septate 480
    uterus 25, 323*f*
Septic shock 158
    clinical features of 87*b*
Serologic tests 411
Serosa-bladder interface,
    hypervascularity of 45
Serum beta-human chorionic
    gonadotropin 164
Serum bile acid 153
    levels 118
Serum bilirubin 151
    tests 151
Serum glutamic pyruvic transaminase 118
Serum integrated prenatal screening 129
Serum lactate dehydrogenase 153, 173
Serum transaminases 152
    elevation of 152
Sex
    characters, secondary 418
    cord tumor 353
    hormone-binding globulin 430
Sexual abuse 343
Sexual assault 462, 469*b*
    abdominal examination 467
    anal examination 468
    assessment of survivor of 462
    examination 465
    forensic evidence kit
        components of 463*f*
        contents of 469*b*
    genital examination 467
    history of 464, 465, 465*b*
    sample collection 468
    survivor of 462
    treatment 469
    victim of 470*fc*
Sexual characteristics development,
    secondary 434*t*
Sexual dysfunction, female 334
Sexual experience, traumatic 336

Sexual history 292, 337, 346, 392, 408, 417
Sexual intercourse, unprotected 599
Sexual maturity rating 434, 444, 446
Sexual reproduction, ability of 434
Sexual stimulation 290
Sexual violence 462, 467
    management of 463
Sexually transmitted
    disease 33, 337, 404, 583, 589
    infection 26, 292, 314, 404, 408, 408*t*, 410*t*, 413, 613
Shaw's classification system 366
Sheehan's syndrome 417
Shielding abdomen 165
Shigella 80
Shirodkar cervical clamp 540, 540*f*
    disadvantage 540
    during tuboplasty, use of 540*f*
    indications 540
Shirodkar hook 540
Shirodkar needle 541, 541*f*
Shirodkar sling 540
Shirodkar test 531
Shock
    anaphylactic 158
    cardiogenic 158
    hemorrhagic 50, 157
    neurogenic 158
    nonhemorrhagic 158
    septic 158
    signs of 41
Shoulder dystocia 496
Sickle cell 164*f*, 165
    disease 158, 163, 192
Silicone
    catheter 527*f*
    titanium clip 617
Sim's double bladed vaginal speculum 285*f*
Sim's lateral position 286, 286*f*, 380
Sim's position for visualizing
    vesicovaginal fistula 380*f*
Sim's speculum 286, 286*f*, 379*f*, 477, 479, 487, 538, 543, 544*t*, 545
    advantages 545
    disadvantages 545
    double-bladed 543*f*
    indications 544
    technique of use 544
    use of 545*f*
Sjögren's syndrome 336
Skeletal
    muscle development 317
    skiagrams 422
Skene's gland 338
Skin 162
    lesions, presence of 113
    repair of 495
    squamous hyperplasia of 399
    stretching of 111
Sneezing 62

Sodium 117
    serum 257
    valproate 428
Soft markers 132*f*, 133*fc*
    interpretation of 134*b*
Somatic stigmata 418
Sonography, transvaginal 297
Speculum examination 18, 63*f*, 258
Spermicides 585
Sperms 318*f*
    granuloma 622
Spherocytes 165
Spherocytosis 163
    hereditary 158
Sphincter
    external 497
    injury, risk factors for 496
    internal 389, 497
Spina bifida 139
Spinal cord 390
Spirometry 106
Spironolactone 433
Spleen
    ruptured 50
    traumatic rupture of 50
Splenic rupture 50
    traumatic 158
Spondylolysis 343
Sponge-holding forceps 541, 541*f*
    indications 541
Squamocolumnar junction 508
Squamous cell 504, 506
    carcinoma 408, 504
Squamous intraepithelial lesion,
    low-grade 504*f*
Squamous metaplasia 507
Starvation ketosis 77
Steatohepatitis, non-alcoholic 150, 152
Sterilization 612
    hysteroscopic 618
Steroids 73, 260
    anabolic 428
    topical 402
Still birth 119
Stomatitis 162, 193
Stool
    examination 117, 165
    impaction 375
    microscopic examination of 82
    microscopy 82*f*
Strawberry cervix 293
Stress 302, 399
    urinary incontinence 62, 263, 284, 284*f*, 364, 365*f*, 374, 377, 379, 379*f*, 387, 527
    history of 361
    postpartum 262
Stroke 101, 270, 390
    ischemic 593
Stromal cell tumor 353
Strychnine 92

Subfertility 313, 610
Submucous fibroid 25, 343
    diagnosis of 153
    hysteroscopic view of 483f
Subpubic arch 20
    assessment of 20f
Suction cannula 555f
    color coding of 608t
Suicidal behavior 248
Sulphonamides 409
Surakshit Matritva Aashwasan 632
Surgery, history of 181
Swelling 248
Swine flu 86
Swollen feet 161f
Sympathomimetic drugs 335
Symphysis pubis, posterior surface of 19
Symphysis-fundal height 13, 190
    measurement of 14f
Sympto-thermal method 583, 584
Syncopal attacks 102
Syncope 180
Synechia, intrauterine 25
Syphilis 25, 28, 29, 31, 280, 339, 408, 410
    primary 290, 291
Syringomas 399
Systemic lupus erythematosus 25,
    28-30, 33, 92, 170, 175, 192

T

T sign 214f
Tabes dorsalis 390
Tachycardia 28, 34, 87, 103, 182, 565
Tachypnea 87
    presence of 103
Tacrolimus 413
Talipes equinovarus, bilateral 140f
Tampons 62, 63
Tanner's stages 434
Tear
    first degree of 496
    fourth-degree 497
    second-degree 496
    third-degree 496
Telescope 561
    diameter of 562
Tenaculum 542, 542f
Tenderness, calf 94
Tension
    pneumothorax 235
    premenstrual 343
Tension-free
    obturator tape 387
    vaginal tape 387
Teratogenesis, risk of 607
Termination of pregnancy 32, 199, 603
    after stabilization 98
Testicular sperm aspiration 326
Testosterone 423, 428
    serum 318
Tetanus toxoid 5
Tetracyclines 409

Thalassemia 21, 158, 163, 220
    diagnosis of 153
    screening for 21
Theca lutein cyst 353
Thelarche 415
Theophylline 73
Thermal balloon ablation 417
Thiamine deficiency 77
Thiazides 400
Thighs, hysterical hyperesthesia of 336
Threadworm 399
Throat swabs 89
Thrombocytopenia 172
Thromboembolism 235
    risk of 77
Thrombophilia 25
    genetic 29
    screen 29
Thrombophlebitis
    septic 252
    superficial 253f
Thrombosis 50, 92
Thrombotic thrombocytopenic
    purpura 94, 172
Thyroid 111
    disorders 21, 25, 29, 415
        screening for 21
    dysfunction 25, 77, 399
    enlargement 162
    function tests 75, 105, 117, 174,
        175, 445, 460
    stimulating hormone 21, 29, 164,
        174, 212, 420-423, 431,
        438, 445, 446
Thyrotoxicosis 101, 117, 170
Thyrotropin-releasing hormone 423
Thyroxine 29
Tinea 111, 406f
Tinidazole 402
Tocolysis 101
Tongue 54
    inspection of 9f
    pale 160f, 280f
Torn
    anal mucosa, repair of 497
    perineum 364f
Total leukocyte count 70, 117, 151
Toxic neuropathy 390
Toxicity 235
Toxins 270
Toxoplasma gondii 130, 131
Toxoplasmosis 21, 25, 92, 137
    other agents, Rubella
        Cytomegalovirus, and
        herpes simplex 191
    serology 137
Transabdominal scan 46
Transaminases 150
Transcutaneous electrical nerve
    stimulation 332
Transdermal patch 596

Transformation zone
    large loop excision of 518
    types of 511f
Transfusion, intrauterine 31, 220,
    223, 224
Transient respiratory morbidity,
    risk of 206
Transvaginal scan 45f, 332
    examination 44
Transvaginal technique 493f
Transverse diameter of outlet,
    assessment of 21f
Trauma 92, 226, 232fc, 260
    abdominal 50
    previous 335
    severe 227b
    sonography for 230
Tremors 28
Treponema pallidum 411
    hemagglutination assay 297
Triamcinolone 412
Trichomonas
    vaginalis 62, 64, 69t, 290, 296f,
        402, 489, 504
    wet smear 295f
Trichomoniasis 64, 65, 67, 69, 294, 399
Triiodothyronine 29
Triploidy 192
Trisomy 13 139f, 192
Trisomy 18 192
Trisomy 21 127f, 192
Trocars 553, 553f
Trophoblastic disease 310
Tropical sprue 158
Tubal factor 326
Tubal ligation
    Kroener technique of 616f
    Pomeroy's technique of 616f
Tubal occlusion, methods of 617
Tubal patency test 322
Tuberculoma 270
Tuberculosis 86, 92, 101-103, 147, 158,
    160, 252, 278, 291, 302, 354,
    415, 418, 589
    evidence of 89
    history of 93
    ileocecal 354
    pulmonary 165
Tumor 92, 354
    adrenal 428
    epithelial 353
    intracranial 424
    metastatic 353
    pituitary 425
Turner's syndrome 415, 418, 425t
Twinning, type of 210
Twins
    acardiac 216f
    dizygotic 209t
    fetus, labeling of 214
    gestation 206
    monitoring of 564

Index

monochorionic 215
monozygotic 209t, 210t
pregnancy, management of 215
to-twin transfusion syndrome 209, 216t, 220
Typhoid 147
Tzanck smear 410

U

Uchida technique 616
Ulcer 162, 512
    aphthous 409
    decubitus 306f, 369f
    differential diagnosis of 409
    disease 50
    traumatic 409
Ulcerative colitis 80, 343
Ultrasensitive immunofluorometric assays 444
Ultrasonic scalpel 558
Ultrasound 4, 57f-59f, 125, 137, 175, 194, 221, 223, 357
    abdominal 75
    examination 82, 137
    postmenstrual 432
    transabdominal 44f
    transvaginal 319, 331, 348f
Umbilical artery 190, 191, 196f, 199, 215
    Doppler 195
    feeding abdominal stump 216f
    single 192
Upper abdominal pain 147
    history of 114
Upper limb, flexor aspect of 115f
Urachal cyst 354
Ureaplasma urealyticum 326
Uremia 73, 101, 270
Ureteric calculi 50
Ureterovaginal fistula 384
Urethral caruncle 336
Urethral diverticulum 529
Urethral hypermobility, test for 365, 380
Urethral meatus 409
Urethral orifice 284
Urethral syndrome 343
Urethral tone 377
Urethritis 336
    atrophic 375
Urethrovaginal fistula 384
Urethrovesical angle, normal 381f
Urge urinary incontinence 374
Urinalysis 56, 75, 173
Urinary bladder, invasion of 45
Urinary complaints 250, 261
Urinary incontinence 62, 263, 370, 374, 386fc
    differential diagnosis of 375t
    management of 385, 387fc
    mixed 374, 387
    postpartum 262
    types of 374, 374t, 375

Urinary pregnancy test 422
Urinary problem, nature of 262, 263
Urinary protein concentration 173
Urinary retention
    overt 262
    postpartum 262
Urinary tract 40, 302, 342, 485
    infection 86, 117, 159, 160, 165, 230, 250, 251, 254, 270, 335, 343, 398, 399, 585
    history of 63
    recurrent 361
Urine
    acute retention of 343
    albumin 89, 150
    analysis 230, 382
    cultures 89
    dipstick test, interpretation of 173t
    dribbling 248
    examination 57, 105, 117, 165, 184
    microalbumin 29
    porphyrins 75
    pregnancy test 4, 230, 310, 468
    production, excessive 375
    protein estimation 29
    routine 257
    toxicology 75
Uroflowmetry 383
Urogenital fistula 381, 384
Urography, intravenous 385
Ursodeoxycholic acid 120
Urticaria 111
Uterine
    activity 569f
    anomalies 29
        anatomical 29
    artery 499
    cancer 291
    cavity 609f
        assessment of 324
        irregular contracted 481f
        normal panoramic view of 483f
    curette 532, 532f
        complications 532
        indications 532
        technique of use 532
    defects, acquired 478
    enlargement 347
    fibroid 212
        degeneration of 344
    inversion 361
    leiomyoma 73
    lumps 355
    manipulators 559, 560f
    masses 212
    perforation 485, 610
        signs of 610b
    prolapse, early stages of 343
    rupture 157, 158
    septum 31, 484
    sound 541f, 542, 543b
        complications 543

        contraindications 543
        indications 542
        technique of use 542
Uterovaginal prolapse 304
    diagnosis of 371
Uterus 13, 286, 348f, 598
    cut section of 309
    D12 scan of 320f
    D15 scan of 321f
    height of 162
    posterior wall fibroid of 348f, 349f
    postpartum 245f
    retroverted 336
    rupture 40, 50
    surgical removal of 416
    tone of 162
    unicornuate 323f

V

Vagina 63, 302, 390, 466
    appearance of 258
    erythema of 64
    lacerations of 498
    surgery on 290
    tumors of 40
    visualization of 286f
Vaginal adhesion 335
Vaginal agenesis 419f
Vaginal bleeding, excessive 248
Vaginal caliber 585
Vaginal cancer 291
Vaginal candidiasis 63, 292
    treatment of 69t
Vaginal delivery 186, 240, 535
    instrumental 496
    trial of 201
Vaginal diaphragm 585
Vaginal discharge 61, 65, 86, 290, 297, 339, 383, 400
    causes of 62t, 64, 294t
    differential diagnosis of 65t, 67t, 290, 290t
    Gram stain of 65, 295
    management of 69
    pathological 290
Vaginal examination 17, 384, 450
    steps of 18
Vaginal growth 35
Vaginal infections 32, 488
Vaginal intraepithelial neoplasia 510
Vaginal lacerations 498
Vaginal length, total 366
Vaginal lesions 544, 544t
Vaginal mucosa 369f, 419
    atrophic 368f
    normal well-estrogenized 381f
    repair of 495
Vaginal muscles 381
Vaginal opening 409
Vaginal pathology 588

Vaginal pH 67
  testing of 295
Vaginal route 611
Vaginal secretions
  abnormal 489
  normal 489
Vaginal septum, transverse 329, 335
Vaginal smear 488
Vaginal speculums 543
Vaginal tear 491
Vaginal tubal ligation 618
Vaginal tumors 32
Vaginal wall 467
  defect, lateral 367f
Vaginal wet mount 488
  complications 488
  indication 488
  prerequisites 488
  procedure 488
Vaginismus 336, 338
Vaginitis 35, 335
  atrophic 375, 399
Vaginoplasty 376
Vaginoscopy 384
Vaginosis, bacterial 65
Valproate 193
Valsalva maneuver 63, 365, 366, 379
Valvular dysfunction 108
Vancomycin, oral 84
Vanillylmandelic acid 175
Varicella 111
  zoster 137, 142
Varicocele 317, 326
Varicosities 11, 40, 210
Vas deferens 317
  congenital bilateral absence of 317
Vas dissection forceps 621
Vasa previa, ruptured 40
Vasculature, examination of 513
Vasculopathy 192
Vasectomy 619
  conventional 620
  failure of 623
Vasomotor symptoms, history of 415
Vasovagal attack 622
Vasovagal reaction 481
Vasovagal syncope 588, 610
Vault cap 586
Velamentous cord insertion 192
Venereal Disease Research
  Laboratory 26, 29, 137, 468
  Test 21, 212, 401, 411
Venous thromboembolism 107
  high-risk of 433
Ventilation perfusion scan 107
Ventouse delivery 575, 578
  complications of 580, 580t
  indications 579
  instrument 578
  technique 579
Ventouse kiwi omnicup 579f
Ventouse silastic cup 578f

Ventricular fibrillation 236
Ventricular tachycardia 236
Ventriculomegaly 132
Veress needle 552f
Vesical calculi 40, 343
Vesicovaginal fistula 376, 385f, 386, 527
  repair of 540
Vesicular mole 50
Vestibular disorders 73
Vestibulitis 335
Vibrio cholerae 82
Viral hepatitis 117, 151
  active 145, 150
  acute 146, 147
Viral infections 163
Viral serology 153
Viral warts 290, 291
Virilism, symptoms of 427
Visual disturbance 418, 437
  history of 415
Visual field 438
  defects 437
Visual inspection 501, 506-508
  advantages of 509t
  disadvantages of 509t
Vital parameters 281
Vitamin
  B12 163
    deficiency 158, 163
    levels 117
  D analogs 402
Vitiligo 407f
Voice, deepening of 415
Volvulus 354
  intestinal 50
Vomiting 53, 72, 72fc, 75b, 345
  differential diagnosis of 73b
  history of 73, 114, 415
von Willebrand disease 302
Vulsellum 546, 546f
  indications 546
Vulva 338, 390, 408f
  appearance of 258
  hysterical hyperesthesia of 336
  inaccessibility of 336
  inspection of 338
  soiling of 399
Vulval diseases 400
Vulval dystrophy 408f
Vulval growth, differential diagnosis
  of 405t
Vulval hematoma 246f
Vulval infections 335
Vulval intraepithelial neoplasia 399
Vulval lesion 412fc
Vulval lipoma 407f
Vulvar intraepithelial neoplasia 401,
  409, 510
Vulvar irritation 399
Vulvar lesions 404, 413
  history of 405
  management of 411

Vulvar lichen sclerosus 413
Vulvar skin dermatoses 404
Vulvar soreness 400
Vulvar varicosities 399
Vulvodynia 335, 399
Vulvovaginal candidiasis 111, 294, 402
Vulvovaginal varicosity 35

W

Warfarin 192
Warmth, feeling of 606
Warts, vulval 407f
Water intoxication 97
  oxytocin-induced 92
Weight
  assessment of 74
  gain 302
  loss 302
Wernicke's encephalopathy 73, 77
Wertheim's vaginal clamp 546, 547, 547f
Wet mount 64
Wet smear 67, 293
  candida 67f
  examination 489, 489t
  preparation 65
  test 475
  with potassium hydroxide 295
  with saline 293
Wheeze 102, 182
Whiff test 64, 65, 67, 295
  positive 68
White blood cells 67, 82, 88
White discharge 68
Widal test 89
Wilson's disease 146, 153
World Health Organization 589
  growth charts 191f
Worm infestation 117
Wound 89
  sepsis 622
Wright's stain 410
  methods 411

X

Xerosis 111
X-ray 57, 230
  chest 89, 97, 165

Y

Y chromosome 424
Yeast
  cell 295f
  mycelia 489f
Yersinia 80
Yolk sac 36f
Young syndrome 316

Z

Zuspan regime 98